# The Complete Guide to
# Alternative Cancer Treatments

A Publication of The Alternative Cancer Research Institute

# The Complete Guide to Alternative Cancer Treatments

A publication of The Alternative Cancer Research Institute

Website: www.cancerdefeated.com
Email: custserv@cancerdefeated.com

> "...never take defeat. When all is lost, try something new. Life is too precious to let it slip away from lack of initiative or plain inertia."
>
> - Hulda Regehr Clark, Ph.D.,N.D. *The Cure for All Advanced Cancers*

## Important Note:

Do not delay in seeking advice from a qualified, licensed medical professional regarding treatment for your cancer. The information presented here is in no way meant to discourage you from seeking medical care. Rather, the hope is that it will support you and your doctor as you undertake smarter, more effective approaches to beat your cancer.

The information is provided for educational and informational purposes only, and is not intended to be a substitute for the diagnosis, treatment, and advice of a qualified, licensed medical professional. The information is provided to support your informed consent to any treatment program you may decide to undertake. Self-treatment for clinical cancer is not advised.

Statements regarding alternative treatments for cancer have not been evaluated by the FDA. Please consult your qualified, licensed medical professional or appropriate health care provider about the applicability of any opinions or recommendations with respect to your own symptoms or medical conditions.

The researchers, writers and editors at Online Publishing & Marketing, LLC, and Cancer Defeated are not doctors, and shall have neither liability nor responsibility to any person or entity with respect to any loss, damage, or injury caused or alleged to be caused directly or indirectly by the information provided. They believe the information provided herein to be accurate but its accuracy is not guaranteed. No representations or warranties of any kind are made with regard to completeness or accuracy of the information. Quotations are used as 'fair use' to illustrate various points made. Quoted text may be subject to copyright owned by third parties.

ISBN 978-1-4675-1524-5

Published in the United States of America

# Table of Contents

# Herbal Treatments . . . . . . . . . . . . . . . . . . . . . . . . . . . . . . . . . .43

# Plant-Based Treatments . . . . . . . . . . . . . . . . . . . . . . . . . . .83

# Greens . . . . . . . . . . . . . . . . . . . . . . . . . . . . . . . . . . . . . 130

# Mushrooms and Yeast Treatments . . . . . . . . . . . . . . . . . 140

# Introduction

## Purpose

This book is a comprehensive compilation of over 350 natural and alternative cancer treatments. It is a result of extensive research of the methods cancer victors have used to make themselves cancer free. Read their stories in *I Beat Cancer!*, a directory of nearly 1,000 people who beat their cancer using the treatments described in this e-book. The objectives of the book are to:

- Encourage you to be open-minded and seek ALL the information about your choices of treatments

- Be a starting point for your discussions with your doctor or with the qualified, licensed physicians who use these treatments in their practices, or your chosen natural therapist. Please do not delay in consulting a licensed physician for an opinion if you suspect you have cancer.

- Be a launching point for your own research so you can make the best-informed decisions about your treatment plan. The consensus of the majority of alternative cancer therapists is that the chance of full recovery using alternative therapies is very high with a newly diagnosed condition of early cancer, before any traumatic or toxic treatments have been received. Unfortunately, by the time most patients consider alternative treatments, they have already undergone other treatments. In fact, most patients are late-stage or deemed terminal before they turn to alternatives.

The e-book does not advise you which treatments to choose. It simply provides you with information that you are unlikely to obtain from your doctor or find by yourself. You can make use of the information from the experts who developed these treatments as well as by speaking with licensed physicians, therapists, and clinics who use them in their practices.

## Background

The "war on cancer" has been a colossal failure despite hundreds of billions of dollars spent on research and treatment. Each year, approximately one and a half million Americans will learn they have cancer. Two out of three cancer patients will die of the illness (or related therapy) within five years of diagnosis.

For more information, read your free bonus report, *How Successful are Conventional Cancer Treatments?*

## Local Therapy or 'Whole Body' Therapy?

Cancer is a biologic puzzle. There is no unanimous agreement on what makes cells grow abnormally in endless, uncontrolled multiplication. There could be many different valid ways to treat cancer.

To conventional physicians (also called allopathic physicians), cancer is a localized disease, to be treated in a localized manner. By cutting out the tumor, irradiating it, or flooding the body with toxic (and often carcinogenic) drugs, the conventional physician hopes to destroy the tumor and thus save the patient. But all too often, the cancer is still present and has metastasized (spread to other sites in the body), or is present at an undetectable level re-occurs months or years later. In contrast, the alternative physician regards cancer as a systemic disease, one that involves the whole body. In this view, the tumor is merely a symptom and the therapy aims to correct the root causes.

Dr. Josef Issels, who successfully treated many "incurable" cancer patients, stated:

"Those who believe cancer is a local disease [that is, conventional physicians] think that the tumor comes first and only afterwards is followed by the generalized illness. Those who think it is a generalized disease of the body [alternative physicians] believe that first comes the illness, and only afterwards the tumor … from this basically different way of looking at cancer, [the two types of physicians] take separate paths towards the solution to cancer.

"Cancer is a general disease of the whole body from the outset. The tumor is a symptom of that illness.

"It is my contention, based on twenty-five years of clinical experience with over eight thousand cancer patients, that only by recognizing the disease is, and always has been, one affecting the whole body from the outset, can it be more effectively arrested. By adopting that principle, the statistics of survival can be improved from the present grim position where eight out of every ten patients die having received all possible surgery, radiotherapy, and chemotherapy."

## What Will My Doctor Say About These Treatments?

He or she may not be interested. You may be asked for published articles about the treatments in peer-reviewed medical journals. Even if those articles exist (and they often do), you will most likely be told that if the treatments in question were effective, the FDA would have approved them; if a treatment is not approved, it cannot be a good and beneficial therapy. The trouble with this answer is that obtaining FDA approval takes many years and can cost hundreds of millions of dollars. <u>The simple fact is that there is no money to spend to do these trials on treatments that are often un-patentable and therefore unprofitable</u>. There is little profit in natural remedies because nobody "owns" them.

As far as publishing is concerned, it is against the policy of all mainstream medical journals to publish any research that comes from anything other than allopathic (mainstream) sources. It is not common knowledge that many such therapeutic categories exist. For example, none of the medications used by homeopathic and naturopathic doctors are regulated by the FDA. Chemotherapy drugs are regulated by the FDA and you may well ask the question, "If chemotherapy is not only harmful, but has been statistically shown to be almost useless, as indicated in *How Successful are Conventional Cancer Treatments?* and by many others like Ralph W. Moss in their books, then why does my doctor insist that I should take it?" You should ask your doctor that question.

## Why Doesn't My Doctor Know about These Treatments?

The reason alternative cancer treatments are not more widely known has little to do with their alleged therapeutic ineffectiveness and far more to do with political control and the therapy marketplace.

Many of the best alternative treatments are on the "Unproven Methods of Cancer Management" list maintained by the American Cancer Society, which is effectively a 'blacklist'. Also, your doctor will not know about most of these treatments because:

- Medical schools don't teach alternative treatments.

- Medical journals rarely contain articles about alternative treatments. Medical journals are published for the allopathic establishment, and they are mostly financed by advertisements from pharmaceutical companies.

- Doctors receive a lot of negative information about alternative treatments from the American Medical Association (AMA) and the pharmaceutical industry.

- Internet 'Quackwatches' and so forth decry alternative therapies even when there is significant evidence of their effectiveness. (See **Quackwatch** below.)

- The American Cancer Society (ACS), the National Cancer Institute (NCI) and other Government cancer bodies will not investigate or promote alternative treatments.

- Your doctor can only prescribe treatments that are Food and Drug Administration (FDA) approved. If your doctor prescribes treatments that are not FDA approved, he or she can be sued or may lose his or her medical license.

- Doctors' state medical boards may fine them heavily, suspend their license to practice or even revoke it if they recommend non-FDA approved treatments.

- The federal government can close them down and confiscate their property.

- They may lose their right to see patients in hospitals.

- Other doctors (their peers) openly ridicule and criticize them.

## How Can the American Medical Association Ignore These Alternative Treatments?

The AMA is not a scientific body. That is a widespread misconception. It is the professional association of a special interest group of allopathic medical doctors. The AMA is their "trade union", their political lobbying group, and their disciplinary board. Its task is to protect the financial and other interests of its members and at the same time to control them. The AMA has as much to do with medical science as the Teamsters' Union has to do with automotive engineering.

## Hope for the Future

Yes, there is hope. Ever so slowly, the medical scene is being revolutionized. According to the American College for Advancement in Medicine, physicians (in many cases) are showing an eagerness to learn more about natural medicine and how to best implement it into their practice. Scientists, teaching at nutritional seminars, report that attendees are often medical doctors, a radical change from years past.

The references attached to many of the treatments demonstrate that non-toxic alternative treatments are now passing from the fringes of medicine into the mainstream. They are increasingly being adopted and authenticated by conventional scientists around the world. Ralph W. Moss, Ph.D., a respected cancer industry analyst, states:

"In more than thirty years of studying and chronicling developments in the field of cancer therapy I have seen many useful alternative treatments at first mercilessly vilified and driven underground, only to resurface years later when science eventually confirms that the active principle of such a treatment really does have some recognizable, quantifiable effect against cancer cells."

For example, hyperthermia or heat therapy, once branded as a "worthless remedy" and "quackery" by the ACS in 1967, was removed years later from the Unproven Methods list. Today, hyperthermia has been hailed by some oncologists as the fifth modality in cancer treatment after surgery, radiation, drugs, and immunotherapy.

## Quackwatch and Quackbusters

One mechanism by which people are 'frightened off' from alternative treatments today is so-called 'quackbuster' organizations like Quackwatch. Dr. Elmer Cranton, in defending chelation therapy (see **Chelation**), writes about them:

"There exist a small number of self-styled medical thought-police who call themselves 'quack-busters.' This organization has the mission of attacking alternative and emerging medical therapies in favor of the existing medical monopoly. They even have their own Quackwatch Internet website. It would be interesting to trace the funding for this group back to its original source. One investigator alleges that funding comes indirectly, through a number of cutouts, from pharmaceutical manufacturers.

"For years, these so-called quack-busters have attacked nutritional supplementation and high potency multi-vitamins as 'quackery.' ... Recent scientific studies now prove that virtually anyone can benefit from nutritional supplementation. With egg on their faces from this recent vitamin research, those same critics continue to attack chelation therapy. I will answer below, point by point, a critical article on the Quackwatch website by Dr. Saul Green entitled 'Chelation Therapy: Unproven Claims And Unsound Theories,' in which Dr. Green attempts to discredit EDTA chelation using half-truths, speculation, and false statements." (See http://www.asakpa.com/busting_the_quackbusters.html for Dr. Cranton's report.)

Dr. Robert Atkins, inventor of the highly-popular Atkins Diet, stated:

"There's a war going on ... The 'War Against Quackery.' It is a fight against the carefully orchestrated, heavily endowed campaign sponsored by extremists holding positions of power in the orthodox hierarchy ...

"The multi-million-dollar campaign against quackery was never meant to root out incompetent doctors; *it was, and is, designed specifically to destroy alternative medicine* ... Millions were raised and spent because orthodox medicine sees alternative, *drugless* medicine as a real threat to its economic power. And right they are ... the majority of the drug houses will not survive."

The research team that created this book found the warnings of the Quackbusters website very helpful in their research, but in a way opposite to what you'd expect. The more agitated and vociferous Quackbusters was about particular treatments or individuals, the more our team knew it was something that should be looked into and may very well have been proven effective!

"It is estimated that if people had a choice, lack of demand would shrink Doctors and Drugs to less than 10% of its current size, with the remainder almost entirely related to trauma medicine. That would be a $900,000,000,000.00 (nine hundred BILLION dollar) loss to them. They are not going to take this loss without a good fight." - Dr Richard Shulze, N.D.

Many perceive an organized, worldwide movement to eliminate alternative remedies in favor of pharmaceutical drugs. Will consumers accept the fear and anxiety promoted by news items that natural nutrients such as Vitamin E and A in larger-than-RDA dosages can damage one's health? Or will they realize that the methodology of such research is flawed and limited in scope and so is the way it's reported?

See **Erosion of Your Health Freedom is Happening NOW** a few pages further on for more information.

Rather than rushing (or being rushed) into selecting a treatment plan, please take a while to make up your own mind about what will help you overcome your cancer. Your life may depend on it. In particular, read what other people have said has helped them get rid of their cancer. You can find stories of many cancer survivors and winners in your free bonus report, *I Beat Cancer!*

# Take Control of Your Own Health!

Many say that the Cancer Establishment's system is largely designed to protect the financial interests tied to chemotherapy, radiation, and surgery. Keep an open mind about all the other available options.

This e-book is not meant to provide medical advice. The only advice we wish to give you is this: do not surrender your independent thinking. Reason things out and make your own decisions. Network with other patients. Consult with researchers and innovative doctors. Search out different opinions. Do not let arrogance, based on fancy titles and institutional authority, dictate your most important decisions. Do you know how many thousands of cancer patients have been sent home to die, who later completely recovered thanks to alternative treatments? We are not talking about "spontaneous" remissions, but natural healing, achieved with non-toxic holistic treatments.

Become your own Health Detective! For example, go to Pubmed at http://www.ncbi.nlm.nih.gov/ entrez/query.fcgi and search the title *"Beta-glucan inhibits the genotoxicity of cyclophosphamide, adriamycin and cisplatin."* An article will come up that describes how beta-glucan pretreatment approximately cuts in half the damage done by chemotherapy drugs. Why not ask your doctor about it if you have decided to receive chemotherapy? This valuable supplement, available over the counter without a prescription, is described later in this book.

If you become aware of any factual errors in this book, sources not given due recognition, or additional information you believe should be included in this book, please write to custserv@cancerdefeated.com Thank you in advance for your feedback.

Please be aware that because most of these treatments have not been rigorously tested, there is no guarantee that they are safe or will work for you. No treatment works for every patient and a treatment that has been highly successful for hundreds of patients may still fail in a significant number of cases. Keep in mind that for conventional chemotherapy, the failure rate is estimated at roughly 97-98 percent for advanced cancer patients – and this is the "safe, recommended, approved approach!"

It is beyond the scope of this e-book to provide fool-proof safety advice and warnings. Please determine these for yourself. Work with your doctor to identify treatments that, at the least in his/her eyes, will "do no harm". Also, talk with people who have used the treatments successfully. Be aware that a treatment that may work for one person may not work for another because of differences in our genetic make-up and unique circumstances.

Take control of your own health! There is no one on the face of the earth who has more interest in your welfare and well-being than you yourself do. You must take control of your own destiny and not leave it to others who have their own vested interests.

# How To Get the Most From This E-book

Several links have been provided for you throughout this e-book with the goal of helping you access more information about the treatments in which you're interested. Though we have done our best to provide active links with live sites, there is no guarantee that these third-party sites will remain published. We encourage you to use the links provided. Should you come across a webpage that has been taken down, try using a search engine such as Google to locate more information on the topic in which you're interested.

The Index includes an alphabetical listing of all the treatments and the different names under which they are known. This is useful if you wish to locate a treatment quickly. Print out any treatment that you might want to discuss with your doctor or research further.

Books recommended for further reading can be ordered online or from your regular bookshop.

# Glossary of Common Cancer Terms

Understanding a few simple definitions and acronyms that repeatedly crop up in this e-book will be helpful to you.

**Term Definition**

| | |
|---|---|
| **acidosis** | A condition characterized by excessive acid in the body fluids. See **alkalization** and **pH**. |
| **alkalization** | Blood serum pH never changes – it is maintained by the body at around 7.37. It does this by excreting with the urine either more acid or more alkali. However, body tissue pH will fluctuate constantly based on diet. Most cancer patients tested apparently will show a pH of 4 – 5 which is very acidic. This acidity of body tissue drives out oxygen. Low oxygen creates an environment ripe for cancer. As two-time Nobel Prize winner, Otto Warburg, pointed out, cancer thrives in an oxygen-deficient environment. Alkaline tissue holds 20 times more oxygen than does acidic tissue and this oxygen-rich environment is critical for maintaining health and eliminating anaerobic bacteria, viruses, fungi, etc. that are harmful. This is why wellness practitioners recommend eating green foods (these foods are rich with alkaline elements to keep the pH balanced) and to avoid eating processed foods which contain numerous acid elements. See **pH**. |
| **alopecia** | The loss of hair, which may include all body hair as well as scalp hair. |
| **AMA** | American Medical Association |
| **anaerobic** | Does not require oxygen. |
| **angiogenesis** | (an-je-o-JEN-uh-sis). The growth of new blood vessels feeding the tumor. Cancer patients want to disrupt this process by whatever means possible (consistent with safety). |
| **angiogenesis inhibitor** | An agent that prevents the growth of new blood vessels to a tumor in an attempt to starve the tumor of necessary nutrients. |
| **antioxidant** | Antioxidants are substances that may protect cells from the damage caused by unstable molecules known as free radicals. Free radical damage may lead to cancer. Antioxidants interact with and stabilize free radicals and may prevent some of the damage free radicals otherwise might cause. Examples of antioxidants include glutathione, lipoic acid, catalase, superoxide dismutase, melatonin, betacarotene, lycopene, and vitamins C, E, and A. |
| **apoptosis** | Natural cell death. Cancer patients want apoptosis to happen to their cancer cells as soon as possible. |
| **cachexia** | (ke-KEK-se-uh). A wasting away of normal body tissue. |
| **cancer** | Any malignant growth or tumor caused by abnormal and uncontrolled cell division; it may spread to other parts of the body through the lymphatic system or the blood stream. |

| | |
|---|---|
| **carcinogenic** | Cancer-causing. |
| **carcinoma** | A form of cancer made up of epithelial cells. Epithelial cells line body cavities, cover internal organs and line the internal portions of organs and the skin. |
| **chemotherapy** | ( kee-mo-THER -a-pee). Chemotherapy is the use of drugs to try to stop or slow the growth of cancer cells. It often is used in combination with other treatments (radiation therapy or surgery). Chemotherapy can be administered orally (capsule, pill, or liquid), by injection into a vein, artery, or muscle, or by intravenous (IV) drip. Chemotherapy affects rapidly growing cells, which may be cancerous or normal (such as hair cells, bone marrow). Short-term side effects of chemotherapy include pain, fatigue, hair loss, mouth sores, nausea, vomiting, suppression of the immune system, infection, fungus, shearing off of intestinal villi, memory loss and heart damage. Longer-term side-effects include permanent damage to ovaries and testes, and an increased risk of secondary cancers, as chemotherapy agents are carcinogenic. |
| **cytoxic** | Toxic or poisonous to cells. |
| **debulking** | Surgical removal of the major portion of a tumor. |
| **enzymes** | An enzyme is a protein, or protein complex, that catalyzes a chemical reaction. Enzymes are essential to living organisms, and a malfunction of even a single enzyme out of several thousand present in our bodies can lead to severe or lethal illness. There are two classes of enzymes recognized:<br><br>1. Metabolic enzymes - These are responsible for repair, formation and function of each cell within each and every tissue of the body.<br><br>2. Digestive enzymes - These are necessary for the proper breakdown of ingested foods to allow effective absorption of the nutrients to occur.<br><br>Raw foods contain varying quantities of the following four basic types of plant enzymes: protease for protein digestion, amylase for carbohydrate digestion, lipase for fat digestion, and cellulase for fiber digestion. Every raw food contains exactly the right quantities and types of enzymes necessary to digest that particular food. Although enzymes are present in all raw foods, they become devitalized in cooked or highly processed foods. Temperatures greater than 118° F. kill enzymes. Even steaming vegetables kills enzymes, as does irradiating or microwaving them. Freezing, however, does not affect enzymes. When the body receives foods deficient in enzymes, it increases its number of white blood cells as a defense mechanism. Enzymes are then released from these cells as well as from the lymphatic tissue and spleen, where they also are stored, into the blood to digest toxins resulting from eating processed foods. When white blood cells are continually elevated due to a diet high in processed food, the immune system is weakened. This is because enzymes, normally held in reserve to help fight infection, are instead pulled out of storage from white blood cells and other storage sites to digest the processed food. See **pancreatin**. |
| **FDA** | Food and Drug Administration (United States) |
| **fermentative** | Carry out metabolic processes anaerobically, that is, without oxygen. |

| | |
|---|---|
| **fibrin** | Fibrin is naturally occurring in the body and is involved in the clotting process of blood. Fibrin covers cancer cells with a protective coat, hindering recognition by the immune system. In addition, fibrin relays a signal to the cancer cell to start angiogenesis, the growth of new blood vessels. Once their fibrin coating is removed, for example, by fibrin-eating enzyme formulas, the cancer cells are exposed and our bodies' killer cells can destroy them. And angiogenesis and cancer growth and spread is inhibited. |
| **flavonols** | A class of flavonoids with a 3-hydroxyflavone backbone. |
| **flavonoids** | Compounds that are formally derived from flavones that have antioxidant properties and are found in fruits, vegetables, tea, legumes, and red wine. Flavonoids may help reduce the risk of chronic disease such as heart disease or cancer. They are brightly colored plant pigments known for giving fruits and vegetables their colors. |
| **free radicals** | Highly unstable molecules that interact quickly and aggressively with other molecules in our bodies to create abnormal cells. They are capable of penetrating into the DNA of a cell and damaging its "blueprint" so that the cell will produce mutated cells that can then replicate without normal controls. Free radicals are unstable because they have unpaired electrons in their molecular structure. This causes them to react almost instantly with any substance in their vicinity. Oxygen, or oxyl, free radicals are especially dangerous. Free radicals accelerate aging and contribute to the development of many diseases, including cancer and heart disease. See **oxidative stress**. |
| **immune system** | Our immune system is a complex network of cells and organs that work together to defend the body against attacks by "foreign," or "non-self," invaders. It comprises an army of white blood cells -- NK cells, T and B cells -- which travel around inside us destroying the millions of intruding microbes that penetrate our bodies every day, as well as the thousands of newly infected or abnormal body cells that develop. The immune system is one of the body's main defenses against disease. Cancer may develop when the immune system breaks down or is not functioning adequately. A side-effect of conventional cancer treatments is also depletion of the immune system. |
| **immunotherapy** | A form of therapy that uses your body's immune system to treat a disease. |
| **incidence** | The number of new cases of cancer within a defined group and time frame. |
| **inoperable** | Unsuitable for treatment by surgery. Also called unresectable or nonresectable. |
| **in vitro** | A procedure conducted in an artificial environment outside of a living organism such as a test tube or a Petri dish. |
| **in vivo** | A procedure conducted within a living organism as opposed to an in vitro controlled environment. |
| **isoflavones** | A class of naturally-occurring organic compounds that act as phytoestrogens in mammals commonly found in soybeans and other legumes. They are known to strengthen bones, counter the effects of chemotherapy, and regular excess estrogen. |

| | |
|---|---|
| **leukemia** | (loo-KE-me-uh). Cancer of the blood-forming tissues, such as bone marrow and lymphatic systems. This type of cancer results in the uncontrolled production of abnormal white blood cells. |
| **lymphocytes** | A type of white blood cell distributed throughout the body by way of the lymphatic system. The lymphatic system consists of lymph nodes and vessels, the thymus, spleen and bone marrow. |
| **lymphoma** | A type of cancer that begins in lymphatic tissue and may spread to other parts of your body. |
| **macrophage cells** | Immune cells that trap and engulf foreign cells and particles, scavenge cellular debris, and destroy infectious agents such as viruses, parasites, bacteria, and fungi. |
| **melanoma** | A tumor of the melanocytes — cells that produce skin pigment. |
| **metastasis** | (Muh-TAS-tuh-sis). Spreading of a disease from one part of the body to another, usually referring to the movement of cancer cells through the lymph or blood. Also called distant cancer. |
| **metastasize** | To spread from the first cancer site; for example, breast cancer that spreads to the bone. |
| **mortality rate** | The number of people in a population group who die of cancer within a set period of time, usually one year. A cancer mortality rate usually is expressed in terms of deaths per 100,000 people. |
| **multiple myeloma** | (MUL-tih-pul mi-uh-LO-muh). A cancer of the plasma cells — the part of the immune system that produces antibodies. |
| **NCI** | National Cancer Institute (United States) |
| **natural killer cells** | White blood cells that attack tumor cells and body cells that have been invaded by foreign substances. |
| **neoplasm** | A new growth of tissue or cells; a tumor that is generally malignant. |
| **NIH** | National Institutes of Health (United States) |
| **Non-Hodgkin's lymphoma** | A cancer of the lymphatic system. Non-Hodgkin's lymphoma is related to Hodgkin's disease but is made up of different cell types |
| **oxidative stress** | Destruction caused by free radicals. It occurs when the available supply of the body's antioxidants is insufficient to handle and neutralize free radicals. The result is massive cell damage that can result in cellular mutations, tissue breakdown and immune compromise. It is also the mechanism by which cancer treatments such as radiation therapy and photodynamic therapy exert their anti-tumor effects. See **free radicals**. |

| | |
|---|---|
| **pH** | pH is the abbreviation for potential hydrogen. The pH range is from 0-14, with 7 being neutral. Above 7 is alkaline and below 7 is acidic. The higher the pH reading, the more alkaline and oxygen rich are tissues. The lower the pH reading, the more acidic and oxygen deprived are tissues. The internal environment of a normal healthy body is slightly alkaline, maintaining a pH of just above 7. See **alkalization**. |
| **pancreatin** | The pancreas is a gland that resides behind the stomach. It secretes insulin into the blood to regulate blood sugar. It also makes digestive enzymes which flow into the intestinal tract. These enzymes are necessary to break down protein, carbohydrates and fats so they can be digested. Pancreatin is a mixture of the fat dissolving enzyme, lipase, the protein enzymes such as protease, and those that break down carbohydrates such as amylase. See **enzymes**. |
| **phagocytosis** | The process by which a cell engulfs particles such as bacteria, other microorganisms, aged red blood cells, foreign matter, etc. The principal phagocytes (cells that can engage in phagocytosis) include the neutrophils and monocytes (types of white blood cells). One of the ways to fight cancer is the use of agents to stimulate macrophage production and activity. |
| **phytochemicals** | Chemical compounds that occur naturally in fruits, vegetables, beans, grains, and other plant foods. Many have antioxidant properties which may protect cells against damage and reduce the risk of developing certain types of cancer. |
| **phytosterols** | Phytochemicals that occur naturally in plants. They occur naturally in small quantities in vegetable oils such as corn and soybean oil. There are also known as plant sterols and are a group of steroid alcohols. |
| **pleomorphism** | Pleomorphism is a theory that holds that the human body houses symbiotic, primitive microorganisms which can change in form. When the body's internal environment is healthy, the symbiotic relationship is maintained. However, when the internal environment becomes imbalanced through influences such as poor diet, stress and toxins, the symbiosis shifts. This microbial form changes through several stages to a virulent, pathogenic form, which has been associated with cancer. |
| **prostate-specific antigen (PSA)** | A protein made by the normal prostate gland. Elevated levels of PSA in the blood may indicate the presence of infection, inflammation, prostate enlargement or cancer. |
| **proteolytic** | A catch-all term referring to enzymes that digest protein. Supplemental forms can incorporate any of a wide variety of enzymes including trypsin, chymotrypsin, pancreatin, bromelain, papain, and a range of fungal proteases. In the body, proteolytic digestive enzymes are produced in the pancreas, but supplemental forms of enzymes may come from fungal or bacterial sources, extraction from the pancreas of livestock animals (trypsin/chymotrypsin) or extraction from plants (such as papain from the papaya and bromelain from the pineapple plant). The primary uses of proteolytic enzymes in dietary supplements are as digestive enzymes, anti-inflammatory agents and pain relievers. See **enzymes**. |

| | |
|---|---|
| **radiation therapy** | (ray-dee-AY-shun THER-a-pee). Use of high-energy electromagnetic waves (radiation) — from outside the body or implanted into the tumor or body — to kill cancer cells. Sources of radiation include X-ray, cobalt, strontium, radium and linear accelerators. Possible side-effects are headache, nausea, vomiting, loss of appetite, constipation and infection. Longer-term side-effects include an increased risk of secondary cancers. Adverse side effects of radiation for prostate cancer may include diarrhea, colitis, problems associated with urination and a degree of impotence. |
| **relative survival rate** | Measures survival rates of one group of patients treated one way against those of another group that was treated differently. Usually used to assess if one form of treatment is better than another. |
| **sarcoma** | A malignant tumor of muscles or connective tissue such as bone and cartilage. |
| **sterols** | Organic molecules that occur naturally in plants, animals, and fungi. The most familiar type of sterol in animals is cholesterol, which is vital to cellular function. Sterols are also steroid-based alcohols with a hydrocarbon side-chain of between 8 and 10 carbons at the 17-beta position, along with a hydroxyl group at the 3-beta position (making it an alcohol). |
| **surgery** | In cancer surgery, all or part of the tumor may be cut out. The most common side effects of surgery are scarring, damage to the healthy areas around the tumor, bleeding and infection during healing. Other side-effects may be pain, disfigurement and loss of function. |
| **survival rate** | Commonly defined as the measure of the percentage of people who develop cancer and survive for five years after diagnosis. |
| **systemic** | Affecting the entire body. |
| **testosterone deprivation** | Also known as ablation. A form of prostate cancer therapy involving either surgically removing the testicles or taking medications to block the production of male hormones, specifically testosterone, which encourages prostate cancer growth. An adverse side-effect is memory loss. |
| **tumor** | A tissue growth that can be benign or malignant; a neoplasm. |
| **white blood cells (WBC)** | General term for a variety of cells responsible for fighting invading germs, infection, and allergy-causing agents. Specific white blood cells are: neutrophils 40 - 75%, eosinophils 5%, basophils 0.5%, lymphocytes 20 - 50 %, monocytes 1 - 5%. The figures show the relative proportions of the different types of white blood cell. The reason for the range of figures shown is that the requirement for different types of white blood cell will vary from time to time. Neutrophils, eosinophils and basophils are collectively known as granulocytes due to prominent granules in their cytoplasm. Lymphocytes and monocytes are classed as white blood cells because they are a constituent of blood and ultimately originate from the bone marrow. |

# Erosion of Your Health Freedom is Happening NOW

The 2002 European Union (EU) Food Supplements Directive was big news because it set the stage to make the RDA's (recommended daily requirements of vitamins and minerals) far lower than their ideal therapeutic range. This means that individuals face not being able to purchase Vitamin C in doses higher than 200 mg, folic acid not higher than 1 mg, niacin not higher than 32 mgs, Vitamin $B_6$ not higher than 10 mg, just to name a few examples. In effect, the goal of the EU Directive is to classify vitamins and minerals as medical drugs rather than dietary supplements, which means these supplements would be subject to government regulation in terms of dosage and bioavailability.

To make matters worse, nutrients that are not on the RDA list including chromium picolinate, lysine and selenium, will be banned from over-the-counter sale and will be illegal to buy without a prescription. The Directive only allows supplements to be made from a list of 15 minerals and 13 vitamins, leaving out another 40 that are important to human metabolism. As a result, around 5,000 safe formulas that have been on the market for decades may be banned in Europe.

This will affect those in North America because once legislation is passed in Europe, due to the larger form of legislation called CODEX Alimentarius, it has the potential to become global. The remedies we have come to rely on may no longer be available. And if they are, it will be by prescription only and at a much greater cost than we pay today!

# What People Have Done to Get Rid of Their Cancer

Based on an analysis of the free bonus report *I Beat Cancer!*, a compendium of 1,000 cancer survivor testimonials, the following is a summary of several successful approaches.

Most cancer survivors did a combination of things and did not just rely on a single 'silver bullet' to get themselves well. This seems very important in achieving successful outcomes. For example, combining a treatment that kills cancer cells with a treatment that boosts immunity and another treatment that detoxifies the body appears to raise the odds of recovery to a much higher level than any single treatment could achieve on its own. In combining different approaches, people have not tried to do everything at once but instead have just addressed each priority before adding the next treatment.

As stated above, it seems imperative to use a combinations-approach. Another important aspect is that most natural and alternative treatments are non-specific. In other words, they work with any cancer.

Following are some examples of successful combination-approaches that people have undertaken. We have not attempted to verify all the claims made.

### Dr. Clark's 21 Day Curing Program

"The success rate for advanced cancer is about 95%. So you can count on this method, not merely hope it will work for you. It is a total approach that not only shrinks tumors, but also normalizes your blood chemistry, lowers your cancer markers, and returns your health. The small failure rate (5%) is due to clinical emergencies that beset the advanced cancer sufferer. However, if you combine the advice in this book [The Cure for All Advanced Cancers] with access to hospital care, even "hopeless" patients can gain the time necessary to become well again." All the supplies for this program can be bought very simply by ordering online at https://www.drclark.com/.

### Dr. Budwig Flaxseed Oil and Cottage Cheese (FOCC) Approach

"What she (Dr. Johanna Budwig) has demonstrated to my initial disbelief but lately, to my complete satisfaction in my practice is: CANCER IS EASILY CURABLE, the treatment is dietary/lifestyle, the response is immediate; the cancer cell is weak and vulnerable; the precise biochemical breakdown point was identified by her in 1951 and is specifically correctable, in vitro (test-tube) as well as in vivo (real)... " (Dr. Dan C. Roehm, "Townsend Letter for Doctors", July 1990)

In 1967, Dr Budwig broadcast the following statements during an interview over the South German Radio Network, describing her incoming patients who had experienced failure with operations and radiation therapy: "Even in these cases it is possible to restore health in a few months at most, I would truly say 90% of the time... This has never been contradicted, but this knowledge has been a long time reaching this side of the ocean, hasn't it? Cancer treatment can be very simple and very successful once you know how. The cancer interest-groups don't want you to know this ... May those of you who have suffered from this disease (and I include your family and friends in this) forgive the miscreants who have kept this simple information from reaching you for so long." The approach involves flaxseed oil and cottage cheese and the avoidance of margarine and other hydrogenated oils that are found in processed food and restaurant meals. A typical testimonial is from this stage IV prostate cancer survivor at http://www.beckwithfamily.com/Flax1.html.

### The Four Corners approach with Poly-MVA

This involves taking Poly-MVA (8 tsp/day), Biobran/MGN-3 (3 grams/day), Coral Calcium (9 capsules/day), Liver Support (6 capsules/day) and 9 capsules of Q-gel for a total of 135 mg a day (equivalent to 450 mg of CoQ10). More information about Poly-MVA including video testimonials for breast cancer, multiple myeloma, bladder cancer, non-small cell lung cancer, Stage IV brain cancer, prostate cancer, and leukemia is at http://www.polymvasurvivors.com/. MGN-3 is no longer available, but see the sections on Mushrooms and Yeast Treatments and Immune Therapies for good substitutes.

### Dr. Rosy Daniel's Integrated Self-Help Approach

Reports a 30-40% success rate involving Carctol, a low-acid diet, dietary inclusions such as Chinese mushrooms and turmeric, coriander, cumin seed, other supplements such as Vitamin $B_{17}$ and shark liver oil, and a mind/ body approach such as spiritual healing. See Dr. Rosy Daniel's Health Creation website at http://www.healthcreation.co.uk/. Testimonials at the Health Creation website include: "Pancreatic cancer: Alive 4 years on. Astounding since this is one of the most aggressive cancers." "Secondary melanoma: Alive 2 years on. This case has shocked the medical world." "Grade 4 brain tumor: Alive 2 years on. Doctors are gobsmacked."

### An Example Of A Combination-Protocol that A Woman With Breast Cancer Created For Herself

(Described at http://health.groups.yahoo.com/group/FlaxSeedOil2/message/16293.) "Daily, I took the 3 Tablespoons oil in 1/2 cup cottage cheese [Referring to Dr. Budwig's treatment]. I added other things to make a smoothie out of it. I felt this was a very important part of the things I was doing. I added these things every day:

- 10 or more glasses of water. I added some oxygen enhancing liquid to it. I can't remember the name of it.

- No colas of any kind. (I have been cola-free for 1 year now. Yah!)

- No sweets of any kind.

- Daily doses of pancreatin at each meal and before bedtime. I felt this was another extremely important part of the protocol.

- Primal defense

- RM-10

- Wipe-out

- FOS and Multidophilus

- Alka-Trace and Coral Calcium to balance pH

- Cell Food

- D-Lenolate

The other important part was the Black Salve that I put on my tumor. It basically took out the tumor and created an eschar. I had to do this twice to remove the entire tumor. It created quite a scar but even that seems to be slowly improving. This took about 1 to 2 months to totally remove the tumor. It finally was healed over about 7 months later. Now I am working on making the scar less noticeable as the area was on my chest, easily above the swimsuit line."

With respect to the above-mentioned salve, excellent results have reportedly been obtained with the Cansema black salve, particularly for all skin cancers. Photographs, video testimonials and extensive written testimonials for basal, squamous cell and even advanced melanoma cancers used to be available at the Alpha Omega Labs information site but have been taken down.

Regarding the use of the Cansema salve for breast cancer, Alpha Omega Labs stated: "Unless you are under the care of a CAM (complementary and alternative medicine) physician; or a good naturopath, osteopath, chiropractor, or other licensed health care professional, we do not advise the use of Cansema Salve in the treatment of breast cancer. Pattie's growth was small [referring to a testimonial on the site], so it apparently worked for her. But had her breast cancer been of a larger size, the use of Cansema Salve to remove it could have been excruciatingly painful. You can get good narcotic-grade analgesics (pain-killers) from a good physician — a real 'must' if you're going to tackle a sizeable growth." Cansema can be ordered at http://health.centreforce.com. The product is called Black Salve and is officially sold only for use on animals.

## Mexican Cancer Clinics

Many effective treatments are not available in clinics or doctors' offices in the US, so people have often traveled to clinics in Mexico and beyond for these treatments (For more information, see the Special Report *Adios, Cancer!* available at www.cancerdefeated.com). These treatments include highly successful protocols that were developed by Dr. Josef Issels, Dr. Ernesto Contreras, Sr., Dr. Max Gerson, and other distinguished cancer doctors.

## Helpful Source

A helpful source of high quality and leading-edge natural products beneficial in treating cancer is the Wolfe Clinic at http://www.thewolfeclinic.com/. You can arrange a telephone consultation from anywhere in the world (follow-up consultations are free after the initial consultation) and products can be ordered at http://www.shopthewolfeclinic.com/. The Wolfe Clinic stocks hard-to-find products.

## What to Address

As contained in the free bonus report *I Beat Cancer!*, treatment strategies that cancer winners have employed include

- Treating pain and cachexia

- A change of diet to one incorporating raw food and eliminating sugar, white flour, and processed foods

- Inhibiting tumors by stopping the growth of cancerous cells, or by killing them with the introduction of a cytotoxic (cell-killing) substance

- Lowering the voltage of the cells

- Raising the oxygen content of the cells to create an environment that is lethal to cancer cells or which causes them to revert to normal

- Debulking by surgery (but ensuring that any 'escaping' cancer cells are destroyed before they re-colonize elsewhere in the body)

- Eliminating parasites in the body

- Reversing acidosis (low pH in the body) to increase alkalinity and oxygenate the tissues

- Detoxification to eliminate underlying toxicity as well as toxicity from dying cancer cells

- Building or rebuilding the immune system

- Repairing damage to affected areas and organs

Also, cleaning-up the personal environment to help eliminate the cancer and insure against its recurrence has proven important. For example:

- Doing a dental cleanup to remove dead teeth including root-canaled teeth, mercury and cavitations

- Eliminating parasites and yeast

- Removing suspect substances from everyday life such as deodorants, body lotions, sprays, talcum powder, fragrances, conventional cleaning materials, fluoride, isopropyl alcohol, benzene, industrial emissions, etc

- Minimizing the dosage and the effects of conventional treatments by protecting against heart damage, stroke, hair loss, immune system destruction, etc.

- Forming a support network, or at least having one other person helping

- Addressing the emotional aspects and resolving the possible trigger factors for a person's cancer

- Gaining a feeling of more control in life

## Underlying Theme

An underlying theme with many of the treatments people have used is the need to get more oxygen into the tissues. Two-time Nobel Prize winner Dr. Otto Warburg proved that cancer cells cannot survive in an oxygen rich environment because they have an anaerobic, fermentative metabolism, that is, in simplified terms - they require sugar, not oxygen, to survive. They die in an oxygen-rich environment.

"... for cancer, there is only one primary cause. Summarized in a few words, the cause of cancer is the replacement of the respiration of oxygen in normal body cells by a fermentation of sugar.

"... Because no cancer cell exists in which the respiration is intact, it cannot be disputed that cancer could be prevented if the respiration of the body cells would be kept intact."

Alkaline tissues can apparently hold around twenty times more oxygen than can acid tissues. Cancer patients' tissues are invariably acid. So many treatments deal with raising pH and getting oxygen into the body's tissues to eradicate the cancer.

"Introduce oxygen, they go away. The key is to figure out how to re-establish oxygen uptake of infected cells. It's not rocket science. Remove the toxins and metals, restore missing elements of nutrition and raise the oxygen potential. Then cancer goes away. No surgery, no chemo, no radiation."

(The Prime Cause and Prevention of Cancer, lecture delivered by Dr. Otto Warburg to Nobel Laureates on June 30, 1966 at Lindau, Lake Constance, Germany; http:///www.ozonetherapy.co.uk/articles/ Warburg_The_Prime_Cause_of_Cancer.htm )

## Additional Accessible and Relatively Inexpensive Treatments

The following list merely touches on a score or so of the over 350 treatments described in this e-book, to illustrate the gentle healing power of natural and alternative cancer treatments.

Accessible and relatively inexpensive treatments that cancer victors have used include:

- **Insulin Potentiation Therapy (IPT)** if you decide to have chemotherapy — it makes the chemotherapy you receive many times more powerful, so you only need a small dose of the chemotherapeutic agent which means you avoid major side-effects.

- **DMSO** also may support a reduction in the dosage needed of the chemotherapeutic agent, and also promotes remission. It also helps with side effects such as hair loss, nausea, and dry mouth.

- **Dr. Nagourney's Ex-Vivo Apoptotic Laboratory Assay (EVA)** to identify which chemotherapy will be most effective for you.

- **Radiofrequency Ablation (RFA)** for inoperable tumors when chemotherapy and radiation have failed — to cook the tumors to death without affecting surrounding tissue.

- **Hydrazine sulfate** to reverse cachexia and kill off cancer cells.

- **High pH Therapy With Cesium Chloride** to eliminate pain within 12-24 hours, and raise the pH of tissues to stop the growth of cancer cells.

- **Oncolyn** to regress tumors.

- **CoQ10** – around 500mg daily with fat, to regress tumors.

- **Vitamin E** (in a mixed form that includes succinate, gamma tocopherol and tocotrienols) to inhibit cancer growth, and protect against hair loss and heart damage if you have chemotherapy.

- **Immpower/AHCC** - optimizes the immune system and helps eliminate cancer.

- **Beta-glucan** – optimizes immune function particularly through the activation of macrophage cells. Inhibits the adverse side-effects of chemotherapy.

- **Vitamin C** - some people have experienced a complete remission after following the guidelines in *Cancer and Vitamin C: A Discussion of the Nature, Causes, Prevention, and Treatment of Cancer with Special Reference to the Value of Vitamin C* by Ewan Cameron and Linus Pauling.

- **Dr. Matthias Rath 'Vitamin C, l-proline and l-lysine Epigallocatechin from Green Tea'** – to stop the spread of cancer.

- **Artemisinin** to deliver a knockout oxidative stress to cancer cells.

- **Hydrogen Peroxide** to introduce oxygen.

- **Germanium (GE-132)** to normalize physiology and introduce oxygen.

- **IP-6** to reduce and eliminate tumors.

- **Ellagic acid** to stop cancer growth and promotes apoptosis.

- **Essiac tea** to normalize physiology, counteract the side-effects of chemotherapy and radiation, and promote remission.

- **Dr Robert Jones' gentle phenergan protocol** to knock out the mitochondria (energy centers) in the cancer cells to kill them.

- **Poly-MVA** to replace nutrients, rebuild strength and reverse cancer.

- **Prebiotics and probiotics** — for a healthy immune system.

- **Enzymes** to properly digest food, strengthen the immune system, rid the body of malignant tumor cells, and improve the response rate and counter the adverse side effects of chemotherapy and radiation.

- **Pawpaw** – its papain enzymes break down fibrin on cancer cells, stop cancer cell growth and prevent metastasis.

- **Melatonin** to put cancer cells to sleep and to prevent damage to cells that can lead to cancer.

- **Selenium** to reduce the risk of developing cancer.

- **Nutrition and Diet**

    - Avoidance of sugar (sugar is like 'fertilizer' for cancer) and artificial sweeteners –

    - using xylitol or stevia instead

    - Avoidance of colas and soft drinks

    - Avoidance of margarine and other harmful, hydrogenated oils that are found in

    - processed food and restaurant meals

    - Avoidance of white flour and all processed and refined foods

    - Including an abundance of uncooked vegetables, vegetable juices, and fruit

    - (organic if you can afford it)

- **Dental cleanup** – removal of devitalized (dead) teeth including root-canaled teeth, removal of mercury amalgams, and cleanup of cavitations – to reclaim a healthy immune system and reverse degenerative changes.

- **Dr. Clark Cleanups** for diet, body, and home to remove cancer-causing parasites and pollutants at their source, and allow the body to start healing itself.

- **A Rife-based frequency device** such as the Bare device, to shatter cancer cells and associated parasites.

- **Meditation, massage and exercise to reduce stress** – to improve immune system functioning, and make the body less acidic so tissues can hold more oxygen.

- **Behavioral therapy** to modify characteristics typical of a 'cancer personality'.

- **EFT** to address the trigger factors and other emotional factors connected with cancer.

Of course, discuss these treatments with your doctor, and other health professionals. Self-treatment is not recommended. If you decide to undertake conventional treatments, there may be interactions between natural treatments and the conventional treatments that need to be identified.

Work with a physician or therapist to design a treatment plan. Schedule testing to be done at regular intervals to assess your progress. Keep a diary or record of your treatment and other aspects of your environment that you change so that you can relate these to the improvements you experience.

## Additional Reading

This e-book is only one of the e-books, printed softcover books and special reports available from www.cancerdefeated.com.

# Diets

## Binzel Nutritional Program

Philip E. Binzel, Jr., M.D., is the creator of the Total Nutritional Program and is generally regarded as one of the pioneers in the clinical use of laetrile, a natural food extract. His program consists of vitamins, minerals, enzymes, and laetrile, which must be supplemented by an enzyme-rich diet of raw, non-cooked fruits and vegetables and regular cleansing of the bowels. Dr. Binzel stresses the toxic effects of animal proteins in the diet and their degenerative impact on pancreatic enzymes.

Binzel said he began looking for alternatives to standard treatments in the 1970s after watching a lot of his cancer patients die. He was attracted to studies performed by medical researchers in the 1950s and 1960s that, he said, identified a group of key cancer preventers called nitrilosides, found in roughly 1500 foods including blackberries, strawberries, bean sprouts, and the kernels of apricots and peaches.

When ingested, nitrilosides serve as the body's second line of defense against cancer thanks to a toxic effect they have on cancerous cells. The most common clinical use of nitrilosides is in the form of amygdalin (laetrile), administered via tablets or intravenously.

The objective of the Binzel program is to increase the efficiency of the human immune system. Patients are urged to eat lots of fiber, raw foods, and whole grains like pasta and brown bread. The diet discourages sugar, fat, and anything that comes from an animal.

Dr. Binzel states out of 180 patient cases that spanned 18 years, 87% survived after following his program. This contrasts sharply with the American Cancer Society statistic stating that 85% of cancer patients will die within the first five years of being diagnosed.

### Further Reading & References

- *Alive & Well: One Doctor's Experience with Nutrition in the Treatment of Cancer Patients* by Philip E. Binzel

- Cancer – The Survivor's Battle Plan: http://www.campaignfortruth.com/Eclub/310103/ cancersurviversbattleplan.htm

## Diana Dyer

Diana Dyer, a former hospital dietitian who decided to learn everything she could about cancer and nutrition after her third diagnosis of cancer, published a 120-page cancer and nutrition booklet called *A Dietitian's Cancer Story*.

Cancer sufferers find her advice extremely valuable and see her as someone who relates to their pain. Dyer offers unique perspectives on various complementary approaches to improve the quality of life in cancer patients.

These approaches include lifestyle changes such as diet, exercise, and meditation, as well as other techniques that should be viewed not as alternatives to conventional medicine, but rather as complementary. Dyer herself underwent surgery and chemotherapy for her cancer but used her supplemental treatment to heal herself emotionally and spiritually, as well as to aid in physical healing.

Dyer described feeling abandoned by the conventional medical system following her aggressive treatment schedule and wished for guidance on how to incorporate multiple lifestyle changes. Though she navigated her changes on her own, her book serves as a beacon of guidance for others. By becoming active participants in their own lifestyle changes, as Ms. Dyer has done, cancer survivors can better regain control of their lives and improve their quality of living.

Dyer presents herself as a conventionally-trained dietitian who, prior to her third cancer recovery, had never cooked with tofu and had only tasted soy milk once. Her diet plans are thus an offering of healthful, cancer-fighting foods that anyone can incorporate into their kitchen and lifestyle.

She has developed dozens of healthful, easy-to-fix meals for patients. Especially popular are her "SuperSoy" and "PhytoChemical" shakes. Ms. Dyer, a mother of two, credits diet and daily exercise with keeping her free of cancer for the past fifteen years.

Ms. Dyer also suggests using additional, non-food approaches to supplement cancer healing and prevention, including meditation, prayer, shiatsu, and gardening. She offers insight and tips on how to integrate the diet and life-changes she recommends so they're acceptable to the rest of a cancer survivor's family.

### Further Reading & References

- Diana Dyer, MS RD: http://www.cancerrd.com

- *A Dietician's Cancer Story* by Diana Dyer

# Dr. Dana Flavin-Koenig

Dana Flavin-Koenig, MD, serves as president and founder of the Foundation for Collaborative Medicine and Research. She is considered an expert in multiple targeted therapies, including cancer therapies that use all natural substances. Although there are several treatments based on diet to battle cancer, this one has been in focus worldwide as Dr. Flavin-Koenig is an advisor to the National Cancer Institute (NCI) in the U.S.

To prevent and fight cancer, Dr. Flavin-Koenig recommends following a regimen of vitamins and enzymes. Her recommendations are based on her observations of cancer cell activity in the biological lab and 23 years of treating cancer patients.

This regimen includes:

- Beta Carotene: this is Vitamin A in plant form and is non-toxic. Dosage: 200 mg per day. She calls this the most important treatment (after stopping smoking) which she uses. It inhibits the "bcl-2" gene and makes cells more sensitive to immune therapy, as well as chemo and hyperthermia. Dr. Flavin-Koenig uses low-dose chemo, but only to treat lung and colon cancer. She says "it is not enough alone."

- Vitamin A: from cod liver oil, which also has Vitamin D. Dosage: one gram a day. This "limits the rate of DNA synthesis and causes apoptosis (programmed cell death) in most tumors — colon, prostate, sarcoma, lung, breast, etc." Note: Synthetic Vitamin A and that found in fish oils, like cod liver oil, can be toxic if taken in excess.

- Soy Products: (a controversial subject) "inhibit the receptors for hormones" and are therefore effective in the treatment of prostate cancer.

- Fish Oil: Dosage: 4 grams a day. It inhibits angiogenesis and the "ras" gene that feeds tumor growth.

- N-Acetylcysteine: Dosage: 600 mg, 3 times a day. It inhibits angiogenesis, transforms "bcl-2" into "bax" [another gene], which "makes it pro-apoptosis. It also increases T-killer cells and binds with [gets rid of] nitric oxide which suppresses the immune system and stimulates tumor growth."

- Sodium Selenite: Dosage: 400 micrograms a day. It inhibits the protein kinase C (PKC). It should not be taken at the same time as Vitamin C.

- Vitamin C: Dosage: 3-5 grams a day spread through the day or 3 grams a day combined with 5-7 grams by IV twice a week. It increases hydrogen peroxide in the tumor cells [which kills them].

- Lactoferrin: Dosage: 1 gram dissolved slowly in mouth at bedtime. It inhibits angiogenesis and binds with iron to decrease tumor growth. It also has antiviral activity.

- Bromelain: Dosage: 1 capsule 4 times a day. It also inhibits angiogenesis. It is an enzyme extracted from pineapples.

- Wobe Mugos: An enzyme mixture, which enhances the immune system and helps block tumor growth, especially in colon cancer.

- Indomethacin: May require a prescription. It blocks the Prostaglandin E2 (PGE2) and ornithine decarboxylase. Both of these play a major role in angiogenesis and tumor growth plus metastases.

- Devil's Claw: A somewhat less effective substitute for above. Take 3 times a day.

- Thuja: For cervical cancer. It is an anti-viral plant, which comes in tincture form.


Dr. Flavin-Koenig also promotes a series of general guidelines for treating prostate cancer which include:

- Green tea and soy products to reduce hormone receptors and melatonin (9 mg, at night).

- No Vitamin E except "succinate." Other types of Vitamin E protect tumors.

- No iron, no B complex, or zinc.

- Eat lots of fish (no shellfish -- too much cholesterol), limited eggs, chicken, turkey and all vegetable dishes, with olive oil.

- No red meat.

- No unsaturated fatty acids. Instead, use olive oil and butter. Butter has butyric acid that prevents DNA synthesis. This is also found in wheat bran and figs.


Dr. Flavin-Koenig is constantly searching internationally for treatments including chemo, plants, teas, vitamins, hyperthermia, etc. Because of her encyclopedic knowledge, she often consults with colleagues in hospitals all over Europe and with MD Anderson and others in the U.S. She recently tested a tea from Turkey, which cured liver metastases from kidney cancer.

Dr. Flavin-Koenig often consults and speaks on the topic of cancer treatments, including the integration of therapies such as chemotherapy with other healing methods like teas, vitamins, and plants.

### Further Reading & References

- Dr. Flavin Recommends Nutrients: http://www.annieappleseedproject.org/drflavrecnut.html

- CollMED: http://www.collmed.org/2010/09/causes-of-cancer-interview/

- Foundation for Collaborative Medicine & Research: http://stefansargent.clients.neteverything.com/media/collmed/causes.html

## Dr. Kristine Nolfi

Danish doctor Kristine Nolfi stated that she cured her own cancer of the breast by consuming a pure, raw food diet, wherein the highest nutritional value lies. Dr. Nolfi claims raw foods are easy to digest and therefore easy on the body.

After curing her cancer the first time, Dr. Nolfi resumed a diet with cooked food and found that her cancer came back. She again reverted to a raw food diet and again got rid of the cancer.

Dr. Nolfi founded a cancer cure center, called the "Humlegaarden" sanatorium where she puts patients on a 100% organic and vegetarian raw-food diet. She cured many patients in this way.

Unfortunately, Dr. Nolfi lost her medical license for purportedly using 'dangerous' and unapproved methods but her fame nevertheless spread throughout Scandinavia.

Dr. Nolfi wrote a book, *My Experiences with Living Food*, that contains all her recommendations for consuming vitamins and nutrients through raw vegetables and fruits.

### Further Reading & References

- *Raw Food Treatment of Cancer* by Kristine Nolfi

- *My Experiences with Living Food* by Kristine Nolfi

## Dr. Maud Tresillian Fere's Self-Cure

Dr. Maud Tresillian Fere was a conventional medical doctor in all ways except for her view of cancer treatment. She strongly believed in the power of dietetic control combined with simple supplementary medication. In fact, using these methods was how she claimed to have healed her own cancer of the bowel.

Dr. Tresillian Fere stresses the importance of understanding exactly what goes into the food and drink you consume on a daily basis. She shares vital information on water, sources of the best carbohydrates and proteins, and what she calls "cleansing foods," which are raw vegetables and fruits. In addition, she held that excessive sodium, along with breaking the Laws of Good Health as she describes them, were the most common cause of cancer development.

She also touts health habits such as getting plenty of fresh air, having enough sleep and relaxation, and maintaining a generally cheerful attitude.

Dr. Tressillian Fere's cancer treatment also included a constant regimen of medicine made up of treatments such as iodine, stock vinegar, and acidulated water. She points out that these things are natural chemicals as opposed to drugs.

### Further Reading & References

- *Does Diet Cure Cancer?* by Maud Tresillian Fere

# Dr. Johanna Budwig/Flaxseed Oil & Cottage Cheese (FOCC)

Dr. Johanna Budwig, a German physician and seven-time alternative Nobel Prize nominee, created what is now called the "Budwig Protocol" as a way to cure cancer. It mainly consists of a three-month flax oil-quark program, which is a combination diet of whole flaxseeds, flaxseed oil, and low-fat organic cottage cheese (known in Europe as "quark").

The Budwig diet includes a long list of other recommended foods such as herbs, nuts, cocoa, and tea. She also provided a list of foods to stay away from, which include hydrogenated oils, hard-shell seafood, white breads, and soy products.

The Budwig program replenishes cells that are devoid of essential fats and oils, thereby allowing them to function once again. In turn, this leads to healing and recovery from a number of degenerative diseases including cancer.

Dr. Budwig held that cancer was caused by one of four things: a weak immune system, toxins, an improper diet, or oxygen deprivation (or a combination of any of these things).

Dr. Budwig states in her book, *Flax Oil As a True Aid Against Arthritis, Heart Infarction, Cancer, and Other Diseases*:

"I often take very sick cancer patients away from hospital where they are said to have only a few days left to live, or perhaps only a few hours. This is mostly accompanied by very good results…in the hospital it was said that they could no longer urinate or produce bowel movements. They suffered from dry coughing without being able to bring up any mucous. Everything was blocked. It greatly encourages them when suddenly the …fats with their wealth of electrons, start reactivating the vital functions and the patient immediately begins to feel better."

After three decades of research Dr. Budwig, a seven-time Nobel Prize nominee, found that the blood of seriously ill cancer patients was always, without exception, deficient in certain important essential ingredients such as phosphatides and lipoproteins. The blood of a healthy person always contains sufficient quantities of these essential ingredients. However, without these natural ingredients cancer cells grow wild and out of control.

In the course of her research, blood analysis showed a strange greenish-yellow substance in place of the healthy red oxygen carrying hemoglobin that belongs there. This explained why cancer patients weaken and become anemic. This startling discovery led Dr. Budwig to test her theory. She found that when these natural ingredients were replenished over approximately a three-month period, tumors gradually receded. The strange greenish elements in the blood were replaced with healthy red blood cells as the phosphatides and lipoproteins almost miraculously reappeared. Weakness and anemia disappeared and life energy was restored. Symptoms of cancer, liver dysfunction and diabetes were completely alleviated.

Dr. Budwig then discovered an all-natural way for people to replace those essential ingredients in their bodies. Eating organic flaxseed oil & cottage cheese together made for an effective natural remedy since each triggers the release of the healing properties of the other.

In the mid 1950's, Dr. Budwig began her long and meticulous research on the importance of essential fatty acids (linoleic and linolenic) in the diet.

Her subsequent discoveries and announcements sparked mixed reactions. While the general public was eager for this information, German manufacturers of commercial dietary fats (margarine, hard shortening, vegetable oils) went to extremes to prevent her from publishing her findings.

Dr. Budwig preached against the use of these fats, which she called "pseudo" fats. In order to extend the shelf life of their products, manufacturers use chemical processes that render their food products harmful to the body. These harmful fats go by a number of names, including "hydrogenated," "partially hydrogenated," and even "polyunsaturated."

More than 50 years later, it has now become widely accepted that the hydrogenated "trans fats" made by these manufactures are profoundly harmful. There is no question that Dr. Budwig was right about this subject, yet her other findings, especially those concerning the benefit of the flaxseed oil/cottage cheese mixture, have not gained acceptance despite the testimony of many patients who controlled or reversed their cancers using the Budwig Protocol.

The chemical processing of fats destroys the vital electron cloud within the fat. Once the electrons have been removed, these fats can no longer bind with oxygen, and they actually become a harmful substance deposited within the body. The heart, for instance, rejects these fats and they end up as inorganic fatty deposits on the heart muscle itself.

Chemically processed fats are not water-soluble when bound to protein. They end up blocking circulation, damage heart action, inhibit cell renewal, and impede the free flow of blood and lymph fluids. The bioelectrical action in these areas slows down and may become completely paralyzed. The entire organism shows a measurable loss of electrical energy which is replenished only by adding active lipids to the diet. These nutritional fats are vital.

Science has proven that fats play an important role in the functioning of the entire body. Fats (lipids) are vital for all growth processing, renewal of cells, brain and nerve functions, sensory organs (eyes and ears), and for the body's adjustment to heat, cold, and quick temperature changes. Our energy resources are based on lipid metabolism. To function efficiently, cells require true polyunsaturated, live electron-rich lipids, present in abundance in raw flaxseed oil. True polyunsaturated fats greedily absorb proteins and oxygen and pump them through the system.

Lipids are only water-soluble and free-flowing when bound to protein; thus the importance of protein-rich cottage cheese. When high quality, electron-rich fats are combined with proteins, the electrons are protected until the body requires energy. This energy source is then fully and immediately available to the body on demand, as nature intended.

Dr. Roehm, an oncologist, stated in the July 1990 issue of the *Townsend Letter for Doctors*:

"What Dr. Johanna Budwig has demonstrated to my initial disbelief but lately, to my complete satisfaction in my practice is: CANCER IS EASILY CURABLE, the treatment is dietary/lifestyle, the response is immediate; the cancer cell is weak and vulnerable; the precise biochemical breakdown point was identified by her in 1951 and is specifically correctable."

Dr. Roehm further claimed:

"… this diet is far and away the most successful anti-cancer diet in the world."

General Rules for the Budwig Diet:

- The patient has no nourishment on Day 1 other than 250 ml (8.5 oz) of flax oil with honey plus freshly squeezed fruit juices (no sugar added!). In the case of a very ill person, champagne may be added on the first day in place of juice and is taken with the flax oil and honey. Champagne is easily absorbable and has a serious purpose here.

- Sugar is absolutely forbidden. Grape juice may be added to sweeten any other freshly squeezed juices.

- Other forbidden foods are:

  - All animal fats.

  - All Salad Oils (this includes commercial mayonnaise)

  - All Meats (chemicals & hormones)

  - Butter

  - Margarine

  - Preserved Meats (the preservatives block metabolism even of flax oil)

- Freshly squeezed vegetable (and certain fruit) juices are fine - carrot, celery, apple, and red beet.

- Three times daily a warm tea is essential - peppermint, rose hips or grape tea - all sweetened as desired with honey. One cup of black tea before noon is fine.

Daily Plan:

- Before breakfast - a glass of acidophilus milk or sauerkraut juice is taken.

- Breakfast - Muesli (regular cereal) is topped with 2 tablespoons (30 ml) of flax oil and honey and fresh fruit according to season - berries, cherries, apricots, peaches, grated apple. Vary the flavor from day to day. Use any nuts except peanuts. Herbal teas as desired or black tea. A 4 oz (120 g) serving of "The Spread" (directions below). This is fine to eat straight like a custard, or add it to other foods taken in the day as you will see.

- Morning snack (10am) - A glass of fresh carrot juice, apple, celery, or beet-apple juice is taken.

- Lunch - Raw salad with yoghurt-flax oil mayonnaise (directions below).

- In addition to green salads, use grated turnips, carrots, kohlrabi, radishes, sauerkraut, or cauliflower. A fine powder of horseradish, chives, or parsley may be added for flavor.

- Cooked meal course - steamed vegetables, potatoes, or such grains as rice, buckwheat, or millet may be served. To these add either "The Spread" (see below) or "The Mayo" (see below) - for flavor and to increase your intake of flax oil. Also, mix "The Spread" with potatoes for an especially hearty meal. Add caraway, chives, parsley, or other herbs.

- Dessert - Mix fresh fruit other than those used for breakfast with "The Spread," this time (instead of honey), flavor using cream of lemon, vanilla, or berries.

- Afternoon snack (4pm) - a small glass of natural wine (no preservatives) or champagne or fresh fruit juice with 1-2 tablespoons of honey-coated flax seeds.

- Dinner - have this early, at 6pm. Make a hot meal using buckwheat, oat, or soy cakes. Grits from buckwheat are the very best and can be placed in a vegetable soup, or in a more solid form of cakes with herbal sauce. Sweet sauces & soups can always be given more healing energy by adding "The Spread." Only honey or grape juice can be used for sweeteners. NO white sugar (or brown!) Only freshly squeezed juices and NOT reconstituted juices (preservative danger) may be used. These must be completely natural.

How to prepare The Spread:

- Place 250 ml (8.5 oz) flaxseed oil into a mixer bowl and add one pound (450 g) of 1% cottage cheese (i.e. low fat Quark) and add 4 tablespoons (60 ml) of Honey. Turn on the mixer and add just enough low fat milk or water to get the contents of the bowl to blend in together. In 5 minutes, a preparation of custard consistency results that has NO taste of the oil (and no oily 'ring' should be seen when you rinse out the bowl).

- Alternatively, you can use yogurt instead of cottage cheese in proportions of 1 oz (30 g) of yogurt to 1 tablespoon (15 ml) each of flaxseed oil and of honey and blend as above. Note: When flaxseed oil is blended like this, it does not cause diarrhea even when given in large amounts. It reacts chemically with the (sulphur) proteins of the cottage cheese, yoghurt, etc.

How to prepare the Mayonnaise:

- Mix together 2 tablespoons (30 ml) flaxseed Oil, 2 tablespoons (30 ml) milk, and 2 tablespoons (30 ml) yogurt.

- Then add 2 tablespoons (30 ml) of lemon juice (or apple cider vinegar) and add 1 teaspoon (2.5g) of mustard plus some herbs such as marjoram or dill.

- Next, add 2 or 3 slices of health food store pickles (no preservatives - read the label) and a pinch of herbal salts.

You will have to remain on this diet for a good five years, at which time your tumor may have disappeared. Persons who break the rules of this diet, Dr. Budwig reports, (i.e., eating preserved meats, candy, etc) will sometimes grow rapidly worse and cannot be saved after they come back from their spree.

In 1967, Dr. Budwig broadcast the following statement during an interview over the South German Radio Network, describing her incoming patients with failed operations and x-ray therapy:

"Even in these cases it is possible to restore health in a few months at most, I would truly say 90% of the time.

"This has never been contradicted, but this knowledge has been a long time reaching this side of the ocean, hasn't it? Cancer treatment can be very simple and very successful once you know how. The cancer interests don't want you to know this. May those of you who have suffered from this disease (and I include your family and friends in this) forgive the miscreants who have kept this simple information from reaching you for so long."

It is believed Dr. Budwig was referring to people above who had NOT previously been treated with radiation or chemotherapy. Flaxseed oil is readily denatured by oxygen, heat, and light. That's why it is used in paint. Rancid oil is bad for health, so the flax oil MUST be carefully produced, packed under nitrogen in lightproof containers, refrigerated until used, used as fresh as possible, and promptly stabilized with protein once the container is opened.

Flaxseeds may also be used. Seeds need only be cracked in a food blender, or they may be ground in a coffee grinder. One needs three times the amount of seeds to get the oil equivalent. The seeds are also high in soluble fiber, so blending with liquid tends to produce ever-hardening "jellies." Fresh-cracked seed sprinkled on muesli & eaten promptly tastes great.

At one time, Dr. Budwig served as the Central Government's Senior Expert for fats and pharmaceutical drugs in Germany, therefore giving her a reputation during her life as one of the world's leading authorities on fats and oils. She held that the trans fats used in most deep-fried and processed foods actually work to suffocate cells. By depriving those cells of life-giving oxygen, the result is chronic or terminal disease.

Dr. Budwig held very strongly that her treatment regime could successfully treat cancer. Her views on trans fats, once controversial, are now accepted everywhere. She had 50 years of successes spanning over 2,400 people with cancer and other diseases to back up her claim.

There are variations of the above protocol which are reportedly effective, and some leading alternative cancer clinics and doctors will encourage their patients to use the flaxseed oil/cottage cheese mixture along with other therapies.

Bill Henderson, perhaps North America's leading advocate of the Budwig Protocol, offers this recipe:

"One-third of a cup of flaxseed oil mixed with two-thirds of a cup of cottage cheese. Add berries, almonds and walnuts and a little stevia [optional] in the blender. Add a little fresh water. Adjust to taste. Blend on the 'liquefy' setting. Eat it as soon as it's blended. Order flaxseed oil from Barleans at 800-445-3529 or www.barleans.com. When you've gotten rid of your cancer you can scale back to a maintenance dose, which cuts the amount of flaxseed oil and cottage cheese in half." He adds that "Stirring isn't good enough. To mix it properly, you have to blend it. . .You may have heard that dairy products are bad for cancer patients, and I would agree with that. But when you mix cottage cheese with flax oil, it loses its dairy property. Dozens of people I know who are lactose-intolerant eat the Budwig protocol every day without any problems whatsoever." Henderson's Special Report, *How to Cure Almost Any Cancer at Home for $5.15 a Day*, is available at www.cancerdefeated.com.

### Further Reading & References

- *Flax Oil As a True Aid Against Arthritis, Heart Infarction, Cancer, and Other Diseases* by Dr. Johanna Budwig

- *Cancer: The Problem and the Solution* by Dr. Johanna Budwig

- *The Oil Protein Diet Cookbook* by Dr. Johanna Budwig

- Budwig Center: http://www.budwigcenter.com/

- Health and Well-Being, featuring Dr. Johanna Budwig: http://www.lightsv.org/bud1.htm

- Roehm, *Townsend Letter for Doctors*, July 1990

- "Promotion and Prevention of Tumour Growth Effects of Endotoxin, Inflamation, and Dietary Lipids", by Raymond Kearney, Ph.D, Department of Infectious Diseases, The University of Sydney, Sydney, N.S.W. 2006 Australia. *International Clinical Nutrition Review*, October, 1987 Vol. 7, No. 4.

# Dr. Max Gerson: Gerson Therapy

Gerson Therapy is a whole-body, natural treatment designed to heal the body against cancer, heart disease, allergies, and other illnesses. It was established more than seventy-five years ago by Dr. Max Gerson, and described in detail in his book *A Cancer Therapy: Results of Fifty Cases and the Cure of Advanced Cancer.*

Gerson Therapy requires that fresh, organic juices be consumed on a daily basis. The goal is to provide the body with ultra-heavy doses of enzymes, minerals, and other nutrients. This gives the body the ability to break down and eradicate diseased body tissues.

A typical daily treatment includes thirteen glasses of fresh, raw fruit and vegetable juice, three vegetarian meals, and ample amounts of fresh fruit for dessert and snacks. Medications are included as part of the therapy, all of which are considered organic, biological materials (e.g., Vitamin $B_{12}$, potassium compound, and pancreatic enzymes, just to name a few). Finally, the therapy includes an important detoxification protocol.

The diet also includes potassium/iodine supplements. Dr. Gerson stressed the importance of a high potassium content that is more in the skins or outer part of root vegetables than in the centers. Sodium, on the other hand, was to be severely restricted - the diet was completely without added salt but with added potassium salts instead. Dr. Gerson believed an imbalance between sodium and potassium in each cell also contributed to the development of cancer. Therefore, his therapeutic diet excludes sodium and provides abundant potassium.

Other forbidden foods include salt, oil, berries, nuts, and all bottled, canned, refined, preserved, and processed foods. No aluminum utensils are used, and juices must be pressed.

In addition, Gerson prescribed hydrochloric acid with pepsin, pancreatin, high doses of Lugol's solution (an iodine supplement) together with freeze-dried thyroid, niacin, royal jelly, and injections of vitamin B12 with crude liver.

In addition, raw liver juice was used for its high content of enzymes. Later, with increasing chemicalization of agriculture, the liver juice was omitted while linseed/flax oil was belatedly added to the list of supplements.

Liver detoxification with frequent coffee enemas is a cornerstone of the Gerson Therapy; otherwise, patients with advanced cancer might die despite reduction in the size of tumors. Some patients are also given castor-oil enemas and oral and/or rectal hydrogen peroxide and rectal ozone treatment. Dr. Gerson pioneered the use of coffee enemas, which are now widely used in other alternative cancer treatment protocols. Until the 1970s, coffee enemas were listed in the *Merck Manual* as an accepted mainstream medical treatment. The treatment was apparently removed because the editors lost interest in it, not because it was found to be unsafe or ineffective.

Dr. Gerson stated:

"Cancer *is not a single cellular problem; it is an accumulation of numerous damaging factors combined in deteriorating the whole metabolism, after the liver has been progressively impaired in its functions. This slow poisoning of the entire organism, a lowering of the electrical activity in vital organs, and the weakening of the liver, the prime organ of detoxification, creates a cancerous body that is anergic.*"

Gerson Therapy is based on the view that malignant growths result from metabolic dysfunction within cells. This was to be countered by diet and detoxification. Gerson felt that, in order to be healed, the body needed to be detoxified with agents that rendered it hypersensitive to abnormal substances (including bacilli and cancer cells), which the body will then eliminate. The more malignant the cells, the more effective the therapy. The Gerson Institute, still open under the direction of Max Gerson's daughter

Charlotte, claims to "cure half of the patients who have a month to live, and 90% of patients with any early cancer."

The Cancer Guide Website *Third Opinion* refers to Gerson Therapy in the following way: "*Especially excellent results are observed in advanced cancers of all types, including: inoperable lymphoma; spreading melanoma; metastasis to the liver; aggressive ovarian cancer; and pancreatic cancer.*"

Advocates of this therapy state it brings no damaging side effects and has been successfully used for over 60 years.

Max Gerson was a medical doctor from Germany who befriended Nobel Prize winner Albert Schweitzer after curing Schweitzer's wife of lung tuberculosis when all other treatments had failed. Gerson published many papers on his theories, treatments, and results treating cancer patients naturally. He remains greatly respected in the history of medicine.

Dr. Gerson died in 1959. The Gerson Institute was established as a non-profit organization in 1978; the Gerson Therapy hospital in Tijuana has been open since 1977. More than 8,000 patients have been treated. Although most arrive in terminal condition, yet many have recovered. Dr. Gerson's daughter continues her father's work by consulting at the Gerson Institute.

### *Further Reading & References*

- *A Cancer Therapy: Results of Fifty Cases and the Cure of Advanced Cancer* by Dr. Max Gerson

- *The Gerson Therapy: The Proven Nutritional Program for Cancer and Other Illnesses* by Charlotte Gerson, et al.

- *Dr. Max Gerson - Healing the Hopeless* by Howard Straus

- *Healing Cancer and Other Degenerative Diseases With the Gerson Therapy : The Complete Guide to Home Use* by Charlotte Gerson

- *Gerson Diet Therapy for Women's Cancers: Breast Cancer, Ovarian Cancer, Cervical Cancer* by Charlotte Gerson

- Gerson Institute/Cancer Curing Society: http://www.gerson.org/

- CHIPSA: The 'Official' Gerson Hospital: http://chipsa.com/gerson.html

- Cassileth BR. *Alternative medicine handbook: the complete reference guide to alternative and complementary therapies.* New York: W. W. Norton & Co., 1998:186-188.

- Diamond WJ, et al. *An Alternative Medicine Definitive Guide to Cancer.* Tiburon, California: Future Medicine Publishing, Inc., 1997:772.

- Weitzman S. Alternative nutritional cancer therapies. Int J Cancer 1998;11(Suppl):69-72.

- Third Opinion: An International Resource Guide to Alternative Therapy Centers for Treating and Preventing Cancer, Arthritis, Diabetes, HIV/AIDS, MS, CFS, and Other Diseases by John M. Fink, http://www.thirdopinion.net/support_services.html

# Dr. Moerman's Anti-Cancer Diet

Dr. Moerman, a physician from Holland, developed his anti-cancer diet in the 1930s. He brought a fresh perspective to the nutrition-based idea of cancer treatment and prevention. His work stemmed from observing the instinctive eating patterns of pigeons afflicted with cancer. Gradually, he worked with human patients who voluntarily went through his treatment plans.

Like several other alternative cancer treatments, it was developed on a trial-and-error basis. His research covered around 50 years, from the early 1930s to his death in 1988. From his observations, he created a unique nutrition program that was gradually adopted by other physicians throughout the Netherlands.

The key nutrients of the diet include Vitamins A, D, the B complex, C, and E, as well as citric acid, iodine, iron, and sulfur. Foods include vegetables and fruits, certain whole grains, egg yolks, and dairy products, among other things.

The theory behind the anti-cancer diet is that the natural defenses of the human body are far more sophisticated than anything manufactured in a laboratory setting. Because of that, Dr. Moerman thought it was more important to focus on enhancing the body's immune system rather than just focusing treatment on a cancerous tumor.

By taking this approach, Dr. Moerman believed the body could heal itself. Nobel Prize winner Linus Pauling, who wrote the forward to the book on Dr. Moerman's diet, described his theory in this way:

"...Persons with good vitality might fight cancer more effectively than those with low vitality."

Essentially, the diet creates a hostile environment for cancer cells while simultaneously creating a friendly environment for healthy cells.

This diet is an immune-system-building, "metabolic balancing," diet and is designed to stop the spread of cancer. It is not designed to kill cancer cells directly, but is designed to support various aspects of the immune system and build collagen fibrils so that the cancer does not spread.

Like many other alternative doctors, he considered that "cancer was [caused by] a malfunctioning of the immune system that manifested itself outwardly on the body's weakest organ as a tumor."

There are eight key nutrients in this diet:

- Vitamin A (requires Vitamin D as a catalyst)
- Vitamin B complex
- Vitamin C
- Vitamin E
- Citric Acid
- Iodine
- Iron
- Sulfur

Dr. Moerman identified 17 symptoms of cancer, each of which can be addressed by one or more of the eight key nutrients.

The diet basically consists of most vegetables, most fruits, some whole grains, butter, some other dairy products, egg yolks (not egg whites), and some other items. The diet is designed to supplement the eight key nutrients. The diet is very strict regarding foods that cannot be consumed (e.g., table salt - even iodized table salt, and meat are not allowed). The complete diet, along with recipes, can be found in the book, *Dr. Moerman's Anti- Cancer Diet - Holland's Revolutionary Nutritional Program for Combating Cancer* by Ruth Jochems (with a Forward by Linus Pauling).

More than fifty years later, the Ministry of Health in the Netherlands approved Dr. Moerman's diet as an officially recognized treatment for cancer.

### Further Reading & References

- *Dr. Moerman's Anti-Cancer Diet: Holland's Revolutionary Nutritional Program for Combating Cancer* by Ruth Jochems

- Dr. Moerman's Anti-Cancer Diet: http://www.cancertutor.com/Cancer/Moerman.html

# Dries Cancer Diet

It's a widely accepted medical fact that dietary and nutritional changes can help treat and cure cancer and other illnesses, and it is on this premise that the Dries Cancer Diet is based.

The Dries Cancer Diet is mostly fruit-based and focuses on the bio-energetic properties of certain foods. (The bio-energetic value of a food is determined by its ability to absorb light.) Developed by German researcher and nutritionist Jan Dries, this approach is meant to be used as a supplement to regular treatment. A major premise behind this approach is about keeping life bearable throughout the grueling process of regular oncology treatments.

Dries believes cancerous tumors develop when cells depolarize as a result of a drop in bio-energy and subsequent loss of ability for the body to resist cancer. He points out that certain foods have a high bio-energetic value that exists on the same frequency as the body's innate ability to resist cancer. Because of that, they can restore the energy balance of the body.

Dries divides food into seven groups, based on bio-energetic value. Groups I, II, and III contain the foods of primary importance, which include pineapples, honeydew, raspberries, and avocado (Group I), kiwi, cherries, apricots, and mango (Group II), and blackcurrants, strawberries, and fresh lychees (Group III).

The Dries Diet is low in calories and relatively simple to follow. It's also said to be highly digestible and easy to switch over to.

### Further Reading & References

- *The Dries Cancer Diet: A Practical Guide to the Use of Fresh Fruit and Raw Vegetables in the*

- *Treatment of Cancer* by Jan Dries

- *The Dries Cancer Diet: A Practical Guide to the Use of Fresh Fruit and Raw Vegetables in the*

- *Treatment of Cancer* by Jan Dries

- *The Cancer Handbook: What's Really Working (What Doctors Don't Tell You)* by Lynne McTaggart

- Every Diet Website on the Dries Cancer Diet: http://www.everydiet.org/diet/dries-cancer-diet

# Fruitarian Diet

Fruitarianism is the practice of eating a diet that consists of fruits, seeds, and nuts. Neither vegetables nor grains are eaten, and animal products are completely avoided. Fruitarianism can be considered a specialized form of veganism.

People who practice this diet believe that it was the original diet intended for mankind and think of it as a holistic approach to health. There is also a compassion element involved in the diet because fruitarians avoid killing anything, including plants.

Concerns over the fruitarian diet include the fact that it is highly restrictive and doesn't supply adequate amounts of vitamins, such as $B_{12}$. It is also high in fructose, a form of sugar that is under increasing scrutiny as being toxic to the liver and a possible cause of diabetes and cardiovascular disease as well as cancer.

On the other hand, some studies suggest that lipid profiles and glucose tolerance improve on fruitarian diets.

Australian Dr. O.L.M. Abramowski, M.D., wrote a book called A Raw-Food Doctor's Cure where he states the fruitarian diet saved his life and healed him from age-related problems and disease. He claims to have used the diet to heal patients at his sanitarium.

### Further Reading & References

- *A Raw-Food Doctor's Cure* by Dr. O.L.M. Abramowski

- Fruitarianism: http://en.wikipedia.org/wiki/Fruitarianism

# Rev. George Malkmus: Hallelujah Diet

The Hallelujah Diet is a vegetarian approach to eating that consists of 85% raw, plant-based food and 15% cooked, plant-based food. It was developed by the Rev. George Malkmus after he was diagnosed with colon cancer and has apparently helped people with a wide variety of diseases.

Instead of pursuing radiation and chemotherapy, which had not been able to save his mother from dying of the same disease, Rev. Malkmus changed his diet to raw foods. He consumed significant amounts of raw fruits and vegetables and carrot juice in particular. Gradually, all his symptoms and his tumor disappeared.

The Hallelujah Diet is primarily based on eating fruits and vegetables, drinking lots of water, avoiding saturated fats and hydrogenated oils, taking in more fiber, and steering clear of stress. Exercise is also a crucial element of the program. It's touted to relieve the symptoms of cancer, obesity, and acid reflux.

Hallelujah Acres proclaims the simple message of God's original plan for the care of the physical body. This plan includes the lifestyle features of humanity's first home in paradise: a living plant-food diet, vigorous exercise, fresh air, pure water, sunshine, proper rest, and those other factors that promote physical well-being.

Dr. Malkmus writes:

"After more than 20 years of personal experience and research, I consider BarleyGreen the single most important food I put into my body each day. It is the most nutritionally dense food I know of on earth today, and it provides my body cells with all the nutrients they need to remain strong and healthy. I personally consume three to four tablespoons of BarleyGreen daily.

"The second most important food in my diet is carrot juice. Presently I consume an average of 16 ounces of freshly extracted carrot juice from a Champion Juicer daily. During my bout with cancer more than 20 years ago, I consumed one to two quarts daily, as BarleyGreen did not exist at that time. At the Gerson Clinic today, they give eight 8-ounce servings of carrot juice daily to their patients along with 4 glasses of a green drink similar to BarleyGreen.

"Using this juice therapy along with a cleansing program, they are healing 'incurable' diseases, such as lung cancer, brain cancer, spreading melanoma and more. The third most important food I put into my body is the raw fruits and vegetables, which are consumed at the noon and evening meals. I eat no breakfast and haven't for over 20 years. (A glass of BarleyGreen is my only breakfast food.) Thus, my average daily food intake consists of approximately 85% raw food. I do allow myself some cooked food at the end of the evening meal, which might consist of a baked white or sweet potato, brown rice or steamed vegetables, but this is more for its taste than nutritional value.

"On this basically raw food diet, which has included large amounts of raw vegetable juices, I have not only been able to remove all my physical problems and keep them gone for over 20 years, but also experience abundant energy, great enthusiasm, wonderful clarity of mind, freedom from stress (even though I am in a potentially stressful ministry), and have marvelous physical endurance. What more could anyone ask or want from their body? And my desire is that everyone might be able to know how they too can experience the same … thus the reason for Hallelujah Acres!"

### Further Reading & References

- *The New Cancer Survivors: Living with Grace, Fighting with Spirit* by Natalie Davis Spingarn

- Hallelujah Acres: http://www.hacres.com/

- "Why Juice?" by Reverend/Dr. George Malkmus, http://www.all-creatures.org/cb/a-whyjuice.html

# Jethro Kloss, Back to Eden

Jethro Kloss was a well-known early 20th century American herbalist and promoter of natural healing. Jethro Kloss's cancer treatment is based on natural foods, herbs, water, fresh air, massage, sunshine, exercise, and rest.

Kloss always believed that simple, natural diets could both save money and prevent suffering. He was an advocate of returning to "God's original plan for maintaining health," which meant returning to natural habits of living.

Kloss wrote a book, called <u>Back To Eden</u>, which was originally published in 1939 and has been expanded and revised multiple times, most recently in 2009. Kloss's book has actually been credited with helping to create the natural foods industry. Today, it serves as a groundbreaking text on herbs, natural diet, and holistic health. Jethro Kloss has earned especially high regard among cancer survivors and his work serves as a treasury of legendary formulas and programs.

In his book, Kloss wrote about what causes different kinds of cancers, how to prevent cancer, and how to cure it. Kloss also shares personal success stories in healing others and lists his recommended herbs for healthful living. He talks about food preparation, how to preserve the vitamins in food, which foods are health-destroying, the importance of water, and shares tips in caring for those who are ill.

His book includes a section on documented proof that his treatment works. No drugs are used, just herbs and a health regimen.

### Further Reading & References

- *Back To Eden* by Jethro Kloss

- *Back To Eden Cookbook* by Jethro Kloss

# Johanna Brandt Grape Diet

Johanna Brandt, a naturopathic doctor from South Africa, created her Grape Diet as a contribution toward solving the cancer problem. She states the diet is founded on personal experience and presents it more as a way to prevent cancer than to cure it, though she also says advanced cancer cases have been cured using her methods.

The diet itself starts with a fast that lasts two to three days and includes consumption of cold water. It also includes the administration of a daily enema mixed from lukewarm water and pure white soap. The point of the fast is to clear the stomach of possible poisons.

Following that, a meal of grapes is to be eaten every two hours for twelve straight hours. This process is to be repeated for one or two weeks and as much as a month for serious cases. The process should not continue for longer than two months.

The fasting has a significant purpose: It makes cancer cells hungry, and when the cells do get food, what they get is grape juice, which contains numerous major cancer killing nutrients, such as:

- Ellagic acid

- Catechin

- Quercetin

- Oligomeric proanthocyanidins (opc) or procyanidolic oligomers (pco), originally called pycnogenol (from the grape seeds)

- Resveratrol (skin coloring of purple grapes)

- Pterostilbene

- Selenium

- Lycopene

- Lutein

- Laetrile (amygdalin or vitamin b17) (from the seeds)

- Beta-carotene

- Caffeic acid and/or ferulic acid (together they kill cancer cells) and

- Gallic acid

In other words, the fasting is used to "trick" the cancer cells into consuming the first thing that comes along. The grapes become a great "transport agent" for getting the poisons into the cancer cells, meaning the grape juice carries the cancer killing nutrients into the cancer cells as they feed on the grape juice.

Compared to healthy cells, cancer cells consume about 15 times more glucose and other sugars as well as more minerals and more of some other nutrients. The 1931 Nobel Prize in medicine was awarded to Dr. Otto Warburg for this discovery. This means a sugary grape cure diet can propel several times more of certain cancer-killing nutrients into the cancer cells than into normal cells. Thus, the combination of consuming high levels of glucose, minerals, and other nutrients, plus the fasting, makes the purple grapes an exceptional cancer-fighting food, according to Brandt. The fasting is critical to this diet, and should not be taken lightly.

Brandt is reported to have used the now famous grape cure to cure herself of stomach cancer in the 1920's. For six weeks she ate nothing but grapes and she regards black varieties as the best. Thousands of former cancer victims have testified to the effectiveness of her method. Because it is now so difficult to obtain unsprayed grapes, commercially sprayed grapes have sometimes been used after thorough washing in warm soapy water and careful rinsing. Concord grapes are a recommended variety.

There are many other facets to the diet including a six-month treatment plan and the gradual introduction of vegetables, other fruits, and buttermilk.

To ensure the patient gets all of the main killer nutrients, the grape juice should include crushed seeds and the nutrients from the purple skins (to get the critical resveratrol). The purple color, such as in Concord purple grapes, has a critical cancer killing nutrient not found in other grapes. Back when she wrote her book, in the 1920s, the advantage of purple grapes was not known.

Also, if the patient eats or processes whole grapes, the recommendation is to buy grapes with the seeds, not seedless grapes. This is another aspect that Johanna Brandt could not have known about in the 1920s. The darker the purple grapes the better. Note: Because purple grapes and red grapes are so frequently confused with each other, it is not clear exactly how beneficial red grapes are. This is why it's recommended to look for the word "Concord" on packages of grapes, although there are purple grapes other than Concord grapes that are just as good.

Keep in mind if considering this diet:

Packaged, processed grape juice, even when it is organic, is generally pasteurized as required by law. Pasteurization destroys an unknown number of nutrients in the grape juice and could neutralize a significant portion of those nutrients. Avoid premixed grape juice.

Unfortunately, most, if not all, frozen grape juice is also pasteurized. Frozen grape juice also may have a small amount of tap water added to it. Some organic grape juices are processed with spring water, but even these may be pasteurized.

Only fresh purple grapes, pesticide-free and totally unprocessed, qualify for this diet. As stated in Johanna Brandt's book, *The Grape Cure*:

"It is safe to say that the first seven to ten days on grapes only would be required to clear the stomach and bowels of their ancient accumulations. And it is during this period that distressing symptoms often appear. Nature works thoroughly. She does not build on a rotten foundation. The purification of every part of the body must be complete before new tissue can be built. Also, a person on the Brandt diet will probably lose significant weight during the first few weeks. I mention this because a person, who begins this diet at 120 pounds or less, may need to watch their weight closely in order to keep from getting too low in weight. To keep their weight up, they might want to favor the Wortman Diet (to be discussed next). During the 8 hours they can eat on the Wortman diet, they can make sure they eat enough solid foods to keep their weight from dropping too much. "

Similar custom modifications can be made to address any other potential health problem a person might have. The Wortman Diet allows a great deal of individual flexibility to deal with specific issues.

The Wortman Grape Diet (as described in *The Grape Cancer Cure* by J.F. Goodavage) tells the story of Fred Wortman of Albany, Georgia, who developed an inoperable malignancy of the intestine. He faced the prospect of long treatments with radiation therapy. "*The doctors,*" Mr. Wortman said, "refused to operate when they discovered the condition of my bank balance."

Being a well-read man, he remembered a simple remedy for cancer that was detailed in a book by a Mrs. Brandt and looked it up. It was rather involved and cumbersome to follow, so he reduced it to its essentials, took the "cure," and was completely cancer-free within a month.

Wortman then had his experience published in "The Independent" and received hundreds of replies. Over 200 cancer sufferers reported complete recovery.

The grape treatment cured lung cancer in two weeks, he reported. Cancer of the prostate took a little longer - about a month. Only four cases of leukemia (cancer of the blood) were treated, but the judicious usage of grape juice cured them all. The treatment went like this:

- Begin with a 24 oz. bottle of (dark Concord) grape juice the first thing in the morning. Take a couple of swallows every 10 or 15 minutes (Do not gulp it down all at once). Do not eat until noon.

- After 12 o'clock, live the rest of the day normally, but do not eat anything after 8 o'clock in the evening...food seems to carry off the curative agent in the grape juice, which may be magnesium [sic], so stick to the fast between 8 p.m. and noon the following day.

- Keep this up every day for two weeks to one month.

Whereas Brandt claimed a 100% cure rate of exclusively terminal cancer patients, Wortman claims a "nearly 100%" cure rate of cancer patients in undefined condition.

In the description of her diet, Dr. Brandt takes into consideration the importance of what she calls the seven doctors of nature: fasting, air, water, sunshine, exercise, food, and a healthy mind.

She also explains that the science behind her diet has to do with the ability of the proteins in the grapes to help build new tissues with extraordinary speed. Naturally, she gives high praise to the medicinal properties of grapes.

**Further Reading and Reference**

- *The Grape Cure* by Johanna Brandt (1971)

- *How to Conquer Cancer, Naturally* by Johanna Brandt (1996)

- *The "Grape Cancer Cure"* by J.F. Goodavage (2000)


# Michio Kushi: Macrobiotic Diet/Zen Macrobiotics

Michio Kushi is credited with introducing modern macrobiotics to the United States in the early 1950s. The macrobiotic diet is an eating regimen than includes grains as a primary staple supplemented by natural foods such as fresh vegetables and beans. The diet stays away from refined and highly processed foods and recommends that each bite of food a person takes be chewed thoroughly.

The diet is also based on the view that humans are continually influenced by the environment around them, which includes not only food but also regular social interactions, climate, and geography.

The concept of macrobiotics reflects the writings of a Japanese physician, Sagen Ishizuka (1850-1910). He cured himself of cancer by abandoning the refined diet of modern Japan and reverting back to the unpurified Japanese diet of brown rice, soybeans, fish, miso soup, sea vegetables, and other traditional Oriental foods - the ancestral diet.

Kushi stated in his book, *The Macrobiotic Path To Total Health,* that "The macrobiotic diet is a mainly vegetarian diet consisting of 50% whole cereal grains, 20 to 30% locally grown vegetables, small amounts of soups, beans and sea vegetables, white meat, fish and fruit in limited amounts. Potatoes, sweet potatoes, tomatoes, eggplants, peppers, asparagus, spinach, beets, zucchini, avocados, mayonnaise, tea, coffee, and red meat are to be avoided."

The macrobiotic diet based on cooked brown rice and only a minimum of raw food is very different from all the other anti-cancer diets.

*"Although a relatively recent creation, the macrobiotic diet is based in large part on the yin-yang principle of balance, a fundamental component of ancient Chinese medicine. Yin and Yang are opposite forces believed to describe all components of life and the universe. Here the world view of balance is embodied in diet, including the selection, preparation, and consumption of foods,"* states Kushi.

Some proposed reasons why the macrobiotic diet helps some cancer patients:

- Low in fat

- High in fiber

- High vegetable intake

- Improved sodium to potassium ratio

- Ability to change an acid (cancer) environment back toward alkaline (healthy)

- Potent anti-cancer agents found in soybeans, sea vegetables and other fresh produce

- Thyroid stimulating substances found in sea vegetables.

Michio Kushi established a macrobiotic center in Boston in 1978 and has gained a noteworthy following. He has publicly encouraged cancer patients to continue with conventional care. His program includes cotton clothes, fresh air, and exercise. Earlier in the 20th century, Are Waerland became famous for a successful diet that consisted of sour milk and similar products, whole grains, raw or only partly cooked, as well as fruits and vegetables. There are still many active Waerland groups in Germany and Scandinavia. Bircher-Benner advocated a similar lacto-vegetarian raw-food diet. He invented the by now famous but greatly compromised muesli.

Anthony J. Sattilaro, MD, an anaesthesiologist at Methodist Hospital in Philadelphia has become a vocal proponent. He believed the macrobiotic diet was the reason he was able to heal his metastatic prostate cancer.

According to Kushi, cancer is the result of a person's behavior, largely due to improper diet but also to his or her thinking and lifestyle. Improper diet produces a "chronically toxic blood condition." He considers cancer to be a natural mechanism that localizes the toxic condition and relieves the rest of the body of the toxic load.

Kushi writes, "Of primary importance in dealing with cancer, then, is not to disturb this natural mechanism by taking out or destroying the cancer." The standard macrobiotic diet in cancer treatment is varied depending on the type of cancer.

According to Kushi, the recovery of cancer patients treated macrobiotically is hindered if they have undergone conventional treatments. He believes the conventional treatments of radiation therapy, chemotherapy, and surgery are "violent or artificial" as well as "toxic and unnatural." He states that compared with cancer patients treated only macrobiotically, conventionally treated patients who are then treated macrobiotically "often take longer to recover... and their recovery is often more complicated and difficult."

The macrobiotic diet is said to have helped thousands of people prolong their lives by recovering from a wide range of illnesses, including cancer, diabetes, and heart disease. The macrobiotic approach can be used in partnership with both conventional and alternative therapies. It is not to be thought of as a strict, set diet, but rather as a flexible dietary approach that differs according to personal need.

True macrobiotic healing comes not only from eating optimal quantities of the recommended foods but also from following way-of-life suggestions, which include things like going to bed before midnight and getting up with the sunrise, keeping your home in good order, walking outside for a half hour each day, wearing cotton clothing, avoiding perfumed cosmetics, avoiding the use of electric cooking devices and microwave ovens, and singing a happy song every day.

Kushi's work has been honored at the Smithsonian Institution's National Museum of American History and he has authored more than 40 books on the topic of macrobiotics and alternative health.

### Further Reading & References

- *The Macrobiotic Path To Total Health* by Michio Kushi and Alex Jack

- *The Cancer Prevention Diet: Michio Kushi's Macrobiotic Blueprint for the Prevention and Relief of*

- *Disease* by Michio Kushi, Alex Jack

- *Macrobiotic Approach to Cancer* by Michio Kushi, Edward Esko

- *Zen Macrobiotics for Americans* by Roger Mason

- *The Book of Macrobiotics: The Universal Way of Health, Happiness, and Peace* by Michio Kushi

- Kushi Institute: http://www.kushiinstitute.org/

- *The Macrobiotic Path To Total Health* by Michio Kushi and Alex Jack

- "Zen Macrobiotics Diet" by Hulda Clark, http://www.huldaclarkzappers.com/?page_id=210

# Arnold Ehret: Mucusless Diet Healing System

Professor Ehret was a German health educator in the early 20th century who devoted his life to the study of diet, detoxification, and healing illness through food. His message put heavy emphasis on the practice of fasting as the quickest route to healing. He states one cannot heal disease without eliminating the foods which produce disease, most of which are found in the modern diet.

He created the Mucusless Diet Healing System, which consists of water fasting and a type of raw food vegan diet, with an emphasis on certain fruits. Like all vegan diets, if one is using this diet for the treatment of cancer, it is often recommended there should be a strong emphasis on the allowable foods that are known to treat cancer.

Ehret believed the natural food for mankind to be fruits and starchless, green-leaved vegetables. He believed mucus to be a significant substance in the development of disease, which is why his food recommendations focus on non-mucus inducing foods.

Ehret also promoted the use of an herbal laxative he termed the "Intestinal Broom" and emphasized the need for individuals to make up for unhealthy living and eating habits by providing their bodies with proper, healthful compensation.

### Further Reading & References

- *Mucusless Diet Healing System* by Arnold Ehret

- *Rational Fasting* by Arnold Ehret

- *The Story of My Life* by Arnold Ehret

- Arnold Ehret Health Club: http://www.arnoldehret.org/

# Dr. Norman Walker/Jay Kordich: Raw Food Diet

Dr. Norman Walker is credited with pioneering the raw foods, juicing, and vegetarian movements. He was among the first to promote a raw foods diet and live-vegetable/juice therapy, contending that it healed people of "incurable" diseases. He was an English-American who led the way in the field of vegetable juicing and nutritional health.

Dr. Walker advocated drinking fresh, raw vegetable and fruit juices as a means to heal disease and maintain good health. He also advised against milk and milk products, meat, and refined flour products.

Dr. Walker's specific recommendations were:

- Drink plenty of raw vegetable juices, particularly carrot juice.

- Stop consuming milk and milk products, refined flour products, and meat.

Dr. Walker was particularly adamant about the power of raw foods to unclog the colon. In his book *Colon Health: The Key to a Vibrant Life*, Dr. Walker stated:

"The very best of diets can be no better than the very worst, if the sewage system of the colon is clogged with a collection of waste and corruption."

Walker also invented the Norwalk Hydraulic Press Juicer, which has been in use for over 75 years and is still sold today. The present popularity of juicing can be traced back to him, as can the practice of achieving vibrant health through a raw foods juice diet.

Jay Kordich, at the age of twenty, became ill with cancer and was told he might not live. After finding inspiration from the Gerson diet, he began drinking thirteen glasses of carrot-apple juice every day. Slightly more than two years later, he was completely well.

Kordich became known to the world as "The Juice Man". He met and was tremendously inspired by Dr. Walker – and in due course worked with Dr. Walker beginning in the 1940s up until Dr. Walker's death in 1984 at the reported age of 118.

During their time working together, Kordich and Walker promoted the health benefits of the Raw Food Diet and juice therapy, particularly in relation to cancer. They spread their message that the consumption of enzymes through fresh, raw vegetable juices was one of the most vital and effective ways to nourish the body.

Anne Wigmore, who pioneered wheatgrass treatment, observed that cancer cells thrived on cooked food but could not survive on raw food, thus supporting the claims of Kordich and Walker.

### Further Reading & References

- *Fresh Vegetable and Fruit Juices: What's Missing in Your Body?* by N. W. Walker

- *Become Younger* by Dr. Norman W. Walker

- *The Vegetarian Guide to Diet and Salad* by Dr. Norman W. Walker

- *Colon Health: The Key to a Vibrant Life* by Dr. Norman W. Walker

- *The Juiceman's Power of Juicing* by Jay Kordich

- *The Juice Advantage* by Jay Kordich

# Richardson Cancer Prevention Diet

The Richardson Cancer Prevention Diet is said to prevent cancer and other degenerative diseases by employing fundamental nutrition and appropriate vitamin and mineral supplementation.

Dr. Richardson was a medical doctor whose approach to treating cancer was to effectively turn back time and look to the way humans used nutrition and natural medicine before the advent of heavy pharmaceuticals. He was convinced that vitamin $B_{17}$ (also known as laetrile or amygdalin), arrested, contained, and even prevented cancer. He also contended that a lack of nutritional enzymes was at the root of cancer.

Dr. Richardson's Cancer Prevention Diet consists of eating a large proportion of fresh fruits and vegetables along with seeds, nuts, and grains. It also includes Vitamin $B_{17}$ tablets, pancreatic enzymes, Vitamins C and E, Vitamin $B_{15}$, amino acid tablets, chelated minerals and other vitamins, and liquid protein.

Dr. Richardson wrote in 1977:

"Instead of patients spending their final days or years butchered in surgical theaters or microwaved in chemotherapy and radiation rooms, I have witnessed my patients experiencing an improved quality of life and enjoyment in their remaining time."

Laetrile/vitamin $B_{17}$ is a natural compound that contains cyanide. It only gives up this cyanide portion of its chemical makeup when exposed to the enzyme group beta glucosidase secreted by cancer cells. No harmful side effects are known for $B_{17}$, nor does the cyanide in it appear to affect non-cancerous cells. Its proponents claim it's harmful only to cancer cells, and many decades of successful clinical use of this treatment suggest they're right.

Dr. Richardson never stopped believing that it is not the cancer that kills, but the breakdown of the body's own defense mechanism. If the body's pancreatic enzymes and vitamin and mineral levels are adequate, according to Dr. Richardson, the immune system can keep cancerous cells in check.

According to Dr. Richardson, any cancer that forms in the body is immediately surrounded and sealed-off by non-cancerous cells in an effort to protect healthy cells. When pancreatic enzymes and vitamin and mineral levels in the body are adequate, the immune system is able to stave off cancer growth.

In many cases, Dr. Richardson's patients recovered and went on to lead happy, healthy lives. When total healing was not possible, as in the cases where cancer had already spread too far before Dr. Richardson was consulted, he was at least able to improve quality of life substantially so that the patient's final days would not be painful or humiliating.

### Further Reading & References

- *Richardson Cancer Prevention Diet* by Dr. Janet Starr Hull

- Dr. Janet Starr Hull's Alternative Health & Nutrition Site: http://www.alternativecancerdiet.com/

# Rudolf Breuss/The Breuss Cancer Cure

The Breuss Cure, which originated in Germany, is a modified fasting treatment for cancer. It was created by Rudolf Breuss, a self-taught healing practitioner. The diet includes a 6-week regimen of natural juices and herbal teas. A maximum of 500 ml of freshly pressed vegetable juices is used, mainly beetroot with some carrot, celery, and radish. In addition, herbal teas, potato-peel tea, and onion broth are recommended. The treatment is claimed to have cured thousands.

The treatment is based on the premise that patients suffering from large tumors need very little, if any protein, and benefit instead from a diet of vegetable juices. Breuss has convinced many doubting medical doctors, thanks to a large number of healed and surviving patients, that it is indeed possible to live on juice for 42 days.

Breuss also claims that cancer itself can only live on solid foods, so by drinking only vegetable juice and tea, the cancer will die while the patient thrives.

Patients reportedly feel more alert and energetic after following the treatment plan. This is a sign that the Breuss fast, unlike radiation and chemotherapy, leaves the body healthy and strong. In fact, people not suffering from cancer but rather wishing to prevent illness or lose weight have tried and felt well using this diet.

This "Total Cancer Treatment," as named by Rudolf Breuss, is offered at a clinic in Hannoversch Muenden, Germany, where patients follow the fast while under medical supervision.

### Further Reading & References

- *The Breuss Cancer Cure: Advice for the Prevention and Natural Treatment of Cancer, Leukemia and Other Seemingly Incurable Diseases* by Rudolf Breuss

- Breuss Total Cancer Treatment: http://www.cancertutor.com/Cancer/Breuss.html

- The Breuss Cancer Cure: http://breusscancercure.blogspot.com/

# Herbal Treatments

## African Bush Willow/Combretastatin (CA4P)

African bush willow has been found to kill cancerous cells by disrupting angiogenesis, which cuts off the blood supply to the cells. Combretastatin, which is found in the bark of the African bush willow tree (*Combretum caffrum*), has delivered promising results as a cancer treatment when used with a sophisticated form of radiation therapy.

Combretastatin works by destroying the blood vessels that supply the tumors with vital nutrients, making it what's termed a vascular disruptive agent. However, it has no damaging effect on healthy tissue. The destruction of the tumors is completed through attack by a sophisticated form of radiation carried into the cells by antibodies.

This process is similar to the way the body's immune system manages infection by seeking out and destroying disease-causing substances. For example, when Combretastatin and radiation enter the body, they trigger the production of antibodies (specialized proteins that lock onto foreign substances in the body). These antibodies then carry the drug to where it needs to go, *i.e.* to the cancerous tissue. From there, the radiation destroys the tumor and the Combretastatin cuts off the blood vessel supply.

In essence, the drug attacks the tumor from the inside out while the radiotherapy attacks from the outside in. If administered alone, each treatment could never completely destroy all the cancer cells.

This combination therapy destroyed cancerous tumors in 85% of mice in a controlled experiment by British scientists. Better yet, more than nine months after the treatment was stopped the animals were still clear of cancer.

The research team was led by Professor Richard Begent, head of oncology at the Royal Free Hospital. He reported it was not effective enough to completely cut off the blood supply of a tumor because part of the tumor would continue to be sustained by the body's normal blood supply. But, with the radioactive antibodies used in the new treatment, the tumor would become starved.

He also said, "This does not necessarily mean that we would be able to cure people, but it does make it worth exploring this further and seeing if it can be of benefit to people with cancer."

Dr. Lesley Walker, Director of Cancer Information at the Cancer Research Campaign, reported that this was the most recent step in a growing volume of encouraging findings regarding this drug. She believes, "… that treatments that directly target cancers and spare normal tissue will be the cancer therapies of the future."

Along with proving to be an effective treatment, Dr. Walker reported the combination therapy should also greatly reduce side effects for the patient.

The drug has since been employed against human tumor cells of breast, ovarian and AIDS-related Kaposi's sarcoma that had been injected into animals.

Additional combretastatin research has been conducted at the University of Florida. Dr. Dietmar Siemann, professor of radiation oncology in UF's College of Medicine, says "We previously had shown that the drug was effective when combined with radiation therapy, but now we have shown that it performs well with traditional anti-cancer drugs. It does well on its own, but it's also a way to enhance the effectiveness of chemotherapy."

In breast and ovarian tumor models, combretastatin with cisplatin or cyclophosphamide, both chemotherapy drugs, caused a dramatic increase in tumor cell death (a 10- to 500-fold increase) over any of the medications by themselves.

Combretastatin alone will not eradicate an entire tumor because it attacks only new blood vessels that have developed to support the cluster of cancerous cells. It appears a tumor's outer rim is nourished by blood vessels that supply normal tissue, and so survives.

Human trials exploring the combination effect of radioimmunotherapy and CA4P on advanced solid tumors took place from 2004 to 2007 at University College London Hospital/University College London. The results were promising, but further study is needed to determine optimal dose and timing of Combretastatin.

### Further Reading & References

- "New Anti-Tumor Drug Promising In Animal Studies, UF Research Shows," http://news.ufl.edu/2000/04/06/cancer-dr/

- Cancer 'cure' breakthrough, http://news.bbc.co.uk/2/hi/health/1390664.stm

- "Cancer cure from African traditional medicine found" by Versi, Anver http://www.allbusiness.com/africa/917543-1.html

- "A Phase I Trial of Radioimmunotherapy with 131I-A5B7 Anti-CEA Antibody in Combination with Combretastatin-A4-Phosphate in Advanced Gastrointestinal Carcinomas," http://clincancerres.aacrjournals.org/content/15/13/4484.full

# Aloe Vera/Acemannan

Aloe, an African indigenous succulent related to the lily family, is cultivated throughout the world. The most popular species is aloe vera, which is used medicinally to treat cuts and burns. It has also been known to be used internally for intestinal problems and for cleansing purposes.

The clinical use of aloe began in the 1930s with reports of successful treatment of X-ray and radium burns. Aloe is also found in many commercial shampoos and skin lotions.

Aloe is generally considered safe to use both topically and orally. It is considered non-toxic, even when injected in high doses. Aloe vera has even been approved by the FDA as a natural flavoring.

In a pair of studies carried out at the Pasteur Institute in Madagascar in 1980 and 1981, researchers found that mice given a hypodermic injection of unrefined aloe extract were protected against infection caused by the bacteria Klebsiella pneumoniae, Listeria monocytogenes, Yersinia pestis, Plasmodium berghei parasites, and Candida albicans fungus.

A 1983 study showed that researchers who examined the effect of a polysaccharide fraction of

aloe as it related to the development of experimental fibrosarcoma and melanoma in mice were impressed to find it slowed tumor growth. According to the authors:

"In the case of the McC3-1 tumor, it is encouraging to note that under different experimental conditions the rate of growth of tumors in animals, which were treated, is slower than in those not treated. Preliminary studies of its action seem to indicate that the fraction acts upon non-specific [immune] response and could possibly stimulate the phagocyte [foreign body ingesting] activity of the peritoneal macrophagus [immune cells]."

In another animal study, S.Y. Peng found that acemannan, a D-isomer mucopolysaccharide extracted from aloe vera leaves, increased survival of sarcoma bearing mice. Acemannan, in both enriched and highly purified forms, was administered intraperitoneally to female CFW mice into which murine sarcoma cells had been subcutaneously implanted. The rapidly growing, highly malignant, and invasive sarcoma grew in 100% of implanted control animals, resulting in mortality in 20 to 46 days, dependent on the number of cells implanted. Approximately 40% of animals treated with acemannan at the time of tumor cell implantation (1.5 x 10(6) cells) survived.

Roberts and Travis tested whether a wound dressing gel that contained acemannan extracted from aloe leaves might affect the severity of radiation-induced acute skin reactions in C3H mice and compared the effect to other commercially available gels such as a personal lubricating jelly and a healing ointment.

They found that the average peak skin reactions of the acemannan-treated mice were lower than those of the untreated mice at all radiation doses tested. The average peak skin reactions for mice treated with personal lubricating jelly or healing ointment were similar to irradiated control values. Reduction in the percentage of mice with severe skin reactions was greatest in the groups that received wound dressing gel containing acemannan for at least two weeks beginning immediately after irradiation. There was no effect if gel was applied only before irradiation or beginning one week after irradiation.

Aloe also decreases thromboxane production by platelets in vitro. Thromboxane is produced by platelets and enhances platelet aggregation, which under normal circumstances is the process by which blood clots and wounds begin to heal. But this same coagulation process can also thicken the blood and promote the arrest of cancer cells that have broken loose from tumors to become lodged at distant sites, which is a critical step in the metastatic process. As an anticoagulant, or blood thinner, aloe might inhibit tumor cell arrest at potential metastatic sites.

This research on the ability of aloe to treat skin irritation and radiation burns makes it a significant treatment for patients undergoing radiation therapy. Some practitioners advise patients to take aloe orally for mouth and gastrointestinal damage from radiation. This practice is considered safe because of aloe's lack of toxicity. Some research even shows that aloe may be of use to the significant minority of cancer patients who experience cachexia, or wasting.

Note that side effects from the use of aloe have been reported. A bitter yellow substance in the bundle sheath is a purgative and laxative and should be removed during processing. It creates the risk for skin and intestinal irritation.


*Further Reading & References*

- Aloe, http://www.cancer.org/Treatment/TreatmentsandSideEffects/ComplementaryandAlternativeMedicine/HerbsVitaminsandMinerals/aloe

- "Herbal Therapies for Cancer" by Vivekan Don Flint and Michael Lerner, http://www.commonwealhealth.org/herbs.html

- *Cancer Can Be Cured* by Father Romano Zago (2008)

- *Aloe Isn't Medicine, and Yet … It Cures!* By Father Romano Zago (2009)

# Astragalus/Huang-qi

Astragalus is a well-known immune-boosting herb. Astragalus strengthens the body's resistance and invigorates and promotes tissue regeneration via photochemicals in the plant such as polysaccharides, especially astragalan I, II, and III, and saponins and triterpenes.

Astragalus is not cytotoxic as it does not appear to have any effect on malignant cancers. However, it seems to improve the immune system to a point where cancer is not as difficult to deal with.

Astragalus has been used to improve T-cell counts to relatively normal ranges, which is an important aspect of the immune system. T-cells are a specific type of white blood cell that is part of the lymphocyte family.

It is also used as an adjunctive support for persons undergoing chemotherapy. Astragalus contains numerous components, including flavonoids, polysaccharides, triterpene glycosides (e.g. astragalosides I-VII), amino acids, and trace minerals. Research conducted by the M.D. Anderson Cancer Center in Houston, Texas, confirms this herb's immune-potentiating actions.

It was 5000 years ago when Chinese Emperor Shen Nung first discovered astragalus. Westerners began to realize its medicinal importance during the 1800s. Dr. Alexander van Bunge, a Russian physician who studied East Asian plants, first described the species for the West in 1868.

Astragalus is slowly becoming one of the better-known Chinese herbs. Some of its popularity may be attributed to extensive scientific study that began in the 1970s confirming the herb's ability to stimulate the immune system, fight bacteria, viruses, and inflammation, protect the liver, and act as a diuretic.

In Traditional Chinese Medicine, astragalus is often used in daily doses of 9 g to 15 g of the dried sliced root, simmered for several hours in a quart of water (the decoction is ready when the water is reduced down to a pint).

Though astragalus does not directly attack cancers, it does strengthen a cancer patient's immune system, allowing the patient to recover significantly faster and live longer. Researchers believe on the basis of cell studies that astragalus augments those white blood cells that fight disease and removes some of those that make the body more vulnerable to it. In these same studies, both in the laboratory and with 572 patients, it also has been found that astragalus promotes adrenal cortical function, which also is critically diminished in cancer patients.

Astragalus also ameliorates bone marrow compression and gastrointestinal toxicity caused by chemotherapy and radiation. Astragalus has been considered as a possible treatment for people living with AIDS and other viral conditions as it also increases interferon production and enhances NK and T-cell function. Astragalus shows support for peripheral vascular diseases and peripheral circulation.

Astragalus is available in capsule, tablet, and fluid extract form, and as dried root and prepared tea.

In tablets or capsule form, it is typically combined with ginseng in doses of up to 500mg taken 3 times a day.

Astragalus appears to have no known adverse side effects. As it stimulates the immune system, it may be unwise for patients with autoimmune diseases. It reportedly acts as a diuretic.

### Further Reading & References

- *8 Weeks to Optimum Health* by Andrew Weil M.D. Excerpt from page 135 "... from the immunosuppressive effects of the latter. I commonly recommend astragalus to cancer patients; it will not interfere with the conventional therapies. ..."

- Cancer Treatment Strategies at IEP, http://www.itmonline.org/arts/iepcancer.htm

- "White Blood Cells and Immunity," Cancer Salves, http://www.cancersalves.com/checklist/white_blood.html

# Beetroot/Beet Juice Crystals

The beet juice crystals from red beets are known for multiple nutritional properties. Red beet juice has been an important part of human nutrition for centuries. In modern times, French nutritionists have tested the value of beet juice, using diets that include up to 6 pints of beet juice daily. Often, beet juice is used in combination with other juices.

Many people follow a beet juice diet for cleansing purposes, which may or may not include other types of juices. Many juice diets have widely recognized benefits. Researchers such as Norman Walker D.Sc Ph.D., and Dr. Bernard Jensen have been investigating the effects of making vegetable juice a part of the daily diet since the early part of the 20$^{th}$ century.

Three juices seem to be fundamental to any effective juice program. These are carrot juice, a green vegetable juice, and beet juice. Beetroot juice appears to be high in cancer fighting phytochemicals as well as vitamins $B_1$, $B_2$, $B_6$, beta carotene, vitamin C, folic acid, and vitamin E, as well as the minerals sodium, potassium, magnesium, calcium, manganese, iron, cobalt, copper, zinc, chromium, selenium, and numerous enzymes.

Red beets are also well-known for their high levels of anti-carcinogens and antioxidants. They help the body fight certain types of cancer as well as heart disease. In addition, red beets contain an amino acid called betaine that has anti-cancer properties. A therapy known as "red beet therapy" has been reported to aid in cases of leukemia and tumor growth.

Other research has shown that beet juice helps stop the development of colon and stomach cancer. The preferred method of taking beet root therapy, besides ingesting it as a juice, is to mash up and consume two pounds of raw beets daily.

### Further Reading & References

- *Dr. Jensen's Juicing Therapy : Nature's Way to Better Health and a Longer Life* by Bernard Jensen (2000)

- *Raw Vegetable Juices: What's Missing in Your Body* by N.W. Walker (2003)

- "Health Benefits of Red Beets," http://hubpages.com/hub/Health_Benefits_of_Red_Beets

# Black Seed Oil/Black Cumin/Nigella Sativa

Nigella sativa is an annual flowering plant native to Asia with delicate white or pale blue flowers. The Nigella sativa seed is known as black seed, black caraway, black cumin, or fennel flower.

The seeds have been used in Southeast Asia and the Middle East for centuries to treat inflammatory diseases such as asthma, bronchitis, and rheumatism.

More recently, black seed oil has been found to kill prostate cancer cells. A study conducted at Tulane University showed the oil contained the natural anti-cancer compound Thymoquinone, which suppresses the growth and leads to the death of prostate cancer cells.* Thymoquinone operates in a manner similar to co-enzyme Q10 (CoQ10), which is made naturally by the body. It has also been shown to kill pancreatic cancer cells, colon cancer, and potentially breast cancer.

The study also found that cancer cells resistant to chemotherapy treatment seem to shrink when exposed to black seed oil.

### *Further Reading & References*

- *Black Seed Oil Compound Kills Prostate Cancer Cells in Lab Study, http://www.emaxhealth. com/1020/6/36767/black-seed-oil-compound-kills-prostate-cancer-cells-lab-study.html

- Black Seed Oil Can Help Pancreatic Cancer, http://www.worldwidehealth.com/health-article-Black-seed-oil-can-help-pancreatic-cancer.html

- Black Seed Oil Has Been Shown To Fight Cancer, http://www.sweetsunnah.com/mas_assets/ images/cancer.pdf

# Boluses

A bolus is similar to a suppository and can be used vaginally or anally. Another definition to be aware of regarding the word *bolus* is "A single dose of drug usually injected into a blood vessel over a short period of time."

Boluses can be made into suppositories by mixing several herbal ingredients together and freezing them. In such a form, a bolus is primarily used to treat cervical problems. Some of the herbs that would be used include squaw vine herb, slippery elm bark, goldenseal root, yellow dock root, comfrey root, marshmallow root, chickweed herb, mullein leaf, garlic bulb, and coconut and tea tree oil.

There is a Dr. Schulze who highly recommends the use of boluses to treat cervical, uterine, ovarian, colon cancer, and any lower abdominal cancers (and for cysts). He claims the herbs are cleansing and have anti-tumor properties. When absorbed anally they can help fight many cancers.

Some research has shown this approach to be successful in the treatment of cervical dysplasia.

Dr. Schulze recommends inserting the bolus at night and leaving it there for as long as two days if no discomfort occurs.

Another approach is that of Dr. John R. Christopher, who actually mentored Dr. Schulze. He recommends yellow dock tea as a douche. Do this for six days; rest on the seventh. The routine is to be carried out for a period of six weeks to six months.

Cocoa butter is considered an excellent binding agent for powdered herbs. The directions are to stir the herbs in with melted cocoa butter and then refrigerate.

### *Further Reading & References*

- Boluses, Herbal, http://www.mnwelldir.org/docs/cancer1/altthrpy.htm#Boluses

- *The Way of Herbs* by Michael Tierra (1998)

- National Cancer Institute, http://www.cancer.gov/dictionary/?CdrID=45620

# Burdock Root/Arctigenin

Burdock root is often found in well-known herbal formulas for cancer such as the Hoxsey Therapy and Essiac tea. It is also a staple in some macrobiotic diets.

Burdock root consists of carbohydrates known as inulin, mucilage, starches, and some sugar. Inulin is considered to be the active agent in the burdock root because of its known curative abilities. Certain lab studies have shown that inulin can help strengthen organs and regulate blood sugar metabolism. It is considered a powerful immune system regulator and works quite well when paired up with Echinacea.

It is believed inulin can attach itself to the surface of white blood cells and that it can similarly activate T-cells meant to attack cancer.

Burdock has historically been used to combat tumors for sick people in several countries: China (in a

record from 502 A.D.), Japan, Italy (in the twelfth century), Spain, and Chile. The Potawatomi Indians in the American Midwest used a related species, lesser burdock, as an antitumor agent.

Arctigenin, a lignin found in the greater burdock, has been found to be a potent weapon against certain leukemia cell lines.

Studies have shown burdock can promote anti-tumor behavior in animal tumor systems. Japanese researchers tested burdock and nine other vegetable juices for their ability to prevent chemically induced chromosomal mutations in rat bone marrow cells. Significant suppression of the incidence of mutations was found using the fresh or boiled juice from onion, burdock, eggplant, cabbage, and welsh onion. (See also: **Essiac**; **Hoxsey Herbal Treatment**)

### Further Reading & References

- *Herbal Medicine, Healing & Cancer* by Donald R. Yance, Arlene Valentine (1999)

- *Essiac: A Native Herbal Cancer Remedy* by Cynthia Olsen (1998)

- *Beating Cancer With Nutrition* by Patrick Quillin, (2005)

- *Essiac Essentials: The Remarkable Herbal Cancer Fighter* by Sheila Snow, Mali Klein (2000)

- Herbal Therapies for Cancer, http://www.commonwealhealth.org/herbs.html

- Burdock Root, http://www.countryherbal.com/ingredients.shtml

# Cannabis/Medical Marijuana/Tetrahydrocannabinol (THC)

Marijuana has been found to be most effective as a supportive aid for those battling cancer. Many cancer victims experience significant nausea and vomiting induced by chemotherapy. Smoking marijuana as a medicinal treatment has been found effective in battling the nausea. Research shows the THC, a chemical within marijuana that helps with nausea, is more quickly absorbed when inhaled as a smoke as opposed to taken orally as a pill.

One study found compounds close to those found in cannabis were able to successfully halt the growth process of prostate cancer cells. Two compounds in particular, MET and JWH-015, stopped prostate tumor growth in human prostate cells when tested in Petri dishes. Cell division was halted and the cells were killed. The most effective change was seen in more aggressive prostate cancer cells.

These compounds are not gained from smoking cannabis, but there is hope the compounds tested in the study can be developed into synthetic chemicals.

In another study, researchers announced success destroying incurable brain cancer tumors in rats. They injected them with THC, the active ingredient in cannabis.

In 1974, researchers at the Medical College of Virginia, funded by the National Institutes of Health, were attempting to find evidence that marijuana damages the immune system. Instead, they found that THC slowed the growth of three kinds of cancer in mice: lung and breast cancer and a virus-induced leukemia.

### Further Reading & References

- Marijuana Use in Supportive Care for Cancer Patients, http://www.cancer.gov/cancertopics/factsheet/Support/marijuana

- Briefing: Cannabis compounds fight prostate cancer, http://www.newscientist.com/article/dn17636-briefing-cannabis-compounds-fight-prostate-cancer.html

- Pot Shrinks Tumors: Government Knew in '74, http://americanmarijuana.org/pot.shrinks.tumors.html

- Cancer Treatment & Marijuana Therapy: Marijuana's Use in the Reduction of Nausea and Vomiting and for Appetite Stimulation in Cancer Patients, edited by R.C. Randall (1990)

- Marijuana Medical Handbook: Practical Guide to Therapeutic Uses of Marijuana by Gregory T. Carter, M.D., Dale Gieringer Ph.D., and Ed Rosenthal (2008)

- DVD: What If Cannabis Cured Cancer, directed by Len Richmond

# Chaparral/Larrea/NDGA/M4N

Chaparral (Larrea tredentata) is a type of heathland plant community found mostly in California and the northern part of Mexico. It is drought-tolerant with evergreen leaves. There are more than a hundred varieties of plants called chaparral, though the one used for medicinal purposes is Larrea divaricata.

Chaparral tea is a long-standing Native American medicinal treatment sometimes used as a remedy for cancer. It originated among the tribes of the desert Southwest.

Chaparral tea, which contains a potent antioxidant, nor-dihydroguiaicetic acid (NDGA), has been found to have anti-tumor activity. It is prepared by grinding the leaves and twigs of an evergreen desert shrub known as the creosote.

Chaparral tea has been used to treat a wide variety of ailments, from arthritis, venereal disease, tuberculosis, and colds to rheumatism, bowel cramps, and cancer.

Most researchers attribute the effects of chaparral to NDGA. This is an antioxidant that is often added to oils to prevent rancidity, but it seems to have other benefits. This includes protecting tissue from damage when exposed to carcinogens.

Studies show that NDGA may also inhibit cell proliferation as well as DNA synthesis. Chaparral may also be useful in combating certain bacteria and viruses and has shown much promise with herpes.

Dr. William Kelly from the Kelly Research Foundation states, "I've found that chaparral is very effective in 7% of the cases of malignancy. The action is not as many researchers believe — a specific activity against the cancer cell, but rather an indirect one. In about 7% of the cases of malignancy, the pancreas and the liver as well as other tissues of the body are so congested with poisons such as medications, sprays, drugs, metallic poisons, and pollutants that these tissues cannot carry on normal activity.

"This is basically an antagonist to the enzyme and vitamin and mineral metabolism that goes on in the body. In cancer specifically, we find that the pancreatic enzymes are locked with the antagonists and are rendered totally ineffective. By chelating these antagonists from the pancreatic enzymes, we find that normal activity takes place and the person's own cancer defenses take over and destroy the tumor in malignant conditions."

Dr. Kelly went on to say that chaparral works well when it comes to chelating toxins from drug addicts if two chaparral tables are consumed prior to each meal.

M4N is derived from chaparral. Long derided by medical authorities as both ineffective and dangerous, for the past dozen years its sale has been virtually banned by the Food and Drug Administration (FDA). Yet now chaparral is turning out to be the source of a scientifically validated medicine to fight cancer. In a Phase I study:

"South Carolina doctors have announced that a drug called M4N shrinks inoperable tumors of the head and neck region. Researchers injected M4N directly into the tumors of eight such patients who were not eligible for surgery. According to press releases, they saw evidence that the agent killed the tumors in these patients, all of whom had advanced, otherwise untreatable forms of the disease." (Reuters 2004).

Chaparral is considered toxic to the liver. Larrea should be used with caution in persons who have a history of liver disease. Other potential side effects are allergic reactions to chaparral and its resin.

### Further Reading & References

- Complementary and Alternative Therapies for Cancer Patients: Chaparral, http://cancer.ucsd.edu/outreach/PublicEducation/CAMs/chaparral.asp

- BBC Reports on Beneficial Cancer Treatment Based on Native American Tradition, http://www.wanttoknow.info/chaparralforcancer

- *The Sir Jason Winters Story: Killing Cancer*, by Sir Jason Winters (1980)

# Cayenne Pepper/Capsaicin

Cayenne pepper, also known as red pepper, is used both to flavor dishes and for medicinal purposes.

In several clinical studies with cayenne pepper, capsaicin was found to cause apoptosis (cell death) in cancer cells. Capsaicin is a compound found in cayenne pepper. Capsaicin has also been found to kill leukemic, lung, prostate, and pancreatic cancer cells.

Researchers from the Samuel Oschin Comprehensive Cancer Institute at Cedars-Sinai Medical Center and colleagues from UCLA Medical School conducted animal studies on the pepper component and found that 80% of human prostate cancer cells injected into living mice underwent apoptosis (cell death).

Capsaicin also dramatically slowed the development of prostate tumors in human cell lines grown in mouse models, according to Sören Lehmann, M.D., Ph.D., a visiting scientist at the Cedars-Sinai Medical Center and the UCLA School of Medicine.

Capsaicin has also been found to reduce cancer cell production of prostate specific antigen (PSA), a protein found in abundance in prostate tumors. This means eating capsaicin could lower PSA levels, although scientists are beginning to question the overall efficacy of PSA tests in general.

Says Sam Biser, in his video *Curing With Cayenne,* "Hot chili peppers not only fire up your food, they may also put the heat on cancer cells and force them to self-destruct. A new study shows a natural substance found in chili peppers kills cancer cells by starving them of oxygen. Researchers tested the chili pepper substance (known as capsaicin) along with a related compound (resiniferatoxin) on human skin cancer cells to analyze how the cells reacted. Both compounds are natural substances known as vanilloids. They found that the majority of the skin cancer cells exposed to the substances died. The researchers say these substances seem to kill cells by damaging the cell membranes and limiting the amount of oxygen that reaches the cancer cells."

Capsaicin can be taken in a warm glass of water, in capsule form, or used regularly as a spice in food. It can also be purchases as a cream, gel, or patch.

### *Further Reading & References*

- Can Cayenne Pepper Cure Cancer? http://www.cayennepepper.info/can-cayenne-pepper-cure-cancer.html

- Health benefits of Cayenne Pepper, http://www.healingcancernaturally.com/cayenne-pepper-healthbenefits.html

- *Curing With Cayenne and It's Herbal Partners* by Sam Biser (VHS)

- Mori, A; Lehmann S, O'Kelly J et al. (March 2006). "Capsaicin, a component of red peppers, inhibits the growth of androgen-independent, p53 mutant prostate cancer cells". Retrieved January 7, 2010 from http://cancerres.aacrjournals.org/cgi/content/full/66/6/3222

- American Association for Cancer Research (2006). "Pepper Component Hot Enough to Trigger Suicide in Prostate Cancer Cells." Retrieved January 7, 2010 from http://www.aacr.org/home/public--media/aacr-press-releases/press-releases-2006.aspx?d=583

# Chicory Root

Chicory root is a perennial bush plant. It is cultivated for salad leaves and is used as a coffee substitute. When used medicinally, the roots of the plant are dried along with the foliage from the plant.

Chicory can be used for several ailments such as constipation, upset stomach, gallbladder problems, and cancer. It works as a tonic to increase urine production and has a mild laxative effect along with being able to decrease swelling.

Chicory contains inulin, which is commonly considered a powerful agent in fighting cancer. (See the section on **Burdock Root**.) According to a review of chicory published in the British Journal of Nutrition, inulin prevented the formation of colon cancer tumors in several animal studies.

Chicory has few side effects and appears safe when taken orally. Handling the root itself may cause skin irritation.

### Further Reading & References

- Chicory Side Effects and Safety, http://www.webmd.com/vitamins-supplements/ingredientmono-92-CHICORY.aspx?activeIngredientId=92&activeIngredientName=CHICORY

- Chicory Root, http://www.buzzle.com/articles/chicory-root.html

## Chinese Bitter Melon/Kuguazi/Karela

Bitter melon is a fruit that belongs to the plant family cucurbitaceae. Also known as bitter gourd, bitter apples, and wild cucumber, it is commonly found in Asia as well as in Southern California, southern Florida and South America. The plant bears fruit that looks like a bumpy cucumber.

Several plant chemicals that are biologically active have been found in bitter melon. One, a protein called momordin, demonstrated anticancerous properties against Hodgkin's lymphoma in animal studies. A chemical analog of several of the proteins in the melon were named MAP-30 and appear to inhibit prostate tumor growth.

Various in-vivo studies have demonstrated the antitumorous activity of the entire bitter melon plant. In one study, a water extract blocked the growth of prostate carcinoma in rats; another study reported that a hot water extract of the entire plant inhibited the development of mammary tumors in mice. Several in vitro studies have also demonstrated the anticancerous and antileukemic activity of bitter melon against numerous cell lines, including liver cancer, human leukemia, melanoma, and solid sarcomas.

Bitter melon can be taken orally in capsules or stewed as a tea.

### Further Reading & References

- http://www.rain-tree.com/bitmelon.htm

- *Herbal Medicine, Healing & Cancer* by Donald Yance, Arlene Valentine (1999)

## Chuchuhuasi Tree

The Chuchuhuasi is an enormous canopy tree of the Amazon rainforest that grows up to 30 meters high. Several botanical names have been given to this species of tree (which has led to confusion), including Maytenus krukovii, M. ebenifolia, M. laevis, and M. macrocarpa. It is characterized by large leaves (10–30 cm), small, white flowers, and extremely tough, heavy, reddish-brown bark.

Tribes of the Amazon rainforest have been using the bark of chuchuhuasi medicinally for centuries for ailments such as arthritis, rheumatism, and back pain. One local Indian arthritis and rheumatism remedy calls for one cup of a bark decoction taken three times a day for more than a week.

Chuchuhuasi is packed with phytochemicals, including triterpenes, flavonols, and sesquiterpene alkaloids. Two of the more well-known phytochemicals in chuchuhuasi are mayteine and maytansine. These alkaloids have been shown to assist with antitumor activity. Other compounds, including dammarane- and friedelane-type triterpenes, have also been detected in chuchuhuasi bark.

In the Peruvian Amazon, chuchuhuasi is used for arthritis, muscle relaxation, and as an immune stimulant. It is also considered to be an aphrodisiac and analgesic with expectorant, emetic, diuretic, and anti-inflammatory properties. It is commonly used for adrenal support. Some tribes even use it for menstrual balance and regulation.

In Peruvian herbal medicine systems, chuchuhuasi alcohol extracts are used to treat osteoarthritis, rheumatoid arthritis, bronchitis, diarrhea, and hemorrhoids. In Brazil, herbal medicine practitioners use the bark in a preparation used topically on skin cancers.

A pharmaceutical company in the United States studied chuchuhuasi's anti-inflammatory and anti-arthritic properties and determined that these alkaloids can effectively inhibit enzyme production of protein kinase C (PKC). PKC inhibitors have attracted much interest worldwide, as there is evidence that excess levels of PKC enzymes contribute to a wide variety of disease processes such as brain tumors, cancer, and cardiovascular disease.

In the mid-1970s, Italian researchers identified antitumor-like properties in a chuchuhuasi extract that worked against skin cancers. They gave credit to the two chemicals in chuchuhuasi known as tingenone and pristimerin.

In 1999, three other research groups found new and different sesquiterpene compounds, two of which showed marginal (i.e., limited) antitumor activity against four cell lines. Other researchers found four more chemicals in the roots of chuchuhuasi (named macrocarpins) in 2000—three of which were documented as cytotoxic to four tumor cell lines.

The traditional remedy is to take one to two cups a day of a standard bark decoction or three to six milliliters a few times daily of a standard tincture.

### Further Reading & References

- Tropical Plant Database: Chuchuhuasi, http://www.rain-tree.com/chuchuhuasi.htm

- Perupedia: Chuchuwasai, http://www.karikuy.org/perupedia/index.php?title=Chuchuwasai

- NautralPedia: http://www.naturalpedia.com/C/Clinical-active.html

- *The Healing Power of Rainforest Herbs: A Guide to Understanding and Using Herbal Medicinals* by Leslie Taylor, ND

## Cocoa

Cocoa is derived from a plant called 'cacao', a word derived from the Aztec "cacahuatl." This is an evergreen tropical American tree that bears leathery ten-ribbed fruits on the trunk and older branches. Cocoa powder is made from cacao seeds, which have been fermented, roasted, shelled, ground and freed of most of their fat. Mexicans prize chocolate as an unsweetened food and use it in their famous chicken dish, mole poblano.

The darker the chocolate, the better it is for you, according to Professor Joe Vinson of the University of Scranton. Weight for weight, he said, milk chocolate has twice as many antioxidants as blueberries and dark chocolate has five times as many. And cocoa powder contains twice as much antioxidant activity as dark chocolate and is almost devoid of fat. Researchers at the University of California, Davis found that chocolate inhibits the clumping of platelets. "Cocoa consumption had an aspirin-like effect," they wrote. Cocoa butter is mainly steric triglyceride, which is less well-absorbed than other fats, and is excreted. Thus, cocoa butter has a minimal effect on serum cholesterol.

The eminent food researcher John Weisburger, PhD concluded: "The cocoa bean, and tasty products derived from the cocoa bean such as chocolate, and the beverage cocoa, popular with many people worldwide, is rich in specific antioxidants." The regular intake of such products, he continued, would increase the level of antioxidants, prevent the oxidation of "bad" LDL cholesterol, and probably prevent heart disease. "It would seem reasonable to suggest inhibition of the several phases of the complex processes leading to cancer," Weisburger said.

A report from France in January 2002 showed that certain substances in cocoa powder inhibit 70% of cancer cells during a critical phase of their growth cycle. Japanese researchers have shown that tiny amounts of a cacao bean extract (called polycaphenol) are more toxic to human tumor cells than to normal cells. In some regards, polycaphenol was even more effective than vitamin C. Pretreatment of mice with polycaphenol also protected them from lethal E. coli infections.

Cornell University food scientists say: "Cocoa teems with antioxidants that prevent cancer." Comparing the chemical anti-cancer activity in beverages known to contain antioxidants, they have found that cocoa has nearly twice the antioxidants of red wine and up to three times those found in green tea.

Led by Chang Y. Lee, the Cornell researchers say the reason that cocoa leads the other drinks is its high content of compounds called phenolic phytochemicals, or flavonoids, indicating the presence of known antioxidants that can stave off cancer, heart disease and other ailments.

Their research showed a single serving of cocoa contained 611 milligrams of the phenolic compound gallic acid equivalents (GAE) and 564 milligrams of the flavonoid epicatechin equivalents (ECE). Examining a glass of red wine, the researchers found 340 milligrams of GAE and 163 milligrams of ECE. In a cup of green tea, they found 165 milligrams of GAE and 47 milligrams of ECE.

### Further Reading & References

- "Cocoa froths with cancer-preventing compounds, better than red wine or green tea, Cornell food scientists say," http://psa-rising.com/eatingwell/cocoa122003.htm

- *The What to Eat if You Have Cancer Cookbook* by Daniella Chace, Maureen Keane (1996)


# Comfrey/Symphytum Officinale/Dr. H. E. Kirschner

Comfrey is a perennial plant classified as an herb. It has a black root similar to that of a turnip and bears broad leaves with bell-shaped flowers.

Comfrey has a long history of medicinal uses such as promoting the healing of wounds and broken bones as well as treating other illnesses such as arthritis and ulcers. Comfrey has been used in China medicinally for over 2000 years.

Internal use is not suggested because comfrey may contain chemicals which have been linked to liver damage and the possible initiation of cancer. Instead, it should be used as a skin wash to relieve irritation. Regardless, some herbalists advocate the internal use of comfrey leaves.

One physician, Dr. H.E. Kirschner M.D., promoted comfrey in his medical practice. He stated he personally observed the powerful anticancer effects of comfrey on a patient of his who was dying from advanced, externalized cancer. He prescribed fresh, crushed-leaf comfrey poultices throughout the day.

He wrote that, "Much to the surprise of the patient and her family, there was obvious healing within the first two days of treatment, with continued visible improvement over the next few weeks. He also said, "Much of dreadful pain that usually accompanies the advanced stages of cancer disappeared," and there was a dramatic decrease in swelling." The leaves should only be used externally.

### Further Reading & References

- Herbal Remedies Info: Comfrey, http://www.herbalremediesinfo.com/COMFREY.html

- Cancer, Wounds, and Comfrey, http://www.doctoryourself.com/comfrey_herb.html

# Coriander/Cilantro

Coriander and cilantro are the same plant, known by two different names. Remains of this popular herb were found by archeologists in Egyptian pharaoh Tutankhamen's tomb. It was used for centuries by ancient Greeks and Romans to flavor food and wine, has been known in Asian countries for thousands of years, and is even mentioned in the Bible's Book of Exodus.

Treasured for its medicinal value, coriander was used by Hippocrates, the "father of medicine," and other physicians. Herbalists use it as a digestive tonic, sleep aid, antibacterial ointment, and more.

New research published in August, 2011 showed that coriander oil has the ability to combat serious bacteria such as E. coli, MRSA, salmonella and Bacillus cereus. Of the 12 tested strains, all the bacteria showed reduced growth -- and most were killed – by solutions containing up to 1.6% coriander oil.

Coriander oil works by damaging the membrane of the bacterial cell, causing cell death – according to the *Journal of Medical Microbiology* study.

In 2004, a study published in the *Journal of Agriculture and Food Chemistry* showed the compound dodecenal was twice as effective as the commonly used antibiotic drug, gentamicin, at killing salmonella.

This discovery clarified something that's been known for a while: salsa has antibacterial properties. Scientists didn't know precisely what ingredient in salsa was killing off microbes until they found that dodecenal -- a component found in cilantro leaves -- provides that benefit.

Fresh coriander is both an herb and a spice – since both leaves and seeds are used. The leaves resemble parsley, and are known as cilantro in the U.S. The seeds are generally known to Americans as coriander. (Elsewhere all parts of the plant are referred to as coriander.) It is used in the cuisine of many different cultures, notably those of Mexico and India.

The fruit of the plant consists of two seeds, which smell of citrus and sage in their dried form. Seeds can be purchased whole and crushed with mortar and pestle, or in powdered form.

The abundant phytonutrients in coriander/cilantro have anti-cancer and anti-inflammatory properties which confer many health benefits. It reportedly helps control blood sugar levels, fight cancer, and combat signs of aging.

In Europe coriander is called the anti-diabetic plant. The people of India use it as a potent anti-inflammatory. And in the U.S., it's been studied for its ability to lower cholesterol.

Studies support these claims. When coriander was added to the diet of diabetic mice, their insulin secretion was stimulated, and their blood sugar lowered. Rats fed coriander had reduced amounts of damaged fats in their cell membranes.

Rats given a high-fat, high-cholesterol diet -- plus coriander -- lowered both their total and LDL (bad) cholesterol numbers, while boosting HDL. Apparently coriander's linoleic acid, oleic acid, palmitic acid, stearic acid and ascorbic acid (vitamin C) are effective in reducing blood cholesterol levels and reducing cholesterol deposits along the inner walls of the arteries and veins.

Cilantro is rich in vitamin K, which plays a role in building bone. Vitamin K is synergistic with vitamin D. Most knowledgeable nutritionists now urge patients to supplement with vitamin K or make sure they get enough in their diets.

In addition, cilantro has an established role in the treatment of Alzheimer's disease by limiting neuron damage in the brain.

Further, the seeds of coriander have been used:

- As a folk medicine for the relief of anxiety and insomnia

- In traditional Indian medicine as a diuretic

- To help improve GI-tract upsets such as indigestion, diarrhea and flatulence

- For colic relief when used as a mild, safe tea for children under age 2

- To promote gastric secretions and stimulate appetite

- For relief of toothache and bad breath when made into a tea and gargled

- In Arab and Chinese medicine as a natural aphrodisiac


The leaves and seeds contain eleven components of essential oils, are rich in polyphenolic flavonoids such as quercetin and epigenin, and contain six types of acids, minerals and vitamins – each with its own beneficial properties. Coriander contains the vitamins folic acid, riboflavin, niacin, vitamin A, beta carotene, and a generous dose of vitamin C – all essential for optimal health. It's a source of the minerals potassium, calcium, manganese, iron, and magnesium.

Because phytonutrients act synergistically, and may interact with compounds science has yet to even define, coriander/cilantro is best consumed as just one part of a diet rich with other fruits and vegetables. It should not be viewed as a standalone cancer treatment.


**Environmental Caution**

An annual study by the Environmental Working Group (EWG) names the year's "Dirty Dozen" – fruits and vegetables that are so contaminated with pesticide residue it's important to buy organic. Their June 2011 study showed that conventional cilantro tested positive for not one, but a whopping 30 different pesticides.

Consumers are advised not to cancel out the benefits of coriander (cilantro) by buying <u>conventionally</u> grown varieties contaminated with damaging pesticide residues.

### *Further Reading & References*

- Coriander Oil Could Tackle Food Poisoning and Drug-Resistant Infections, *Science Daily*, Aug 23, 2011, www.sciencedaily.com/releases/2011/08/110823193857

- Filomena Silva, Susana Ferreira, Joao A. Queiroz, and Fernanda C. Domingues. Coriander (Coriandrum sativum L.) essential oil: its antibacterial activity and mode of action evaluated by flow cytometry. *Journal of Medical Microbiology*, August 23, 2011 DOI: 10:1099/jmm.0.034157-0

- Random USDA Testing Finds 34 Unapproved Pesticides on Cilantro, www.TreeHugger.com/green-food/random-usda-testing-finds-34-unapproved-pesticides-on-cilantro.html

- USDA Testing Found Unapproved Pesticides on Cilantro, http://news.agropages.com/Feature/FeatureDetail---1084.htm

# Curcumin/Turmeric

Curcuma longa is a ginger-like plant that grows in tropical regions. The roots contain a bright yellow substance (turmeric) that contains curcumin and other curcuminoids. It's a common household spice.

"Imagine a natural substance so smart it can tell the difference between a cancer cell and a normal cell; so powerful it can stop chemicals in their tracks; and so strong it can enable DNA to walk away from lethal doses of radiation virtually unscathed. Curcumin has powers against cancer so beneficial that drug companies are rushing to make drug versions. Curcumin is all this and more."*

So say researchers who advocate the use of curcumin as an anti-cancer treatment.

Turmeric has been used in Ayurvedic and Chinese medicine for centuries. In India, turmeric has been recognized as a key balancing and detoxifying herb. In Indonesia, Japan, and China people embrace turmeric for its powerful yet safe liver detoxification and in the Western medical and herbal traditions, turmeric is considered by many to be one of the most important healing herbs.

It is only within the past few years that the extraordinary actions of curcumin against cancer have been scientifically documented. Among its many benefits, curcumin has at least a dozen separate ways of interfering with cancer.

Extensive trials have been conducted to ascertain its value as an anticancer drug. Turmeric launches a multiple attack on cancerous cells. Scientists at M. D. Anderson Cancer Center, Texas, wrote in January 2003: "Extensive research over the last 50 years has indicated [curcumin] can both prevent and treat cancer. The anticancer potential of curcumin stems from its ability to suppress proliferation of a wide variety of tumor cells, down-regulate transcription factors NF-kappa B, AP-1 and Egr-1; down-regulate the expression of COX2, LOX, NOS, MMP-9, uPA, TNF, chemokines, cell surface adhesion molecules and cyclin D1; down-regulate growth factor receptors (such as EGFR and HER2); and inhibit the activity of c-Jun N-terminal kinase, protein tyrosine kinases and protein serine/threonine kinases."

In the latest of a series of reports, M.D. Anderson scientists say: "Curcumin can suppress tumor initiation, promotion, and metastasis."

Pharmacologically, curcumin is considered safe. Human clinical trials indicated no dose-limiting toxicity when administered at doses up to 10 g/day. All of these studies suggest that curcumin has enormous potential in the prevention and therapy of cancer.

Researchers at the University of Leicester, UK, began investigating dietary agents including curcumin, genistein, and the vitamin A analogue 13-cis retinoic acid for tumor-suppressing properties. They observed that curcumin slows the rate at which hormone-responsive prostate cancer cells become resistant to hormonal therapy. Antioxidant, anti-inflammatory and anti-carcinogenic properties of turmeric and curcumin are undergoing intense research.

Tests in Germany, reported in July 2003, found that "All fractions of the turmeric extract preparation exhibited pronounced antioxidant activity...." Turmeric extract tested more potent than garlic, devil's claw, and salmon oil as quoted in J Pharm Pharmacol. 2003 Jul; 55(7):981-6.

Several studies indicate that curcumin slows the development and growth of a number of types of cancer cells. In Japan recently researchers defined curcumin as a broad-spectrum anti-cancer agent.

Its induction of "detoxifying enzymes," researchers say, indicates its "potential value ... as a protective agent against chemical carcinogenesis and other forms of electrophilic toxicity. The significance of these results can be implicated in relation to cancer chemopreventive effects of curcumin against the induction of tumors in various target organs".

Several breast tumor cell lines, "including hormone-dependent and -independent and multidrug-resistant (MDR) lines," respond to antiproliferative effects of curcumin. Aggarwal et al examined cell lines "including the MDR-positive ones," and found they were all "highly sensitive to curcumin. The growth inhibitory effect of curcumin was time- and dose-dependent. Overall our results suggest that curcumin is a potent antiproliferative agent for breast tumor cells and may have potential as an anticancer agent."

Some researchers say curcumin inhibits angiogenesis, i.e. formation of new blood vessels,

which tumors use to nourish themselves as they grow. As an anti-inflammatory, turmeric triggers heat-shock stress response. Heat shock proteins stimulate the immune system. "The mechanism of the stimulation by curcumin of the stress responses," Japanese researchers say, "might be similar to that of salicylate [aspirin and similar substances], indomethacin and nordihydroguaiaretic acid [an anti-oxidant that interferes with arachidonic acid metabolism]."

Research at Memorial Sloan-Kettering Cancer Center (New York) a few ago back indicates that it makes sense to drink green tea along with a meal spiced with turmeric for double-boosted anti-cancer protective effects.

### Further Reading & References

- *"A Report on Curcumin's Anti-Cancer Effects" by Terri Mitchell, http://www.lef.org/magazine/mag2002/jul2002_report_curcumin_01.html

- *Beating Cancer With Nutrition* by Patrick Quillin (2005)

- Turmeric, by Jacqueline Strax, http://psa-rising.com/eatingwell/turmeric.htm

- Aggarwal, BB et al, Anticancer Res. 2003 Jan-Feb; 23(1A):363-98.

- Br J Clin Pharmacol 1998 Jan;45(1):1-12; update Toxicol Lett 2000 Mar 15;112-113:499-505.

- Molecular Vision 2003; 9:223-230, full text free online

- Iqbal M, et al. Pharmacol Toxicol. 2003 Jan;92(1):33-8.

- Anticancer Drugs. 1997 Jun;8(5):470-81.

- Ramachandran C, Miami 1999; Hidaka H, Japan, 2002 (human pancreatic cells lines);

- Elattar TM, University of Missouri-Kansas City, 2000(oral cancer cell-line.

- Mol Med 1998 Jun;4(6):376-83).Cell Stress Chaperones 1998 Sep;3(3):152-60

## Echinacea

Echinacea is a flowering herb that comes from the daisy family. One of the more common species of Echinacea is called purple coneflower. These herbs grow in eastern and central North America and are considered to have several positive medicinal effects.

An in vitro study suggested Echinacea supplements may offer antitumor properties. Other studies report Echinacea can greatly enhance the immune system. It is thought that Echinacea may build immunity during cancer treatments and possibly protect against certain forms of cancer.

Rotating echinacea with extracts of medicinal mushrooms also appears to help strengthen overall immunity during cancer treatments. While additional research is needed to define the potential role of echinacea in fighting cancer, a small German study showed that in patients with advanced colon cancer the herb appeared to prolong survival in those who took it in conjunction with standard chemotherapy. The herb presumably boosted the immune system's ability to fight invading cancer cells.

"Echinacea stimulates the white blood cells that help fight infections in the body. Research has shown that echinacea enhances the activity of particular white blood cell macrophages. A particular glycoprotein in echinacea was found to significantly increase the killing effect of macrophages on tumor cells."*

### Further Reading & References

- *Natural Herbal Remedies for Immunity, http://www.holistic-online.com/cancer/Cancer_ echinacea-1.htm

- *Beating Cancer With Nutrition* by Patrick Quillin (2005)

## Essiac/Flor' Essence/Lasagen/Ojibway Indian Tea/Transfer Factor

Essiac is an herbal cancer treatment developed by a Canadian nurse, Renée Caisse (1888-1978). (Essiac is Caisse spelled backwards.) Ms. Caisse claimed that the formula had been given to her in 1922 by a patient whose breast cancer had been cured by a traditional Native American healer in Ontario.

Thousands of patients have since been treated with this herbal mixture, most of them at Caisse's own Bracebridge Clinic in Ontario. The clinic became a virtual pilgrimage destination for cancer patients and Caisse became a revered figured. Reportedly, Essiac received sympathetic consideration from conventional Canadian doctors and came close to becoming an accepted mainstream treatment.

In 1937, Dr. Emma Carson spent 24 days inspecting the Bracebridge Clinic in Ottawa where Caisse did most of her work. In reviewing 400 cases of cancer patients, she declared, "The vast majority of Miss Caisse's patients are brought to her for treatment after [conventional treatment] has failed and the patients are pronounced incurable. The actual results from Essiac treatments and the rapidity of repair were absolutely marvelous and must be seen to convincingly confirm belief."

Although the Bracebridge clinic ceased operations in 1942, Essiac has remained in continuous use as an alternative cancer treatment. Charles Brusch, MD (President John Kennedy's physician) said that Essiac 'cures cancer'. Dr. Brusch in fact treated his own colon cancer successfully with Essiac.

A company in Ontario is allowed to provide Essiac to Canadian patients under a special arrangement with health officials there. It's safe to say the vast majority of Essiac users do not rely on this approved, prescription version of the herbal blend. But for those who prefer the "unofficial" version, it's a problem that Ms. Caisse never made the formula public in her lifetime. A number of companies now sell competing "original" Essiac formulas in the form of a tea, but the authenticity of some of these formulas is open to question. The authors of this article have not attempted to sort out the competing claims. As will be seen shortly, it's not urgent to have the exact formula used by Ms. Caisse.

Since Essiac is now a very well known treatment, it is important to point out that while Caisse did provide the herbs for oral use, most of her greatest success seems to have involved the injectable form of the herbs. They would obviously be more potent and fast-acting if administered in this way. Caisse actually felt quite strongly that this method of delivery was the only way to assure that the body could resist malignancy. Nonetheless, a large number of patients anecdotally report success using the tea.

As with many who explore the frontiers of knowledge, Caisse speculated about questions still remain unresolved today. She felt there was an undiscovered gland that was affected by Essiac, one that acts to inhibit the supply of the substances that nourish cancer cells. Everyone, even her strongest defenders, is quick to point out that while no one has disproved her theory, no one has corroborated it either. This said, the four herbs that everyone agrees are the cornerstones of the Essiac formula are fairly well understood.

Many users of Essiac believe that Essiac can and does improve the body's ability to fight cancer and that Essiac is effective at reducing the side effects of chemotherapy and radiation treatments. Users have reported that with the reduction in chemotherapy/ radiation side effects, they are much better able to handle the full course of their treatments - eliminating interruptions and delays in treatment.

But Essiac was tested at both Memorial Sloan-Kettering (MSKCC) and the US National Cancer Institute (NCI) in the 1970s and was said by these mainstream research centers to have no anticancer activity in animal systems. That conclusion is suspect not only because of the wealth of anecdotal evidence supporting Essiac but also because most of its identifiable ingredients have individually shown anticancer properties in independent tests.

The four core ingredients of Essiac are

- Burdock (Arctium lappa) (see the earlier section about Burdock)

- Indian rhubarb (Rheum palmatum): This plant has been demonstrated to have antitumor activity in the sarcoma 37-test system. Certain chemicals in Indian rhubarb, such as aloe emodin, catechin, and rhein have shown antitumor activity in animal test systems.

- Sorrel (Aloe emodin, isolated from sorrel, shows "significant antileukemic activity")

- Slippery elm: Slippery elm contains beta-sitosterol and a polysaccharide, both of which have shown anti-cancer activity.

According to the providers of the best-known version of the formula, "All four herbs normalize body systems by purifying the blood, promoting cell repair, and aiding effective assimilation and elimination. When combined, their separate beneficial effects are synergistically enhanced."

Homemade, this treatment costs only a few cents per day. No wonder, in the era of $150,000 bone marrow transplants, Essiac is becoming more popular.

The recipe below makes a year's worth of Essiac for roughly $5. It's important to note that most users purchase the preblended herbs that are marketed as Essiac rather than mixing their own.

- Burdock root (4.25 ozs. or 120g), pea-size cut

- Sheep sorrel (2.8 ozs. or 80g), powdered

- Slippery Elm bark (0.7 ozs. or 20g), powdered

- Turkey rhubarb root (0.18 oz. or 5g), powdered


Mix the herbs together very, very thoroughly. Use 1 cup of herb mix per 2 gallons distilled water each time you brew.

To make 1 cup of mix to brew with 2 gallons of distilled water, gather:

- Burdock root (cut) = 1/2 cup

- Sheep Sorrel (powdered) = 3/8 cup

- Slippery Elm bark (powdered) = 2 tablespoons + 2 teaspoons

- Turkey rhubarb (powdered) = 1 teaspoon


Directions:

- Thoroughly mix these dry ingredients in a bowl.

- Pour the dry mixture into a wide-mouth glass jar and shake well.

- Mix 1½ quarts of distilled water to every ounce of the dry mixture and boil it up in a stainless steel, lidded pot.

- After boiling hard for 10 minutes, turn off the heat.

- Scrape down the sides of the pot, and stir well.

- Let the pot sit for 10-12 hours.

- To preserve a supply, sterilize the implements and reheat the liquid until it is steaming hot, but not boiling.

- Strain the mixture and put it in bottles.

- Tighten caps of the bottle and then and set aside to cool. Once the bottles are opened, they should be refrigerated, but not frozen.

General consumption instructions:

Take one ounce of Essiac with two ounces of hot water every second day at bedtime, on an empty stomach two or three hours after supper. Do not eat or drink anything for at least one hour after taking Essiac. Continue the treatment every other day for thirty-two days, and then take the treatment every three days. Always keep Essiac refrigerated, but never place it in the freezer.

Always double check on the source and authenticity of the herbs. There are over 100 species of "sorrel" but it is important to make sure one is getting real sheep sorrel (Rumex acetosella), and not a substitute, such as ordinary garden sorrel (Rumex acetosa).

The final product looks somewhat like apple cider or light honey. It has a mild, earthy aroma and a flavor that some patients describe like dry, decayed wood.

Occasionally, patients complain of nausea and/or indigestion after taking Essiac, says Sheila Snow, author of *Essiac Essentials*. This may be because they take it on a full stomach. Large doses of burdock root tea have also been found toxic in certain cases. Essiac should not be used if you have renal (kidney) problems because it contains two herbs that are contraindicated for such cases.

### *Further Reading & References*

- *The Essiac Report: The True Story of a Canadian Herbal Cancer Remedy and of the Thousands of Lives It Continues to Save* by Richard Thomas (1993)

- *Essiac: A Native Herbal Cancer Remedy* by Cynthia Olsen (1998)

- *Essiac Essentials: The Remarkable Herbal Cancer Fighter* by Sheila Snow, Mali Klein (2000)

- *The Essiac Handbook* by James Percival (2006)

- Foldeak S and Dombradi G. Tumor-growth inhibiting substances of plant origin. I. Isolation of the active principle of Arctium lappa. Acta Phys Chem.1964;10:91-93.

- Dombradi C and Foldeak S. Screening report on the antitumor activity of puriÞed Arctium lappa extracts. Tumori.1966; 52:173.

- Morita K, et al. A desmutagenic factor isolated from burdock (Arctium lappa Linne). Mutat Res.1984; 129:25-31.

- WHO. In vitro screening of traditional medicines for anti-HIV activity: memorandum from a WHO meeting. Bul. WHO (Switzerland), 1989;67:613-618.

- Belkin M and Fitzgerald D. Tumor damaging capacity of plant materials. 1. Plants used as cathartics. J Natl Cancer Inst.1952;13:139-155.

- US Congress, Office of Technology Assessment (OTA). Unconventional cancer treatments. Washington, DC: US Government Printing Office, 1990.

- Kupchan SM and Karim A. Tumor inhibitors. Aloe emodin: antileukemic principle isolated from

- Rhamnus frangula L. Lloydia.1976; 39: 223-4.

- Morita H, et al. Cytotoxic and mutagenic effects of emodin on cultured mouse carcinoma FM3A cells. Mutat Res.1988; 204:329-32.

- Pettit GR, et al. Antineoplastic agents. The yellow jacket Vespula pensylvanica. Lloydia.1977;40: 247-52.

- Rhoads P, et al. Anticholinergic poisonings associated with commercial burdock root tea. J Toxicol.1984-85;22: 581-584.

- Walters, R. *"Essiac" Options: The Alternative Cancer Therapy Book*, 110

# Garlic

The history of garlic dates back 3,500 years. Hippocrates, the father of medicine, was the first to write that garlic was an excellent medicine for eliminating tumors.

Garlic is frequently used as a supporting remedy in the treatment of cancer. It has proven anti-cancer properties. Not only does it protect against the formation of tumors, including metastases, it also inhibits the growth of established tumors. In addition, it strengthens the immune system and improves the detoxifying ability of the liver.

According to researchers Dausch and Nixon, "One possible beneficial effect of garlic or its components may be their ability to enhance the body's mechanism for eliminating exogenous substances including

carcinogens. In some studies, garlic has been shown to have a stimulating effect on certain enzymes that are known to be involved in removing toxic substances. Antihepatotoxic [liver detoxifying] activity of garlic sulfur components have been described in vitro and vivo."

The liver detoxification capacity is potentially of great interest to cancer patients undergoing chemotherapy, since liver eliminates the toxic chemotherapy from the body. Garlic stimulates the production of an enzyme called glutathione S-transferase (GST), which, naturally occurring in the body, protects against cancer by detoxifying potent carcinogens. There is no data in the National Toxicity Program on garlic, but the ancient Chinese classified garlic as a moderately toxic herb because high doses can lead to stomach upset and intestinal gas. However, a cold-aged extract from Japanese whole-clove garlic allows some of the active components to be converted to less irritating compounds with less odor.

Researchers used to believe that the single beneficial element in garlic was Allicin, the compound formed when the bulb is crushed. Allicin is an unstable compound that is strongly antibacterial and mainly responsible for garlic's characteristic odor. Now, researchers have discovered other sulfur compounds in garlic, along with 17 amino acids, germanium, calcium, selenium, copper, iron, potassium, magnesium, zinc, and small amounts of vitamins A, B1, and C. The main active components in garlic seem to be the various sulfur compounds.

Li and colleagues at the Strang-Cornell Cancer Research Laboratory describe the research on garlic in a 1995 article in Oncology Reports: "Based on experimental and epidemiological evidence, garlic could be classified as an anti-carcinogen. The specific phase(s) of the carcinogenic process, i.e., initiation, promotion, or progression at which garlic or its constituents may exert its biological effect, however, remains to be determined in many cases."

According to Boik (See References), "Theoretically, garlic may inhibit cancer by a variety of mechanisms, including reduced angiogenesis, reduced platelet aggregation, and increased fibrinolysis."

Dutch researchers found that compounds in garlic inhibit endothelial umbilical cell proliferation in vivo, an indication that they might also inhibit tumor angiogenic activity. The anti-angiogenic effect of thiols, compounds found in garlic, may be related to their ability to inhibit free-radical production by macrophages.

Macrophages (immune system cells) are found in great numbers in solid tumors, and can comprise 10 to 30% of the cells in a tumor. It may sound odd that these normally desirable cells can be a problem. The reason is that under the low-oxygen conditions found in the interiors of solid tumors, macrophages secrete large amounts of angiogenesis factors, perhaps because the stimuli are similar to those found in situations where wound healing is required. In other words, the macrophages interpret the cancer to be a wound trauma in healthy tissues.

Israeli scientists have destroyed malignant tumors in mice using a chemical that occurs naturally in garlic, the Weizmann Institute reported. The key to the scientists' success lies in a unique, two-step system for delivering the cancer-wrecking chemical to the tumor cells.

Allicin is composed of an enzyme, alliinase, and an inert chemical called alliin. Scientists attached alliinase to an antibody that was programmed to be attracted to a gastric tumor's characteristic receptors. Then they injected that alliinase-antibody combination into a cancerous mouse. Once the alliinase-antibody had settled on the tumors, the scientists introduced alliin into the mouse. The combination of alliinase and alliin - at the site of the tumor - created the toxic allicin, which cured the mouse of its gastric tumors.

Pruthi showed that unstable sulfur compounds undergo loss of therapeutic properties if garlic is heated above 60 degrees centigrade. Cooked garlic loses medicinal value.

### *Further Reading & References*

- Alternative Cancer Therapies continued, http://www.cancure.org/choice_of_therapies_continued.htm

- *Tell Me What to Eat to Help Prevent Breast Cancer: Nutrition You Can Live With* by Elaine Magee (2000)

- *The Cancer Survivor's Guide: Foods That Help You Fight Back* by Jennifer K. Reilly (2009)

- *User's Guide to Garlic: Learn How This Remarkable Food and Reduce Your Risk of Heart Disease and Cancer* by Stephen Fulder (2005)

- Draft, "Status Report of Year One Operations," University of Texas Center for Alternative Medicine Research, September 9, 1996, 45.

- Dausch and Nixon, "Garlic: A Review."

- Boik, Cancer and Natural Medicine, 29., http://www.sciencedirect.com/science/article/pii/037887419601416X

- E. Lee, M. Steiner and R. Lin, "Thioallyl Compounds: Potent Inhibitors of Cell Proliferation," Biochimica et Biophysica Acta 1221(1):73-7 (10 March 1994) Boik, Cancer and Natural Medicine, 30.

- J.S. Pruthi, L.J. Singh and G. Lag, "Determination of the Critical Temperature of Dehydration of Garlic," Food Science 8:436-41 (1959).

- Judith G. Dausch and Daniel W. Nixon, "Garlic: A Review of Its Relationship to Malignant Disease," Preventive Medicine 19:346-361 (1990), 350.

- S. Nakagawa et al., "Effect of Raw and Extracted-aged Garlic Juice on Growth of Young Rats and Their Organs after Per Oral Administration," Journal of Toxicological Sciences 5:91-112 (1980).

# Hoxsey Herbal Treatment

The Hoxsey herbal treatment is administered by the Bio Medical Center in Tijuana. They state, "In general, we have seen a 50-70 percent success rate in the treatment of cancer. The best types of cancer to respond to Hoxsey Therapy have been: breast cancer, kidney cancer, lymphomas, melanoma, prostate cancer, skin cancer and thyroid cancer."

Harry M. Hoxsey, a controversial and colorful figure who said he obtained the formula from his grandfather, first used it in 1924. The elder Hoxsey was a farmer who observed one of his horses cure itself of cancer by instinctively eating certain plants. Some sources cast doubt on this. The truth will probably never be known. But, it's a fact that many plants, which animals seek when they are ill, contain nitrilosides. Amygdalin (laetrile) is classified as a nitriloside.

Born in Illinois, the charismatic practitioner of herbal folk medicine faced unrelenting opposition and harassment from a hostile medical establishment. Nevertheless, two federal courts upheld the "therapeutic value" of Hoxsey's internal tonic. Even his 'arch enemies', the American Medical Association and the Food and Drug Administration, admitted that his treatment could cure some forms of cancer. A Dallas judge ruled in federal court that Hoxsey's therapy was "comparable to surgery, radium, and x-ray" in its effectiveness, without the destructive side effects of those treatments.

But in the 1950s, at the tail end of the McCarthy era, Hoxsey's clinics were shut down. The AMA, NCI, and FDA organized a "conspiracy" to "suppress" a fair, unbiased assessment of Hoxsey's methods, according to a 1953 federal report to Congress. Hoxsey's Dallas clinic closed its doors in 1960, and three years later, at Hoxsey's request, Mildred Nelson, R.N., his long-time chief nurse, moved the operation to Tijuana, Mexico, where it still remains.

According to eminent botanist James Duke, Ph.D., of the United States Department of Agriculture, all of the Hoxsey herbs have known anticancer properties.

They are cited in *Plants Used Against Cancer*, a global compendium of folk usage of medicinal plants compiled by NCI chemist Jonathan Hartwell. Furthermore, Duke noted, the Hoxsey herbs have long been used by Native American healers to treat cancer, and traveling European doctors picked up the knowledge and took it home with them to treat patients.

Medical historian Patricia Spain Ward reported "provocative findings of antitumor properties" in many of the individual Hoxsey herbs when she investigated the Hoxsey regimen in 1988 for the United States Congress's Office of Technology Assessment. The basic ingredients of Hoxsey's internal tonic are potassium iodide and such substances as licorice, red clover, burdock root, stillingia root, barberis root, pokeroot, cascara, prickly ash bark, and buckthorn bark.

Support comes from two Hungarian scientists who, in 1966, reported "considerable antitumor activity" in a purified fraction of burdock. Japanese researchers at Nagoya University in 1984 found in burdock a new type of desmutagen, a substance that is uniquely capable of reducing mutation in either the absence or the presence of metabolic activation. This new property is so important; the Japanese scientists named it the B-factor, for "burdock factor."

Hoxsey himself believed that his therapy normalized and balanced the chemistry within the body. Like many other holistic healers, he considered cancer to be a systemic disease, not a localized one. Cancer, he wrote, "Occurs only in the presence of a profound physiological change in the constituents of body fluids and a consequent chemical imbalance in the organism."

His herbal medicines are intended to restore the original chemical balance to the body's disturbed metabolism, creating an environment unfavorable to cancer cells, which cease to multiply and eventually die. The herbal remedies are said to strengthen the immune system, cause tumors to necrotize (i.e., die), and help carry away the resulting wastes and toxins.

In 1954, an independent team of ten physicians from around the United States made a two day inspection of Hoxsey's Dallas clinic and issued a remarkable statement. After examining hundreds of case histories and interviewing patients and ex-patients, the doctors released a signed report declaring that the clinic "... is successfully treating pathologically proven cases of cancer, both internal and external, without the use of surgery, radium, or x-ray."

They went on to say, ""Accepting the standard yardstick of cases that have remained symptom-free in excess of five to six years after treatment, established by medical authorities, we have seen sufficient cases to warrant such a conclusion. Some of those presented before us have been free of symptoms as long as twenty-four years, and the physical evidence indicates that they are all enjoying exceptional health at this time.

"We as a Committee feel that the Hoxsey treatment is superior to such conventional methods of treatment as x-ray, radium, and surgery. We are willing to assist this Clinic in any way possible in bringing this treatment to the American public."

At the Bio-Medical Center in Tijuana, Hoxsey Therapy is administered in two forms. One is taken orally and the other is a salve (containing bloodroot) which, if the tumor is on or close to the surface of the skin, is applied topically. The Hoxsey therapy is reportedly effective in alleviating pain in many cases. The clinic's patient brochure includes case histories of patients successfully treated.


### Further Reading & References

- Bio-Medical Center (Hoxsey Clinic), http://www.cancure.org/hoxsey_clinic.htm

- *You Don't Have to Die* by Harry Hoxsey (1985)

- *When Healing Becomes a Crime: The Amazing Story of the Hoxsey Cancer Clinics and the Return of Alternative Therapies* by Kenny Ausubel (2000)

- Cancer Herbal Extracts/Plant Products, http://www.alternativehealth.co.nz/cancer/herbs.htm

- Ken Ausubel, "The Troubling Case of Harry Hoxsey," *New Age Journal*, July-August 1988, p. 79. Surgery, Gynecology and Obstetrics, vol. 114, 1962, pp. 25-30; and see Walter H. Lewis and Memory

- P.F. Elvin- Lewis, *Medical Botany: Plants Affecting Man's Health* (New York: John Wiley and Sons, 1977).

- F.E. Mohs, "Chemosurgery: A Microscopically Controlled Method of Cancer Excision," Archives of Surgery, vol.42, 1941, pp. 279295, cited in Patricia Spain Ward, "History of Hoxsey Treatment," contract report submitted to U.S. Congress, Office of Technology Assessment, May 1988, pp. 2-3. Ward, op. cit., p. 8.

- Kazuyoshi Morita, Tsuneo Kada, and Mitsuo Namiki, "A Desmutagenic Factor Isolated From Burdock (Arctium Lappa Linne)," Mutation Research, vol. 129, 1984, pp. 25-31, cited in Ward, op. cit., p. 7.

- *Plants Used Against Cancer: A Survey* (Bioactive Plants, Vol 2), by Jonathan L. Hartwell (1984)

# Jason Winters Tea

Jason Winters was an adventurer throughout the Sixties and Seventies who crossed the Canadian Rocky Mountains in a hot air balloon and sailed the Mackenzie River by canoe. In 1977 he was diagnosed with squamous cell carcinoma after developing a tumor on his neck. After being given only three months to live, he traveled around the world in search of a way to heal his terminal cancer.

Winters gradually came across the right combination of herbs found in a variety of different countries, healed himself, wrote a book about it, traveled on lecture tours, and helped others heal their cancers. You can find this tea in most health food stores.

Winters also became a vocal proponent for herbal healing, much to the chagrin of pharmaceutical companies. He says in his book, "I must tell you that I was scared. I was not prepared to take on the billion-dollar drug companies, the medical associations and doctors, all of whom would chew up and spit out anyone that would dare to even say that possibly, just possibly, herbs can help."

The individual herbs found during his world journey had little effect on Jason, but when he mixed them together in a tea, their synergistic effect caused his tumor to begin to shrink, the cancer to leave his body and he gradually achieved perfect health.

The herbal ingredients in his tea blend seem to act synergistically, each boosting the effect of the others, making an herbal beverage that acts as a powerful natural blood purifier and detoxifier.

According to the Jason Winters website, the tea contains red clover, Indian sage leaf (which the website claims has properties similar to chaparral, Oolong leaf tea (mildly caffeinated), and a trademarked "special spice" called Herbalen Blend, for which the ingredients are not disclosed.

### Further Reading & References

- *The Sir Jason Winters Story: Killing Cancer.* by Sir Jason Winters (1980)

- *Killing Cancer 18 Years Later* by Sir Jason Winters (1996)

- Alternative Cancer Therapies, Page 2, http://www.mnwelldir.org/docs/cancer1/altthrpy2.htm

# Kampo

Kampo is fundamentally a clinical system based on the classical medical literature dating back to the Han Dynasty in ancient China. In Japan today, fully 75% of physicians use at least some of the traditional Kampo formulas, which are available in almost all pharmacies by prescription, or under the advice of specially-trained pharmacists. Kampo is integrated into the national health care system in Japan.

"Western-style" herbology tends to blend individual herbs or their standardized extracts. Kampo, on the other hand, mixes together multiple raw herbs, according to specific ancient formulas. From there, an extraction of the entire mixture is created.

When combined, the specific herbs of the Kampo blend and this specific extraction process create a remedy more effective than the total of each herb extracted individually.

Kampo, the Japanese version of Chinese herbalism, has reported many successes in treating cancer. In Tokyo, many Kampo doctors work in conventional hospitals prescribing drugs, but moonlight to pursue their private herbal practices. Kampo doctors dispense with much of the conceptual framework of traditional Chinese medicine such as the division of the body into yin and yang parts.

One Kampo formula tested for efficacy in non-resectable liver cancer patients by the Memorial Sloan-Kettering Cancer Center included bupleurum root, pinellia tuber, ginger, scutellaria root, jujube, ginseng, and licorice.

For more information on specific Kampo formulas for cancer, the 14th edition of the *Japanese Pharmacopoeia* is an excellent resource.

### *Further Reading & References*

- Research in Japanese Botanical Medicine and Immune Modulating Cancer Therapy, http://www. findarticles.com/p/articles/mi_m0ISW/is_2001_August/ai_78177216

- Japanese Herbal Mix Non-Resectable Hepatocellular CA, http://www.annieappleseedproject.org/ japhermixfor.html

- Kampo Medicine: The Practice of Chinese Herbal Medicine in Japan, http://www.itmonline.org/ arts/kampo.htm

- "Kampo medicine and new immunological parameter." http://www.ncbi.nlm.nih.gov/entrez/query.f cgi?cmd=Retrieve&db=pubmed&dopt=Abstract&list_uids=15206133

- "Preventive effect of Kampo medicine (Hangeshashin-to) against irinotecan-induced diarrhea in advanced non-small-cell lung cancer." http://www.ncbi.nlm.nih.gov/entrez/query.fcgi?cmd=Retri eve&db=pubmed&dopt=Abstract&list_uids=12687289

- "Suppressive effect of Shichimotsu-koka-to (Kampo medicine) on pulmonary metastasis of B16 melanoma cells. Suppressive effect of Shichimotsu-koka-to (Kampo medicine) on pulmonary metastasis of B16 melanoma cells." http://www.ncbi.nlm.nih.gov/entrez/query.fcgi?cmd=Retriev e&db=PubMed&list_uids=12132662&dopt=Abstract

- Kampo: Japan's Herbal Tradition Emerges in US, http://www.holisticprimarycare.net/topics/ topics-a-g/acupuncture-a-oriental-med/14-kampo-japans-herbal-tradition-emerges-in-us

# Licorice root/Glycyrrhiza glabra

According to some herbalists, licorice (or Glycyrrhiza glabra) is one of the two or three most important herbs in the world. To the Chinese, there is no other herb that acts on such a grand scale except, perhaps, ginseng. Licorice root is found in more medicinal combinations in Chinese Medicine than any other herb including ginseng. Many Chinese consider it the key to health.

Licorice root contains both the isoflavone licochalcone-A and triterpenoid saponin. Regarding licochalcone-A, in a scientific study: "Cells from patients with leukemia, breast and prostate cancer that were grown in cultures in the lab were killed when enough of the extract was added."

In addition, triterpenoids may be effective against cancer due to their ability to block prostaglandin, the hormone-like fatty acid potentially responsible for stimulating the growth of cancer cells. Triterpenoids have also been shown in test tubes to stunt the growth of rapidly multiplying cells like cancer cells. It's also possible that they help precancerous cells return to normal.

Note that licorice root is toxic, so further research is needed.

### Further Reading & References

- Wild Licorice (Glycyrrhiza lepidota), http://www.holoweb.com/cannon/wildd.htm

- Licorice, http://www.cancer.org/Treatment/TreatmentsandSideEffects/ComplementaryandAlternativeMedicine/HerbsVitaminsandMinerals/licorice

- Licorice and cancer, http://www.ncbi.nlm.nih.gov/pubmed/11588889

## Lymphotonic PF2

Lymphotonic PF2 is a little-known cancer treatment option with a unique approach to destroying cancer cells. Supporters of the treatment claim cancer actually puts the immune system to sleep so that the cancer can take over weak cells. Cancer growth then manifests itself. Lymphotonic PF2 purportedly "poisons" your system through an herbal, non-toxic drink. This "wakes up" the immune system, thanks to the nature of the invasive attack. Once awake, the immune system goes after the malignant cancer cells.

### Further Reading & References

- A Free Consultant's Report, Dedicated to Ridding the World of Cancer Once and For All, http://www.naturalcancer.net/FreeGuide.htm

## Mangosteen Fruit

Mangosteen should not be confused with mango fruit, as the two are entirely different. Mangosteen comes from a plant related to the Guttiferae family which is made up of tropical trees and shrubs that secrete a yellow, resinous juice. It is a hard-shelled fruit native to southern Asia and is about the size of a small tangerine.

There is some scientific evidence for the fruit's anti-cancer properties.

"We found that antiproliferative effect of CME [crude methanolic extract] was associated with apoptosis on breast cancer cell line by determinations of morphological changes and oligonucleosomal DNA fragments. In addition, CME at various concentrations and incubation times were also found to inhibit ROS production. These investigations suggested that the methanolic extract from the pericarp [skin] of Garcinia mangostana had strong antiproliferation, potent antioxidation and induction of apoptosis. Thus, it indicates that this substance can show different activities and has potential for cancer chemoprevention which were dose dependent as well as exposure time dependent."*

In addition, mangosteen appears to have 43 different antioxidants called xanthones which are biologically active polyphenolic compounds similar to bioflavonoids. Xanthones appear to have "anti-allergic, anti-inflammatory, anti-tuberculotic, anti-tumor, anti-platelet, Beta-adrenergic blocking and … anti-convulsant [properties]" according to professional journals such as *Free Radical Research, Journal of Pharmacology*, and the *Indian Journal of Experimental Biology*.

Xanthones from the mangosteen also appear to inhibit cancerous cell development and the growth of some breast cancer cells and human leukemia cell lines.

Mangosteen offers the most health benefits if the flesh of the whole fruit is consumed. Simply drinking the juice will not offer as many benefits.

### *Further Reading & References*

- *Antiproliferation, antioxidation and induction of apoptosis by Garcinia mangostana (mangosteen) on SKBR3 human breast cancer cell line, http://www.ncbi.nlm.nih.gov/entrez/query.fcgi?cmd=Retrieve&db=PubMed&list_uids=14698525&dopt=Abstract

- A Friendly Skeptic Looks At Mangosteen Ralph W. Moss, http://www.cancerdecisions.com/050904_page.html

- Marona H, Pekala E, Filipek B, Maciag D, Szneler E. Pharmacological properties of some aminoalkanolic derivatives of xanthone. Pharmaxie. 2001;56:567-572. http://rawfoodswitch.com/fruits-vegetables-nuts-and-seeds/king-queen-fruits-durian-mangosteen/

- "Secrets of the Natural Health Benefits of Xanthones from Mangosteen Fruit" by Laurie Kristensen

# Noni Juice

Noni Juice, also known as Tahitian Noni, is a commercially available extract that comes from a South Seas island plant. It has reportedly been used by natives for centuries to treat a wide variety of diseases. There have been many anecdotal, but few published scientific, reports on its ability to greatly assist the body in overcoming cancer.

Like grape juice, Noni juice contains a whole slew of cancer fighting nutrients. It kills cancer cells (the anthraquinone damnacanthal and the trace element selenium), it stops the spread of cancer (beta sitosterol, Noni-ppt and limonene), it stimulates the white blood cells and other parts of the immune system (polysaccharides) and it takes part in a process that enlarges cell membranes so they can better absorb nutrients (proxeronine aids in creating xeronine). And this is only a partial list.

Noni juice is reputed to work quickly. It is regarded by many as a very effective cancer treatment. Notable cases have been reported where terminal cancer patients were completely cured of their cancer in as little as 10-12 days, but this is not necessarily typical. Frequently, patients turn to Noni after orthodox medicine has given up on them.

Noni juice also stimulates the production of nitric oxide, which may be the key to its health benefits. In addition to helping regulate blood circulation and the functions of major organs such as the brain, scientists have discovered that nitric oxide also boosts immune response and reduces tumor growth.

In addition to helping regulate blood circulation and the functions of major organs (including the brain), scientists have discovered that nitric oxide also boosts immune response and reduces tumor growth. For example:

"Recently, researchers found that the main reason Noni juice provides so many benefits is that it stimulates the production of nitric oxide in the body. The 1998 Nobel Prize for Medicine was awarded to three researchers for the discovery of nitric oxide. They found it to be a signaling molecule involved in controlling the circulation of blood, regulating activities of the brain, lungs, liver, kidneys, stomach, and other organs. In addition, they found that it effected a "seemingly limitless" range of functions in the body. They found that nitric oxide reduces tumor growth, and increases the immune response against the radical replication of cells."

Anything that gets enough oxygen to a cancer cell is going to kill the cell. Health Science Institute panelist Jon Barron admits that at first he dismissed multi-level marketing testimonials about Noni benefits. But, Barron describes his reaction as "shocked" once he had a chance to examine the nutrients in Noni juice, which he now describes as a "serious cancer treatment."

In a study done at the Louisiana State University Health Sciences Center, the effects of Noni juice were tested in a three-dimensional fibrin clot matrix model. The concentrations of the juice were found to be highly effective in stopping the growth of new vessel sprouts from placental vein explants and were also effective in halting the growth rate and spread of capillary sprouts. In addition, Noni juice was found to be an effective inhibitor of capillary initiation in explants from human breast tumors.

### Further Reading & References

- *The Noni Phenomenon* by Neil Solomon (1999)

- *Tahitian Noni Juice: How Much, How Often, For What*, by Neil Solomon (2000)

- *76 Ways to Use Noni Fruit Juice* by Isa Navarre (20010

- Noni Juice Treatment for Cancer, http://www.cancertutor.com/Cancer/Noni.html

- "Inhibition of angiogenic initiation and disruption of newly established human vascular networks by juice from Morinda citrifolia (noni)," http://www.ncbi.nlm.nih.gov/entrez/query.fcgi?cmd=Retrieve&db=pubmed&dopt=Abstract&list_uids=14739620

# Olive Leaf Extract

Olive leaf extract offers significant antiviral, antifungal, antibacterial, and anti-parasitic benefits, as well as heart health benefits. It contains an active ingredient called oleuropein that interferes with viruses in

several ways. For starters, it disrupts the viral amino acid production, inhibits replication, and in retro-viruses neutralizes enzymes that are needed to alter the RNA of a healthy cell, whereby the virus would be able to take over those cells.

According to Michael Lam, M.D., a natural medicine researcher, "Olive leaf extract also has a powerful immune system boosting effect by means of increasing phagocytosis in white blood cells (the effect is the destruction of foreign bacteria and viruses that are literally gobbled up)."

Olive leaf extract has a long history of being used against illnesses in which microorganisms play a major role. In more recent years, a drug company discovered that an extract from olive leaf (calcium elenolate), tested in vitro (test tube) was effective in eliminating a very broad range of organisms, including bacteria, viruses, and parasites, as well as yeast, mold, and fungi. The problem with using it in the body was that once in the blood, a protein combined with it and caused it to be inactivated. It's reported that most olive leaf extracts last only 15 minutes in the blood.

In 1995, a U.S. company claimed that if the active molecule in olive leaf extract was rotated around a specific axis by a precise amount, the blood protein no longer inactivated it and it was therefore able to effectively eliminate or control a very broad range of microorganisms and associated conditions in the body, including herpes, Epstein Barr and cytomegalo viruses, chlamydia, cholera, hepatitis (A, B and C), malaria, measles, meningitis, rabies, tapeworm, salmonella, tuberculosis, staphylococcus, polio, vaginitis, thrush, strep throat, whooping cough, pneumonia, ringworm, bacillus cereus, and many others.

### Further Reading & References

- *Olive Leaf Extract* by Morton Walker, Morton, Dr. Walker (1997)

- *Olive Leaf Extract* by Jack, N.D. Ritchason (2007)

- Dr. Lam, Body, Mind, Nutrition, http://www.lammd.com/articles/cancer_and_immunity. asp?page=2

# Oregano Oil

Oil of oregano is made from the leaves and flowers of the oregano plant which is native to the Mediterranean region. The plant has a history of medicinal use stretching back to the ancient Greeks, who first mastered the art of harvesting the oil when the content in the plant was at its highest.

Naringin is one of the substances within oil of oregano that may help with cancer. Studies have shown it can halt the growth of cancer cells as well as ramp up the effect of antioxidants. Rosmarinic acid, an antioxidant found in the oil, has been shown to prevent atherosclerosis and cancer. It acts by reducing fluid retention and alleviating swelling.

Oregano oil has also been reported to have the power to halt or even reverse skin destruction caused by cancer.

### Further Reading & References

- Oil of Oregano Research, http://www.colloidalsilversolutions.com/oreganoresearch.html

- Oil of Oregano: A Powerhouse for the Alternative Medicine Cabinet, http://www.naturalnews. com/024685_oregano_alternative_medicine_health.html

# Pau D'Arco/Taheebo Tea/Lapacho/Lapacho Morado/Ipe Roxo/Ipe/ Trumpet Bush

Also, known as "lapacho," "ipe roxo" and "taheebo tea," pau d'arco is derived from the inner bark of the Tabebuia tree of Brazil and Argentina. It is used in folk medicine in South America for the treatment of a wide variety of illnesses including colds, flu, malaria, gonorrhea, and cancer.

Lapachol, the active ingredient in pau d'arco, is known to produce strong biological responses against cancer. It is said that the pau d'arco tree yields lapachol and 20 other compounds that may be useful in treating cancer.

In some cases, cancer remissions have been achieved; however, it is apparently necessary to continue drinking the tea for the rest of one's life to maintain the remission. The tea is sold widely in health food stores.

Pau d'arco is thought to act by inhibiting the formation of fibrin, which has the effect of preventing the formation of new blood vessels. New blood vessels are necessary for the formation and growth of new tumors. The process of blood vessel proliferation is called angiogenesis. Fibrin also is necessary for the formation of the protein coats, which surround and protect malignant cells.

Pau d'arco also is also employed in herbal medicine systems in the United States for lupus, diabetes, ulcers, leukemia, allergies, liver disease, Hodgkin's disease, osteomyelitis, Parkinson's disease, and psoriasis, and is a popular remedy for candida and yeast infections. The records of European herbal medicine systems reveal that it is used in much the same way as in the United States, and for the same conditions. The chemical constituents and active ingredients of pau d'arco have been well documented. Its use with (and reported cures for) various types of cancers fueled much of the initial research in the early 1960s.

The plant contains a large quantity of chemicals known as quinoids, and a small quantity of benzenoids and flavonoids. These quinoids (chiefly, anthraquinones, furanonaphthoquinones, lapachones and naphthoquinones) have shown the most biological activity and are believed to be the center of the plant's efficacy as an herbal remedy.

In the 1960s, plant extracts of the heartwood and bark demonstrated marked anti-tumor effects in animals, which drew the interest of the NCI. Researchers decided that the most potent single chemical for this activity was the naphthoquinone named lapachol. They concentrated solely on this single chemical in their subsequent cancer research. In a 1968 study, lapachol demonstrated highly significant activity against cancerous tumors in rats. By 1970, NCI-backed research already was testing lapachol in human cancer patients. The institute reported, however, that their first Phase I study failed to produce a therapeutic effect without side-effects—and they discontinued further cancer research shortly thereafter.

These side-effects were nausea and vomiting and anti-vitamin K activity (which caused anemia and an anticoagulation effect). Interestingly, other chemicals in the whole plant extract (which, initially, showed positive anti-tumor effects and very low toxicity) demonstrated positive effects on Vitamin K and, conceivably, compensated for lapachol's negative effect.

As often happens in mainstream study of plant remedies, instead of pursuing research on a complex combination of at least 20 active chemicals in a whole plant extract (several of which had anti-tumor effects and other positive biological activities), research focused on a single, patentable chemical - and it didn't work as well as the whole-plant extract.

Despite NCI's abandonment of the research, another group developed a lapachol analog (which was patentable) in 1975. In one study, they reported this lapachol analog increased the life span of mice inoculated with leukemic cells by over 80%.

In a small, uncontrolled 1980 study of nine human patients with various cancers (liver, kidney, breast, prostate, and cervix), pure lapachol was reported to shrink tumors and reduce associated pain —and three of the patients realized complete remissions.

The phytochemical database housed at the U.S. Department of Agriculture has documented lapachol as being anti-abscess, anti-carcinomic, anti-edemic, antiinflammatory, anti-malarial, antiseptic, antitumorous, anti-viral, bactericidal, fungicidal, insecticidal, pesticidal, protisticidal, respiradepressant, schistosomicidal, termiticidal, and viricidal. It's not surprising that pau d'arco's beneficial effects were seen to stem from its lapachol content. But another chemical in pau d'arco, beta-lapachone, has also been studied closely recently and a number of patents have been filed on it.

In a 2002 U.S. patent, beta-lapachone was cited to have, "significant antineoplastic activity against human cancer cell lines . . . [including] promyelocytic leukemia, prostate, malignant glioma, colon, hepatoma, breast, ovarian, pancreatic, multiple myeloma cell lines and drug-resistant cell lines." In another U.S. patent, beta-lapachone was cited with the in vivo ability to inhibit the growth of prostate tumors.

In addition to its isolated chemicals, a hot water extract of pau d'arco demonstrated antibacterial actions against Staphylococcus aureus, Helicobacter pylori (the bacteria that commonly causes stomach ulcers), and Brucella. A water extract of pau d'arco was reported (in other in vitro clinical research) to have strong activity against 11 fungus and yeast strains.

Pau d'arco and its chemicals also have demonstrated in vitro antiviral properties against various viruses, including Herpes I and II, influenza, polio virus, and vesicular stomatitis virus. Its antiparasitic actions against various parasites (including malaria, schistosoma, and trypanosoma) have been confirmed as well. Finally, bark extracts of pau d'arco have demonstrated anti-inflammatory activity and have been shown to be successful against a wide range of induced inflammation in mice and rats.

Pau d'arco is an important resource from the rainforest with many applications in herbal medicine. Unfortunately, its popularity and use have been controversial due to varying results obtained with its use. For the most part, these seem to have been caused by a lack of quality control—and confusion as to which part of the plant to use and how to prepare it. Many species of Tabebuia, as well as other completely unrelated tree species exported today from South America as "pau d'arco," have few to none of the active constituents of the true medicinal species. Pau d'arco lumber is in high demand in South America.

The inner bark shavings commonly sold in the U.S. are actually by-products of the timber and lumber industries. Even mahogany shavings from the same sawmill floors in Brazil are swept up and sold around the world as "pau d'arco" (due to the similarity in color and odor of the two woods). In 1987, a chemical analysis of 12 commercially-available pau d'arco products revealed only one product containing lapachol—and only in trace amounts.

As lapachol concentration typically is 2–7% in true pau d'arco, the study surmised that the products were not truly pau d'arco, or that processing and transportation had damaged them. Most pau d'arco research has centered on the heartwood of the tree.

When buying, read the label, and be sure the tree listed is Tabebuia impetiginosa or Tabebuia heptaphylla.

### Further Reading & References

- *The Healing Power of Pau D'Arco: The Divine Tree of the South American Shamans Provides Extraordinary Healing Benefits* by Walter Lubeck, Christine M. Grimm

- *Pau D'Arco: Immune Power from the Rain Forest* by Kenneth Jones (1995)

- *Pau D'Arco: Taheebo, Lapacho* by Rita Elkins (1997)

- Borino B. 1,000-year-old Inca cancer cure works. Globe 1981 Sept 15;28(37). Diamond WJ, et al. An alternative medicine definitive guide to cancer. Tiburon: Future Medicine Publishing, Inc., 1997:834.

- Fetrow CW, Avila JR. Professional's handbook of complementary and alternative medicines. Springhouse, Pennsylvania: Springhouse Corporation 1999:491-93.

- Santana CF, et al. Preliminary observations with the use of lapachol in human patients bearing malignant neoplasms. Revista da Instituto de Antibioticos 20 1980/81:61-68.

- Herbal Extracts/Plant Products, http://www.alternativehealingtools.com/cancer/herbs.htm

- Dr. Christopher's Herbal Legacy, http://www.herballegacy.com/Maiden_Medicinal.html

# Red Clover/Trifolium pratense

Red clover, also known as *Trifolium pratense*, is a perennial herb native to Europe and Western Asia. The NCI researched the herb and found four anti-tumor compounds in it.

Red clover has been cultivated since ancient times, primarily to provide a favorite grazing food for animals. But, like many other herbs, red clover was also a valued medicine. Although it has been used for many purposes worldwide, the one condition most consistently associated with red clover is cancer. Chinese physicians and Russian folk healers also used it to treat respiratory problems.

In the nineteenth century, red clover became popular among herbalists as an "alterative" or "blood purifier." This medical term, long since defunct, refers to an ancient belief that toxins in the blood are the root cause of many illnesses. Cancer, eczema, and the eruptions of venereal disease were all seen as manifestations of toxic buildup. Red clover was considered one of the best herbs to "purify" the blood. For this reason, it is included in many of the famous treatments for cancer, including the Hoxsey cancer cure and Jason Winter's cancer-cure tea.

Recently, special red clover extracts high in substances called isoflavones have arrived on the market. These isoflavones produce effects in the body somewhat similar to those of estrogen, and for this reason they are called phytoestrogens (phyto indicates a plant source). The major isoflavones in red clover include genistein and daidzein, also found in soy. Two other isoflavones in red clover are formononetin and biochanin.

"The isoflavones isolated from red clover have been studied for their effectiveness in treating some forms of cancer. It is thought that the isoflavones prevent the proliferation of cancer cells and that they may even destroy cancer cells. Laboratory and animal studies have found that red clover isoflavones may protect against the growth of breast cancer cells. This is surprising because estrogens (and isoflavones have estrogenic properties) have generally been thought to stimulate the growth of breast cancer in women."

Red clover also appears to have a positive effect on prostate cancer. In one case, a 66-year-old physician took a concentrated phyto-estrogen derived from red clover. His prostate tumor shrunk. Later surgery showed his tumor had experienced a significant amount of apoptosis, similar to high-dose estrogen therapy.

### *Further Reading & References*

- Prostate Cancer Treatment, http://www.yourhealthbase.com/prostate_cancer_treatment.html

- Stephens, Frederick O., Medical Journal of Australia, Vol. 167, August 4, 1997, pp. 138-40

# Rye Extract/Oralmat

Oralmat is a patented extract of Secale cereale, more commonly known as ryegrass. It is completely non-toxic and pleasant tasting and is administered as a liquid under the tongue. This allows active ingredients to be absorbed directly by the mucous membranes in the mouth.

Researchers are in the process of uncovering the particular nutrient or nutrient combination in rye that is responsible for its overall healing power. To date, they have discovered that individual constituents of rye grass extract possess a significant number of health advantages, proven in clinical and laboratory studies.

These advantages include the ability to strengthen immune function, increase bone marrow production, weaken and destroy infections, boost cell energy, protect against the toxicity of radiation therapy, neutralize free radicals, and act as an anti-inflammatory.

Another interesting effect is the ability to organize the brain's processes. The drops, taken under the tongue like many homeopathic tinctures, act as an anti-trauma agent and can relieve different kinds of pain, such as headache, sunburn and pain from wounds, as well as reportedly providing dramatic relief from asthma and other respiratory conditions. Tests have also shown that the rye extract drops act to normalize blood profiles and can dilate or constrict blood vessels. Some studies have shown positive results in the instance of cancers responding to rye extract drops of different strength.

The latest laboratory or clinical tests on the use of rye extract drops were carried out by Professor Indies Moodily from the Faculty of Health and Sciences at the University of the Witwatersrand in Johannesburg. There, he tested the use of rye extract drops in relation to five types of cancer. The results showed that liver carcinoma was inhibited by 52.3% to 89.3%. Breast cancer and chronic myelogenous leukemia were inhibited by 89.3% and 78.12% respectively, and liver cancer (He 3B) and renal cancer registered 55% and 52.3% in inhibition factors.

The results differed largely because the drops were tested on different cancers in different strengths. Some cancers responded to a greater degree with the lower strength drops while others gave better results with the stronger strengths. However, in all cases, the results were very positive.

Kay Kohnke, wife of John Kohnke, who was involved in work done on Oralmat in wound healing on animals, underwent surgery for breast cancer. David Rudov takes up the story: "She was badly knocked about, ...in considerable pain, was badly bruised and inflamed across the breast and under the arm. The incision was covered by a see-through occlusive plastic covering ........ and the wound was not looking good." On David's suggestion and her Doctor's approval, the occlusive covering was replaced by nonabsorbent gauze and sprayed with ORALMAT Spray.

Kay also took ORALMAT drops, 3 drops sublingually 3 times a day and the next day was "amazed as to how well she felt. There was no pain, the inflammation had gone, and the bruising and swelling were receding."

Neither gluten nor pollen are present in rye extract. To date, there are no known side effects associated with its use.

### Further Reading & References

- Rye Grass Extract, http://www.grainmills.com.au/webcontent38.htm

- "Sodium 1-monolinolenin isolated from Italian ryegrass (Lolium multiflorum Lam) induces apoptosis in human lymphoid leukemia Molt 4B cells,"http://www.ncbi.nlm.nih.gov/entrez/query.fcgi?cmd=

Retrieve&db=pubmed&dopt=Abstract&list_uids=11179505

- Evaluation of Rye Extract for Anti-neoplastic Activity, http://www.oralmat.co.uk/cancer1.html

# Sassafras Tea

Sassafras itself is a species of deciduous trees in the family Lauraceae which can be found in eastern North America and eastern Asia. Sassafras tea is made from the young root of sassafras, Sassafras albidum. It contains up to 9% of a volatile oil, which consists of about 80% safrole, the active ingredient. Safrole is also a component of many essential oils, such as star anise oil, micranthum oil and camphor oil.

Sassafras was always popular in folk medicine, being regarded by rural people as a spring tonic or purifier of the blood. The root bark was used to treat fevers by the natives of Florida prior to the arrival of Europeans in 1512 and formed one of the earliest exports of the New World. It still enjoys a considerable reputation as a stimulant, and as treatment for rheumatism, skin disease, syphilis, typhus, dropsy (fluid accumulation), and so on.

Pharmacologist Daniel Mowrey, who wrote *The Scientific Validation of Herbal Medicine,* tells the story of sassafras tea. According to his account, safrole, an extract of sassafras, can be toxic to the liver when administered in large doses in its pure form. Like many herbs with toxic compounds, the whole plant contains other substances that neutralize the toxic one. No study had ever shown that the herb sassafras was toxic.

There wasn't even anecdotal evidence that the tea posed a danger. But the FDA prohibited its interstate shipment in 1976 based on this reasoning: When sassafras — a food — is added to water — also a food — the substance safrole migrates from the sassafras into the water and therefore becomes a food additive. Once this convoluted reasoning was used to label sassafras a food additive, the FDA was allowed to control it.

"During the entire proceedings, the power of the scientific method, initially utilized to create the controversy, became impotent in resolving the situation. Unasked questions cannot be answered. The question of whether whole sassafras herb or even sassafras tea was toxic to the liver was never experimentally addressed," Mowrey reported.

There is evidence that safrole, at more modest doses, could stimulate the conversion of other carcinogens to non-carcinogenic metabolites, thus potentially being an anticarcinogen. One study shows that Safrole oxide induces apoptosis in human lung cancer cells. Apoptosis is the programmed cell death that's natural in healthy cells but is not found in cancer cells, which continue to divide and multiply indefinitely. It's highly desirable to induce apoptosis in cancer cells.

### Further Reading & References

- "Safrole oxide induces apoptosis in A549 human lung cancer cells," http://www.ncbi.nlm.nih.gov/entrez/query.fcgi?cmd=Retrieve&db=pubmed&dopt=Abstract&list_uids=15524402

- *Country Folk Medicine: Tales of Skunk Oil, Sassafras Tea & Other Old-Time Remedies* by Elisabeth Janos (20040

- Drug Safety Society: Sassafras, http://drugsafetysite.com/herbs/sassafras/

- *The Scientific Validation of Herbal Medicine*, by Daniel Mowrey

# Saw Palmetto/Beta-Sitosterol

Saw palmetto is an herb that has been shown in clinical studies to have beneficial effects in reducing symptoms of benign prostatic hyperplasia (BPH). BPH does not necessarily lead to prostate cancer.

Several compounds are found within the saw palmetto berry including phytosterols (plant sterols). These plant sterols have a chemical structure similar to cholesterol. The most commonly found phytosterols in saw palmetto are beta-sitosterol, campesterol, stigmasterol and cycloartenol.

The best known use of saw palmetto is for the treatment of prostate enlargement. However, there is a possibility that substances in saw palmetto could have an influence on a variety of body tissues. They may even have anti-tumor potential. In one study, treatment with beta-sitosterol resulted in a dose-dependent growth inhibition on human colon cancer cells.

Saw palmetto is best taken with meals since it is fat-soluble. Most of the time, the recommended dosage is one pill, twice a day. However, a higher dosage of 320 mg taken once a day is also an option. It appears that urinary symptoms due to mild to moderate prostate enlargement respond more readily to saw palmetto than do symptoms caused by severe enlargement.

### Further Reading & References

- *Saw Palmetto Nature's Prostate Healer: Natures Prostate Healer* by Ray Sahelian (1998)

- *Saw Palmetto: The Natural Choice for Prostate Health* by Kate Gilbert Udall (1998)

- *Prostate And Cancer: A Family Guide To Diagnosis, Treatment And Survival* by Sheldon Marks (2003)

- "Induction of Bax and activation of caspases during beta-sitosterol-mediated apoptosis in human colon cancer cells," http://www.ncbi.nlm.nih.gov/entrez/query.fcgi?cmd=Retrieve&db=pubmed&dopt=Abstract&list_uids=14612938

- Herbal Therapy for BPH, http://www.itmonline.org/journal/arts/bph.htm

# Sheep Sorrel

Sheep sorrel is taken from the above-ground parts of the plant of the same name. It is one of the ingredients of Essiac Tea. Rene Caisse, the Canadian nurse who popularized Essiac as a cancer cure, felt this herb was the most active cancer fighter among all the herbs present in the old Indian brew. She said on a number of occasions:

"The herb that will destroy cancer… is the dog-eared sheep sorrel, sometimes called sour grass."

Interestingly, for hundreds of years, sheep sorrel has appeared in historical archives in both North America and Europe as a remedy for cancer.

Rene Caisse observed that not only was sheep sorrel effective in attacking and breaking down tumors, it also was effective in alleviating many chronic conditions and degenerative diseases. See **Essiac Tea**.

Patients with a history of kidney stones should not ingest this herb.

### Further Reading & References

- Sheep Sorrel, http://www.mskcc.org/mskcc/html/69375.cfm

- Essiac Tea Cancer Treatment, http://www.cancertutor.com/Cancer/Essiac.html

- Mother Earth Herbs: Sheep Sorrel, http://www.motherearthherbs.com/sorrel.html

# St John's Wort/Hypericin

St. John's Wort is a shrub-like, perennial plant that bears bright yellow flowers and is native to Europe, western Asia, and northern Africa.

Studies by a number of researchers have shown that some cancers can be treated through the administration of hypericin, one of the active constituents of St John's Wort. Hypericin's effectiveness is believed to be in its ability to induce a natural cell death (apoptosis) in cancer cells, essentially converting immortal cancer cells to mortal cells. Couldwell et al (1994) incubated malignant glioma cancer cells with hypericin for 48 hours. Results demonstrated that hypericin inhibited the growth of established tumors in a dose dependent manner.

Hypericin might also be useful as a transport agent to get cancer-killing nutrients into cancer cells. It is already being tested for use with orthodox Photodynamic Therapy (PDT).

In successful, experiments on mice, hypericin performed effectively against tumor-infested tissue. Mice treated with hypericin were irradiated, at which time it was observed that previous tumor growth had been road-blocked. The result of this study and others is to suggest that hypericin can be used as an effective phototherapy tool in the treatment of cancer.

### Further Reading & References

- "St. John's Wort: More Implications for Cancer Patients," http://jnci.oxfordjournals.org/content/94/16/1187.full

- American Cancer Society: St. John's Wort, http://www.cancer.org/Treatment/TreatmentsandSideEffects/ComplementaryandAlternativeMedicine/HerbsVitaminsandMinerals/st-johns-wort

- Hypericin and Cancer, http://angus.bob11.co.uk/cancer/Hypericin%20Cancer.html

# WLA-132 (Concentrated form of Aloe Vera)

Aloe has a long history of therapeutic uses for burns and reduction of pain, as well as anti-viral and anti-bacterial applications. A highly concentrated form of aloe, WLA- 132, seems to provide a strong boost to the body's immune system. WLA-132 appears to increase T lymphocytes and attack cancer, AIDS, herpes, and other viruses. WLA-132 has the attributes of being natural, nutritional, and non-toxic as well as powerful.

WLA-132 builds up the number of T-4 and T-8 lymphocytes in the body. When these increase to sufficiently balanced numbers, they help the body to strengthen itself. It may be also be taken alongside conventional cancer treatment. WLA-132 is reported to be safe. Dr. Wendell Winters, associate professor of Microbiology at the University of Texas Health Science Center in San Antonio, who has been researching aloe vera for the past 16 years, says, ""In fact, WLA-132 probably should be in everyone's household arsenal to become and stay healthy."

The research studies of H. Reginald McDaniel, chief Pathologist at the Dallas/Fort Worth Medical Center, confirm the ability of Aloe Vera to stimulate and dramatically strengthen the natural immune system. According to McDaniel, "The material in this plant turns on the defensive intracellular mechanisms to fight against not only the viruses but also tumors."

In fact, McDaniel, believing that the potential of Aloe extract is unmatched, says, ""The development of the aloe vera extract may be the most important single step forward in the treatment of diseases in the history of medicine."

In a different context, McDaniel said, "Yet, three weeks after having given these three people WLA 132, their T cells were way up and we had three people who were literally jogging around the clinic."

Four months into a study where AIDS patients were treated with WLA-132, all of the cancers that accompanied AIDS began to disappear. The researchers found that when they stimulated the production of the T4 lymphocytes, they were also stimulating the production of interferon, interleukins, and tumor necrosis factor. In essence, the entire immune system was being activated into a major defensive maneuver. The interferon and interleukins were attacking the viruses, and the tumor necrosis factor, in concert with the naturally occurring emodines and lectins in aloe, were destroying the malignant tumors.

Aloe vera also seems to be effective in eliminating liver cancer. In the treatment of liver cancer, WLA-132 has been extremely successful because the liver is highly vascular and there is no problem with feeding nutrients into it. In a film produced by Dr. McDaniel, time-lapse photography was done on a cancer patient who had seventeen liver tumors.

The patient was considered terminal. After seventeen weeks of aloe vera treatment by Dr. McDaniel, those very large tumors all disappeared. "In fact, WLA-132 is effective in the treatment of most malignancies except pancreatic cancer and brain cancers. Prostate cancer, which is slow growing tissue, responds particularly well to treatment with WLA-132. Even patients who have had the gland removed find the aloe solution valuable for removing any last traces of the cancer cells."

WLA-132 is a specially grown, uniquely processed, highly concentrated aloe product, which is substantially different from anything available. In many of the aloe vera products found on store shelves, the manufacturers take two drops, put them in two quarts of water, and then label the product "100% Aloe Vera." The drops may have been pure aloe but the product is highly diluted and mostly water.

In studying over one hundred research articles published in medical and scientific journals, there was a direct correlation between the concentration of aloe vera used, the dosage, and the degree of success. If aloe vera is bought from the store shelves it takes between fifty to sixty-three gallons to equal one teaspoon of the WLA-132 concentrate. It is absolutely necessary to take at least enough aloe concentrate to deliver 500 mg of monosaccharides and 500 mg of polypeptides in order to stimulate T cells. With any less than that amount nothing happens.

To date, WLA-132 has been taken by thousands of people. The only side effect is diarrhea, which affects less than 5% of the users, and usually subsides within two or three days. The diarrhea reaction can be controlled by cutting the dosage back significantly until the body becomes used to the substance. Then, the amount is brought back up to a full dosage and at that point there are no side effects. Safety studies submitted to the FDA show no toxicity in any of the tissues in the body.

See **Aloe Vera**.

### *Further Reading & References*

- The Most Natural and Powerful Way to Boost Your Immune System, http://www.thewolfeclinic. com/wla132.html

- WLA132, http://sylviascreations.com/WLA132-51058.htm

# Plant-Based Treatments

## AGS/Aglycon sapogenins

Aglycolin sapogenin or AGS is a phytochemical found in ginseng and other plants. While relatively rare and expensive, AGS shows great promise in cancer prevention and treatment. The AGS group of sapogenins found in ginseng is also called R-family sapogenins.

Ginseng is an *adaptogen*—a substance that regulates various body functions depending on individual needs. Eastern medical practitioners have used this Chinese herb to:

- Boost the immune system

- Enhance memory

- Normalize blood pressure…

- Reduce stress…

- Restore memory and cognitive abilities…

- Treat pulmonary problems…

Now Western doctors are noticing the growing body of scientific research that proves a specific chemical in ginseng —**aglycon sapogenin** or **AGS**— may be a potent cancer killer.

In some laboratory tests on melanoma tumors, AGS completely destroyed cancer cells within 24 hours of contact with almost no toxicity and no side effects. AGS appears to be very safe, with a number of studies reporting that no side effects were observed.

### Therapeutic AGS not found in ginseng

Ginseng contains substances called ginsenosides. Ginsenosides are the major active ingredients of ginseng root, and commercial ginseng products typically are standardized to contain about 4 to 7 percent ginsenosides. The amount can vary widely depending on the brand. In addition, there are about 30 different types of ginsenoside.

But in any case the benefits of the AGS breakthrough are not available by taking ginseng, no matter how rich it is in ginsenosides. The new treatment is based on the fact that each ginsenoside contains a sugar (glycon) and a non-sugar (aglycon) component.

The glucose-formed components strengthen the immune system and support the formation of healthy cells in the body. They fuel cell growth. Unfortunately, these compounds provide these benefits to healthy cells and cancer cells alike.

Only the non-sugar components of ginsenosides, one of which is AGS, are effective against cancer.

Dr. William Jia, associate professor of research and neurosurgery at the University of British Columbia said AGS attacks cancer cells in several ways, including:

- **Apoptosis**—or self-destruction in cancer cells; Jia said AGS can activate an enzyme that causes apoptosis. It also can increase the levels of free radicals in cancer cells to cause this internal combustion.

- **Increasing absorption of cancer drugs**—AGS can work with other anti-cancer agents to prevent drug resistance in cancer cells.

- **Changing cancer cells to benign cells**—In one Japanese study, AGS not only stopped liver cancer cells from growing, it actually changed them back into normal cells.

Dr. Jia said the AGS attack plan is more effective than standard cancer treatments because cancer cells tend to mutate while they multiply. This means the same tumor can have several different types of cancer cells.

Conventional treatments might be effective for one type of tumor cell—and completely useless for other cancer cells in the same tumor. The idea of "drug resistant" cancer cells is becoming more and more important in cancer research. In this respect AGS appears to be superior to mainstream medical treatments because it can attack <u>all types of cancer cells</u>.

It's significant that Jia was writing about a group of plant compounds known as "dammarane sapogenins," an AGS group obtained from other plants besides ginseng. The dammarane sapogenins are similar to but not identical to AGS sourced from ginseng, but they're less rare and should be less expensive.

AGS can also be useful in cancer prevention. According to sources cited by Dr. Jia, AGS taken in low doses stops cancer cell division, helps remove toxins, and can inhibit the breast cancer-promoting action of excess estrogens.

AGS is a cancer-fighting compound that must be *extracted* from ginseng. It's not available from whole ginseng. The ginsenosides in the herb have to be broken down into their component parts, the AGS or R-family sapogenins have to be extracted, and this active ingredient has to be taken by the patient in large amounts. For best results it appears this natural "drug" should be administered intravenously.

According to one estimate, it takes about 100 pounds of ginseng to make just one gram of AGS. This very likely renders ginseng-sourced AGS unaffordable. The dammarane sapogenins extolled by Dr. Jia offer hope of an alternative source.

One company producing an AGS product is Pegasus Pharmaceuticals Group, Inc. of Canada. Pegasus produces AGS in both liquid and soft gel formulas. Called Careseng, the product contains a combination of ginseng-derived AGS and dammarene sapogenins.

Another AGS product, called Force C, is available at www.HealthSecretsUSA.com without a prescription.

### *References and Further Reading*

- Chen, J. et al. Research on the antitumor effect of ginsenoside Rg3 in B16 melanoma cells. Melanoma Res. 2008 Oct;18(5):322-9. Retrieved from www.ncbi.nlm.nih.gov/pubmed/18781130

- Jia, W. "What is sapogenin?" Dammarane Sapogenin website. Retrieved from www.sapogenin. info

- Odashima, S. et al. "Induction of phenotypic reverse transformation by plant glycosides in cultured cancer cells," Gan To Kagaku Ryoho, 1989 Apr; 16 (4 Pt 2-2):1483-9. Retrieved from www.ncbi.nlm.nih.gov/pubmed/2658830

# Alsihum/Alzium

The plant Alsihum contains extracts that show promising cytotoxic effects on cancer cell lines. Eight of these extracts were studied at the Cancer Pharmacology Laboratory of Children's Mercy Hospital in Kansas City, MO.

The cancer cell lines tested included leukemia, colon, glioma, breast, ovarian, adrenal and lung cancer. The principal researchers were Dr. Albert Levya, PhD., Director of the Cancer Pharmacology Lab; and Dr. Arnold I. Freeman, M.D., the Chief of Hematology and Oncology.

Results of the study indicated a strong likelihood that Alzium had significant cytotoxic effects on specific types of tumor cells. In addition, cell lines that were commonly 100 times more resistant to conventional chemotherapy drugs seemed to be considerably sensitive to Alzium.

### Further Reading & References

- Alternative Cancer Treatments, http://www.cancertutor.com/Other/Big_List.htm

- *Prescription for Herbal Healing*, by Phyllis A. Balch (2002)

# Anvirzel™/Oleander Soup

Nerium oleander is a type of shrub, ornamental in nature, native to the Mediterranean, Southeast Asia, and northern Africa. It's now commonly grown in the tropical and subtropical American South for its beautiful flowers. It has been used for centuries as a traditional treatment for ulcers, hemorrhoids, and leprosy, and more recently, AIDS.

Anvirzel™ itself comes from nerium oleander in the form of a patented extract. Anvirzel was initially thought to work only on cancers found early. More recently, positive results were seen in people given the treatment after having been pronounced to have only a few weeks to live.

Anvirzel appears to be the first cancer remedy to show positive results for leiomyosarcoma, which is one of the deadliest of cancers. It works by crossing the blood-brain barrier (like Poly-MVA) and offers hope to those with brain tumors.

While the oleander plant is very poisonous and very toxic (and must be handled with protective gloves), if a solution of oleander is diluted enough it can reportedly be made safe to drink or made into a cream. Some advocates claim a person can make an effective oleander cancer treatment at home.

At present, Anvirzel is not an approved drug in the United States. Furthermore, the oleander plant in raw, uncooked form is toxic and poisonous to humans. When ingested, as little as one leaf of raw oleander may cause death.

What makes oleander effective at clobbering cancer cells? In 1988, a research team at Munich University Pharmacology Institute set out to answer this question.

The researchers isolated the active components in the oleander extract. They found several polysaccharides—also called cardiac glycosides—that impact immune activity.

The team presented their initial findings at a July 1990 symposium of Biology and Chemistry of Active Natural Substances (BACANS), held in Bonn, Germany. Also, the presentation was published in *Planta Medica* 1990-56:66.

The researchers said no single component of the oleander extract provided all its benefits. Rather, the cancer-fighting properties are activated by a blend of extract components that help regulate the immune system.

More recent studies support this conclusion. A study conducted by researchers at Japan's Niigata University evaluated the effect of 13 oleander compounds against fibroblast, liver and ovarian cancer cells. They concluded:

- Seven oleander compounds showed anti-cancer activity against the fibroblast tumors

- Four compounds selectively slowed the growth of fibroblast tumors

- Three compounds were active against liver tumor cells

- Three compounds showed significant effects on calcein accumulation in MDR human ovarian cancer cells

In fact, one of the oleander compounds proved stronger than the calcium channel blocker Verapamil that doctors use to help kill cancer cells!

In the second study, one of oleander's pregnane compounds was significantly toxic against fibroblasts and liver cancer cells. What's more, researchers found three of the pregnanes were toxic to ovarian cancer cells.

A book called *Cancer's Natural Enemy*, by Tony M. Isaacs, purportedly describes how to make an oleander-based medicine "at home on your stovetop." Given the toxicity of the plant, readers should proceed with extreme caution – if at all.

### *Further Reading & References*

- Anvirzel Update, http://www.mnwelldir.org/docs/Newsletters/03_May.htm#Anvirzel

- Oleandrin, http://www.mskcc.org/mskcc/html/69314.cfm

- Zhao, M., Bai, L. et. al. 2007. Bioactive cardenolides from the stems and twigs of Nerium oleander. J Nat Prod. 2007 Jul;70(7):1098-103. Epub 2007 Jun 27. Retrieved January 10, 2011 from http://www.ncbi.nlm.nih.gov/pubmed/17595134

- Bai, L, Wang, L. et. al. 2007. Bioactive pregnanes from Nerium oleander. J Nat Prod. 2007 Jan;70(1):14-8. Retrieved January 10, 2011 from http://www.ncbi.nlm.nih.gov/pubmed/17253842

# Arjuna

Terminalia Arjuna is a deciduous tree (about 60-70 feet height), found in abundance in India and Ceylon, also in Myanmar and Sri Lanka. The thick, white-to-pinkish-gray bark has long been used in India's native Ayurvedic medicine.

The main constituents in the bark, stem and leaves are tannins, triterpenoid saponins (arjunic acid, arjunolic acid, arjungenin, arjunglycosides), flavonoids (arjunone, arjunolone, luteolin), gallic acid, ellagic acid, oligomeric proanthocyanidins (OPCs), phytosterols, calcium, magnesium, zinc, and copper.

Several of these constituents have been identified to have anti-cancer properties. In one study, the cancer cell line active components were found to be gallic acid, ethyl gallate, and the flavone luteolin. Luteolin has a well established record of inhibiting various cancer cell lines and may account for most of the rationale underlying the use of T. arjuna in traditional cancer treatments.

In another study, a novel naphthanol glycoside was isolated from the stem bark of Terminalia arjuna that showed potent antioxidant activity and inhibited nitric oxide (NO) production in "lipopolysaccharide (LPS)-stimulated rat peritoneal macrophages." These macrophages, normally beneficial, are abundant in tumors and their inhibition could be beneficial to the patient.

### *Further Reading & References*

- Pettit GR, Hoard MS, Doubek DL, Schmidt JM, Pettit RK, Tackett LP, Chapuis JC. Cancer Research Institute, Arizona State University, Tempe 85287-1604, USA.

- Ali A, Kaur G, Hayat K, Ali M, Ather M. Faculty of Pharmacy, Hamdard University, Hamdard Nagar, New Delhi, India., Pharmazie. 2003 Dec;58(12):932-4.

- "Antineoplastic agents 338. The cancer cell growth inhibitory. Constituents of Terminalia arjuna (Combretaceae)." http://www.ncbi.nlm.nih.gov/entrez/query.fcgi?cmd=Retrieve&db=pubmed&dopt=Abstract&list_uids=8844460

- Gupta R, et al. Antioxidant and hypocholesterolemic effects of Terminalia arjuna tree-bark powder: a randomized placebo-controlled trial. J Assoc Physicians India 2001 Feb;49:231-5.

- Ayurveda For You: Arjuna, http://ayurveda-foryou.com/ayurveda_herb/arjuna.html

# Artemisinin/Artemisia/Sweet Wormwood/Qinghaosu/Qinhau

Artemisinin, which is originally from Chinese folk medicine, is a type of chemical compound that comes from the common garden plant artemesia, or wormwood. It has been shown in studies to induce apoptosis (natural cell death) in human cancer cells. During an in vitro study, it successfully killed select cancer cells and slowed the growth of tumors in rats.

In fact, Seattle scientists have shown that a compound extracted from the wormwood plant actually seeks out and destroys invaders such as breast cancer cells while leaving healthy cells unscathed. The substance is used extensively in European alternative cancer clinics.

Artemisinin is considered a safe, non-toxic, and inexpensive alternative for cancer patients. Chinese researchers said the key to its effect was a peroxide linkage (two oxygen atoms hooked together) within the herb's active molecule, which makes this treatment very similar to oxygen therapy. Cancer cells thrive in an oxygen-free (anaerobic) environment and high levels of oxygen are therefore fatal to them.

In laboratory experiments, the compound killed virtually all human breast cancer cells that had been exposed to the compound over a span of 16 hours. These studies were conducted by Dr. Henry Lai and his bioengineering research team at the University of Washington. Dr. Lai also stated that nearly all of the normal cells exposed to the compound remained alive.

In a separate experiment, a dog with severe bone cancer known as osteosarcoma couldn't walk across the room. The animal made a complete recovery within five days of receiving the treatment. X-rays showed the animal's tumor "had basically disappeared," says Lai. He added that the dog survived for at least two more years.

Artemisinin reemerged as a therapy for malaria, for which it was once common, after a "secret recipe" for the treatment was discovered on a stone tablet in the tomb of a prince of the Han Dynasty during an archaeological dig in the 1970s. In fact, a purified form of the plant compound is now the drug of choice for treating malaria.

Experiments into why artemisinin works as an anti-malaria agent led to its being tested as an anticancer drug. The key turned out to be a shared characteristic of the malaria parasite and dividing cancer cells: high iron concentrations.

When artemisinin, or any of its derivatives, meets iron, a chemical reaction ensues. This prompts the creation of free radicals. In malaria, the free radicals attack and bind with cell membranes, breaking them apart and killing the single-cell parasite.

Lai points out that cells need iron to replicate DNA when they divide. Because cancer is characterized by out-of-control cell division, cancer cells have much higher iron concentrations than do normal cells.

"Not only does [the drug] appear to be effective, but it's very selective," Lai says. "It's highly toxic to the cancer cells, but has a marginal impact on normal cells."

On the surface, cancer cells have more so-called transferrin receptors than healthy cells have. Transferrin receptors are cellular pathways that allow iron to enter. In the case of breast cancer, the cells have five to 15 times more transferrin receptors on their surface than normal breast cells, Lai says.

The main strategy, according to Lai, is to pump up cancer cells with even more iron and then introduce artemisinin to kill them selectively. In his experiments, Lai subjected sets of both breast cancer cells and normal breast cells to two substances. The first was a compound known as holotransferrin, which binds with transferrin receptors to transport iron into cells and thus further increases the cells' iron concentrations. The second was a water-soluble form of artemisinin. He also studied a combination of both compounds.

Cells exposed to just one of the compounds showed no noticeable effect, Lai reported. But the response by cancer cells when hit with first holotransferrin and then artemisinin was dramatic, he says.

After eight hours, three-fourths of the cancer cells were obliterated. After16 hours, nearly all the cancer cells were dead. Just as importantly, he says, the vast majority of normal breast cells did not die, showing the safety of the treatment.

The normal breast cancer cells were also resistant to radiation utilized in the experiment, Lai adds. "So that means this approach might work for cancer resistant to conventional therapy." One might expect even more aggressive cancers such as pancreatic and acute leukemia, known for rapid cell division and so much higher iron concentrations, to respond even better.

Further animal testing followed by human trials is expected. In human trials, patients would likely be given iron supplements to raise the iron concentrations in their cancer cells.

Even though human tests are years away, the treatment could revolutionize the way cancer, especially the aggressive, fast-growing kind, is approached.

One study found elevated iron storage in 88% of breast cancer patients, so the application is logical. There's also a wealth of research linking iron and cancer.

Artemisinin is best taken on an empty stomach with some natural fat to enhance absorption. If iron is present from residual food, it may neutralize the peroxides. Milk has a minimal amount of iron, as do cottage cheese and yogurt — and all three have enough fat to enhance absorption. Artemisinin is also administered intravenously in some clinics.

### Further Reading & References

- Chinese remedy 'may fight cancer,' http://news.bbc.co.uk/1/hi/health/1678469.stm

- "Artemisinin induces apoptosis in human cancer cells." http://www.ncbi.nlm.nih.gov/entrez/query.fcgi?cmd=Retrieve&db=pubmed&dopt=Abstract&list_uids=15330172

- Cancer Therapies Page: Artemisia or Sweet Wormword Anti-Cancer Herbs, http://www.huldaclarkzappers.com/php2/sweetwormwoodtherapy.php

## Aveloz

Aveloz is also known as the pencil cactus or pencil tree. It is a shrub native to South America and has previously been called "kill-wart" because of its ability to destroy wart growth. This ability to destroy growth drew attention from several doctors.

Five to ten drops of an Aveloz solution, taken once an hour (depending on size and density of the malignancy), has been known to eliminate cancerous growths in one week. The hard tumor appears to collapse after treatment.

What appears to happen is that the cancer suffers from the escharotic (tissue tearing) properties of the solution. The only reported side effect to taking Aveloz is possible irritation of the kidneys. The treatment's advocates say a patient can alleviate that side effect by taking extra Vitamin C.

### Further Reading & References

- Tropical Plant Database: Aveloz, http://www.rain-tree.com/aveloz.htm

- Aveloz, http://www.cancer.org/Treatment/TreatmentsandSideEffects/ComplementaryandAlternativeMedicine/HerbsVitaminsandMinerals/aveloz

## Avocados

Avocado is rich in the potent antioxidant lutein. This is thought to safeguard the cardiovascular system from atherosclerosis as well as prevent prostate cancer.

Avocados also contain high amounts of carotenoids and significant levels of Vitamin E. An extract of avocado with carotenoids and tocopherols appears to inhibit the growth of prostate cancer cells, as opposed to using just lutein alone.

In the case of oral (mouth) cancer, the phytochemicals within the avocado appear to halt the growth of cancerous cells without harming normal cells.

### Further Reading & References

- "30 Power foods: these foods can help you slow aging, prevent disease, and boost immunity." http://www.findarticles.com/p/articles/mi_m0NAH/is_2_33/ai_97177920

- "Avocado cures prostate cancer, oral cancer, and helps diabetes," http://hubpages.com/hub/avocadocuresprostateoralcancer

- Avocados, http://www.whfoods.com/genpage.php?tname=foodspice&dbid=5

# Azelaic Acid

Azelaic Acid is a dicarboxylic acid occurring in whole grains such as wheat, rye, and barley, and animal products; it has a cytotoxic effect on malignant or hyperactive melanocytes, that is, it kills melanoma cells in the test tube, apparently affecting the energy centers (mitochondria) of the melanoma cells. It is applied topically in the treatment of acne vulgaris.

B.J. Ward *et al.* found that carnitine increased the transport of azelaic acid into the mitochondria thereby increasing the drug's tumor cell killing effect.

It's worth considering whether using azelaic acid and carnitine together with Dr. Robert Jones' protocol may be very effective for melanoma – to deal a powerful blow to the mitochondria within the melanoma cells.

### Further Reading & References

- Journal of Investigative Dermatology, http://www.jidonline.org/cgi/content/abstract/86/4/438

# Beet Juice

The crimson colored pigment in beets known as betacyanin is believed to be the compound in the vegetable that possesses anticancer properties. In studies, beet juice commonly ranks close to the top in preventing cell mutations that commonly lead to cancer.

Beets are high in folate, which is frequently used by pregnant women to prevent birth defects.

Beet juice should not be drunk alone but rather mixed with other vegetable juices or blended with apple juice. Pure beet juice is very potent and can temporarily paralyze your vocal chords, make you break out in hives, increase your heart rate, and cause chills or a fever.

### Further Reading & References

- Beet Juice (Kills cancer cells), http://www.cancertutor.com/Other/Big_List.htm

# Beetroot/Betacyanin/Betaine

Beetroot juice as a cancer therapy was pioneered by Hungarian doctor Alexander Ferenczi, MD. He explored the long-known therapeutic properties of the juice and found that the natural red coloring agent, betacyanin, was a potent cancer fighter.

Beets also contain betaine, an unusual substance that is found in few foods. This phytochemical is important for detoxifying homocysteine and reducing heart disease risk, and is involved in the metabolic pathways involved in fighting cancer.

"The Hungarian Professor Bakay of the University of Budapest carried out experiments in 1939 (long before Dr. Ferenczi) on 72 patients suffering from cancer or leukemia in his clinic in the Hungarian capital. He observed regression of the tumors, increases in weight and improvement in the general condition of his patients."

Dr. Ferenczi's clinical report included administration methods and case studies:

"I diagnosed a man of 50 years of age, with a lung tumor. And subsequently confirmed in a Budapest hospital and also in a country hospital, which corresponded clinically to lung cancer. I started treatment with beetroot in the described manner. After 6 weeks of treatment the tumor had disappeared ... after 4 months of treatment he gained 10 kg. In weight, the erythrocyte [mature red blood cell] sediment rate [E.S.R] was reduced drastically. Thus he represented the symptoms of a clinical recovery."

### Further Reading & References

- Beetroot (juice) as cancer therapy, http://www.karlloren.com/biopsy/book/p14.htm

- Raw Food Treatment for Cancer: Brandt Grape Cure Using Vegetable Juices, http://www.cancertutor.com/Cancer/RawFood.html

# Beta Sitosterol/Saw Palmetto

Beta-sitosterol is a plant sterol that has been shown through research to induce cell death in breast cancer cells. As far as phytosterols go, beta-sitosterol is commonly found in the human diet and throughout the plant kingdom. It is present in saw palmetto, pumpkin seeds, and the herb Pygeum africanum.

It has also been found to reduce the growth of human prostate and colon cancer cells. It also acts against lymphocytic leukemia. It is a common constituent of formulas marketed to reduce the symptoms of prostate enlargement and promote general prostate health.

### Further Reading & References

- Beta-sitosterol, http://www.greatvistachemicals.com/nutritional-supplements/beta-sitosterol.html

- "Beta-sitosterol, a plant sterol, induces apoptosis and activates key caspases in MDA-MB-231 human breast cancer cells." http://www.ncbi.nlm.nih.gov/entrez/query.fcgi?cmd=Retrieve&db=pubmed&dopt=Abstract&list_uids=12579296

# Boswellic Acids

Boswellic acids can be found in the resin of the plant that secretes them. They are molecules that come from plants in the genus *Boswellia*. They've been indicated as effective in prompting apoptosis, the death of cancer cells. In particular, they are effective as treatment for brain tumors, leukemia, and cells affected by colon cancer.

Boswellic acids have been used to treat inflammatory diseases for years in the Far East. Now that they have been identified as having apoptotic qualities, they show significant promise as natural "drugs" for the future.

### *Further Reading & References*

- "Keto- and acetyl-keto-boswellic acids inhibit proliferation and induce apoptosis in Hep G2 cells via a caspase-8 dependent pathway." http://www.ncbi.nlm.nih.gov/entrez/query.fcgi?cmd=Retrieve&db=PubMed&list_uids=12239601&dopt=Abstract

- "[Boswellic acids (components of frankincense) as the active principle in treatment of chronic inflammatory diseases]," http://www.ncbi.nlm.nih.gov/pubmed/12244881

- Boswellia, http://www.mskcc.org/mskcc/html/69149.cfm

# C-Statin/Bindweed

C-Statin comes from a group of proteoglycan molecules (PGM) isolated from Bindweed (Convolvulus arvensis) a common garden weed. C-Statin is an anti-angiogenesis substance. Essentially, it stops the growth of new blood vessels so cancer cannot feed and grow.

No toxicity has been detected when C-Statin is taken at physician-recommended doses.

### *Further Reading & References*

- Alternative Medicine: Supplement called C-Statin, http://en.allexperts.com/q/Alternative-Medicine-991/Supplement-called-C-Statin.htm

- Improving Health of Cancer Patients - July 16, 2010 by Richard Loyd, Ph.D., http://www.royalrife.com/cancer.html

# Canthaxanthin

Canthaxanthin, a less well-known carotenoid, has been shown to inhibit growth and to induce apoptosis (cell death) in human cancer cell lines. Because of its reported efficacy as an anti-tumor agent both in vivo and in vitro, scientists ran experiments to see whether it still remained effective with dietary administration. It was found to be satisfactory as a preventive and therapeutic agent.

### *Further Reading & References*

- "Canthaxanthin induces apoptosis in human cancer cell lines," http://carcin.oxfordjournals.org/content/19/2/373.full.pdf

- Carcinogenesis. 1998 Feb;19(2):373-6.Palozza P, Maggiano N, Calviello G, Lanza P, Piccioni E,

- Ranelletti FO, Bartoli GM.Institute of General Pathology, Catholic University, Rome, Italy.

- "Mitogenic and Apoptotic Signaling by Carotenoids: Involvement of a Redox Mechanism,"

- http://onlinelibrary.wiley.com/doi/10.1080/15216540252774810/pdf

# CARESENG® Cancer Therapy/Ginseng

CARESENG® is a product produced from ginseng that contains greater than 99% anti-cancer ginsenosides. The two main compounds are Rh2 and aglycon sapogenins that have been shown in initial clinical trials to have strong cancer-inhibitory effects. Laboratory data and preliminary clinical observation strongly indicate that in combination with conventional chemotherapy, the ginsenosides dramatically sensitize cancer cells to conventional treatments.

The compounds found within CARESENG® are useful for multi-drug resistant cancer cells, which are common in late stage cancer patients. Scientific data strongly support that Careseng is a non-toxic natural supplement for cancer patients, especially for those with late stage and drug resistant cancer of various types.

Laboratory studies on cultured cancer-cells resulted in rapid cancer-cell death. Clinical observation I with 40 patients with various types of cancer including lung, colon, liver, and breast after 60 days resulted in 75% tumor inhibition and no toxicity. Clinical Observation II in 15 patients with breast, colon, brain, liver and ovarian cancer showed 80% inhibition with no adverse side-effects.

CARESENG® is produced by Pegasus Pharmaceuticals by patented technology. (Note: this is not an endorsement.) It contains >99% anti-cancer ginsenosides, an amount equivalent to greater than 100 lbs of ginseng.

See: **AGS**

*Further Reading & References*

- PPG Inc. http://www.pegasuspharm.com/

# Carnivora®

Carnivora® was discovered and developed by Helmut G. Keller, MD, oncological investigator at Klinik Winnerhof in Bad Wiessee, Germany. It enhances the immune system response. Carnivora® is comprised of the pressed juices of Dionaea Muscipula, a concentrated extract of the Venus-flytrap plant. It is supplied as drops for oral ingestion and inhalation, and as Carnivorain injections for intravenous and subcutaneous administration.

Carnivora® capsules are now available in the U.S. as a food supplement. Carnivora externally applied has helped with skin cancers and when taken in capsules. It may stop or reduce tumor growth. The active component of carnivora is plumbagin, a powerful immunological booster.

Dr. Helmut Keller stated: "Carnivora®, a patented phytonutrient and extract of the Venus flytrap plant, Dionaea muscipula, has been used clinically for over 25 years."

Biologically active compounds in the extract are essential to healthy immune systems and to support healthy cardiovascular functions in the body. At higher doses, the extract has been shown to have immodulatory, tumoricidal, antimicrobial, antiviral, antiparasitic and antibiotic properties.

The pharmacology of Venus flytrap extract has been extensively studied and evaluated in both animal and human studies.

Professor D.K. Todorov, MD, PhD, DSc, and Chief of Oncopharmacology at the National Oncological Center of Bulgaria performed clinical studies on Carnivora for over two decades. He has conducted cancer research at Heidelberg University in Heidelberg, Germany. His findings involving various cell lines show that cancer cells were destroyed within a matter of hours when exposed to Carnivora.

Dr. Todorov's initial studies of sarcoma show the dramatic reduction of human sarcoma cells from 2500 to 880 over a 72-hour period. Additionally, Todorov found that 400 nanograms per milliliter (ng/ml) of Carnivora® had caused a diminution of 2200 multidrug resistant sarcoma cells to 1130 cells in just 72 hours.

As a result of these in vitro findings, some doctors began to employ the protocol in vivo, treating patients with sarcoma tumors. Despite previous treatment with toxic therapies, some patients achieved remission.

Professor Todorov performed a study on brain cancer by administering 200 ng/ml of Carnivora to human glioblastoma cells and achieved the destruction of 50% of these cells during a seven-day period.

To study the effects of Carnivora against leukemia, Todorov used 200 ng/ml of Carnivora® to destroy human T-lymphoblastic leukemia cells. Thirty-one hundred of these cells were reduced to 1820 in 72 hours. He then took multi-drug resistant human leukemia cells and exposed them to 200 ng/ml of Carnivora to achieve remarkable results; within 72 hours, 2250 leukemic white blood cells were demolished to just 570 cells.

Doctors have treated patients who suffer from chronic myeloid leukemia, as well as chronic lymphocytic leukemia with long-term Carnivora® therapy with great success. The key in this instance seems to be prolonged treatment. A majority of CML and CLL patients reported positive findings.

And in the case of ovarian cancer, studies showed fifteen hundred ovarian cancer cells were dramatically reduced to 435 cells in a rat model in vivo when treated with 200 ng/ml of Carnivora® within forty-eight hours. Seventeen hundred eleven cells of human ovarian cancer were again dramatically reduced to a mere 359 cells upon exposure to 200 ng/ml of Carnivora® in just 48 hours. It was shown that despite this cancer's chemotherapeutic resistance, Carnivora® had nearly destroyed this entire cell line.

Carnivora® should not be used in conjunction with chemotherapy.

### Further Reading & References

- *German Cancer Therapies: Natural and Conventional Medicines That Offer Hope and Healing* by Morton Walker (2003)

- http://www.carnivora.com/

- Townsend Letter for Doctors and Patients, Nov, 2001 "Carnivora: Pharmacology and Clinical Efficacy of a Most Diverse Natural Plant Extract" http://the-medical-dictionary.com/chenodeoxycholic_acid_article_4.htm

- "Carnivora fights Lyme," http://www.mail-archive.com/silver-list@eskimo.com/msg25524.html

# Cherries

Cherries contain high levels of melatonin, which is used by the body to regulate sleep. It may also have cancer fighting properties. The body produces melatonin to facilitate a deep night's sleep. It's also an immune system regulator.

A 2003 research study revealed that higher melatonin levels in women slowed the progression of breast cancer by 70 percent (*Journal of the National Cancer Institute*). In general, patients with cancer have lower than average levels of melatonin. It's a reasonable hypothesis that foods rich in melatonin have an anticancer effect.

Cherries are also known to treat pain, due to the fact that 25 milligrams of anthocyanins, an antioxidant, can be found in only twenty cherries. This substance helps shut down the enzymes that cause tissue inflammation. In short, cherries are anti-inflammatory.

Anthocyanins were also found to inhibit intestinal tumor growth.* In laboratory experiments conducted on mice, those who consumed a cherry diet had fewer adenomas than those consuming a different diet. Based on these results, it is believed cherries could significantly reduce the risk of colon cancer.

Cherries are also rich in quercetin, a potent flavonoid that's also found in apples, potatoes and garlic. Quercetin has anti-inflammatory and antioxidant properties that can kill cancer cells while leaving healthy cells unharmed.

A study published in the *British Journal of Cancer* found that quercetin rapidly killed off abnormal cells, specifically in prostate and skin cancers. There's evidence this flavonoid also helps prevent cataracts, bronchitis, allergies and heart disease.

The dark color of cherries is an excellent source of other antioxidants as well. In fact, the antioxidant activity of tart black cherries is greater than that of vitamin E, the benchmark antioxidant. Dark-colored Balaton cherries are particularly rich in nutrients, with a total of 37.5 mg of anthocyanins in every 100 grams of fruit.

"Cherries can prevent and treat many kinds of pain," said Muraleedharan Nair, the lead researcher of a Michigan State University project exploring the health benefits of cherries.

Michigan produces 80% of America's tart cherries. Depending on the variety, two teaspoons to two tablespoons per day of concentrated cherry juice is a reasonable dose. No adverse side effects are known.

### *Further Reading & References*

- The Moss Reports:" A Bowl of Cherries," http://www.cancerdecisions.com/120301.html

- *"Tart cherry anthocyanins inhibit tumor development in Apc(Min) mice and reduce proliferation of human colon cancer cells." http://www.ncbi.nlm.nih.gov/pubmed/12706854?dopt=Abstract

- Wong, Cathy. "What are Tart Cherries?," June 2006. http://altmedicine.about.com/od/completeazindex/a/tart_cherry.htm.

- "Cherries for Cancer?" May 2006. http://curezone.com/blogs/fm.asp?i=982194.

- "Cherries Prevention for Cancer." http://fasting.ws/cancer/cherries-prevention-cancer.

- "Increasing Melatonin Levels To Heal From Cancer." http://www.alternative-cancer-care.com/Melatonin_Cancer.html.

- "Cancer Prevention: Anthocyanin," Cancer Quest. http://www.cancerquest.org/cancer-prevention-anthocyanin.

- Lee YK, Lee WS, Kim GS, Park OJ., Anthocyanins are novel AMPKα1 stimulators that suppress tumor growth by inhibiting mTOR phosphorylation. Dec. 2010. http://www.ncbi.nlm.nih.gov/pubmed/21042741.

- McCune LM, Kubota C, Stendell-Hollis NR, Thomson CA., Cherries and health: a review. Jan 2011. http://www.ncbi.nlm.nih.gov/pubmed/21229414.

# Cranberry Juice

In a study funded by Ocean Spray Cranberries, researchers at the University of Western Ontario uncovered potential cancer-fighting properties. They found that consistent consumption of cranberry products may inhibit the development of breast cancer tumors in animals.

Cranberries offer a rich source of flavonoids, as well as a variety of other compounds that have been investigated for their anti-cancer activity.

Cranberry juice is also a popular holistic way to combat urinary tract infections. It is believed cranberry juice may also help in the prevention of bladder cancer.

### Further Reading & References

- Urinary Tract Infections, http://www.healthatoz.com/healthatoz/Atoz/dc/caz/kidn/utri/alert05202000.jsp

- Potential Additional Health Benefits of Cranberries, http://www.medscape.com/viewarticle/411791

# Croton Treatment

The croton is a tropical plant widely popular for landscaping lawns and gardens. This shrub can give you a rash like poison ivy; but it may also stop prostate cancer. Croton oil, derived from the seeds, shows promise for the treatment of this dreaded disease. The oil has long been used as a purgative in traditional Chinese medicine, but is said to be very harsh.

An active ingredient found in the oil of the Southeast Asian croton plant--12-Otetradecanoylphorbol- 13-

acetate, commonly known as TPA - may inhibit the growth of new prostate cancer cells, according to researchers at Rutgers University.

"We demonstrated TPA could simultaneously stop the growth of new prostate cancer cells, kill existing cancer cells, and ultimately shrink prostate tumors," said Allan Conney, Ph.D., one of the study's authors. The researchers also tested the effect of TPA in combination with all-trans retinoic acid (ATRA), a vitamin A derivative that has been shown to treat leukemia effectively.

"We knew that ATRA is an effective synergist with TPA in treating leukemia cells in the laboratory, but prostate cancer is a different situation, probably involving different molecular mechanisms," Conney said.

The studies by Zheng and Conney are the first to show a synergy between TPA and ATRA in inhibiting the growth of cultured prostate cancer cells and the first to assess their combined effects, and the effects of TPA alone, on human tumors grown in mice. Scientists, intrigued by the skin-irritating property of croton seed oil, demonstrated more than 50 years ago that croton oil and its constituent TPA promoted tumors in laboratory animals following the introduction of a strong carcinogen at a low dose. Subsequent laboratory tests, however, produced dramatically different outcomes.

"It turned out that extremely low concentrations of TPA had an extraordinarily potent effect on myeloid leukemia cells, causing them to revert to normal cell behavior," Conney explained. However, it was a long time before anyone acknowledged that TPA could actually do good things for people, Conney observed. Investigators at China's Henan Tumor Research Institute and Rutgers, interested in the potential beneficial effects of TPA, began a collaborative study in 1995. When TPA was administered to terminally ill myeloid leukemia patients in China, the number of leukemia cells in the blood and bone marrow decreased and there were remissions of the disease.

According to Conney, "We are clearly encouraged by our laboratory results with TPA and ATRA on prostate cancer cells. Our studies are an important early step in a long process, and we are planning additional testing in humans. Further research with these compounds and others could provide hope for the half million new cases of prostate cancer each year."

### Further Reading & References

- "Can a plant that acts like poison ivy cure prostate cancer?" http://www.innovations-report.de/html/berichte/medizin_gesundheit/bericht-27076.html

- "Mutagenic and antioxidant activities of Croton lechleri sap in biological systems." http://www.ncbi.nlm.nih.gov/entrez/query.fcgi?cmd=Retrieve&db=pubmed&dopt=Abstract&list_uids=15507372

# D-limonene/Limonene

D-limonene or limonene is a colorless compound found in plants. It is classified as a monoterpene (a type of organic compound) and smells like oranges. It is a solvent often used in cleaning agents. One of the best sources of d-limonene is the oil found in orange peels, which can be accessed by juicing an orange with its peel (preferably from oranges grown organically).

Scientists at the University of Wisconsin contend that adding d-limonene to the diets of rats with tumors caused 90% of the tumors to disappear entirely.

Monoterpenes have the characteristics of an ideal chemopreventive agent. This includes efficacious anti-tumor activity, commercial availability, low cost, oral bioavailability, and low toxicity, all of which make it feasible to begin considering them for human cancer chemoprevention testing.

D-limonene, which comprises more than 90% of orange peel oil, has chemopreventive activity against rodent mammary, skin, liver, lung, and fore-stomach cancers. D-limonene also has chemotherapeutic activity against rodent pancreatic tumors.

In addition, monoterpenes stimulate apoptosis, a cellular self-destruction mechanism triggered when a cell's DNA is badly damaged. This safety feature is generally activated before a cell becomes cancerous. Finally, monoterpenes inhibit protein isoprenylation. The cell uses this process to help a particular protein involved in cell growth find its proper location within the cell. If the protein is not in the right place, it becomes overactive and can spur cancerous cell growth. Thus, monoterpenes would appear to act through multiple mechanisms in the chemoprevention and chemotherapy of cancer.

Several dietary monoterpenes also display anti-tumor activity, meaning they can prevent the formation or progression of cancer and possibly even halt existing malignant tumors.

### Further Reading & References

- Alternative Cancer Therapies continued, http://www.cancure.org/choice_of_therapies_continued.htm

- *Cancer: The Complete Recovery Guide,* by Jonathan Chamberlain (2008)

- Limonene Acts as Chemo, http://www.howcurecancer.com/limonene.htm

- Elson CE, Yu SG. The chemoprevention of cancer by mevalonate-derived constituents of fruits and vegetables. J Nutr 1994;124:607-14.

- Gould MN. Cancer chemoprevention and therapy by monoterpenes. Environ Health Perspect 1997;105:S977-9.

- Mills JJ, et al. Induction of apoptosis in liver tumors by the monoterpene perillyl alcohol. Cancer Res 1995; 55:979-83.

- Hohl RJ. Monoterpenes as regulators of malignant cell proliferation. In: American Institute for Cancer Research. Dietary Phytochemicals in Cancer Prevention and Treatment. New York: Plenum Press;1996.

## Dandelion Plant

Dandelion, also known as Taraxacum, is a large genus of flowering plants. It has high levels of potassium and iron and is a rich source of vitamins and carotene. Dandelions also have roughly 7,000 units of Vitamin A per ounce, an important fact for cancer sufferers as they are commonly deficient in this vitamin.

The dandelion plant also contains high levels of potassium, which is a rich source of iron and vitamins. Ounce for ounce, dandelions contain more carotene than carrots.

The dandelion has shown promise in treating cancer as an adjuvant, especially in the case of liver cancer. It stimulates growth of healthy liver cells and helps eliminate toxins and bile. It is both a diuretic and a laxative.

In addition, one of the major chemicals in dandelion known as inulin is being studied for immune-stimulatory ability. In tests against cancer, it shows promise in stimulating white blood cells and actively fighting two tumor systems.

The Chinese have used dandelion to treat breast cancer for more than a thousand years. It is often taken as a tea, or sometimes the roots of the dandelion plant are eaten raw.

### Further Reading & References

- Dandelion, http://www.self-healing-herbs.com/dandelion.html

- Dandelion, http://www.mskcc.org/mskcc/html/69200.cfm

- *Help Nature to Heal You From Cancer: A Guide on Cancer Prevention, and Natural and Alternative Therapies* by Danuta Ryduchowski (2006)

- Eat More Herbs. http://eatmoreherbs.com/zine/dandelion.html

# D-Glucarate (Phytonutrient)

The supplement known as calcium D-glucarate can be useful in treating cancer because of its ability to inhibit the size and metastatic potential of colon and other intestinal cancers. In a rat study, D-glucarate inhibited adenocarcinoma formation at the initiation stage of cancer formation, following the injection of a carcinogen known to cause intestinal cancer in rats.

D-glucarate may be effective in the prevention and treatment of cancer by inhibiting the beta-glucuronidase enzyme and by inhibiting cancer cell proliferation induced by chemical carcinogens.

It can be found naturally in grapefruit, apricots, cherries, apples, Brussels sprouts, broccoli, lettuce, cabbage, and alfalfa sprouts.

### Further Reading & References

- *D-Glucarate* by Rita Elkins (1999)

- *D-Glucarate : A Nutrient Against Cancer* by Thomas Slaga and Judi Quilici-Timmcke (1999)

- Calcium D-Glucarate Supplement Can Reduce Your Risk Of Cancer, http://www.thehealthierlife.co.uk/natural-health-articles/cancer/calcium-d-glucarate-supplement-reduce-risk-cancer-00081.html

# DIM (Diindolylmethane)

DIM is an anticarcinogen compound found in plants from the mustard family such as broccoli, cauliflower, and collard greens.

The National Cancer Institute has begun clinical trials of DIM as a therapy for various forms of cancer as well as viral infections like HIV (the cause of AIDS), HPV, and hepatitis.

The growth of breast cancer, pancreatic, colon, ovarian, and bladder cancer cells have been shown to be inhibited by DIM in laboratory studies.

Eating fresh vegetables from the mustard family (also known as the *Brassica* family) is the best and easiest way to consume DIM, although it can be purchased in supplement form.

### Further Reading & References

- "DIM, from green vegetables that prevent some cancers, may eventually yield cures, Texas researcher says," http://psa-rising.com/eatingwell/broccoli_DIM_jan_2004.htm

- *Indoles: Psilocybin, Tryptophan, Iprindole, Sunitinib, Indometacin, Yohimbine, Sumatriptan, 3,3'-Diindolylmethane, Alpha-Amanitin, Roxindole* by Books LLC (2010)

# Ellagic Acid

Ellagic Acid is based on a natural extract from fruits and nuts that has the power to stop cancer cells from mutating. Specifically, it has antiproliferative properties that allow it to inhibit the replication of DNA within certain cancer cells.

It is widely found in plants such as strawberries, blackberries, cranberries, walnuts, and pecans – with the greatest amounts observed in raspberries. Ellagic Acid also has two special functions - it maintains apoptosis and protects DNA.

Healthy cells in the body have a normal life cycle of approximately 120 days before they die. This process is called apoptosis (programmed cell death). The body normally replaces these dying cells with healthy cells. Cancer cells, however, do not die this way. Inducing apoptosis is one of the principal goals of cancer treatment.

With the help of ellagic acid, cancer cells appear to go through normal apoptosis, without damaging healthy cells. Chemotherapy, radiation, and most conventional treatments, on the other hand, cause the death of both cancer cells and healthy cells indiscriminately, sometimes destroying the entire immune system in the process.

At the Hollings Cancer Institute, a nine year, double-blind study on the properties of ellagic acid, involving 500 cervical cancer patients, demonstrated the following:

- Ellagic acid stops cancer cells from dividing in 48 hours

- Ellagic acid causes normal cell death (apoptosis) within 72 hours in cases of breast, pancreas, esophageal, skin, colon, and prostate cancers

- Ellagic acid prevents the destruction of the p53 gene that leads to cancer

- HPV (human papilloma virus) exposed to ellagic acid from red raspberries experienced apoptosis (normal cell death)

- Consuming one cup (150 grams) of red raspberries per day prevents the development of cancer cells

In its *Complementary and Alternative Cancer Methods Handbook*, the American Cancer Society indicated that ellagic acid:

" … prevents the binding of carcinogens to DNA and strengthens connective tissue, which may keep cancer cells from spreading."

Additionally, the American Cancer Society pointed out that studies demonstrated ellagic acid inhibited tumor growth and protected against chromosome damage from radiation therapy.

Ellagic acid is available in supplement form but can also be ingested by eating large amounts of berries and other natural sources.

### Further Reading & References

- *American Cancer Society's Complementary and Alternative Cancer Methods Handbook* (2002)

- Ellagic Acid & Cervical Cancer, http://www.annieappleseedproject.org/studelaccerc.html

- Ellagic Acid Cancer Treatment, http://cancertutor.com/Cancer/EllagicAcid.html

- Ellagic Acid, http://www.cancer.org/treatment/treatmentsandsideeffects/complementaryandalternativemedicine/dietandnutrition/ellagic-acid

- About Herbs: Ellagic Acid, http://www.mskcc.org/mskcc/html/69212.cfm

# Fucoidan

Scientists have discovered that brown seaweeds contain a compound called **fucoidan** that shows promise as a natural cancer killer.

In Japan, edible brown seaweeds such as bladder wrack, kombu and wakame are often used in soups and other dishes. Their widespread use is thought by some experts to contribute to the remarkable longevity of the Japanese. Besides their use as foods, seaweeds also have a long history of use in Oriental medicine.

For example, bladder wrack has long been a rich source of iodine, and was used extensively to treat swelling of the thyroid gland (goiter), a deficiency disease caused by lack of iodine.

Wakame, another type of seaweed, has been used to purify the blood, promote intestinal function, and improve skin and hair. Some recent Japanese studies identified the wakame compound known as fucoxanthin as an efficient way to burn body fat. Now the cancer-fighting benefits of fucoidan are attracting attention.

Research into fucoidan started around 1970, and since then fucoidan has been cited in about 700 studies indexed in the National Library of Medicine's database.

Fucoidan is a type of carbohydrate called a *polysaccharide* that's found in the cell walls of brown seaweed. It has a high nutritional value—given that it's rich in calcium, iodine, zinc, iron, selenium and vitamin A.

These nutrients are essential to ensure the circulatory, immune and neurologic systems function properly. In addition, scientific studies confirm that fucoidan causes certain types of rapidly growing cancer cells to die.

Fucoidan induces *apoptosis,* or natural cell death, in cancer cells. Cells reproduce themselves by dividing and becoming two cells. The two "daughter cells" eventually divide again and make four cells. But the process doesn't go on forever: Healthy cells die off after dividing and dividing again for a certain number of generations.

But cancer cells generally escape this fate unless something is done to induce it. Getting cancer cells to undergo apoptosis is one of the Holy Grails of cancer therapy. Fucoidan appears to trigger the mechanism that causes cancer cells to undergo apoptosis. Scientists are still researching how this happens.

An animal study* suggests there may be a second way that fucoidan acts to clobber cancer cells. This study showed it enhances the activity of natural killer (NK) cells. These cells play a crucial role in killing tumor cells. Stimulating NK cells is another major goal of cancer therapy (more so in alternative medicine than in mainstream medicine).

Mice in the study ate a diet containing 1 percent fucoidan for 10 days. During this time, they were also injected with leukemia cells. Afterwards, the rodents continued to eat the diet containing fucoidan for 40 additional days. Researchers found that in the mice receiving fucoidan, tumors were inhibited by an impressive 65.4 percent.

What's more, NK cell activity significantly increased in the fucoidan-fed mice compared to animals who did not receive the nutrient.

So far, scientists have found examples of self-destruction in several types of cancer cells, including:

- Cancer cells of the descending colon

- Human colon cancer cells

- Human stomach cancer cells

- Leukemia cells


Fucoidan induced apoptosis only in cancer cells, with no damage to normal cells.

Another fucoidan's significant health benefits lies in its ability to strengthen the immune system. Several studies in vitro (*i.e.* in lab cultures) as well as in animals show it has restrained so-called "coated viruses" such as herpes, HIV and a type of herpes virus called *human cytomegalovirus* that can cause blindness and fatal pneumonia in people with compromised immune systems.

Scientific experiments suggest fucoidan may act in two ways:

- It stops the virus from attaching to and penetrating host cells, and

- It prevents the virus from duplicating after cell penetration.**


A University of Chicago pilot study*** found that fucoidan provided significant protection when human subjects took it orally. Fifteen patients with active herpes infections (including herpes simplex virus types 1 and 2, herpes zoster or Epstein-Barr virus) and six subjects with latent infections took fucoidan orally.

Researchers noted increased healing rates in patients with active infections. What's more, patients with latent infections continued to show no symptoms of illness while taking fucoidan.

Fucoidan also confers significant cardiovascular benefits. It's a natural blood thinner, helps lower cholesterol and blood pressure, and provides overall protection to the blood vessels, heart and other organs.

Fucoidan is available in supplements from a variety of online and retail providers.

### Further Reading and References

- *Maruyama, H. et al. Antitumor activity and immune response of Mekabu fucoidan extracted from Sporophyll of Undaria pinnatifida. In Vivo. 2003 May-Jun;17(3):245-9. Retrieved from http://www.ncbi.nlm.nih.gov/pubmed/17054048

- **Hoshino T, Hayashi T, Hayashi K, Hamada J, Lee JB, Sankawa U. An antivirally active sulfated polysaccharide from Sargassum horneri (TURNER) C. AGARDH. Biol Pharm Bull. 1998 Jul; 21(7): 730-4.

- ***Thompson KD, Fitton JH, Dragar C, et al. GFS, a Preparation of Tasmanian Undaria pinnatifida, is Associated with Healing and Inhibition of Reactivation of Herpes. BMC Complementary and Alternative Medicine. 2002;2:11.

# Genistein/Isoflavones/Soy

Much research supports the theory that a soy-rich diet may prevent cancer. Research indicates that soyfoods help protect against several types of cancer, including lung, colon, rectal, stomach, and prostate cancer. Advocates maintain that in countries where soy is heavily consumed, such as Japan, people are less likely to develop cancer.

For example, mortality rates for breast cancer mortality are much lower in Asia, where soy is a main diet staple, than in the U.S., where soyfoods are consumed less often. Comparatively, U.S. women are four times more likely to die of breast cancer than Japanese women. These striking facts, however, are not proof that soy accounts for lower cancer rates, since American and Asian lifestyles and environments differ in many other ways as well.

Soyfoods are rich in compounds called phytochemicals. One particular family of phytochemicals, known as isoflavones, may fight cancer in a variety of ways. Isoflavones are found in significant amounts only in soybeans and in soyfoods, such as tofu, soy milk, tempeh, and textured soy protein.

One isoflavone, genistein, has attracted the most attention. Genistein is an isoflavone found only in soy among our daily foods. It blocks a process in the body called angiogenesis, the growth of new blood vessels that nourish malignant tumors. Once a tumor grows beyond a millimeter, it must foster the growth of new blood vessels to support its growth. An increase in tumor size must be accompanied by an increase in blood vessel formation.

Genistein is also believed to inhibit certain enzymatic processes that would otherwise allow normal cells to convert to cancer cells. It may also work against cancers that depend on hormones for growth stimulation.

It is also thought that genistein keeps new tumors from growing because it inhibits blood vessel growth. Tumors do well only when tiny networks of new blood vessels supply them with nutrients and oxygen.

Laboratory tests show live cancer cells stop growing once genistein is added. More than 100 studies on a variety of cancer cells have demonstrated the effectiveness of genistein.

It is believed that genistein acts against cancer in other ways as well. For example, scientists believe certain enzymes in the body convert normal cells to cancer cells and that certain cancer drugs simply inhibit these enzymes. Genistein apparently also has inhibitory properties.

In addition, genistein may work against cancers that depend on hormones to grow, such as breast and prostate cancer. By interfering with the hormones, it inhibits the development of cancer cells and tumors. Research indicates that genistein also interferes with the process by which tumors receive nutrients and oxygen.

Researchers at the University of Minnesota attached genistein to antibodies and injected them into mice with leukemia. All injected mice survived, while a control group of mice that did not receive genistein died within three months.

These finding have positive implications in the treatment of solid tumors such as malignancies of the breast, prostate, colon, and brain.

Regarding prostate cancer in particular, isoflavones may have a significant role. Beneficial effects include:

- A decrease in blood androgen (testosterone) levels by increasing the level of SHBG (sex-hormone binding globulin). SHBG binds to testosterone. Therefore, less testosterone is available to help the cancer grow.

- Binding to androgen receptors. As a result, more potent sex hormones (testosterone, dihydrotestosterone) are blocked from binding to the receptors and stimulating cancer growth.

- Inhibition of alpha-5 reductase, an enzyme that converts testosterone to its most potent form (dihydrotestosterone).

- Restriction of other enzymes associated with cancer cell growth.

- Inhibition of tumor blood vessel formation. Blood vessel growth within the tumor allows the cancer to grow and spread.

- Decrease in insulin growth factor-1 (IGF-1), which may be a marker for increased prostate cancer risk.

Prostate cancer, which is linked to diet as a major factor, is also much lower in Asian countries than in the United States. As with breast cancer, research suggests a potential reason for the difference may be soy protein intake. In East Asian countries like Japan, Korea, China, and Taiwan, the estimated isoflavone mean daily intake is between 10-50 mg per day, as compared to 1-3 mg per day for Americans.

Certain animal studies have shown genistein to be effective in inhibiting tumor growth. In one study, a group of human prostate cancer cells was treated with genistein and another group was left untreated. Prostate cancer cell growth was inhibited only in the cells treated with genistein. In another study, prostate cancer cells were transplanted into animal models. These animals ate either a soy-free diet or a soy-based diet. The progression of prostate cancer was reduced by 25% in the animals on the soy-based diet versus the animals on the soy-free diet.

Despite the impressive evidence for the benefits of soy, the food is a source of controversy in the alternative health community because soy is rich in phytoestrogens, which are similar although not identical to human estrogen hormones. While most associated with female sexuality, estrogens are present in both sexes. Critics of soy consumption believe the phytoestrogens in soy mimic human estrogens when ingested and introduce profound hormonal imbalances. The controversy is unresolved, but casts doubt on the benefits of soy.

Recommendations for battling prostate cancer as stated by the Louis Warschaw Prostate Cancer Center at Cedars-Sinai include:

- Daily intake of 35 to 40 grams soy protein per day. Note: A good way to add soy protein to your diet is by having a soy-protein smoothie with breakfast. Some soy protein isolate powders have up to 20 grams of soy protein and 20 mg of isoflavones per serving. (This is half of the recommended intake.)

- Avoidance of soybean oils. Soybean oil does not contain beneficial isoflavones. It is best to get isoflavones as they occur in soy products, such as soy protein isolate powder, tofu, and soy meat substitutes. Avoid isoflavone supplements, which may not provide the proper balance of genistein to daidzein.

- Gradual increase of soy intake. Large amounts of soy contain high amounts of soluble fiber, which can cause gastrointestinal discomfort.

As mentioned earlier, because the incidence of breast cancer in Japan is far lower than in Western countries, and because the soy intake of Japanese women has historically been several hundred times higher than Western women, a great deal of speculation has been devoted to the role that soy may play in preventing breast cancer.

When researchers isolated statistics about the intake of isoflavone-rich foods (particularly soy foods and miso soup) and measured them against the breast cancer information, three results stood out significantly:

- Consumption of isoflavone-rich foods and miso soup was associated with a decreased risk of breast cancer.

- Consumption of soy foods alone was NOT associated with a decreased risk of breast cancer.

- The decreased risk of breast cancer was strongest among postmenopausal women.

### Further Reading & References

- *Soy Smart Health: Discover The Super food That Fights Breast Cancer, Heart Disease, Osteoporosis, Menopausal Discomforts and Estrogen Dominance* by Neil Solomon, Rita Elkins, and Richard Passwater (2004)

- *Cancer: Fight It with the Blood Type Diet (Eat Right for Your Type Health Library)* by Peter J. D'Adamo and Catherine Whitney (2004)

- "Influence of genistein isoflavone on matrix metalloproteinase-2 expression in prostate cancer cells." http://www.ncbi.nlm.nih.gov/pubmed/17201635

- Soy Rich, Anti Cancer Diet, http://www.huldaclarkzappers.com/php2/soyadiet.php

- Soy, www.cedars-sinai.edu/Patients/Programs-and...**Cancer**/.../Soy.aspx

- Louis Warschaw Prostate Cancer, http://www.cedars-sinai.edu/Patients/Programs-and-Services/Prostate-Cancer-Center/

# Geraniol

Chemically, geraniol is both an alcohol and a monoterpenoid. It occurs naturally in essential oils such as rose, citronella, and palmarosa. It has been found to be effective as a plant-based mosquito repellant and has also been used as an additive to cigarettes to improve flavor.

Some research shows geraniol is helpful in inhibiting certain types of cancer cell growth and that it may also effectively block cancer cell differentiation.

The combined administration of geraniol and 5-FU to mice with human colonic tumor cells showed a 53% reduction in tumor size after seven days.

Geraniol appears to be most promising in the area of colorectal cancer chemotherapy.

### Further Reading & References

- "Geraniol, a Component of Plant Essential Oils, Inhibits Growth and Polyamine Biosynthesis in Human Colon Cancer Cells." http://jpet.aspetjournals.org/content/298/1/197.full

- Geraniol: Essential Oil/5FU & Human Colon Cancer, http://www.annieappleseedproject.org/geroil5fuhum.html

- "Inhibition of pancreatic cancer growth by the dietary isoprenoids farnesol and geraniol." http://www.ncbi.nlm.nih.gov/pubmed/9075204

# Ginger Root

Ginger root has long been used to ease nausea, making it particularly helpful for cancer patients undergoing chemotherapy. This is important since it means chemotherapy patients may eventually have an easier way to take drugs and keep them ingested, by pairing them with some form of ginger.

The root itself is native to Southeast Asia and is often used as a cooking spice and to combat morning sickness in pregnant women. Ginger has also been shown to stop blood clots, help with addictions, and halt the growth of ulcers.

Some studies even show that topical application of ginger may help ward of skin cancer and help repair the oxidative damage caused by other cancers.

University of Minnesota researchers found that mice that were fed the main active component in ginger root three times a week had slower cancer growth rates than control animals.

Ginger can be consumed as a tea, a supplement, or as a spice in a variety of foods.

### Further Reading & References

- Scientific American: "Green Tea and Ginger Show New Cancer-Combating Abilities," http://www.

sciam.com/article.cfm?articleID=0002329D-E1EF-1F9E-A1EF83414B7F0000

- Bloomberg: "Ginger Root Eased Nausea in Study of Chemotherapy Patients," http://www.bloomberg.com/apps/news?pid=newsarchive&sid=ap4Lx_.1Dd4o&refer=home

- Ginger Root (Zingiber officinale), http://www.herbwisdom.com/herb-ginger-root.html

# Goji Berries/Wolfberries/Goji Juice/Lycium/Chinese Boxthorn

Goji berry is the commercial name for the fruit of the wolfberry along with two other related species, the *Lycium barbarum* and *Lycium chinense*. Native to Southeastern Europe and Asia, the goji berry is bright orange-red, runs one to two centimeters across, and has anywhere from 10 to 60 small yellow seeds.

Hundreds of U.S. companies have capitalized on this fruit and market it as nutritional support against a variety of maladies from depression to cancer. It likely contains healing antioxidant properties much like those of many other small, colorful fruits. One chemical in the berry is cyperone, which helps the body maintain normal blood pressure and has been linked to effective treatment for cervical cancer. Goji berries may also play a role in stopping and reversing the growth of cancerous cells.

### Further Reading & References

- *Goji: The Himalayan Health Secret* by Earl Mindell, Rick Handel (2003)

- *The Super Antioxidant Diet and Nutrition Guide: A Health Plan for the Body, Mind, and Spirit,* by Robin Jeep, Sherie Pitman Ellington, and Richard Couey PhD (2008)

- Columbia News Service: "Goji berries: the new miracle fruit?" http://jscms.jrn.columbia.edu/cns/2007-02-27/rosenberg-gojiberries.html

- Goji Berry Properties, http://www.health-report.co.uk/goji_berry.html

# Grains/Whole Grains

Whole grains consist of cereal-like grains that contain bran and germ along with endosperm. This is in contrast to refined grains, which only contain endosperm. Whole grains include wheat, oats, barley, brown rice, rye, spelt, quinoa, amaranth, and teff, among others.

These grains have fiber that may assist in isolating and removing cancer-causing compounds from the body. This means that a person who consumes whole grains on a regular basis has a significantly lowered risk of developing cancer.

Other agents within whole grains appear to help stabilize insulin and blood sugar, which also helps ward off developing cancer. Whole grain foods are high in fiber, which contributes to bowel regularity and thereby help prevent colon cancer.

### Further Reading & References

- Linus Pauling Institute, Micronutrient Information Center, http://lpi.oregonstate.edu/infocenter/

foods/grains/

- Whole Grains, Fiber, And Breast Cancer Risk, http://envirocancer.cornell.edu/factsheet/diet/ fs36.grain.pdf

- Prostate Cancer, http://clem.mscd.edu/~boettner/CancerTutor/Other/Prostate_Cancer.html

- Foods That Fight Cancer? Whole Grains, http://www.aicr.org/site/PageServer?pagename=food sthatfightcancer_whole_grains

## Grape Seed Extract and Grape Skin Extract

Grape seed extracts have high concentrations of flavonoids, vitamin E, and linoleic acid, among other healthy nutrients. They are recognized as a significant source of polyphenols and antioxidants.

Grape seed extract is particularly helpful in treating conditions like atherosclerosis, high blood pressure, and poor circulation.

Several studies are underway by the National Cancer Institute and the National Center for Complementary and Alternative Medicine to determine whether grape seed extract can help with breast cancer, colon cancer, or other forms of the disease.

You can consume grape seed extract in capsule and tablet form. It is prepared, of course, from the seed and skin of grapes.

See **Brandt Grape Cure** for more information.

### Further Reading & References

- National Center for Complementary and Alternative Medicine: "Grape Seed Extract," http://nccam. nih.gov/health/grapeseed/

- Grape Seed Extract, http://www.grapeseedextract.com/

- *All About Grape Seed Extract* by Dallas Clouatre (2004)

- *The Flavonoid Revolution: Grape Seed Extract and Other Flavonoids Against Disease* by Michael Colgan (1997)

## Graviola/Annona reticulata

Graviola, which is the common name for *Annona reticulata*, is a fruit also known as soursop, guanabana, and custard apple. It comes from a tree common to South America and the Caribbean region. The leaves of the tree are commonly used in traditional medicine treatments to treat diarrhea and eliminate worms.

Proponents claim it is more effective at killing colon cancer cells than common chemotherapeutic drugs because it seeks out and destroys prostate, lung, breast, colon, and pancreatic cancers while leaving healthy cells unharmed. It is also said to provide an immune system boost.

The National Cancer Institute included graviola in a plant-screening program that showed its leaves and stems were effective in attacking and destroying malignant cells. Strangely, the results were never released to the public and remained part of an internal NCI report.

There have been several promising cancer studies on graviola since 1976, when it was first introduced, but the tree's extracts have yet to be tested on cancer patients. No double-blind clinical trials exist.

Regardless, graviola has been shown to kill cancer cells in vitro (i.e., in laboratory cell cultures) in as many as 20 laboratory tests. A study conducted at Catholic University of South Korea demonstrated two chemicals extracted from graviola seeds were selective in cytotoxicity and comparable with Adriamycin (a common chemotherapy drug) for targeting and killing malignant breast and colon cancer cells.

Perhaps the most significant result of this study and others is that Graviola was shown to selectively target only cancer cells, leaving normal, healthy cells untouched.

By comparison, chemotherapy indiscriminately seeks and destroys all actively reproducing cells, including normal hair and stomach cells, which leads to the devastating side effects of hair-loss and severe nausea.

Another study, published in the *Journal of Natural Products*, showed that graviola also outperforms Adriamycin in laboratory tests. One chemical found in graviola selectively killed colon cancer cells at 10,000 times the potency of Adriamycin.

Research from Purdue University detailed the active components of the tree, which may be potent in inhibiting the growth of cancer cells. The Purdue studies found the active components to be effective against multi-drug-resistant (MDR) cancer cells, those cells that survive chemotherapy and cause cancer to return.

Purdue researchers also found that leaves from the graviola tree killed cancer cells "among six human-cell lines" and were especially effective against prostate and pancreatic cancer cells.

In a separate study, Purdue researchers showed that extracts from the graviola leaves are extremely effective in isolating and killing lung cancer cells.

Graviola looks to be a promising alternative or supplement to mainstream treatments. Graviola and N-Tense (an anti-cancer formula featuring graviola and seven other rainforest herbs) are completely natural substances. No side effects have been reported except for possible mild gastrointestinal upset at high dosages (in excess of 5 grams) if taken on an empty stomach.

See **N-Tense**, a patented substance that contains 50% graviola.

### *Further Reading & References*

- Memorial Sloan-Kettering Cancer Center: Graviola, http://www.mskcc.org/mskcc/html/69245.cfm

- Weil: Graviola: A Worthwhile Botanical Against Cancer? http://www.drweil.com/drw/u/QAA400299/graviola-a-worthwhile-botanical-against-cancer

- *The Healing Power of Rainforest Herbs: A Guide to Understanding and Using Herbal Medicinals* by Leslie Taylor (2005)

- Graviola Leaf For Cancer (Soursop), http://www.fasting.ws/juice-fasting/disease-treatments/graviola-leaf-for-cancer-soursop

- Graviola Tree and Paw Paw Treatments, http://www.cancertutor.com/Cancer/Graviola.html

# Haelan/Haelan 951

Haelan is an anti-cancer agent made from liquid soybean extract. It contains mass quantities of single cell proteins and their metabolites thanks to a fermentation process that hydrolyzes the soybean proteins into amino acids and other compounds.

The reported benefits of Haelan include blocking cancer-cell blood supplies, while at the same time supporting enzymatic activity, tumor reduction, and the immune system. It has also been found to help relieve the side effects of conventional cancer therapies.

When the immune system operates properly, cancer cells can exist in the body without causing harm. They are dissolved by T-cells, a type of immune cell that converts nitrogen into nitric acid and releases it onto the cancer cells. Healthy cells are coated in the enzyme superoxide dismutase (SOD) so they are protected (this coating is absent in cancer cells).

Because cancer cells seek out the nitrogen in the body's protein, they deplete the nitrogen that the T-cells need to work their protective actions. This nitrogen comes from protein stored in the muscle tissue and is a target for cancer cells.

Consuming specific formulations of soy can provide cancer-fighting phytochemicals (natural plant compounds), which penetrate the cancer cell and cause the cancer to self-destruct. Fermented and nitrogenated soy hydrolyzes the soybean proteins into bioactive amino acids. These acids are small components, better able to permeate the walls of cancer cells.

Cancer cells absorb nitrogen in their normal foraging for this element. They take in the nitrogenated soy proteins that carry with them undetected, immune-supporting compounds consisting of isoflavones, protease inhibitors, saponins, phytosterols, and phytic acids. Once within the cancer cell, the anticancer components set out to reprogram the part of the cell that affects its reproduction and life span.

Research shows that the use of nitrogenated, fermented soy along with chemotherapy and/or radiation treatments results in a greater number of cancer cell deaths by apoptosis (natural cell death) than either chemotherapy and/or radiation produces when used alone.

Researchers at the Department of Pathology, Karmanos Cancer Institute, Wayne State University School of Medicine have determined that the soy isoflavone genistein, together with other cellular effects of genistein, completely shut down the NF-kB activity survival mechanism that cancer cells employ. Cisplatin, docetaxel, and adriamycin were the chemotherapeutic agents used with the soy isoflavone pretreatment. The combination resulted in increased cancer cell growth inhibition and increased apoptosis induced by the chemotherapy drugs in prostate, breast, and pancreatic cancer cells.

Many oncologists do not recommend the use of antioxidants by patients undergoing chemotherapy and/or radiation treatments because they are concerned that antioxidants may protect cancer cells, resulting in lower cancer cell death rates. Research and case studies apparently show this is not a valid concern for cancer patients who are considering the use of the nitrogenated fermented soy beverage along with their chemotherapy and/or radiation treatments.

Other studies show that isoflavones such as genistein can have antitumor benefits in cancers of the breast and prostate as well as sarcoma and retinoblastoma cell lines.

### Further Reading & References

- Memorial Sloan-Kettering Cancer Center: Haelan, http://www.mskcc.org/mskcc/html/69251.cfm

- Haelan Products, http://www.haelanproducts.com/

- *Beating Cancer with Nutrition* by Patrick Quillin (2005)

- *The World of Soy (The Food Series)*by Christine M. Du Bois, Chee-Beng Tan, and Sidney Mintz (2008)

- Sage, Donna, M.S.S.A., "Interview," Townsend Letter for Doctors, Oct. 7, 1998.


# Indole-3-carbinol (I3C)

Indole-3-carbinol (I3C), is a chemical found in cruciferous vegetables such as cabbage, broccoli,

brussels sprouts, cauliflower, kale, kohlrabi, and turnips. It appears to have anticancer properties. Early studies show it has the potential to partially block the effects of estrogen on cells as well as facilitate the conversion of estrogen to a less cancer-promoting form.

I3C is being studied as a chemopreventive agent: a substance that helps prevent cancer. Numerous animal studies suggest that I3C might help reduce the risk of estrogen-sensitive cancers as well as other types of cancer. A 4-week, double-blind, placebo-controlled trial of 57 women found that a minimum dose of 300 mg of I3C daily may reduce the risk of estrogen-promoted cancers. Another study found benefits with 400 mg of I3C per day. In addition, a double-blind, placebo-controlled study in humans suggests that it can help reverse cervical dysplasia, a precancerous condition. Still other studies (referenced below) suggest I3C has the ability to induce apoptosis (natural cell death) in breast cancer cells.


### Further Reading & References

- "Inactivation of akt and NF-kappaB play important roles during indole-3-carbinol-induced apoptosis in

- breast cancer cells." http://www.ncbi.nlm.nih.gov/entrez/query.fcgi?cmd=Retrieve&db=pubmed&dopt=Abstract&list_uids=15203382

- *The Breast Cancer Prevention Diet: The Powerful Foods, Supplements, and Drugs That Can Save Your Life* by Jim Arnosky (1999)

- *Keeping aBreast: Ways to PREVENT Breast Cancer* by Khalid Mahmud (2008)

- Indole-3-carbinol: http://www.mbmc.org/healthgate/GetHGContent.aspx?token=9c315661-83b7-472d-a7ab-bc8582171f86&chunkiid=21757

# Laetrile/Amygdalin/Vitamin B17/Sarcarcinase/Nitriloside/ Mandelonitrile/Hydrocyanic Acid

Laetrile is the commercial name for a modified form of amygdalin, which is also known as bitter almonds. Chinese doctors allegedly used this substance, which is highly concentrated in the pits of apricots and other fruits, some 3,500 years ago for the treatment of tumors. Dioscorides of Anazarbos, 2000 years ago, was perhaps the first to document it. It was usually administered in the form of bitter almonds.

Modern laetrile is usually derived from apricot kernels where it comprises about 2-3% of the kernel, a relatively large amount. It's also found in the kernels of other fruits, such as plums, cherries, peaches, nectarines, and apples. All fruit seeds have a healthy form of organic cyanide in them, from apple seed to apricot seed, although laetrile treatments have been alleged to cause cyanide poisoning.

The fruit kernels or seeds generally have other nutrients as well -- some protein, unsaturated fatty acids, and various minerals. Although often called B17, laetrile is not found with other B vitamins in yeasts. Many plants do contain some laetrile, with the sprouting seeds, especially mung bean sprouts, containing the highest amount.

The diet of primitive man and most fruit-eating animals was very rich in nitrilosides. They regularly ate the seeds (and kernels) of all fruits, since these seeds are rich in protein, polyunsaturated fats, and other nutrients. Seeds also contain as much as 2% or more nitriloside. When civilized humans eat less than the whole fruit -- for example, by discarding the seed or kernel -- they experience a specific and total deficiency not only in oils and proteins but also in minerals and such vitamins as B17 (nitriloside) because it is found only in the seed, not in the flesh of the fruit.

Several other foods are naturally rich in nitriloside, including lima beans, succotash containing nitriloside-rich chick peas, plum jam, elderberry wine, bean sprouts, millet sprouts, sorghum molasses, wild berries, raspberries, macadamia nuts, and nitriloside-rich bamboo sprouts.

Nitriloside was "rediscovered" in 1920 by a California physician, Ernest Krebs while experimenting with flavorings for bootleg whisky. His son, Dr. Ernest Krebs, Jr., purified it and coined the name 'laetrile' in 1952. Krebs's studies showed that when a human or animal system ingests sufficient amounts of laetrile (or in its natural form, hydrocyanic acid), this substance becomes selectively toxic to cancer cells.

In the early seventies, Dr. Harold Manner of the Biology Department at Loyola University, Chicago, conducted a study on a strain of mice using a combination of enzymes, Vitamin A, and laetrile. He reported in his book, *Death of Cancer*:

"After 6-8 days, an ulceration appeared at the tumor site. Within the ulceration was a pus-like fluid. An examination of this fluid revealed dead malignant cells. The tumor gradually underwent complete regression in 75 of the experimental animals. This represented 89.3% of the total group." (quoted in Moss, 1982).

Laetrile needs to be taken with vitamin A and enzymes to be most effective.

Pure laetrile has been illegal in the U.S. for decades and was pulled from the shelves in Britain.

Challengers claim it is potentially toxic and leads to cyanide poisoning. As late as the end of the 1970s, between 50,000 and 100,000 cancer patients were ingesting close to 1 million grams per month. Only between two and three deaths were reported from accidental overdose. Considering these statistics, laetrile does not seem as toxic or dangerous as opponents make it out to be.

Laetrile has been described as a parcel that contains poisons that are only released once the parcel is unwrapped. It has an effect on cancer cells because those cells secrete the enzyme beta-glucosidase that releases the cyanide, which then poisons the cancer cells. In contrast, normal cells have the enzyme rhodanase which effectively renders the cyanide molecule inactive. In the absence of cancer cells, the toxic cyanide is not released.

Laetrile/amygdalin is not digested in the stomach by hydrochloric acid. Instead, it passes into the small intestine where it is acted on by enzymes that split it into various compounds, which are then absorbed.

Laetrile can be separated by appropriate enzymes, in the presence of water, into glucose, benzaldehyde, and hydrocyanic acid. The last two substances are each, individually, a poison, but together they work synergistically and become more powerful when combined than when used separately.

In the treatment of cancer, laetrile is used to reduce tumor size and further spread of the disease, as well as to alleviate the sometimes severe pain of the cancer condition.

Laetrile does not make tumors grow smaller, so the question of tumor regression is sometimes brought up as evidence that laetrile is ineffective. Laetrilists argue that tumor size is not a good indicator of anti-cancer activity because a tumor does not just consist of malignant cells. Tumors also contain normal cells.

When chemotherapy is used, all cells are attacked so it's not unusual to see short-term tumor regression (because both malignant and normal cells are killed). Unfortunately, the long-term result of such treatment is for the tumor to become more aggressive due to the chance of increasing the ratio of malignant cells. In the case of laetrile, however, normal cells are not affected and so tumors do not decrease in size. Instead, they become benign.

According to pathologist Gerald Dermer, "There is a marked discrepancy between ostensible tumor response and actual patient survival. In only about 32% of the clinical trials that reported significant tumor responses to new drugs was survival also prolonged." In other words, tumor "response" or shrinkage may be largely irrelevant to controlling cancer, and the charge that laetrile doesn't shrink tumors may be likewise irrelevant.

Nearly all laetrile supporters advocate a diet of raw vegetables in conjunction with the therapy, partly because such a diet contains a large amount of dietary laetrile. Indeed, one of the things that makes the laetrile controversy so bizarre is that laetrile is a very common component of food.

Between 1,200 and 2,500 plants contain laetrile. This includes most cereals and fruits and many vegetables. A diet that contains high quantities of the following will also be high in laetrile: chickpeas, bean sprouts, nuts, mung beans, blackberries, raspberries, and the seeds of apples, apricots, cherries, plums, and pears.

Laetrile's safety was demonstrated in an experiment with mice undertaken at a leading US cancer research institution (Memorial Sloan-Kettering Cancer Center). For thirty months, mice were injected daily with laetrile at a rate of 2 grams per kilogram of body weight (equivalent to giving a human a quarter of a pound a day). At the end of the period, the mice were healthier and exhibited greater well-being than the control group that did not get any laetrile.

Refer to *The Cancer Syndrome* by Ralph Moss for more details.

In addition, it should be noted that some young plants develop their own naturally occurring pesticides to provide some protection against insects and rodents. These pesticides are rich in nitrilosides, which are similar in chemical structure to laetrile. This presents the question that a diet high in young fresh plants such as alfalfa sprouts is like undergoing continuous non-toxic chemotherapy that kills pockets of cancer cells before they divide and grow.

Laetrile authority Elson M. Haas M.D. says, "When used, laetrile is administered at 250-1,000 mg. (a gram is a thousand milligrams) daily. Higher amounts, up to 3 grams per day, have been used, but divided into several smaller dosages, each usually limited to 1 gram. If the source is whole apricot kernels, the quantity is usually about 10-20 kernels per day; 1-2 cups of fresh mung bean sprouts may provide an equivalent amount. If apricot kernels are blended or pulverized, it is suggested that they be consumed immediately."

### *Further Reading & References*

- *The cancer syndrome: With an afterword to the 1982 edition* by Ralph W. Moss (1982)

- *World Without Cancer: The Story of Vitamin B17* by G. Edward Griffin (2010)

- *Death of Cancer* by Harold Manner (1979)

- *Alive and Well: One Doctors Experience With Nutrition in the Treatment of Cancer* Patients by Philip E. Binzel Jr. (1994)

- *Laetrile Control for Cancer* by Glenn D. Kittler (1963)

- *Politics, Science and Cancer: The Laetrile Phenomenon* by Gerald Markle (1980)

- *The Little Cyanide Cookbook; Delicious Recipes Rich in Vitamin B17* by June De Spain (2000)

- *Vitamin B-17- Forbidden Weapon Against Cancer: The Fight For Laetrile* by Michael L Culbert (1974)

- *Laetrile Control for Cancer* by H. Knaus (1963)

- *Too Young to Die: Dramatic Use of Laetrile to Conquer Terminal Cancer* by Rick Hill (1979)

- *An Alternative Medicine Definitive Guide To Cancer* by W. John Diamond and W. Lee Cowden, (1997)

- Vitamin B17 — Laetrile, http://www.healthy.net/scr/article.aspx?Id=1926

- "Amygdalin," Memorial Sloan-Kettering Cancer Center, http://www.mskcc.org/mskcc/html/11790. cfm?Disclaimer_Redirect=%2Fmskcc%2Fhtml%2F69118.cfm

# Lycopene

Lycopene is a carotenoid in the same family as beta carotene. It is also the phytochemical that gives tomatoes and other red fruits their deep color. Lycopene is a powerful antioxidant that has shown remarkable fighting power against degenerative diseases. Tomatoes are the only major dietary source of lycopene.

Tomatoes may help reduce the risk of certain types of cancer, according to a study presented at an annual meeting for the American Association for Cancer Research. Scientific evidence has already established that carotenoids are not only essential to human nutrition, but may play an important role in preventing degenerative conditions through enhancement of the function of the immune system, inhibition of mutagenesis and reduction of induced damage to the cell's nucleus.

The antioxidative properties of lycopene are well documented. Lycopene is present naturally in human plasma in greater amounts than beta carotene and other dietary carotenoids. This indicates its extensive biological significance in the human defense system.

In a trial conducted at the Karmanos Cancer Institute at Wayne State University, researchers looked at the impact of short-term lycopene supplements on men who were facing surgery for newly diagnosed prostate cancer. The 26 patients in this study were randomly assigned to receive either a tomato extract (containing 30 milligrams of lycopene) or no supplement for 3 weeks before undergoing radical prostatectomy.

Men who received the lycopene supplement had lower prostate-specific antigen (PSA) levels and less aggressive tumors than the non-supplemented control group. Their tumors were smaller (80% of the tumors were under 4 milliliters (ml) in volume, compared to 45% in the control group). Results showed those who received the lycopene had cancer much more likely to be within normal surgical margins and/or confined to the prostate gland (73%, compared to 18% of the control group). The invasion of the prostate gland by cancer-like "PIN" cells was completely prevented in this group, compared to a 33% incidence of "PIN" cells in the control group.

"This pilot study suggests that lycopene may have beneficial effects in prostate cancer," concluded researcher Omer Kucuk, MD, and colleagues. They called for larger clinical trials in an effort to investigate the potential preventive and therapeutic role of lycopene in prostate cancer.

Another benefit to lycopene is that it may also help prevent liver cancer, as stated in findings from a study presented at the American Association for Cancer Research meeting in October 2002. Hoyoku Nishino, MD, of the Kyoto Prefectural University of Medicine, Japan, presented the results of this five-year clinical study examining the protective role of lycopene and other nutrients in people who demonstrated high risk of liver cancer.

A 50% decrease in hepatocellular carcinoma (HCC or liver cancer) was demonstrated in participants who consumed 10 milligrams of tomato lycopene daily along with other tomato phytonutrients. These phytonutrients included 10 milligrams of carotenes (30% alpha, 60% beta carotene), 50 milligrams of alpha tocopherols – a form of vitamin E -- and another form of vitamin E, tocotrienols. These results suggest that a mixture of natural tomato extract, carotenes and vitamin E has clinical promise.

P&S and Harlem Hospital researchers evaluated the association between lycopene and lung cancer. In a case-control study, investigators collected blood samples from 93 individuals with non-small cell lung cancer and from 102 matched controls. The researchers tested the samples for levels of certain micronutrients, including lycopene, retinol, and beta carotene.

They found no significant differences between subjects with lung cancer and control subjects in most of the micronutrients for which they tested. However, they found that lung cancer patients had significantly lower concentrations of lycopene.

After adjusting for age, sex, race, smoking, drinking, occupational exposure, vitamin supplements, and season, the investigators found that the group with the lowest lycopene levels had nearly a three-fold increased risk for cancer compared with the group with the highest lycopene levels. In African-Americans, subjects with the lowest level of lycopene demonstrated an eight-fold increase in cancer risk.

When the investigators evaluated current smokers, they found that the group with the lowest blood levels of lycopene had four times the risk of cancer than the group with the highest lycopene levels.

According to principal investigator Dr. Jean G. Ford, Assistant Professor of Medicine, "We concluded from our findings that low intake of lycopene may be a risk factor for lung cancer, especially for smokers. Even though our findings are preliminary, they add to the growing body of evidence that diets rich in tomatoes and tomato products are strongly linked to a reduced risk of certain types of cancer."

A study from North Carolina showed that drinking just one can (5.5 ounces) per day of the popular vegetable drink V-8 raised levels of lycopene in the lungs by 12%. It also decreased ozone-induced DNA damage to the lungs by 20%. Blood lycopene levels were raised 192% by a daily serving of tomato sauce, 122% by tomato soup, and 92% by V-8 juice.

### Further Reading & References

- *The Cancer Lifeline Cookbook: Recipes, Ideas, and Advice to Optimize the Lives of People Living with Cancer* by Kimberly Mathai and Ginny Smith (2004)

- *Lycopene may help prevent liver cancer.* (Research.: An article from: Food Processing (2005)

- *Tomatoes gain strength in cancer battle: new studies boost the resume of lycopene and fellow carotenoids*: An article from: Food Processing by Steve Ennen (2005)

- *Unlock the Power of Lycopene* by David Yeung and Venket Rao (2001)

- *Tomato Power: Lycopene : The Miracle Nutrient That Can Prevent Aging, Heart Disease and Cancer* by James F. Scheer, James F. Balch (1999)

- REF.: Stahl, W. and Sies, H. lycopene: a biologically important carotenoid for humans? Arch.

- Biochem. Biophys. 336: 1-9, 1996

- Gerster, H. The potential role of lycopene for human health. J. Amer. Coll. Nutr. 16: 109-126, 1997

- Arab L et al. Lycopene and the lung. Exp Biol Med (Maywood) 2002;227:894-9.

- Giovannucci E et al. Intake of carotenoids and retinol in relation to risk of prostate cancer. J Natl Cancer Inst 1995;87:1767-76.

- Kucuk O et al. Effects of lycopene supplementation in patients with localized prostate cancer. Exp Biol Med (Maywood) 2002;227:881-5.

- V8 Juice and Cranberry Juice, http://www.judgerc.org/nutrition/Articles/v8juice.html

# Modified Citrus Pectin/MCP/PectaSol

PectaSol is the brand name for modified citrus pectin. More specifically, it is a carbohydrate derived from citrus fruit peel. Pectin is found in several other plants as well, but especially in citrus fruit. Normally used for making jellies, it is also an ingredient in some anti-diarrhea medicines.

Grocery store pectin contains a long-chain molecule that is not absorbed by the body. Modified citrus pectin, on the other hand, is made from shorter molecular chains and is readily absorbed in the intestinal tract.

PectaSol is beneficial to cancer sufferers because of its ability to stop the adhesion of cancer cells. By doing that, it prevents or inhibits metastases. Cancer cells are particularly susceptible to having Modified Citrus Pectin attach to them because of the nature of their cell membranes. Once the modified citrus pectin has attached itself to the cancer cells floating in the blood stream, the cancer cells become coated and unable to attach themselves to the lining of blood vessels or other potential metastatic sites.

Cancer cell metastasis is the mechanism of disease progression that greatly increases the systemic harm caused by cancer and eventual death of most cancer patients. "A special pH-altered form of citrus pectin has been shown to inhibit cancer cell metastasis by interfering with the transport and proliferation of tumor cells to secondary sites in the body, specifically by inhibiting the ability of cancer cells to adhere to other cells."

Research on modified citrus pectin shows it also enhances the activity of natural killer (NK) immune cells that are required to destroy cancer cells which are migrating in the bloodstream.

While the research on modified citrus pectin is still preliminary, the results of the published research indicate that it is completely safe and should be considered for use by any cancer patient who can afford it.

There is a special manufacturing process required to turn regular citrus pectin into the pH-altered citrus pectin that's clinically effective, so the consumption of pectin as it naturally occurs in citrus fruits is not an alternative.


### Further Reading & References

- Fernandez ML J Lipid Res 1995 Nov; 36(11):2394-404, 9.

- Fernandez ML, et al. Am J Clin Nutr 1994 Apr; 59(4):869-78, 11.

- Hexeberg S, et al. Br J Nutr 1994 Feb; 71(2):181-92, 12.

- Inohara H, et al. Glycocon/ J 1994 Dec; 11(6):527-32.

- Matheson HB, et al. J Nutr 1995 Mar; 125(3):454-8, 9.

- Naik, H et al. Proc Ann Meet Am Assoc Cancer Res; 36:A377 1995.

- Pienta, KJ et al. J Natl Cancer Inst 1995 Mar 1; 87(5):331-2.

- Platt D. J Natl Cancer Inst 1992 Mar 18; 84(6):438-42.

- Veldman FJ, et al. Thromb Res 1997 May 1; 86(3):183-96, 7.

- Zhu HG, et al. J Cancer Res Clin Oncol 1994; 120(7):383-8.

- Alternative Cancer Therapies continued, http://www.jhsnp.com/store/pectin.html

- PectaSol® Modified Citrus Pectin Can Slow Progression of Prostate Cancer, http://www.newsdial.com/health/nutraceuticals/petasol.html

# N-Tense®

N-Tense is a commercial combination of medicinal plants from the rainforest. Makers of the supplements claim it is an all natural cancer remedy. Ingredients include graviola, mullaca, guacatonga, espinheira santa, cat's claw, mutamba, vassourinha, and bitter melon.

As a dietary supplement, N-Tense is taken at 6 to 8 capsules daily.

See **Graviola**.

*Further Reading & References*

- Clinical documentation of N-Tense can be found at: http://www.healthyheartht.info/N-tense.pdf

- To locate and purchase this remedy, conduct an Internet search. [Note: this information is provided for informational purposes only and is not intended to be an endorsement of this product.]

# Oncolyn®

Oncolyn is a patented extract of edible plants created by Dr. Arthur D'Jang, MD, PhD. Together with a team of other physicians and scientists, Dr. D'Jang developed this mixture of more than ten ingredients shown to have excellent antioxidant and anticancer capability. The ingredients are: Proanthocyanidins (100 mg), Plant saponins (100 mg), Plant polyphenols (100 mg).

The developers of the product claim that Oncolyn targets free radicals and helps to enhance the immune system. The ingredients listed are merely general categories of phytochemicals and do not permit a detailed assessment of these claims.

### *Further Reading & References*

- Cancer Treatment Registry: Oncolyn, http://cancer-treatment-registry.org/cancer-treatment/Oncolyn.php

- Sante International: What is Oncolyn? http://www.santelink.com/faq.html

- To locate and purchase this remedy, conduct an Internet search. [Note: this information is provided for informational purposes only and is not intended to be an endorsement of this product.]

# Oligomeric Proanthocyanidins (OPC)/Grape Seed Extract

OPC (oligomeric proanthocyanidins) is a group of plant-based compounds named after the flavonoids from which they are derived. They come from many different sources, but the highest concentration of OPCs is found in beans, red wine, the nuts of many plant types, and the leaves and fruits of several plant species. The highest concentrations for supplement use are found in grape seed extract, entire grape extract, and pine bark extract.

Enzymes are involved in converting cancer-causing chemicals to active forms in the cells, which can initiate cancer. Flavonoids in OPC's can interfere with the activity of these enzymes, thus providing an ameliorative effect.

It is believed the flavonoids can influence key enzymes to interfere with free-radical production, thus abolishing tumor promotion and growth in the body. Also, several studies have shown dietary administration of certain flavonoids may significantly halt the growth of cancers; such as been proven with laboratory animals.

Huynh, et al., showed that Pycnogenol® inhibits nitrogen- containing compounds from causing cancer in the gastro-intestinal tract of rats. Nitrogen compounds are known to increase risk in humans for both gut and lung cancers. It was also shown to protect DNA single and double strands from breaking in the presence of oxygen free radical species. This breakage of genetic material is thought to be a possible factor in carcinogenesis (creation of cancer). See **Pycnogenol**.

As a potent antioxidant, OPC is a scavenger of free radicals. OPC contains multiple electron donor sites (hydroxyl sites) that allow it to bind to unstable molecules called free radicals by donating its hydrogen atoms. OPC also recycles other antioxidants such as Vitamin C and glutathione by removing the free radicals they bind with which frees them to interact again with other free radicals.

### *Further Reading & References*

- Oligomeric Proanthocyanidins

- PCs: http://www.herbs2000.com/h_menu/opc.htm

- OPC Antioxidant Reference Guide, http://www.opc.cc/opc-prostate.html

- OPC & Resveratrol, http://greenwoodhealth.net/np/opc.htm

# Omegasentials

Omegasentials is a nutritional supplement based on research by Johanna Budwig. The ingredients include flax seeds, rice bran, inulin, sage, rosemary, fish powder, riboflavin, folic acid, vitamins B-6, B-12, C, and E, niacin, and calcium.

The supplement comes in a powder mix and may be blended with juice, water, or mixed into a smoothie.

Note that Omegasentials is not intended to replace the Budwig Protocol, but rather to be used as a supplement to it. See **Dr. Johanna Budwig**.

### *Further Reading & References*

- Johanna Budwig Revisited, http://www.mnwelldir.org/docs/cancer1/budwig.htm

- Label to Omegasentials, http://www.mnwp.org/omega/label.htm

- Omegasentials Advantage Fact Sheet, http://www.mnwp.org/omega/advantages.htm (Note: for informational purposes only; not an endorsement)

# Pao Pereira/Dr. Mirko Beljanski

Pao pereira is a tree native to Brazil with compounds that apparently have therapeutic benefits. Dr. Mirko Beljanski gets credit for first discovering the therapeutic action of pao pereira and isolating alkaloid compounds from pao pereira called flavopereirines.

In vitro tests by Dr. Beljanski show that extract from the pao pereira may suppress the spread of diseased cells, including those of HIV, herpes viruses, and cancer.

Other studies report that pao pereira extract appears to significantly suppress cell growth as well as induce apoptosis in human prostate cancer cell lines.

Dr. Beljanski's in vitro laboratory tests demonstrated that pao pereira extract effectively suppressed the proliferation of HIV, herpes viruses, cancer, and leukemia cells. Because of such positive results, Doctor Beljanski concluded that pao pereira could be useful in the fight against AIDS, herpes, and cancer.

### Further Reading & References

- Schachter Center for Complementary Medicine, http://www.mbschachter.com/mirko_beljanski1.htm

- "Beta-carboline alkaloid-enriched extract from the amazonian rain forest tree pao pereira suppresses prostate cancer cells." http://www.ncbi.nlm.nih.gov/pubmed/19476740

# Perillyl Alcohol

Perillyl alcohol (POH) is a dietary monoterpene reported to have excellent chemopreventive and chemotherapeutic properties. In an in vivo study, POH effectively prevented the growth of new blood vessels (angiogenesis) and induced apoptosis (natural cell death) of cultured endothelial cells.

POH is derived from the essential oils of various plants, including lavender and peppermint. It can be administered orally. POH is actively used to both prevent and treat cancer. Potential side effects include fatigue, nausea, and early satiety.

"In an article in *Cancer Letters*, perillyl alcohol was shown to reduce the growth of pancreatic tumors injected into hamsters to less than half that of controls. Moreover, 16% of pancreatic tumors treated with perillyl alcohol completely regressed, whereas no control tumors regressed." (Stark et al. 1995).

"Perillyl alcohol and perillic acid are metabolites of limonene. Limonene is only a weak inhibitor of the isoprenylation enzymes of Ras and other proteins, whereas perillyl alcohol and perillic acid are more potent inhibitors." (Hardcastle et al. 1999)

### Further Reading & References

- "Perillyl alcohol is an angiogenesis inhibitor." http://www.ncbi.nlm.nih.gov/entrez/query.fcgi?cmd=Retrieve&db=pubmed&dopt=Abstract&list_uids=15210838

- Memorial Sloan-Kettering Cancer Center: Perillyl Alcohol, http://www.mskcc.org/mskcc/html/69329.cfm

- "Inhibition of protein prenylation by metabolites of limonene." Hardcastle et al., 1999 http://www.ncbi.nlm.nih.gov/pubmed/10075086

- "Chemotherapy of pancreatic cancer with the monoterpene perillyl alcohol," Stark et al., 1995, http://www.sciencedirect.com/science?_ob=ArticleURL&_udi=B6T54-4037W83-P&_user=10&_coverDate=09%2F04%2F1995&_rdoc=1&_fmt=high&_orig=gateway&_origin=gateway&_sort=d&_docanchor=&view=c&_searchStrId=1698752316&_rerunOrigin=google&_acct=C000050221&_version=1&_urlVersion=0&_userid=10&md5=a6effa2d250762ffc51ad5e72e3723bc&searchtype=a

# Papaya/Pawpaw

The papaya is the fruit of a tree native to the tropics of the Americas with orange flesh, dark seeds, and skin with an amber or orange hue. The fruit is rich in an enzyme called papain which is a protease with the ability to break down tough protein molecules.

The juice of the papaya leaf rather than the fruit has been reported to get rid of cancer. Papaya leaf juice is made by boiling papaya leaves and drinking the resulting infusion (tea).

Stan Sheldon, an Australian citizen diagnosed with cancer in 1962, claims drinking this extract healed him. "I was dying from cancer in both lungs when it was suggested to me as an old Aboriginal remedy," he said. "I tried it for two months and then I was required to have a chest x-ray during those compulsory TB checks they used to have. They told me both lungs were clear."

University of Florida researcher Nam Dang, M.D., Ph.D., and colleagues in Japan have documented papaya's dramatic anticancer effect against a broad range of lab-grown tumors, including cancers of the cervix, breast, liver, lung and pancreas. The researchers used an extract made from dried papaya leaves, and the anticancer effects were stronger when cells received larger doses of the tea.

Papaya leaf extract appears to boost the production of key signaling molecules called Th1-type cytokines. This regulation of the immune system, in addition to papaya's direct antitumor effect on various cancers, suggests possible therapeutic strategies that use the immune system to fight cancers. This was documented in a paper published in the Feb . 17, 2010 *Journal of Ethnopharmacology* by Dr. Dang and his colleagues.

Many confuse the papaya with the Pawpaw because the papaya is actually called "paw paw" in Australia and New Zealand. However, it is not related to the North American pawpaw tree.

### *Further Reading & References*

- "Papaya Leaf: The Anti-Cancer Treatment," Dr. Hulda Clark, http://www.huldaclarkzappers.com/php2/papayaleaf.php

- *Papaya The Medicine Tree* by Harald W. Tietze, (2006)

- "Papaya extract thwarts growth of cancer cells in lab tests," http://www.eurekalert.org/pub_releases/2010-03/uof-pet030910.php

# Pawpaw

The pawpaw tree boasts the largest edible fruit native to North America. It's often confused with papaya, a fruit that looks similar but is not related. The confusion stems from the fact that the American papaya is called "paw paw" by many people, because the two resemble one another. It also confuses things that papaya fruit has cancer-healing properties in its own right.

The pawpaw (also called the American pawpaw) is mostly found in the Eastern part of the U.S. It's rich with proteins, beneficial fats, and complex carbohydrates. The pawpaw species *Asimina triloba* has powerful bioactive compounds called annonaceous acetogenins. These compounds have been proven to fight insects, parasites, and most importantly, cancer cells.

Pawpaw takes on cancer cells in a different way than other natural cancer fighters. It's believed to be the single most effective treatment to kill multiple-drug-resistant (MDR) cancer cells.

It has also reportedly been successful in shrinking tumors naturally and preventing the growth of new cancer cells with minimal side effects. When this plant is used in conjunction with chemotherapy, the chemo is more effective at tackling MDR cells. It appears pawpaw can improve the effectiveness of chemotherapy.

The most potent acetogenins are found in an extract of pawpaw tree twigs. The acetogenins, which are fatty acid derivatives, kill cancer by attacking the life energy source of cancer cells, their ATP. ATP, or adenosine triphosphate, fuels the production of DNA and RNA and helps cancer cells multiply. The cancer cells are no longer able to grow. The cells also begin to starve because ATP is no longer present to produce blood vessels as a food source to cells. Without these blood vessels to feed on, cancer cells lose their source of nutrients and either weaken or die.

Lab results show that pawpaw acetogenins focus on cancer cells and don't seem to affect healthy cells. Pawpaw appears to be the only cancer treatment known to effectively stand up to MDR cells. Similar plants like the graviola (also known as the guanabana) have similar acetogenin properties, but are not as potent as pawpaw.

The man credited with discovering the pawpaw cancer treatment is Dr. Jerry McLaughlin. This PhD of Pharmacognosy studied 3,500 botanical extracts for 28 years and found evidence to support pawpaw as a powerful cancer killer. For a clinical trial, McLaughlin led a team of researchers who tested 94 cancer patients. The type of cancer varied in each patient, the stage of cancer varied (but many were at the terminal stage), and the treatment procedure for each patient also varied.

Some patients tried pawpaw in conjunction with chemotherapy and radiation, some tried it after failed attempts at chemo and radiation, and others tried the extract with no other form of treatment.

The constant factor within each test was a daily regimen of four pawpaw pills. Despite all the other variables, the results looked promising:

- A 73-year-old male with stage four prostate cancer that spread to his hip bone, abdomen, and neck, saw an improvement within six weeks of taking pawpaw. A CT scan showed 25% reduction in the tumor masses and his blood levels remained constant. At the end of the 18-month trial, he remained in stable condition.

- A 62-year-old female with breast cancer took pawpaw concurrently with a seven-month chemotherapy treatment. In that time, her tumor nearly disappeared. She underwent a lumpectomy to remove any traces of cancer, but the surgery found no metastatic cancer. The patient experienced complete remission.

- A 66-year-old male participant with terminal lung cancer had already tried two years of chemo. The drugs were unsuccessful due to drug-resistant cancer cells. After two months of pawpaw treatment, his blood tumor markers decreased from 275 to 222, he gained five pounds, and his energy allowed him to walk on his own — something he had not done for many months as a bedridden patient.

- A 59-year-old female with breast cancer decided against chemo, radiation, and surgery altogether. Within four months of taking pawpaw, her blood levels of relevant cancer markers fell to a normal range and the size of her tumor shrank. Her doctor reported improvement in her overall energy level.

The trials showed evidence that pawpaw was effective. It was reported that of 20 terminal cancer patients in the study, 13 survived the 18-month trial and were all in stable condition.

It also appeared that those undergoing chemotherapy in conjunction with pawpaw experienced a reduction in side effects and a noticeable boost in energy.

Apparently, pawpaw can work as an emetic, like ipecac. But, the urge to vomit seems to go away after a couple weeks of use. No other side effects have been reported.

Note: Pawpaw should never be used to prevent cancer. It's only useful as a treatment.

### *Further Reading & References*

- "ImmunoCellular Therapeutics: At the Forefront of Targeting Cancer Stem Cells," http://www.dailymarkets.com/stock/2010/11/09/immunocellular-therapeutics-at-the-forefront-of-targeting-cancer-stem-cells/

- Henderson, B., 13 Nov. 2008. Cancer-Free: Your Guide to Gentle, Non-Toxic Healing, 3rd ed.

- "Introduction to Pawpaw." http://www.pawpawresearch.com/pawpaw-intro.htm

- McLaughlin, J, PhD, G. Benson, and J. Forsythe, MD. 2003. *A novel mechanism for the control of clinical cancer: Inhibition of the production of adenosine triphosphate (ATP) with a standardized extract of pawpaw.* http://www.pawpawresearch.com/pawpaw-trials1.pdf

- Oberlies, N., C. Chang, and J. McLaughlin. "Pawpaw shows promise in fighting drug-resistant tumors." http://www.pawpawresearch.com/purdue-mdr-97.htm

- Winter, Paul. "Pawpaw Alternative Cancer Treatment Comparison." http://alternativecancer.us/pawpaw.htm

# Red Raspberry Capsules

Ellagic acid is a naturally occurring plant phenol found in raspberries, strawberries, cranberries, walnuts, pecans, pomegranates, and other plant foods.

Clinical tests conducted at the Hollings Cancer Institute at the Medical University of South Carolina (MUSC) show that it may be an extremely potent way to prevent cancer.

Dr. Daniel Nixon published work that showed apoptosis occurring within cervical cancer cells after being exposed to ellagic acid. Ellagic acid leads to G1 arrest of cancer cells, thus inhibiting and stopping mitosis (cancer cell division). Ellagic acid prevents destruction of the P53 gene by cancer cells. P53 is regarded as the safeguard of mutagenic activity in cervical cells.

Tests reveal similar results for breast, pancreas, esophageal, skin, colon, and prostate cancer cells. Consuming one cup (150 grams) of red raspberries per day prevents the development of cancer cells. Results were achieved with laboratory animals given ellagic acid from natural sources and also synthetic ellagic acid.

Red-raspberry seed concentrate was used in the clinical studies at the Hollings Cancer Institute. This is commercially available as red raspberry capsules/red raspberry extract.

See **Ellagic Acid**.

*Further Reading & References*

- Red Raspberry Ellagic Acid, http://www.therapure.com/ellagic-acid/

# Resveratrol

Resveratrol is currently a hot topic in many medical circles and has been the subject of several human and animal trials and studies. It is a polyphenol that is produced naturally by several plants when under attack by bacteria or fungi.

According to the National Cancer Institute, resveratrol is one of a category of plant compounds called polyphenols. Resveratrol is a potent, antioxidant-like compound found in the skin of red grapes and in red wine. It is known to reduce oxidative stress and can also stop cancer from forming. It has been shown to kill a variety of existing cancer cells as well as protect healthy cells from damaging free radicals that make individuals more vulnerable to disease, including cancer.

According to a study published in the July 1st, 2008 issue of *Cancer Prevention Research*, Doctors Ercole Cavalieri and Eleanor Rogen of the University of Nebraska Medical Center wanted to determine how resveratrol might impact the formation of cancer cells.

The researchers tested a blend of resveratrol, the amino acid n-acetyl-l-cysteine, lipoic acid, and melatonin. They found that adding resveratrol greatly enhanced the body's natural protective mechanisms. Resveratrol shows definite anti-cancer action when put in direct contact with tumors such as those found in the skin and in gastrointestinal tracts.

These scientists tested the formula with and without resveratrol. They found that adding resveratrol greatly reduced the formation of breast cancer cells.

More studies are underway to see how resveratrol affects the initiation, promotion, and progression of cancer. In addition to killing breast cancer cells, studies have shown so far that resveratrol could be an effective way to treat neuroblastoma, eye cancer, prostate cancer, and skin cancer.

Many other anti-cancer studies of resveratrol have shown success, such as one conducted in 1997 that showed skin cancer development in mice was halted after the animals received resveratrol. In another study, resveratrol reduced the number and size of tumors in rats, specifically in esophageal tumors.

It is unknown how much of a resveratrol concentration is needed to prevent cancer. It is also unknown whether the relationship between alcohol consumption and resveratrol leads to overall good health. Whatever the resveratrol benefits of wine may be, heavy consumption of alcohol carries significant and well-established health risks. Resveratrol supplements would seem to be the safer choice.

Beer and hard liquor do not contain resveratrol.

Resveratrol may be taken orally for anticancer as well as general health benefits, or applied topically for skin cancer.

*Further Reading & References*

- "Role of resveratrol in prevention and therapy of cancer: preclinical and clinical studies." http://www.ncbi.nlm.nih.gov/entrez/query.fcgi?cmd=Retrieve&db=pubmed&dopt=Abstract&list_uids=15517885

- *The Longevity Factor: How Resveratrol and Red Wine Activate Genes for a Longer and Healthier Life* by Joseph Maroon and Joseph Baur (2009)

- *Resveratrol in Health and Disease (Oxidative Stress and Disease)* by Bharat B. Aggarwal and Shishir Shishodia (2005)

- Resveratrol, http://en.wikipedia.org/wiki/Resveratrol

- Lu, F., Zahid, M. et al. 2008. Resveratrol Prevents Estrogen-DNA Adduct Formation and Neoplastic Transformation in MCF-10F Cells. Retrieved 1/28/11 from http://cancerpreventionresearch. aacrjournals.org/content/1/2/135.abstract

# Mucorihicin

Supposedly an "87% effective treatment from Pittsburgh", but no details can be located.

# Myrrh

Myrrh is a type of fragrant sap most often used in incense. Specifically, it is dried gum resin from different trees of the Commiphora species.

"Myrrh has a long history of healing, with many references throughout the ages to its health-giving properties, with virtually no toxicity," says Mohamed M. Rafi, an assistant professor in the department of food science at Rutgers University.

"What makes it such an exciting player in the anti-cancer field is not only how well it kills cancer cells in general, but how it kills those that are resistant to other anti-cancer drugs," Continues Rafi.

"The myrrh compound definitely appears to be unique in this way; it is working where other compounds have failed."

Interestingly, myrrh can "inactivate" a protein called Bcl-2, a natural factor that is overproduced by cancer cells, particularly in the breast and prostate.

### Further Reading & References

- Myrrh as Anti-Cancer Therapy, http://search.store.yahoo.net/annieappleseedproject/cgi-bin/n search?catalog=annieappleseedproject&query=myrrh&.autodone=http%3A%2F%2Fwww. annieappleseedproject.org%2Fnsearch.html

- Memorial Sloan-Kettering Cancer Center: Myrrh, http://www.mskcc.org/mskcc/html/69309.cfm

# Procyanidins

Procyanidins, also known as oligomeric proanthocyanidin (OPC), leucocyanidin, leucoanthocyanin, and condensed tannins, is a class of flavanols that can be extracted from certain plant species. They can be found in grape seed extract, red grapes, the red skins of peanuts, coconuts, and in the skins of apples.

Proanthocyanidins are sold as nutritional supplements in most of the world.

These supplements appear to have anti-cancer effects on colon cancer. The French National Institute for Health and Medical Research found that key chemicals in apples called procyanidins reduced precancerous lesions in laboratory animals by half compared to those without apples in their diet. Procyanidins are polyphenols, mostly concentrated in the skin of the apple. They triggered signals that led to apoptosis (cell suicide), thus thwarting the growth and spread of cancer. Further study in humans is forthcoming.

### Further Reading & References

- American Association for Cancer Research 10/19/2004

- "Eat the Peel: Apples' Anti-Cancer Agents Are in the Skin." http://fruitguys.com/almanac/2010/11/01/eat-the-peel-apples%E2%80%99-anti-cancer-agents-are-in-the-skin

# Pycnogenol/Polybioflavanoids

Pycnogenol® (pronounced pic-nodge-a-nol) is a patented antioxidant from France that is made from a pine tree bark extract. Pycnogenol® describes "an entire class of bioflavanoids that are composed of polyphenols, or Proanthocyanidin complexes." The bioflavanoids may be extracted from pine bark, lemon tree bark, grape seeds, grape skins, or cranberries.

An excess of free radicals in a person's body causes major damage, including cancer. The best free radical killer is reportedly Pycnogenol®.

The normal oxygen atom in your body has four pairs of electrons. However the effects of radiation, sunlight, air pollution, harmful chemicals, food additives, tobacco smoke, infections and stress can rob one of the electrons from the oxygen atom. This atom then becomes a free radical. It tries to replace its lost electron by raiding other molecules. It will rob an electron from a molecule in a cell wall.

This robbed molecule proceeds to replace its lost electron by robbing another molecule, and a chain reaction is created. This leads to disintegration of the cell, and opens the door to cancer and many other ills. It promotes cancer by altering the DNA, thereby damaging the way in which the cells in the body replicate. This leads to aging. Some studies suggest that free radicals are a major cause of aging.

Pycnogenol® is a powerful antioxidant that neutralizes free radicals. An antioxidant has extra electrons, which it can "give up" to the free radicals, thereby rendering them harmless.

Pycnogenol® is reported to have the ability, in a matter of a few months, to destroy all of the excess free radicals that the body has built up over a lifetime. It comes in tablet form. Dr. Lamar Rosquist recommends one mg. of Pycnogenol® daily per pound of body weight during the initial period of eliminating all accumulated free radicals. This means that a 200 pound man would take 200 mg. of Pycnogenol® daily for the first two or three months. Later, a lower maintenance level dosage can be taken.

Pycnogenol® is claimed to treat 60 free radical-related disorders including cancer, Alzheimer's, A105, hemorrhoids, and senility. Pycnogenol® has the capability to bond collagen fibers and reverse tissue damage and injury. It is absorbed into the bloodstream in about 20 minutes. Once absorbed, the maximum protective effect lasts about 72 hours. Proponents claim that Pycnogenol® causes no adverse effects and can also assist vitamin C in entering cells.

Pycnogenol also has the ability to kill breast cancer cells whilst leaving normal cells unharmed. According to an *Anticancer Research* article (2000 Jul-Aug;20(4):2417-20) entitled "Selective induction of apoptosis in human mammary cancer cells (MCF-7) by pycnogenol," the response of human breast cancer cells (MCF-7) and normal human mammary cells to apoptosis in the presence of pycnogenol was compared.

"Pycnogenol is a mixture of flavonoid compounds extracted from the bark of pine trees. …. Apoptosis, as detected by DAPI staining, was significantly higher in MCF-7 cells treated with pycnogenol than the untreated cells. The presence of pycnogenol did not significantly alter the number of apoptotic cells in MCF-10 samples. These results suggest that pycnogenol selectively induced death in human mammary cancer cells (MCF-7) and not in normal human mammary MCF-10 cells."

### *Further Reading & References*

- "Selective induction of apoptosis in human mammary cancer cells (MCF-7) by pycnogenol." http://www.ncbi.nlm.nih.gov/entrez/query.fcgi?cmd=Retrieve&db=pubmed&dopt=Abstract&list_uids=10953304

# Ukrain/Greater Celandine/Chelidonium major

Ukrain™ is a product made up of alkaloids and a synthetic drug called ThioTEPA. It is used to treat cancer, HIV and AIDS, and hepatitis, apparently due to a cytotoxic (cell-killing) effect on cellular oxygen consumption and the ability to induce apoptosis (natural cell death).

Ukrain was first developed in 1978 by Dr. Wassyl J. Nowicky, director of the Ukrainian Anti-Cancer Institute of Vienna. It is a mixture of Greater Celandine (Chelidonium major) and an old long-established cytotoxic (chemotherapy) drug, ThioTEPA. The idea is that the combination of the two makes treatment effective at far lower doses than the usual toxic amounts of ThioTEPA.

Greater Celandine is a poppy-like plant, filled with a bright, orange-colored juice. It has long been stated in the folk literature to have disease-fighting effects. It has been known for centuries in Russia as a cancer treatment. It contains alkaloids with known anti-cancer activity.

Such alkaloids taken by themselves can be irritating or even toxic. What makes Ukrain so unique is that this forced marriage of herb and drug yields a compound that is almost totally lacking in toxicity to normal cells, according to its proponents. Yet it seems to have a strong affinity for killing cancer cells. In hamsters and rats, for example, no clinical signs of toxicity or damage to embryos could be found. The only toxicity was a slight decrease in the average hamster litter size.

In addition, for three years healthy human volunteers in Poland, Austria, and Germany received repeated courses of the new drug. There was some local pain, and a few reported cases of drowsiness as well as increased thirst and urge to urinate. But, there were no other significant side-effects.

Ukrain was first unveiled at the 13th International Congress of Chemotherapy in Vienna in August 1983. Ukrain (spelled like Dr. Nowicky's native country, but without the final "E") is classified as a semisynthetic "reaction product" or "conjugate" created by the merger of the herb and the drug. It is patented in both Europe and the U.S. and has been the subject of many scientific papers.

Clinical studies have shown that this combination of ThioTEPA and a highly effective derivative of a certain plant extract improves the overall health and strength of terminal cancer patients, boosts their immune systems, and blocks tumor growth. It appears to be effective against many types of cancer, except for leukemia and brain cancer.

Ukrain has been shown to stimulate the immune system of mice, which could contribute to cancer prevention. In addition, when Ukrain was given intravenously to mice, it had a pronounced tumor growth inhibiting activity. By day 15, only one out of five such mice had developed tumors, while all five control mice had tumors and were already beginning to show signs of cachexia (wasting), according to doctors at the University of Miami where the study was conducted. This difference was attributed to the stimulation of macrophages, part of the immune system.

Ukrain has been tested against 60 different human cancer cell lines at the National Cancer Institute. A 100% growth inhibition was found in nearly all cell lines. A possible mechanism for this effect is that Ukrain increases the oxygen consumption of both normal and malignant cells. Oxygen is known to be toxic to cancer cells.

Ukrain has also been shown to decrease DNA, RNA, and protein synthesis in malignant cells. This makes it highly toxic to cancer cells, though it shows little or no toxicity to non-cancerous cells in the test-tube (e.g., endothelial cells or fibroblasts).

In another study conducted under contract to the Ministry of Science and Research of Austria, the drug was found to be cytostatic or cytotoxic to human leukemias, non-small and small-cell lung cancers, colon cancers, central nervous system cancer, melanomas, ovarian cancer and renal cancer.

Investigation of Ukrain is now underway not just in Austria, but at many institutions in Canada, France, Germany the Netherlands, Switzerland, Thailand and even Swaziland (in Africa). Currently, Ukrain is only available through unconventional clinics.

It is also believed that Ukrain may extend the survival rate of pancreatic cancer patients. More research is needed.

### Further Reading & References

- Ukrainian Anti Cancer Institute, http://www.ukrin.com

- Memorial Sloan-Kettering Cancer Center: Ukrain: http://www.mskcc.org/mskcc/html/69402.cfm

- "Intriguing New Anticancer Compound from East Europe," The Moss Reports, http://www.ralphmoss.com/html/ukrain.shtml

- "Ukrain: A New Cancer Cure?" Cancer Evolution, http://www.cancerevolution.info/index.php?/cancer-therapy/alternative-therapies/ukrain-a-new-cancer-cure.html

## Yucca glaucoma

The Yucca is a plant native to the Mojave Desert in the southwestern region of the United States. The steroidal saponins within the plant are medicinal ingredients with anti-inflammatory properties.

Only the fresh yucca flower is said to have anti-cancer activity, not the leaves, fruits, roots, or seeds. The activity is lost when the flowers wilt or dry. Yucca appears to also serve as a diuretic, blood purifier, and a cardiac stimulator. Yucca saponins are believed to help with absorption of nutrients while reducing toxins.

The flowers and the fruit are edible but should only be eaten freshly picked from the plant. One source recommends eating only the petals, as the centers of the flower are bitter.

### Further Reading & References

- Over 250 Alternative Cancer Treatments …, http://www.new-cancer-treatments.org/Lists/Big_List_T_.html

- Yucca glaucoma, http://www.encognitive.com/node/2710

# Yuccalive®

Yucca Schidigera is a substance that has been used for thousands of years by Native Americans of the southwest region of the U.S. It has natural healing properties currently under investigation, but at the very least it's known to be high in vitamins A, B-complex, and C. Yucca also contains significant amounts of iron, calcium, potassium, phosphorous, and copper,

The saponin in yucca appears to reduce stress and swelling in joints and helps eliminate toxins from the colon.

Yuccalive is an herbal product manufactured in China and believed to provide, when combined with Chinese herbal formula Cessiac® (Kang Ji), an excellent body cleansing and purification program. Yucca is the main ingredient in the mixture, along with licorice root, fennel seed, clove buds, anise seeds, honey, and cinnamon bark.

### Further Reading & References

- Yuccalive: Yucca Schidigera, http://www.encognitive.com/node/2711

# Greens

## Alfalfa (Medicago Sativa)

Alfalfa is known to contain a large amount of chlorophyll, beta-carotene, vitamin E, and the amino acid L-Canavanine. This particular amino acid is an active anti-cancer agent believed to have significant antibacterial, antiviral, and anti-tumor capabilities.

L-Canavanine is antineoplastic, which means it inhibits and combats the development of cancer. It has been noted to be particularly successful against several animal-bearing carcinomas and cancer cell lines.

This amino acid is abundant in at least ten varieties of commercially-grown spouts. Alfalfa seeds are also rich in this amino acid. This makes alfalfa a significant source of L-Canavanine.

In addition, researchers at Iowa State University detected a chemical in genetically modified alfalfa that may prevent the development of colon cancer.

Modified alfalfa is high in resveratrol glucoside, which is a substance that prevents root rot when soil becomes too wet for the plant. Resveratrol is already known to help prevent skin cancer, so researchers decided to see if putting this substance in a person's diet could prevent colon cancer. Primary research showed the chemical had a preventative effect on early-stage colon cancer.

Alfalfa is most often harvested as hay and used as food for cattle and especially dairy cattle. It has been used as an herbal medicine for over 1,500 years, especially by the Chinese. Alfalfa can be purchased as an herbal tea or extract, or as a nutritional supplement.

### Further Reading & References

- Alfalfa (Medicago Sativa), http://www.encognitive.com/node/2441

- "Phytochemical and pharmacological potential of Medicago sativa: A review." http://www.bioportfolio.com/resources/pmarticle/104289/Phytochemical-And-Pharmacological-Potential-Of-Medicago-Sativa-A-Review.html

- Alfalfa Fights Colon Cancer, http://hayandforage.com/news/farming_alfalfa_fights_colon/

## Barley Grass/BarleyGreen®

Dr. Yoshihide Hagiwara, President of the Hagiwara Institute of Health in Japan, gets credit for the most extensive research on barley grass. Hagiwara reportedly researched over 150 different plants during a span of 13 years. His research indicated that barley contained the highest number of quality nutrients needed by the body for growth, repair, and well-being.

Another scientist, biologist Yasuo Hotta from the University of California, La Jolla, discovered barley grass contains a substance called P4D1. This substance has strong anti-inflammatory capabilities and proved itself up to the task of repairing damaged DNA in the cells of the body. This meant a patient could use barley grass to aid in the prevention of cell death, carcinogenesis, and aging.

Hotta also revealed during a Japan Pharmacy Science Association meeting that P4D1 could suppress or cure illnesses such as pancreatitis, stomatitis, inflammation of the oral cavity, and dermatitis. In addition, he said it could aid in healing lacerations of the stomach and duodenum. In his opinion, barley juice is much stronger than steroid drugs and has the benefit of fewer side effects.

Barley grass extracts have also been found to benefit the body's immune system and protect human fibroblasts against carcinogenic agents. In an unpublished report, Dr. Allan Goldstein, a professor at the George Washington School of Medicine, Washington D.C., claims results showing that a Vitamin E analog isolated from green barley killed a leukemic cell line. He writes:

"Barley grass leaf extract dramatically inhibits the growth of human prostatic cancer cells grown in tissue culture. It may provide a new nutritional approach to the treatment of prostate cancer."*

Dr. Howard Lutz, who is director of the Institute of Preventive Medicine in Washington, D.C., said this about barley grass:

"[Barley grass is] one of the most incredible products of this decade. It improves stamina, sexual energy, clarity of thought, and reduces addiction to things that are bad for you. It also improves the texture of the skin, and heals the dryness associated with aging."**

Those who find they cannot tolerate the flavor of wheatgrass juice may find barley grass juice more palatable. It is milder, although quite bitter, compared to the sweetness of wheatgrass juice.

BarleyGreen® has always been grown and produced by Dr. Y. Hagiwara's company, Green Foods Corporation, the marketing arm of which is now YH International.

Dr. George Malkmus, in his all-raw Hallelujah Diet, used BarleyGreen® as his main raw food. Dr. Francisco Contreras, who runs the Oasis of Hope Cancer Hospital in Mexico, provides BarleyGreen® to his patients. Perhaps the most visible testimonial for BarleyGreen® is provided by Lorraine Day, M.D., who treated her breast cancer with natural herbal remedies that included BarleyGreen®. It also comes highly recommended by Bill Henderson, creator of the Henderson Protocol for self-treatment of cancer, and author of the book *Cancer-Free*.

### Further Reading & References

- *Wheatgrass Nature's Finest Medicine Steve Meyerowitz Sproutman, New Edition 2006, http://www.naturesgreenz.com/sprouts.html

- **Barley Grass, http://www.wellbeingwithnutrition.co.uk/content/index.php/articles/42-super-foods/76-barley-grass

- ***The World's MOST POPULAR Green Juice Drink, http://www.drday.com/barleygreen/index.html

- *Everything I Know About Nutrition I Learned From Barley* by Betty Kamen, et al (2002)

- *Barley Grass Juice: Rejuvenation Elixir and Natural, Healthy Power Drink* by Barbara Simonsohn (2001)

- *Green Leaves of Barley: Nature's Miracle Rejuvenator* by Mary Ruth Swope and David Darbro (1996)

- Lorraine Day, MD discusses… "Natural, Alternative Therapies for all Diseases, including Cancer and AIDS," http://www.drday.com/

- *Cancer-Free: Your Guide to Gentle, Non-toxic Healing* by Bill Henderson (2007)

# Chlorella

Chlorella is a type of single-celled, green algae. It stands apart from other "superfoods" in its ability to efficiently create chemical energy (i.e., photosynthetic efficiency) up to levels of 8%. This means it uses photosynthesis to rapidly multiply plant cells, using only carbon dioxide, water, sunlight, and certain minerals. In short, green algae grow fast, making the plant easy to cultivate in large quantities with little effort.

As a food source, chlorella is known to be high in protein and other nutrients. It also boasts 19 amino acids, several vitamins and minerals, and unsaturated essential fatty acids. The medicinal properties of chlorella include detoxification of the body from heavy metals and other chemical pollutants, many of which are precursors to several degenerative diseases.

Chlorella contains a special phytochemical called chlorella growth factor (CGF) which is believed to be the reason for its therapeutic effects.

Chlorella is not meant to be a quick fix, but rather something that can help one achieve long-term optimal health. It often takes two to three months to feel the benefits of chlorella. The major benefit chlorella offers is a strengthened immune system which goes a long way in preventing or treating cancer.

In Japan, chlorella is one of the most popular nutritional supplements, used daily by millions. This popularity is partly because the Japanese government classifies chlorella as a "functional food," meaning it is a food scientifically proven to be beneficial to humans.

Beyond the documented therapeutic effects of chlorella, many users report increased energy levels,

improved mental clarity, a clearer complexion, a positive sense of wellbeing, and a decrease in stress-induced tension or anxiety.

Some chlorella users may have trouble in the early stages of taking chlorella as they become accustomed to the effects of the supplement, which includes shedding toxins. Examples of reactions to the detoxification process include slight headaches, stomach cramps, nausea, skin blemishes, or bowel irregularity. These symptoms usually diminish and disappear within a week to ten days as the body adjusts and moves closer to biochemical balance.

A 1990 study conducted at the University of Tokushima School of Medicine in Japan showed that chlorella could effectively suppress tumor growth.* Other studies have shown chlorella's ability to raise albumin levels in the body in order to prevent cancerous changes and extend the life span of cells. Still other studies showed chlorella could raise the survival rate of glioblastoma patients by 30%.**

Most chlorella supplements are taken either in pill form or as a powder mixed with liquid.

### Further Reading & References

- *The Green Foods Bible: Everything You Need to Know About Barley Grass, Wheatgrass, Kamut, Chlorella, Spirulina And More* by David Sandoval (2007).

- *Herbal Medicine, Healing & Cancer* by Donald Yance, Arlene (1999).

- *Chlorella* by William C. Y. Lee (1998).

- *Chlorella: The Emerald Food* by Dhyana Bewicke (1993).

- *Oral administration of Chlorella vulgaris augments concomitant antitumor immunity, http://www.ncbi.nlm.nih.gov/entrez/query.fcgi?cmd=Retrieve&db=pubmed&dopt=Abstract&list_uids=2229925

- **Chlorella as a powerful defense against cancer, http://www.naturalnews.com/008527.html

- Chlorella: Small but Mighty, http://ecobites.com/eco-news-articles/herbal-a-natural-remedies/2035-chlorella-small-but-mighty

# Chlorophyll/Chlorophyllin

The antimutagenic effects of chlorophyllin, or chlorophyll, were first made known to the public in 1989 by the Life Extension Foundation. The Foundation recommended supplementation with chlorophyll based on a study from the journal *Mutation Research* that showed the plant extract to be more effective than other food supplements.

A separate study in *Mutation Research* found chlorophyll could suppress the mutagenic activity of carcinogens by more than 90%. This is the highest rate of suppression for deadly gene mutations known for supplements. In fact, most of the health benefits of chlorophyll have to do with its antimutagenic and anticarcinogenic properties.

Unlike other antioxidants which merely quench free radicals, chlorophyll traps heterocyclic hydrocarbon carcinogens by reacting with their backbone, making it impossible for them to form adducts with DNA. An adduct is formed when a carcinogen combines with DNA to form a single reaction product.

Here are just a few of the more than 50 cancer-causing agents chlorophyll can protect against: benzopyrene, dimethylbenzanthracene (DMBA), dibenzopyrene, TRP-P2, aflatoxin B-1 and aflatoxin B-2, 2-aminoanthracene, 2-nitrofluorene, 1-nitropyrene, 1-methyl-6-phenylimidazo [4,5-pyridine] (PHIP), and 2-amino-3-methylimidazo [4,5-f] quinoline (IQ).

The majority of these carcinogens can be found in foods cooked at high temperatures.

One of the worst carcinogens found in the human diet is aflatoxin B-1, which occurs in staple grains like wheat, rice, and rye that get infected with a type of fungus. This fungus is particularly problematic in Third World countries, which is also where farmers tend to have some of the highest liver cancer rates in the world.

In one study, researchers reduced aflatoxin urinary bio-markers by 55% by giving farmers tablets of 100 mg of chlorophyllin three times a day with meals.* The researchers estimated this doubled the time needed for liver cancer to develop, moving from 20 to 40 years. This study underscored the relationship between dietary aflatoxin reduction, DNA adducts, and lower cancer rates for both humans and animals.

In another study, the anticancer properties of chlorophyllin were compared with those of green and black tea. Chlorophyllin was found to be much more potent as an antimutagenic agent with protection that extended to more carcinogens than those affected by tea.

Chlorophyllin was also found to be extremely effective in protecting against DNA adduct formation in human breast cells. It inhibited adduct formation 65% of the time.

In-vitro studies with chlorophyllin show it can capably inhibit cytochrome P-450 liver enzymes. When this enzyme activity was reduced, the result was lower cancer rates and a longer lifespan.

A significant amount of research both through animal and human studies shows that a 100-mg capsule of chlorophyllin should be taken with any meal known to contain a lot of carcinogens, such as a dinner of grilled or barbecued meat. Assuming the main benefit of supplementing with chlorophyllin is to detoxify dietary mutagens, it should always be taken with food.

Known side effects of chlorophyllin include occasional diarrhea, greenish stool, and possibly a pale green color in blood serum. Coloring of the sera is believed to be a good thing, as it shows the likely effect chlorophyllin has as an antioxidant and antimutagenic agent in the bloodstream.

Algae, spirulina, chlorella, wheat grass, barley grass, and dark green leafy vegetables are all good sources of chlorophyllin. Supplements of chlorophyll as powder, capsules, tablets, and drinks are also widely available.

### *Further Reading & References*

- *"Chlorophyllin intervention reduces aflatoxin–DNA adducts in individuals at high risk for liver cancer," http://www.ncbi.nlm.nih.gov/pmc/articles/PMC64728/

- Cancer Prevention, http://www.lef.org/protocols/prtcls-txt/t-prtcl-149.html

- "Dietary modifiers of carcinogenesis," http://www.ncbi.nlm.nih.gov/pmc/articles/PMC1518962/

- Rudolph C. The therapeutic value of chlorophyll. Clin Med Surg 1930;37:119-21.

- Chernomorsky SA, Segelman AB. Biological activities of chlorophyll derivatives. N J Med 1988;85:669-73.

- Gruskin B. Chlorophyll—its therapeutic place in acute and suppurative disease. Am J Surg 1940;49:49-56.

- Hayatsu H, Negishi T, Arimoto S, et al. Porphyrins as potential inhibitors against exposure to carcinogens and mutagens. Mutat Res 1993;290:79-85.

# GC10-100

GC10-100 is an organic medicinal extract that functions in the body by altering the chemistry of cancer cells and converting them back to normal function. The main ingredients for the blends of GC10 through 100 come from natural formulations extracted from specific organic fruits and vegetables and then separated into their respective molecular components. The extract itself is then created by combining these components into one of the 90 different formulations.

The components include these micro-compounds:

- Terpenes

- Organosulfides

- Aromatic isothiocyanates

- Indoles

- Dithiolethiones

- Phenols

- Flavonoids

- Tannins

- Ellagic Acid

- Conjugated Dienoic linoleic acids

- Gluccarates.

- Nerolidol

Several of these micro-compounds work to block or suppress the effects of carcinogens.

GC10-100 is said to offer a chemotherapeutic effect through the fruit and vegetable extracts because of the high concentration of micro-molecular nutrients found in each formulation.

The extract mixtures prompt an anti-tumor effect after reaching specific levels in a patient's blood serum. Most often, this takes at least ten to fifteen days of treatment.

This treatment has been primarily used to treat cancer patients in the advanced stages of the disease. It appears to be most effective when the patient is not taking any other strong medication so that the immune system and other regenerative processes are at their best. The ideal approach is to follow a nutritious diet and avoid unnecessary supplements.

### *Further Reading & References*

- Protocol for Clinical Studies to Evaluate the Chemotherapeutic Effect of GC10-100 in Advanced Cancer, http://www.dietcancer.com/html/patients.html

- Protocol for Clinical Studies to Evaluate the Chemotherapeutic Effect of GC10-100 in Advanced Cancer, http://www.gc100.com/html/protocol_gc100.html

# Green Tea/EGCG/Green Tea Extract

Green tea comes from the leaves of the plant Camellia sinensis. The leaves undergo minimal oxidation in order to be used as a tea or tea extract. Dry green tea leaves are about 40% polyphenols by weight, and the most potent of these is EGCG (epigallocatechin gallate). These polyphenols in green tea are thought to affect enzyme activity in the body. It's believed they can slow the conversion of normal cells into tumor cells.

Green tea polyphenols (GTP), particularly EGCG, curb an enzyme needed for cancer cell growth and thereby kills cancer cells while sparing the healthy cells. Scientists believe that EGCG actually inhibits cancer cell growth and division, leading to apoptosis (programmed cell death). EGCG also has strong free-radical-scavenging (antioxidant) properties.

EGCG is such a potent antioxidant, it's considered by some to be more beneficial than Vitamins E or C. Researchers from the University of Kansas conducted a study in 1997 that showed EGCG to be twice as powerful as resveratrol, a known cancer cell killer.

Drinking green tea may also help protect women from getting breast cancer, according to a study that appeared in the July 2001 issue of the *Journal of Cellular Biochemistry*. The study, which used rats, found a significant reduction in the size and malignancy of breast tumors in those animals that were fed green tea.

Green tea has been used for centuries in Asia both to prevent cancer and as a favored beverage. Dr. Fujiki, a representative of Japan's National Cancer Center, once pointed out that green tea was not a guaranteed way to prevent every cancer but that it is the most cheap and reliable option available to the general public. The typical amount consumed is 1-3 cups per day. Recently, green tea in capsule form has become available, although the clinical benefits of encapsulation are less well-known.

Cell biologist Dr. Stephen Hsu, from the Medical College of Georgia Department of Oral Biology, found that green tea polyphenols actually activate two separate pathways. One is for normal cells and one for cancer cells. The polyphenols apparently act as a guard that separates cancer cells from cells with p57 (which cancer cells lack). He later found that by inserting the p57 gene in the cancer cells, the protective protein they lack was restored and they were spared from destruction.

Dr. Hsu used human cancer cells and found that the polyphenols destroyed the mitochondria (the powerhouse of a cell) of cancer cells while protecting normal cells. Without mitochondria, cells are very vulnerable. The mitochondria are often called the cells' "energy factories."

Oral cancer cells seem to be particularly vulnerable to green tea because of their direct contact with the drink. Oral cancer is known to be hard to treat and has a 50% mortality rate, so these findings are promising. Because those who use tobacco products are at high risk for cancer, Dr. Hsu recommends they drink a few cups of green tea every day.

In 2004, a study was conducted on the molecular and cellular effects of green tea on oral cells of smokers. The study found that green tea and its components inhibited cell growth and lowered the incidence of tumors.

Further studies show that drinking green tea reduced the number of damaged cells in smokers by inducing cell growth arrest and apoptosis, a mechanism similar to that observed in cultured cells and animals.

In addition, green tea may help protect skin from sun damage, according to a review conducted by Hasan Mukhtar, Ph.D., of the Department of Dermatology at Case Western Reserve University in Cleveland, Ohio.

Dr. Mukhtar suggested that green tea polyphenols (GTP) work as powerful antioxidants capable of providing protection from the sun. In other words, it's possible that green tea is protective at all stages of cancer formation, including initiation, promotion, and progression.

Other laboratory studies have shown tea catechins to be powerful inhibiting agents of cancer growth (catechins are flavonoids and potent antioxidants). Not only do they inhibit the growth of tumor cells, they also reduce the incidence and size of those cells and search for oxidants before cell injury can occur.

Green tea's phytonutrients and catechins effectively help the detoxification process, particularly eliminating those toxins that are linked to cancer.

Green tea extract is a concentrated form of green tea available in capsule or tablet form.

### Further Reading & References

- *The Green Tea User's Manual* by Helen Gustafson (2001)

- *Green Tea* by Nadine Taylor (1998)

- *Fight Cancer, Lower Cholesterol, Live Longer: Green Tea* by Kate Gilbert (1998)

- "Molecular and cellular effects of green tea on oral cells of smokers: a pilot study,"http://www.ncbi.nlm.nih.gov/entrez/query.fcgi?cmd=Retrieve&db=pubmed&dopt=Abstract&list_uids=15538715

- Green Tea Cancer Treatment, http://www.cancertutor.com/Cancer/GreenTea.html

- Benefits of Green Tea: Anti Cancer, http://www.greenteabenefits.info/against_ca.php

- "Identification of Green Tea Polyphenol-Targeted Genes," by Stephen Hsu, http://www.experts.scival.com/mcg/grantDetail.asp?id=505224&n=Hsu%2C+Stephen&u_id=2734

# Spirulina/Blue-Green Algae

Spirulina is a microscopic blue-green algae. It is found in both fresh and sea water and grows in the shape of a coil. A significant amount of commercially marketed algae is harvested in Hawaii and is from the species Spirulina Pacifica.

Spirulina is an excellent source of bio-available chlorophyll. This is because spirulina grows in the water and does not have thick cell walls made up of hard-to-digest cellulose like most plants found on land.

Spirulina also has an unusually high protein content that ranges from 55% to 77% by dry weight alone. As a protein source, it has all the essential amino acids along with several fatty acids like gamma-linolenic acid, alpha-linolenic acid, and arachidonic acid. In addition, algae contain high amounts of vitamins $B_1$, $B_2$, $B_3$, $B_6$, $B_9$, C, D, A, and E.

This food source has proven itself effective in treating a variety of illnesses, from allergies to high cholesterol to viral and inflammatory conditions and finally to cancer.

In fact, a 2002 Japanese study of 12 adult males followed the activity of each study participant's natural killer cells (NK cells). After drinking spirulina extract mixed with hot water, researchers found a significant increase in the production of NK cells. The cancer-killing ability of the NK cells was also heightened, as demonstrated by tests following exposure of the NK cells to a bacterial product and testing interleukin-12 production (interleukin-12 is a measure of immune strength).

The study authors concluded that spirulina seems to have a direct effect on NK cells. In addition, the study participants' heightened immunity persisted for up to five weeks after stopping the supplement.

In an Indian study, spirulina was shown to reduce tumors in animals with various types of cancer. In China, spirulina demonstrated potential for diminishing the effects of chemotherapy and radiation. It has been shown to both increase the number of white blood cells as well as the level of red blood cells.

Human clinical studies that took place in India have shown spirulina to be an effective treatment of oral leukoplakia, a precancerous condition characterized by the formation of white patches in the mouth that do not rub off. Often, this leads to oral cancer.

In Kerala, India, a clinical study conducted in the 1990s on tobacco chewers showed that spirulina could reverse oral leukoplakia in this population. Half of the patients received one gram per day of spirulina and the other half received a placebo. There was a complete regression of lesions in 20 of 44 patients (45%) receiving spirulina as opposed to 3 of 43 (7%) in the placebo arm.

Results were even more pronounced, leading to a complete regression in 16 of the 28 study participants, among those who had homogeneous lesions (usually considered less malignant than non-homogeneous lesions). Even after discontinuing use of the spirulina supplements for one year, 55% of participants remained free of the lesions.

Spirulina also contains certain powerful photosensitizers called chlorins. Chlorins interact with red and infrared light to trigger a photodynamic effect, which could kill abnormal cells. It seems more than coincidental that the most prominent reports of benefit come from very sunny climes, such as Hawaii, Latin America, and India.

Spirulina can be purchased as a concentrated food supplement at most natural food stores and from online retailers.

### Further Reading & References

- *The Green Foods Bible: Everything You Need to Know About Barley Grass, Wheatgrass, Kamut, Chlorella, Spirulina And More* by David Sandoval (2007)

- *Achieving Great Health -- How Spirulina, Chlorella, Raw Foods and Ionized Water Can Make You Healthier than You Have Ever Imagined* by Bob McCauley (2005)

- *Spirulina* by Jack Challem (1999)

- "Molecular mechanisms in C-Phycocyanin induced apoptosis in human chronic myeloid leukemia cell line-K562," http://www.ncbi.nlm.nih.gov/entrez/query.fcgi?cmd=Retrieve&db=pubmed&dopt=Abstract&list_uids=15242812

- Spirulina / Blue-Green Algae an Excellent Diet Supplement, http://www.huldaclarkzappers.com/php2/spirulina.php

- Anti-Cancer Effects of Spirulina, http://www.bioalg.com/spirulina-faydalari/PDF%20Dosyalar/spirulina-anti-kanser-abstracts.pdf

## Wheatgrass Juice/Ann Wigmore

Wheatgrass itself comes from the young cotyledons of the wheat plant. Wheatgrass juice therapy was pioneered by Ann Wigmore, who promoted the therapy in conjunction with an organic vegetarian diet after reportedly using it to cure her own cancer.

Fresh wheatgrass is known to be a powerful source of many vitamins, minerals, and plant enzymes. Some consider it one of the most nutrient-dense, green superfoods of all. Research scientist Dr. Charles F. Schnabel has stated that 15 pounds of wheatgrass is the equivalent of 350 pounds of carrots, lettuce, celery and other fresh vegetables.

Wheatgrass is also a good source of living chlorophyll, which is the green pigment and detoxifier found in nearly all plants and algae. Chlorophyll provides an ideal alkaline balance to many of the common acidic foods in the American diet. According to advocates, it also increases the production of hemoglobin and in turn prompts a rise in the amount of oxygen that reaches cancer cells. Though this claim has yet to be proven conclusively, studies show promising results. If true, it's an important finding, since cancer cells cannot thrive in a high-oxygen environment. For example, a 2008 study on tumors in rabbits showed more tumors disappeared after being treated with oxygen as opposed to being treated with nothing at all.

In addition, wheatgrass contains Amygdalin/laetrile, a substance whose cancer-fighting properties are well-established and accepted among alternative cancer treatment experts.

Therapy with wheatgrass is comprised primarily of detoxification through diet while drinking wheatgrass juice several times a day. Wheatgrass also contains selenium which, along with chlorophyll, helps strengthen the immune system.

A scientific study conducted in 1980 by Dr. Chiu Nan Lai of the University of Texas System Cancer Center showed wheatgrass effectively halts the destruction caused by carcinogens in the body. This makes it apparent that wheatgrass is at least useful for *preventing* cancer if not curing it.

Other studies show that applying low levels of wheatgrass extract to cancer-causing agents diminished their activity by up to 99%.

Along with Victoras Kulvinskas, Wigmore went on to form the Hippocrates Health Institute in Boston. Branches of the Institute and related health farms practicing wheatgrass therapy quickly sprouted up across the country.

Wheatgrass supplements can be purchased as a powder or drink.

### Further Reading & References

- *Wheatgrass Nature's Finest Medicine: The Complete Guide to Using Grasses to Revitalize Your Health*, by Steve Meyerowitz (2006)

- *The Wheatgrass Book: How to Grow and Use Wheat Grass to Maximize Your Health and Vitality*, by Ann Wigmore (1985)

- *The Hippocrates Diet and Health Program* by Ann Wigmore (1983)

- Hippocrates Health Institute http://www.hippocratesinst.org/

- Wheat Grass Nutritional Program http://www.huldaclarkzappers.com/php2/wheatgrass.php

- Schultz S, Häussler U, Mandic R, Heverhagen J, et al. Treatment with ozone/oxygen-pneumoperitoneum results in complete remission of rabbit squamous cell carcinomas. Int J Cancer 2008; 122(10): 2360-7.

# Mushrooms and Yeast Treatments

## Agaricus Blazei Murill

Agaricus blazei Murill, also known as cogumelo do sol (sun mushroom), cogumelo de Deus (god's mushroom), Brazil mushroom or Himematsutake, is a mushroom originating from the village of Piedade in the State of São Paulo, Brazil. It flourishes in the hot weather of Brazil. It has been gaining worldwide attention because the population in that area has a lower rate of cancer and other adult diseases.

Agaricus blazei Murill contains the highest levels of beta D glucans of any mushroom known in the world. Beta glucan is a polysaccharide (a chain of sugar molecules formed together to make larger sugars) known to enhance the body's immune system. It is widely recognized for its ability to enhance the function of innate immune cells against a broad range of foreign challenges.

A Japanese-Brazilian farmer first discovered the Agaricus blazei Murill in the summer of 1965. Since 1968, Dr. Takashi Mizuno Ph.D., has studied the bioactive substances in fungi, especially those related to anti-tumor active polysaccharides. At the 12th Symposium of the 7th General Meeting of Technical Discussion Group for Fungi (held at Kinki University in Nara, Japan 1995), Dr. Mizuno presented his results with the following comments:

"A remarkable anti-tumor activity was found in glycoprotein FIII-2-b, isolated from the fruiting bodies of Agaricus blazei Murill. This glucan-protein complex was the first case of an anti-tumor compound found in an edible mushroom."

The graph below shows the result of the cooperative analysis based on the experiment on a mouse model, which was conducted by the Tokyo University Medical School, the National Cancer Institute, Samsung University Medical School, and the Tokyo University School of Pharmacy. The cancerous cells were injected, and multiplied. The mice were expected to survive only three weeks, 5 weeks at the maximum.

During the experiment, 10mg of Agaricus blazei Murill abstract, administered by injection, resulted in a prevention rate of 99% in mice that were first given the mushroom extract before being exposed to cancer. In mice that already had cancer before receiving the extract, 90% completely recovered.

In a 2004 study, further substances were found in Agaricus blazei Murill that inhibit angiogenesis. These substances also, by other actions, inhibit tumor growth and metastases.

Researchers found that the Agaricus blazei inhibited tumor growth by inhibiting tumor-induced neovascularization. From the researchers:

"We isolated further anti-angiogenic substances (A-1 and A-2) from this fungus using an assay system of angiogenesis induced by Matrigel, supplemented with vascular endothelial growth factor, and A-1 was identified as sodium pyroglutamate. Next, we examined the antitumor and antimetastatic actions. The reduction of the numbers of splenic lymphocytes, CD4+ and CD8+ T cells in LLC-bearing mice was inhibited by the oral administration of A-1 (30, 100 and 300 mg/kg). Further, A-1 increased the number of apoptotic cells of tumors and the numbers of CD8+ T and natural killer cells invading the tumors, and inhibited the increase of von Willebrand factor expression (a measure of angiogenesis) in the tumors.

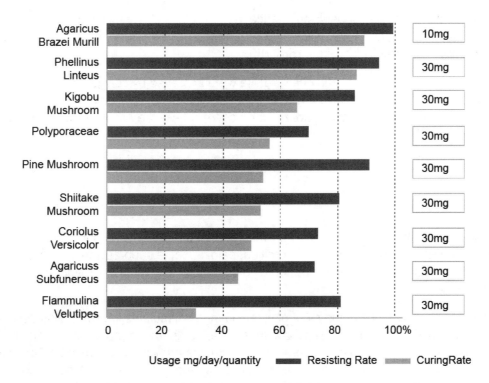

"These results suggest that the antitumor and antimetastatic actions of A-1 (sodium pyroglutamate) may be associated with inhibition of the reduction of immune response caused by the tumor growth and tumor-induced neovascularization. This is the first report showing that sodium pyroglutamate isolated from A. blazei as an anti-angiogenic substance has potent antitumor and antimetastatic actions, as well as immunemodulatory activity, in tumor-bearing mice."*

An additional study in 2004 indicated that Agaricus blazei Murill might be beneficial for patients undergoing chemotherapy:

"Natural killer cell activity and quality of life were improved by consumption of a mushroom extract, Agaricus blazei Murill Kyowa, in gynecological cancer patients undergoing chemotherapy.

"A mushroom extract, Agaricus blazei Murill Kyowa (ABMK), has been reported to possess antimutagenic and antitumor effects. ... One hundred cervical, ovarian, and endometrial cancer patients were treated either with carboplatin (300 mg / m(2)) plus VP16 (etoposide, 100 mg / m(2)) or with carboplatin (300 mg / m(2)) plus taxol (175 mg / m(2)) every 3 weeks for at least three cycles with or without oral consumption of ABMK.

"We observed that natural killer cell activity was significantly higher in ABMK-treated group (ANOVA, n = 39, P < 0.002) as compared with nontreated placebo group (n = 61). ... chemotherapy associated side effects such as appetite, alopecia [hair loss], emotional stability, and general weakness were all improved by ABMK treatment. Taken together, this suggests that ABMK treatment might be beneficial for gynecological cancer patients undergoing chemotherapy."**

### Further Reading & References

- *Medicinal Mushrooms for Immune Enhancement: Agaricus Blazei Murill, Discover the Beta Glucan*

- *Secret* by Beth M. Ley (2001)

- *The Agaricus Blazei Murill Notebook* by Stephen Black (2003)

- *"Isolation of an anti-angiogenic substance from Agaricus blazei Murill: its antitumor and antimetastatic actions." http://www.ncbi.nlm.nih.gov/entrez/query.fcgi?cmd=Retrieve&db=pubmed&dopt=Abstract&list_uids=15471563

- **"Natural killer cell activity and quality of life were improved by consumption of a mushroom extract, Agaricus blazei Murill Kyowa, in gynecological cancer patients undergoing chemotherapy." http://www.ncbi.nlm.nih.gov/entrez/query.fcgi?cmd=Retrieve&db=pubmed&dopt=Abstract&list_uids=15304151

# AHCC®/ImmPower™

The Japanese mushroom extract AHCC (Active Hexose Correlated Compound) is a supplement shown by medical research to reduce nausea, vomiting, pain, appetite suppression, liver damage, hair loss, and immune suppression in patients undergoing chemotherapy, resulting in improved quality of life and overall survival.

AHCC is recognized as one of the most powerful immune stimulants known. It was developed by the Amino-Up Chemical Company of Sapporo, Japan. It is made from a proprietary hybrid of Shiitake, Kawaratake, and Suehirotake mushrooms grown with rice bran in a liquid medium (a controlled environment like hydroponic gardening for mushrooms), that is then fermented to extract a unique, low molecular weight compound, not commonly found in medicinal mushrooms.

More than 29 published studies have focused on AHCC since 1986 and its use in over 700 Japanese hospitals in Japan. There is a great deal of scientific evidence that AHCC not only helps to prevent the side effects of chemotherapy, but enhances its primary effectiveness as well.

Several animal studies provided the ground work for research in humans. A study published in the *Proceedings of the American Association For Cancer Research* in March of 1999 showed that AHCC was able to relieve the side effects of several standard chemotherapy drugs.

Mice treated with the chemotherapy drugs fluorouracil (5-FU), or cyclophosphamide (CY), or both, daily showed decreases in weight, blood count and bone marrow that were "significantly restored" by coadministration with AHCC. Mice treated with Mercaptopurine (6-MP), and methotrexate (MTX) showed decreased body weight, serum albumin, and liver functions, which were significantly improved when AHCC was administered together with the chemotherapic agents.

Hair loss, also known as alopecia and usually caused by cytosine arabinoside (Ara-C), was reduced when AHCC was taken. The protective effects of AHCC in this regard were confirmed in another study where, in a control group of rats treated with the chemotherapy drug cytosine arabinoside (Ara-C)— 5 out of 7 showed severe and 2 of 7 moderate alopecia. Mice given AHCC along with chemotherapy were protected from hair loss.

Liver function damage is often the reason for the unpleasant side effects of chemotherapy. Co-treatment with AHCC and carbon tetrachloride, in a study done on mice, actually prevented decline in liver function. In addition, metabolism was enhanced, thus preventing the buildup of carcinogenic compounds and the development of hormone disorders that often accompany liver failure.

AHCC showed an antioxidant-like protection against free radicals as measured in liver enzyme profiles, protecting the liver itself and the body as a whole.

Besides protecting against adverse side effects, AHCC has also been shown to enhance the effectiveness of chemotherapy. In a study done on rats implanted with a line of breast cancer cells, three groups that were observed for 38 days. There was a control group, a group treated with UFT (an oral form of the chemotherapy drug fluorouracil), and a UFT + AHCC treatment group.

The control group showed the greatest tumor growth. There was a slight, but significant enhancement of tumor suppression in the AHCC group compared to the UFT group. The greatest difference was found in the growth of distant metastases, which were inhibited by the treatment with AHCC + UFT, but enhanced by UFT alone. This is likely because of AHCC's ability to prevent the suppression of immune function that occurs with chemotherapy.

Mice treated only with UFT suffered from suppressed Natural Killer (NK) cell function. NK cells are immune system cells thought to be particularly important in the body's fight against cancer. AHCC restored and enhanced the function of NK cells as well as macrophages, another important type immune system cell. It also improved production of anti-cancer cytokines.

It is important to maintain the immune defense of the host, otherwise distant metastases may occur after primary tumors have been reduced or eradicated. The impaired immune system allows microscopic tumors to grow freely.

More than 130 subsets of white blood cells make up the human immune system. Natural Killer (NK) cells make up roughly 15% of these white blood cells. They are the first line of defense for dealing with invaders. NK cells themselves contain multiple small granules that act as chemical destroyers. Once an NK cell has recognized a cancer cell, for example, it attaches itself to the cell's outer membrane and injects these granules directly into the interior of the cell. The granules then destroy the cancer cell within five minutes. The undamaged NK cell then moves on to other cancer cells and repeats the process.

In a strong immune system, active NK cells take on more than one cancer cell or other infected cells at the same time. Inadequate numbers of NK cells are very rarely a problem, unlike other white blood cells.

Instead, it is the *activity* of the cells that generally determines whether a person is sick or healthy. If NK cells lose their ability to either recognize or destroy an invader, the patient's health can quickly deteriorate. In AIDS and cancer patients, NK cell activity is regarded as probably the primary criterion for estimating the chances of survival. It is commonly accepted that when NK cells cease to function, death will shortly follow.

Individuals with low NK cell activity are significantly more vulnerable to autoimmune diseases, chronic fatigue syndrome, viral infections and the development of cancerous tumors, according to recent research.

Doctors use the NK cell function test to measure NK cell activity. First, a blood sample is taken from the patient and placed in a vial containing live tumor cells. After four hours, a count is taken to determine what percentage of the cancer cells have been destroyed by the NK cells. The higher the percentage, the more active the cells. This test is commonly referred to as the 4 hour 51Chromium-release assay.

NK cell function is particularly heightened after taking AHCC. In addition to an increased susceptibility to cancer metastasis, immune system suppression can also lead to life-threatening opportunistic infections (microbes that prey on people with weakened immune systems). AHCC helps prevent these complications and enhance survival, as demonstrated by a study with mice whose white blood counts were suppressed with the chemotherapy drug cyclophosphamide. The mice were then exposed to Candida albicans, Pseudomonas aeruginosa and Staphylococcus aureus.

Validation of animal research with AHCC is found in controlled studies and case reports with human patients. As mentioned above, AHCC is widely used in Japanese hospitals, and since 1986 doctors have gathered at the annual meeting of the AHCC Research Association to present the results of their clinical experience demonstrating improved appetite, reduced vomiting and pain and other improvements in the quality of life of patients undergoing chemotherapy, radiation and surgery for cancer.

In a study that extended from 1992 to 1999, 70 patients with pathologically confirmed liver cancer who took AHCC orally (3 grams per day) following surgery showed overall survival benefits. A clinically balanced control group of 82 liver cancer patients were followed who had surgery only. As of September 1999, 34 (49%) of the patients in the AHCC group had recurrences, compared to 55 (67%) of the control group.

More significantly, AHCC increased the 50% survival rate from 45 months to 68 months.

AHCC is available in the U.S. and is sold as ImmPower AHCC.

The following dosages reflect what was successful in studies based on repeated NK cell activity tests:

- For cancer, HIV or other life-threatening conditions, 3 grams per day for two weeks, then 1 gram per day until the condition is resolved. Some people continue to take the maintenance dosage even after the problem has been resolved, while others stop taking it and resume if the problem returns. In rare cases it's necessary to take as much as 6 grams daily.

- As a form of prevention, 1 gram per day is recommended.

Taking 3 grams a day resulted in a dramatic increase in NK cell activity within two weeks, according to all studies. At the lower dosage of only 1 gram per day, the same results were reached after four weeks (which is why the 3 grams per day is recommended). Even after the dosage was dropped back to 1 gram per day, NK cell activity continued to increase.

AHCC appears to be completely non-toxic and safe to take long-term when used as directed.

### *Further Reading & References*

- American BioSciences http://www.americanbiosciences.com/abs_immpower.htm#DGP

- AHCC Battles Therapy Unwanted Effects, http://www.annieappleseedproject.org/ahbattherune.html

- *The Science of AHCC: Japan's Medical Breakthrough in Immunotherapy* by Fred Pescatore (2010)

- *AHCC* by Fred Pescatore (2010)

- *AHCC* by Dan Kenner (2001)

- Combination Therapy of Active Hexose Correlated Compound (AHCC) Plus UFT Significantly Reduces the Metastasis of Rat Mammary Carcinoma, Anti-Cancer Dr.ugs 1998, 9, 343-350 K. Matsushita, et al., (University School of Medicine, Laboratory of Pathology, Cancer Institute, Hokkaido) 1998.

- Prophylactic Efficacy of a Basidiomycetes Preparation AHCC against Lethal Opportunistic Infection in Mice, Yakugaku Zassi 2000, 120, 749-753H. Ishibashi et al. (Department of Microbiology and Immunology, Teikyo University School of Medicine).

- Improving Effect of Active Hexose Correlated Compound (AHCC)on the Prognosis of Postoperative Hepatocellular Carcinoma Patients, 34th Congress of the European Society for Surgical Research

(Bern, Switzerland), Y. Kamiyama et al. (First Department of Surgery, Kansai Medical University) 1999.

# Beta Glucan

Beta glucan polysaccharides are found in yeast, mushrooms, bacteria and plants. Beta 1, 3 D Glucan, a non-toxic immune modulator, is emerging as one of the most powerful cancer-fighting agents. It is a naturally occurring compound derived from the cell wall of baker's yeast (Saccharomyces Cerevisiae).

There is no yeast in Beta Glucan, hence almost no danger of an allergic reaction in sensitive individuals. The extracting technology allows for a totally pure extract. Nevertheless, for persons who are extra sensitive to even minute traces of yeast protein, the alternative is a Beta Glucan product made of oat. The oat extract is said to be easier for people with a very sensitive stomach as well. Both types of glucans are well researched and documented.

The fact that the immune system has trouble recognizing and then responding appropriately to cancer tumors is a major contributing factor to the ability of the disease to multiply and spread. Beta glucan works by activating and strengthening the body's own defense mechanism against diseases. Beta glucan is a non-toxic nutritional biomolecule, classified 'generally recognized as safe' (GRAS) by the FDA, that significantly potentiates the activities of the macrophage, the large white immune cell, increasing its ability to recognize cancerous cells.

Renowned immunologist, Dr. Joyce Czop of Harvard Medical School describes Beta 1, 3 D Glucan this way:

"Beta 1, 3 D Glucan is a true miracle of nature. It produces a dynamic immune response by virtue of its unique molecular shape (triple helical). This unique shape allows the Beta 1, 3 Glucan molecules to bond with a perfectly matched activating receptor on the macrophage cell, somewhat like your car is activated only by a uniquely shaped car key. Macrophage cells are one of the most important components of your immune system-- and your first line of defense. Once the Beta 1, 3 D molecule activates them they become awesome disease destroyers. Besides most pathogens, macrophages can recognize and kill a variety of tumor cells. In fact, any cancer is fair game for an activated macrophage..."

"When a single dose of Beta Glucan is administered, the macrophage activity will peak in 72 hours, then the activity level returns to its previous plateau. The immune response of the organism begins when a white blood cell called a macrophage encounters a hostile invader or mutant cell and consumes it.

"Beta Glucan targets the macrophage and keeps it in a more prepared state. With this modulation, all subsequent immune response increases. Let us remember that the Glucan and the macrophage are oblivious to the type of invader. The macrophage knows only self versus non-self.

"But the immune system consists of more than Macrophages; it has an incredible array of weapons designed to defeat anything that threatens our health: T-cells, B-cells, antibodies, and potent chemical messengers (Interferon and Interleukin 1& 2). Once Beta Glucan has activated the macrophage cells, they in turn activate all the weapons of the entire immune system, producing a massive and total immune response. This is what the literature indicates, and the quantity of serious laboratory and clinical documentation on this product is huge."

He goes on to explain that once Beta Glucan has activated the macrophage cells, they end up activating all the weapons of the entire immune system. This produces a massive and total immune response. In addition, macrophage activity peaks 72 hours following a single dose of Beta Glucan.

After that, the activity level returns to its previous plateau. It seems that when a white blood cell called a macrophage encounters a hostile invader, the immune response of the organism begins and then consumes it.

Other experts have made the following comments on Beta Glucan:

Dr. James Shortt, MD., discusses the action of the immune system against disease and how Beta-1, 3-D Glucan can be a prudent course of treatment: "Beta Glucan has been studied in the lab and found to enhance natural killing of tumor cells, bacteria, fungi and virus infected cells. Due to the nature of the immune response to Beta-1, 3-D glucan, resistance does not occur. It triggers the killing of tumor cells and has been shown to be an excellent adjuvant to many types of chemotherapy, radiation, and surgery."

Dr. Joe Brownholtz, Ph.D., a researcher and professor of sports and nutritional medicine, discusses the effect of Beta Glucan on the immune system. He writes, "Researchers have also concluded that Beta Glucan has anti-tumor properties, inhibits the development of diabetes in animals, lowers cholesterol, prevents cancer reoccurrences, is a free radical scavenger and when combined with sulfur, a factor in reducing the probability of HIV carriers contracting AIDS."

According to research by Tulane University, the Armed Services Radiobiology Research Institute and a many other scientific research centers, Beta Glucan extracted from yeast cell wall enhances the immune system's awareness of the cancerous cells and nutritionally aids in the control of cancer.

Results have been particularly dramatic in breast, sarcoma, and melanoma cancers when it comes to potentiating immune response. A particularly potent immune potentiator is an insoluble particulate Beta 1, 3/1, 6 glucan. Potentiated by Beta 1, 3/1, 6 glucan, the immune system is activated against cancer. This enables the macrophages to attack cancer cells with enhanced cytotoxic granules (toxic chemicals) that kill the cancer cell and prevent further multiplication and spreading.

When Beta 1, 3/1, 6 glucan is administered in particularly small particle sizes (microparticulate as distinguished from globular), it shows better absorption and more rapid response and increases protection of the immune cells from the damage of radiation treatments. After treatments, it enhances recovery of platelets and white immune cells. The macrophage is also enhanced to more ably and rapidly remove the toxic debris (phagocytosis) created by radiation and chemotherapy in the body, thus reducing or eliminating the negative side effects such as nausea, hair loss, inability to sleep and skin radiation injury.

In a Research Summary Report issued in 2001 by The University of Nevada School of Medicine and Nutritional Supply Corporation it was found:

"MPG Glucan has been shown to enhance the envelopment and digestion (phagocytosis) of pathogenic microorganisms that cause infectious disease. The Beta- 1,3/1-6 glucans additionally enhance the ability of macrophages, one of the most important immune cells in the immune system, to kill tumor cells. Laboratory studies have revealed the new MPG Glucan is significantly effective at activating macrophages, and via the macrophages, in turn the entire immune cascade including T-Cells and B-Cells."

The results of further studies indicate the following:

"The initial 9 patients studied had malignant carcinoma of the breast. Control and experimental lesions were injected [with Beta Glucan]; subsequently biopsies were performed at varying intervals for histological [tissue] evaluation. Always when glucan or glucan and RF fraction were administered intralesionally, the size of the lesion was strikingly reduced in as short a period as 5 days. In small lesions, resolution was complete, whereas in large lesions, resolutions were partial."*

"Intravenous administration of soluble or particulate glucan resulted in significant reduction in the growth of a syngeneic anaplastic mammary carcinoma and melanoma B16 and enhanced survival."**

"Over the past 11 months I have been able to convince five out of eight breast cancer patients who were undergoing radiation therapy, to consume one capsule of beta 1,3/1,6 glucan (NSC-24 3 mg) three times per day. To date, I have observed that none of the patients using NSC-24 have suffered from any type of radiation injury to the skin, while the three patients who chose not to use NSC-24 all show signs of extensive radiation damage to the skin."***

By supplying a larger amount of Beta Glucan in the body, a higher state of immune response is created. This is the primary pathway by which medicinal mushrooms help the body to fight off invasion by diseases and cancer cells. This is called Immunomodulation - modulation of the immune system. It is perhaps better referred to as stimulation of the body's immune system.

Additionally, the clinical trials at the Zhejiang University in Hangzhou, China found that conventional chemotherapy for lung cancer was approximately 10% effective while the same chemotherapy with 3 grams per day of a Beta-Glucan concentrate (from Maitake mushroom in this case) boosted the efficiency to over 80% cure! This is now the standard treatment for advanced lung cancer in China, and has been since 1994. With a reported 80% cure rate against this dreaded disease, this is most impressive.

It was noted early on in the research that Lentinan (1-3{1-6} Beta-Glucan) was not effective orally and had to be administered by injection. In many cancer patients, digestive function is also impaired. This means that extremely large organic molecules such as Beta Glucan are not readily absorbed in the stomach and intestines but pass through unchanged. However, it has been found that breaking the long-chain molecules into shorter segments makes the substance more readily bioavailable while maintaining its clinical properties.

One approach is to co-administer vitamin C with the mushroom extracts, though the Vitamin C cannot be mixed with the medicine ahead of time because it would launch the breakdown process and leave behind only simple sugar molecules. The addition of 1000 mg (1 gram) of vitamin C at the same time the mushroom or mushroom extracts are taken, is said to logarithmically increase the absorption of the Beta-Glucans, making them much more bioavailable to the system. It is thought that Ginger has this same effect.

### Further Reading & References

- Cancer - Melanoma: DiLuzio N.R. Williams D.L. et al, Comparative evaluation of the tumor inhibitory and antibacterial activity of solubilized and particulate glucan Recent Results Cancer Res 75:165-172. 1980)

- **Cancer - Sarcoma and Melanoma: Williams DL, et al, Therapeutic efficacy of glucan in a murine model of hepatic metastatic disease Hepatology 5(2):198-206. Mar 1985)

- ***Hemopoietic Stimulation: Patchen M.L., McVittie T.J.; Temporal Response of Murine Pluripotent Stem Cells and Myeloid and Erythroid Progenitor Cells to Low-dose Glucan Treatment. Acta Hemat; 70:281-288. Experimental Hematology Dept, Armed Forces Radiobiology Research Inst, Bethesda, MD. 1983.

- *Discover the Beta Glucan Secret: For Immune Enhancement Cancer Prevention & Treatment,*

- *Cholesterol Reduction, Glucose Regulation, and Much More*! : by Beth M. Ley (2001)

- Beta Glucan Research – Saccharomyces cerevisiae, http://www.betaglucan.org/

- *Beta Glucan: Nature's Secret* by Vaclav Vetvicka PhD, Vaclav Vetvicka, and Ph.D. (2009)

- *Beta-Glucan - A Medical Dictionary, Bibliography, and Annotated Research Guide to Internet References* by ICON Health Publications (2004)

- *Medicinal Mushrooms for Immune Enhancement: Agaricus Blazei Murill, Discover the Beta Glucan Secret (Health Learning Handbook)* by Beth M. Ley (2001)

- Disease & Beta-Glucan Chemistry, http://www.corenutritional.com/customer/pages. php?pageid=14&mode=preview


# Coriolus Versicolor/PSK

Coriolus versicolor is a mushroom traditionally used by the Chinese as a tonic. Coriolus versicolor is increasingly referred to as *Trametes versicolor*. "Versicolor" means "several colors," which is true for this rainbow-type polypore mushroom found throughout the world.

The active ingredient of coriolus versicolor is a protein-bound polysaccharide known as Polysaccharide-K (called Krestin or PSK). PSK has been shown to have immunostimulant and anti-tumor properties. It is used primarily in conjunction with chemotherapy, radiation, and surgical treatments for cancer. Commonly, it is used in China, Japan, and some European countries as an immune system enhancer. In Japan, PSK is covered by government health insurance and is approved for use as an adjuvant for cancer therapy.

Clinical studies have demonstrated results that show a 30% vs. 10% disease-free survival for colon cancer patients over an eight-year clinical trial when PSK was used alone and tested against a placebo; 22% vs. 5% survival at five years for stage III lung cancer patients who were given radiation plus PSK as opposed to radiation alone; 81% vs. 64% survival at ten years for breast cancer patients who were given chemotherapy plus PSK as opposed to chemotherapy alone; 73% vs. 60% survival at five years for gastric cancer patients who combined daily PSK use with their chemotherapy as opposed to chemotherapy alone.

MD Anderson, a top-ranked cancer hospital in the United States, has reported that it is a "promising candidate for chemoprevention due to the multiple effects on the malignant process, limited side effects and safety of daily oral doses for extended periods of time."


### Further Reading & References

- Memorial Sloan-Kettering Cancer Center: Coriolus Versicolor, http://www.mskcc.org/mskcc/html/69194.cfm

- Medicinal Mushrooms, http://www.mushroomscience.com/ (not an endorsement; for informational purposes only)

- American Cancer Society, http://www.cancer.org/docroot/ETO/content/ETO_5_3X_Coriolous_Versicolor.asp

- *Complementary/Integrative Medicine Education Resources*. MD Anderson Cancer Center. http://www.mdanderson.org/education-and-research/resources-for-professionals/clinical-tools-and-resources/cimer/therapies/herbal-plant-biologic-therapies/coriolus-versicolor-scientific.html.

# Kombucha/Manchurian Tea/Mo-Gu/Fungo Japon

The "kombucha mushroom" looks like a slippery, rubbery, brownish-gray "pancake" floating on top of a sugared tea. Why sugared tea? Because Kombucha itself is a fermented drink that transforms heavily sugared tea into a health drink over a period of 5-7 days. Japanese, Chinese, and Koreans have known about it for several thousand years. It is said to be widely used in Russia, where communities drinking this tea are credited with extraordinarily long lives.

In reality, the "kombucha mushroom" is not a mushroom at all, but a culture of yeast and bacteria that's classified as a "zoogleal mat."

It is claimed that kombucha discourages cancer, lengthens the lifespan, is good for sleeping, energy, and menopausal problems, and is a good protection from the damaging effects of chemotherapy and radiation. It is also believed to detoxify the body and energize the mind. However, there is little published research on these health benefits. Most of the reputation for the tea comes from the thousands of years of use by the different cultures mentioned above.

Kombucha produces acids similar to those made by the liver, which bind with toxins in the digestive tract, and carry them out of the body via normal waste elimination. It reportedly helps prevent and treat cancer. If prepared properly, it has no known harmful side effects in regular dosage of a cup or two a day.

Kombucha tea contains various bacterial/yeast colonies, metabolites, C and B-vitamins, and up to 1.5% alcohol. The tea tastes like sour cider. Research has been carried out for many years to identify its constituents. Based on the research, some of the known active components in kombucha tea are lactic acid, acetic acid, malic acid, gluconic acid, butyric acid, nucleic acids, amino acids, and enzymes.

Early chemical analysis of kombucha tea shows that glucuronic acid may be the key component and that it works by assisting the liver in a detoxification process. Later studies suggest that glucuronic acid isn't present in kombucha, and that the most active component is glucaric acid, which helps eliminate glucuronic acid conjugates that get produced by the liver. These glucuronic acids, detected in the urine, gave rise to the notion that glucuronic acid was present in the tea itself, but this view may have been mistaken.

Therefore researchers theorize that glucaric acid is the active ingredient, and that it essentially makes the liver more efficient by ensuring that glucuronic acid conjugates are properly eliminated instead of reabsorbed by the body.

Many fruits and vegetables contain glucaric acid, and, aside from its presence in kombucha tea, it's being evaluated on its own as a cancer preventive agent. It has also been discovered that the bacterial beta-glucuronidase enzyme can interfere with proper disposal of a chemotherapeutic agent, and that antibiotics employed as a treatment against gut bacteria can neutralize the toxicity of some chemotherapy drugs. These observations support the theory that glucaric acid is an active component of kombucha.

One Kombucha drinker has said:

"Its overall effect - an extended feeling of well-being - cannot be fully explained by the individual ingredients alone. Kombucha is certainly more than the sum of its parts."

The evidence for kombucha tea appears to be thin. Like many traditional remedies, it has found favor in some quarters because our modern diet is far removed from the natural foods our bodies are designed to consume. Over a period of years, this leads to an accumulation of toxins in the system. Alternative cancer treatment experts almost universally recommend that one of the first things cancer patients do is detoxify the body so its own natural defense mechanisms reestablish themselves. Natural "detoxifiers" are therefore popular – especially among patients who decide on self-treatment -- although their efficacy may not be known.

Kombucha is available commercially to consumers. The tea can be made at home.

### *Further Reading & References*

- *Kombucha – The Miracle Fungus* by Harald Tietze (1996)

- *Kombucha Teaology Over 1001 ways to brew Kombucha for Best Flavour and Maximum Healing* by Harald Tietze (1997)

- *Kombucha Tea for your Health and Healing: The Most In-Depth Guide Available* - Paperback by Alick Bartholomew and Mari Bartholomew (1998)

- Is Kombucha tea the answer to all your health problems? http://www.bdc-canada.com/TEA/Articles/All_Info_about_Kombucha_Tea.htm

- Michael R. Roussin (1996-2003). *Analyses of Kombucha Ferments.* Information Resources, http://www.kombucha-research.com.

- Walaszek, Z. (1990-10-08). "Potential use of D-glucaric acid derivatives in cancer prevention". *Cancer Letters* (Elsevier Science Ireland) **54** (1-2): 1–8. http://www.sciencedirect.com/science?_ob=ArticleURL&_udi=B6T54-4BY9X3F-3FC&_user=10&_coverDate=10%2F08%2F1990&_rdoc=1&_fmt=high&_orig=gateway&_origin=gateway&_sort=d&_docanchor=&view=c&_acct=C000050221&_version=1&_urlVersion=0&_userid=10&md5=112a580fd37506780cbfae0af33c459c&searchtype=a

- Involvement of ß-Glucuronidase in Intestinal Microflora in the Intestinal Toxicity of the Antitumor Camptothecin Derivative Irinotecan Hydrochloride (CPT-11) in Rats, http://cancerres.aacrjournals.org/content/56/16/3752.abstract

- KBBK Kombucha Brooklyn, http://www.kombuchabrooklyn.com/

# Maitake – Grifola frondosa/D Fraction

Maitake (Grifola frondosa) is the Japanese name for an edible fungi with a large fruiting body characterized by overlapping waves. Maitake means "dancing mushroom" in Japanese. In the United States, they also are known as hen-of-the- woods because the mass of mushrooms looks like fluffed-up feathers. The stalks are often fused, massed at the base of tree stumps and on roots. They are common in eastern North America, Europe, and Asia. Maitake is a premier culinary as well as medicinal mushroom.

Laboratory studies have shown that maitake extract can inhibit the growth of tumors and stimulate the immune system of cancerous mice.

In China, sixty-three patients with lung, stomach, or liver cancers or leukemia who took four capsules of maitake extract three times daily before meals for one to three months experienced an anticancer effect. There have also been reports that maitake extracts may help AIDS patients fight Kaposi's sarcoma and other symptoms.

In the late 80s, Professor Hiroaki Nanba, Ph.D., of Japan's Kobe Pharmaceutical University, isolated various fractions or components and came up with the D-Fraction. Dr. Nanba conducted a study in which three groups of mice were injected with cancer cells and then fed a normal diet or one with maitake powder or with injections of D-fraction. The spread of the cancer was not inhibited at all in the mice on the normal diet but was prevented in 81.3% of the maitake-fed group, and in 91.3% of the group given D-fraction.

Dr. Nanba studied 165 advanced cancer patients and while the study was not a blind, placebo-controlled study, the results indicated that breast, lung, and liver cancers respond more favorably to maitake treatment than do bone cancer, stomach cancer, or leukemia. Presenting his results in l995, Dr. Nanba noted:

"Though it cannot be said that Maitake D-Fraction and tablets are the cancer cure, one can safely say they do maintain the quality of life of patients and improve the immune system, resulting in the possible remission of cancer cells with no side effects."

A 44-year old male patient with a brain tumor was given D-fraction for four months. After four months without any other medication, radiation, or chemotherapy, an MRI confirmed that the tumor the size of a chicken egg had disappeared. He had previously received four cycles of chemotherapy.

In the US, over 2,000 practitioners are reportedly dispensing maitake. Using the newer Maitake D-fraction™, a number of natural medicine practitioners in the US have also reported good results with patients with, for instance, uterine fibroids and in prostate cancer cases where chemotherapy didn't work.

The MD-fraction, the most recent development, is a proprietary maitake extract. Its Japanese inventors consider it a notable advance upon the preceding D-fraction. The D-fraction, the MD-fraction, and other extracts, often in combination with whole maitake powder, have shown particular promise as immunomodulating agents, and as an adjunct to cancer and HIV therapy.

A 2002 study looked at how maitake MD-fraction can aid cancer patients:

"Maitake mushroom (Grifola frondosa) MD-fraction containing beta-1,6 glucan with beta-1,3 branched chains has previously exhibited strong anticancer activity by increasing immune-competent cell activity.[1,2] In this non-random case series, a combination of MD-fraction and whole maitake powder was investigated to determine its effectiveness for 22- to 57-year-old cancer patients in stages II-IV. Cancer regression or significant symptom improvement was observed in 58.3 percent of liver cancer patients, 68.8 percent of breast cancer patients, and 62.5 percent of lung cancer patients. The trial found a less than 10-20 percent improvement for leukemia, stomach cancer, and brain cancer patients. Furthermore, when maitake was taken in addition to chemotherapy, immune-competent cell activities were enhanced 1.2-1.4 times, compared with chemotherapy alone. Animal studies have supported the use of maitake MD-fraction for cancer."*

### Further Reading & References

- *Can Maitake MD-Fraction Aid Cancer Patients? Noriko Kodama, PhD, Kiyoshi Komuta, MD PhD, and Hiroaki Nanba, PhD, *Alternative Medicine Review,* Volume 7:3, 2002.

- Medicinal Mushrooms, http://www.suerussellwrites.com/mushrooms.html

- "Can maitake MD-fraction aid cancer patients?" http://www.ncbi.nlm.nih.gov/entrez/query.fcgi?cmd=Retrieve&db=pubmed&dopt=Abstract&list_uids=12126464

- "Effect of Maitake (Grifola frondosa) D-Fraction on the activation of NK cells in cancer patients."

http://www.ncbi.nlm.nih.gov/entrez/query.fcgi?cmd=Retrieve&db=pubmed&dopt=Abstract&list_uids=14977447

- *Maitake Mushroom and D-Fraction (Woodland Health Series)* by Shari Lieberman PhD and Ken Babal CN (2004)

- *Maitake Magic* by Harry G. Preuss (2002)

- *Maitake: King of Mushrooms* by Shari Lieberman (1998)

# MycoSoft®

MycoSoft® Gold Extract, considered an immune system enhancer, is based on several medicinal mushrooms. It is specifically designed to potentiate the immune system with a complex assortment of polysaccharides, precursor nutrients for the immune system.

It is reformulated with thirteen species of polypore mushrooms (Ice Man Polypore, Agarikon, Artist Conk, Reishi, Oregon Polypore, Maitake, Chaga, Shiitake, Mesima, Birch Polypore, Zhu Ling, Suehirotake, and Yun Zhi; 500 mg total per capsule).

Recommended as an adjuvant to conventional therapies, advocates claim that any individual needing potentiation of the immune system may benefit from MycoSoft® Gold. In general, fungal remedies such as MycoSoft® can safely be used during chemotherapy.

### Further Reading & References

- 78 successful natural alternative cancer treatments commonly used worldwide, http://www.alternative-cancer.net/78_alternatives.htm

# Phellinus Igniarius

Phellinus Igniarius is a plant pathogen and a mushroom believed to have anti-cancer properties. A 2003 study showed in vitro selective cytotoxicity (cell-killing capacity) against a human lung cancer cell line and a liver cancer cell line.

This mushroom is also believed to have tumor-inhibitory and live-protecting effects. This conclusion was drawn following a study of the mushroom in mice who were injected with a sarcoma and then given extracellular polysaccharides (EPS) taken from the liquid mycelia culture of the Phellinus Igniarius mushroom. The EPS doses were shown to have antitumor activity and also appeared to protect the liver.

### Further Reading & References

- "Phelligridins C-F: cytotoxic pyrano[4,3-c][2]benzopyran-1,6-dione and furo[3,2-c]pyran-4-one derivatives from the fungus Phellinus." igniarius.http://www.ncbi.nlm.nih.gov/entrez/query.fcgi?cmd=Retrieve&db=pubmed&dopt=Abstract&list_uids=15165144

- "Tumor-inhibitory and liver-protective effects of Phellinus igniarius extracellular polysaccharides." http://www.springerlink.com/content/g8p6553669364560/

# Phellinus Linteus/Mesima

Phellinus linteus is a medicinal mushroom used in Japan, Korea and China. It is shaped like a hoof, has a bitter taste, and grows on wild mulberry trees. In Korean traditional medicine, the mushroom is consumed in the form of hot tea.

Early research has suggested that Phellinus linteus has anti-breast-cancer activity. Phellinus linteus is also reported to significantly reduce the toxicity of chemotherapy and enhance the results. Mesima is the common name of Phellinus linteus.

A 2004 study highlighted the positive impact of this mushroom on a hormone refractory prostate cancer: "Dramatic remission of hormone refractory prostate cancer achieved with extract of the mushroom, Phellinus linteus," according to the study's authors.

The research team of Dr. Chihara in Tokyo National Cancer Research Center in Japan found that hydrothermal extract of Phellinus linteus significantly suppresses solid tumor sarcoma 180. In addition, a paper published by Harvard Medical School reported that Phellinus linteus is a promising anti-cancer agent, but that more research is required to understand the mechanisms behind its anti-cancer activity.

The following table shows results from a study where the sarcoma 180 tumor was transplanted into mice. Following that, 27 different kinds of hot-water-based mushroom extracts were injected into the animals. The rate of tumor proliferation was recorded. Hydrothermal extract of Phellinus linteus displayed predominant suppression effect at 96.7% compared to other mushrooms.

Table. Antitumor activity of hot-water extracts of mushrooms
(Solid Tumor Sarcoma 180 /mouse, ip method)*

| Name of Fungus | Inhibition rate(%) | Complete regression (Tumor free mouse/ No. of treated mice) |
|---|---|---|
| Ganoderma applanatum | 64.9 | 5/10 |
| Coriolus versicolor | 77.5 | 4/8 |
| Coriolus hirsutus | 65.0 | 2/10 |
| Trametes gibbosa | 49.2 | 1/10 |
| Lenzites betulina | 23.9 | 0/8 |
| Daedaleopsis tricolor | 70.2 | 4/7 |
| Fomitopsis cytisina | 44.2 | 3/10 |
| Leucofomes ulmarius | 44.8 | 0/7 |
| Hirschioporus fuscoviolaceus | 45.5 | 1/10 |
| Coriolus pubescens | 59.5 | 0/10 |
| Favolus alveolaris | 71.9 | 0/10 |
| Fomes fomentarius | 5.7 | 2/8 |
| Fomitopsis pinicola | 51.2 | 3/9 |
| Ganoderma tsugae | 77.8 | 2/10 |
| Piptoporus betulinus | 49.2 | 3/9 |
| Trametes dickinsii | 80.1 | 2/10 |
| Phellinus hartigii | 67.9 | 0/7 |
| Phellinus igniarius | 87.4 | 0/8 |
| Phellinus linteus | 96.7 | 1/9 |
| Lentinus edodes | 80.7 | 6/9 |
| Flammulina velutipes | 81.1 | 7/8 |
| Pleurotus ostreatus | 75.3 | 6/10 |

| Pleurotus spodoleucus | 72.3 | 3/10 |
| Tricholoma matsutake | 91.8 | 5/9 |
| Pholiota nameko | 86.5 | 3/10 |
| Agaricus bisporus | 2.7 | 0/10 |
| Auricularia auricula-judae | 42.6 | 0/9 |

### Further Reading & References

- *"What is Mesima?" Han Kook Shin Yak, http://www.hsp.co.kr/eng/mesima/mesima01.html

- "Dramatic remission of hormone refractory prostate cancer achieved with extract of the mushroom, Phellinus linteus." http://www.ncbi.nlm.nih.gov/entrez/query.fcgi?cmd=Retrieve&db=pubmed&dopt=Abstract&list_uids=15331908

- What is Mesima? http://hsp.co.kr/eng/mesima/mesima01.html

- Lee YS, Kang YH, Jung JY, et al. (October 2008). "Protein glycation inhibitors from the fruiting body of Phellinus linteus". Biological & Pharmaceutical Bulletin 31 (10): 1968–72. doi:10.1248/bpb.31.1968. PMID 18827365. http://joi.jlc.jst.go.jp/JST.JSTAGE/bpb/31.1968?from=PubMed.

# Reishi - Ganoderma lucidum

The lingzhi or reishi mushroom has been used as a medicinal mushroom in traditional Chinese medicine for more than 2,000 years, bringing it special renown in East Asia. It encompasses several fungal species of the genus Ganoderma. Reishi is one of the oldest mushrooms known to have been used medicinally. It has few side-effects and is believed to have many health benefits.

The Latin word lucidum means "shiny" or "brilliant" and refers to the varnished surface of reishi's cap, which is reddish orange to black. The stalk usually is attached to the cap at the side. In Japan, 99% of reishi growing in the wild are found on old plum trees, although wild reishi are rare.

Reishi works in the treatment of cancer because it helps cleanse the body from toxins and it helps strengthen the immune system. It enhances liver detoxification, thus improving liver function and stimulating the regeneration of liver cells - making it a potentially valuable supplement for those who have liver cancer.

Reishi can be used as a supplement during chemotherapy or radiotherapy to reduce side effects such as fatigue, loss of appetite, hair loss, bone marrow suppression, and risk of infection. It can also reduce the toxic side effects and mitigate the pain of chemotherapy and radiotherapy, in particular for cancer patients at terminal stages, thereby prolonging their lives and improving their quality of life.

### Further Reading & References

- *The Power of Japanese Red Reishi: the Real Magic Mushroom* by Brad J. King, Dr. Meg Jordan, World Health Publishing Inc., and Robert Brown (2008)

- *Mysterious Reishi Mushroom* (Lifeline book) by K'sai Matsumoto (1979)

- *Reishi: Ancient Herb for Modern Times* by Kenneth Jones (1992)

• Guide to Reishi Mushrooms, http://www.reishi.com/

# Sun's Soup/Sun Farm Vegetable Soup

It has been reported that a treatment developed by Dr. Alexander Sun, a biochemist who once worked in the oncology department at Mt. Sinai School of Medicine in New York, lengthened the survival of patients with advanced non-small cell lung cancer and other types of malignant tumors.

Sun's Soup was first conceived as a treatment for cancer in the mid-1980s. In an effort to help his mother who was diagnosed with stage IV non-small cell lung cancer (metastasis to the left adrenal gland), the developer created a mixture that contained shiitake mushroom, mung bean, Hedyotis diffusa, and Scutellaria barbata in the belief that these plant materials had anticancer and/or immune-system–stimulating properties. Also, it is thought that the shiitake and the mung bean act *synergistically* in this treatment.

After his mother appeared to benefit from this treatment (she was reported to be alive and cancer free more than 13 years later), 3 additional patients (one with stage IV kidney cancer that had metastasized to the lungs, one with stage IV kidney cancer that had metastasized to the liver and to the lungs, and one with stage IV non-small cell lung cancer that had metastasized to the brain) were treated with a variant of the original mixture, i.e., a combination of shiitake mushroom and mung bean. These additional patients were also said to benefit from the treatment.

In June 1992, Dr. Sun filed a patent application for the "Herbal treatment of malignancy," and US Patent # 5437866 was awarded in August 1995. Also in June 1992, Dr. Sun initiated a clinical trial in the Czech Republic to test the soup as a treatment for advanced non-small cell lung cancer. A second clinical study that also involved patients with advanced non-small cell lung cancer was completed in 1997. In both reports of the clinical study results, the authors concluded that patients who received Sun's Soup survived longer.

In 1998, the developer reported at a scientific conference that additional patients with various other types of cancer had benefited from treatment with Sun's Soup. The basic ingredients and preparation of the soup are as follows (see the patent for the quantities involved):

• Shiitake mushroom: Lentinus edodes: the whole plant is macerated in a food processor and is cooked with meat or chicken as soup for at least 5 minutes at 100.degree. C. The plant is known to contain several polysaccharides, which are known to stimulate natural killer cell activity.

• Mung bean: Prepared by boiling to soften the bean, and the whole bean is eaten. A boiled extract is, however, preferred. This is prepared by grinding the beans, e.g., in a coffee grinder and boiling at 100.degree. C. for 5 minutes. Preferably, however, the cooked extract is used. Mung bean is known to contain nucleases (a type of enzyme) as well as protease inhibitors. Nucleases hydrolyze single-stranded DNA; when cancer cells proliferate, their DNA changes to single-stranded DNA first, which could be digested by mung bean nucleases. Proteases could facilitate metastasis of cancer cells. "Mung bean" protease inhibitors may have the effect of preventing cancer metastasis.

• Hedyotis diffusa (wild): The herb should be washed with water, covered with water, and cooked together with 50 g of "Scutellaria barbata" (see paragraph 4), and 10 of the root of Glycyrrhiaz uralensis fisch as a sweetener. This herb is known to inhibit the growth of tumor S-180, U.sub.14 and L1 ascites. The herbs should not be eaten; only the soup should be drunk once or twice a day. The soup should be cooked down to the volume of a coffee cup.

- Scutellaria barbata: This herb should be cooked with "Hedyotis diffusa" (wild). This herb is known to inhibit the growth of tumor S-180, ascites and T22.

The soup is available from Sun Farm Corporation in either freeze-dried or frozen form. It contains additional ingredients besides those listed above, but apparently it was this version of the soup that was used in the following study.

Abstract of the Pilot Study of a Specific Dietary Supplement in Tumor-Bearing Mice and in Stage IIIB and IV Non-Small Cell Lung Cancer Patients:

"Previously, a specific dietary supplement, selected vegetables (SV), was found to be associated with prolonged survival of stage III and IV non-small cell lung cancer (NSCLC) patients. In this study, several anticancer components in SV were measured; the anticancer activity of SV was assessed using a lung tumor model, line 1 in BALB/c mice.

"SV was also used in conjunction with conventional therapies by stage IIIB and IV NSCLC patients whose survival and clinical responses were evaluated. A daily portion (283 g) of SV was found to contain 63 mg of inositol hexaphosphate, 4.4 mg of daidzein, 2.6 mg of genistein, and 16 mg of coumestrol.

"Mouse food containing 5% SV (wt/wt) was associated with a 53-74% inhibition of tumor growth rate. Fourteen of the 18 patients who ingested SV daily for 2-46 months were included in the analyses; none showed evidence of toxicity.

"The first lead case remained tumor free for >133 months; the second case showed complete regression of multiple brain lesions after using SV and radiotherapy. The median survival time of the remaining 12 patients was 33.5 months, and one-year survival was >70%.

"The median survival time of the 16 "intent-to-treat" patients (including ineligible patients) was 20 months, and one-year survival was 55%. The Karnofsky performance status of eligible patients was 55±13 at entry but improved to 92±9 after use of SV for five months or longer ($p < 0.01$).

"Five patients had stable lesions for 30, 30, 20, 12, and 2 months; two of them, whose primary tumor was resected, used SV alone and demonstrated an objective response of their metastatic tumors.

"In addition to the two lead cases, eight patients had no new metastases after using SV. Three patients had complete regression of brain metastases after using radiotherapy and SV. In this study, daily ingestion of SV was associated with objective responses, prolonged survival, and attenuation of the normal pattern of progression of stage IIIB and IV NSCLC. A large randomized phase III clinical trial is needed to confirm the results observed in this pilot study."*

As a link on the Sun Farm Corporation website, Dr. James Lewis Jr. of the Prostate Cancer Exchange says: "Can Sun Soup help prostate cancer patients? I believe it can. I am aware of a prostate cancer patient with hormone refractory disease whose PSA level of 232 ng/ml dropped to an undetectable level of 0.1 ng/ml after having been on Sun Soup for eight months."

Another quote in Asia News-IT 2004: "Dr. Steve Lai, chief consultant of the Hong Kong-based United Asia Medical Network, was one of the first to apply the herbal therapy to cancer patients four years ago.

"More than half of the desperate stage-IV cancer patients had their condition significantly improved after they took it," he said. "This is amazing considering the fact that these are people doomed to die in the eyes of a conventional oncologist."

"In my 20 years experience as a cancer doctor," Dr. Lai added, "Dr. Sun's soup is the best single drug in use for being most effective and least toxic."

*Further Reading & References*

- *Pilot study of a specific dietary supplement in tumor-bearing mice and in stage IIIB and IV non-small cell lung cancer patients. http://www.ncbi.nlm.nih.gov/pubmed/11588907

- National Cancer Institute: Sun's Soup (PDQ), http://www.nci.nih.gov/cancertopics/pdq/cam/vegetables-sun-soup

- Sun Farm Corporation, http://sunfarmcorp.com/index.htm (Note: not an endorsement; for informational purposes only)

- *Sun's soup: An entry from Thomson Gale's "Gale Encyclopedia of Cancer, 2nd ed"* by Lee Paradise (2006)

- Memorial Sloan-Kettering Cancer Center: Sun Farms Vegetable Soup, http://www.mskcc.org/mskcc/html/69391.cfm

- Sun Farms Vegetable Soup, http://cancerguide.org/sun_soup.html

# Shiitake - Lentinus edodes

The Shiitake (Lentinula edodes) is an edible mushroom native to East Asia that is cultivated and consumed in many Asian countries and has become increasingly popular in the West. The caps have nearly ragged gills and an inrolled margin when young, and they are covered with a delicate white flocking. The stem may be central or off center.

Significant research into shiitake's medicinal properties has been undertaken and shows that it has the ability to fight tumors and viruses and enhance the immune system. It has been shown that lentinan, from shiitake, taken orally, inhibits colon cancer cell growth. Lentinan, in pure form (known as D-glucan lentinan), is also the most highly researched bioactive molecule isolated from shiitake.

Lentin is a novel and potent antifungal protein component from shiitake mushroom with inhibitory effects on activity of human immunodeficiency virus-1 reverse transcriptase and the proliferation of leukemia cells. Lentinan, on the other hand, is a polysaccharide isolated from shiitake and has been found to be an immunomodulator.

Lentinan has undergone multiple studies in Japan and is described as a host-mediated anti-cancer drug. It is approved for clinical use in Japan because of its ability to prolong the survival rate of cancer patients. Lentinan is particularly effective in patients battling gastric or colorectal cancer. Quality of life for cancer patients has also been known to improve while taking lentinan.

The mechanism of lentinan's anti-tumor activity is not clear; lentinan is known as a biological response modifier (BRM) which is often taken as a synonym for an immune-modulator. Many claim lentinan can enhance cell-mediated immune responses in vitro and in vivo (that is, in laboratory cultures and in living subjects), which probably plays a part in its anti-tumor activity.

Studies have shown that powdered shiitake fruit bodies, when included in the diet, offer anti-tumor benefits. Some studies suggest a striking difference in the effectiveness of shiitake depending on the strain of cancer treated, with results varying greatly.

Biobran/MGN-3 is a natural immune booster made from rice bran and shiitake mushroom extract. It has been shown to significantly increase immune response, especially NK cells. Clinical studies with MGN-3 and cancer patients have been very positive. See **Biobran/MGN-3**.

According to The Healing Mushroom, the most amazing application of shiitake is in the treatment of HIV. In 1983, lentinan was used to successfully treat a woman with HIV to the point where she no longer had the disease. Although few outside of the AIDS community know of this case, the results were presented to the world in 1985 at the Third International Conference on Immunopharmacology in Florence, Italy.

### Further Reading & References

- Shiitake The Healing Mushroom by Kenneth Jones (1993)

- "Lentin, a novel and potent antifungal protein from shitake mushroom with inhibitory effects on activity of human immunodeficiency virus-1 reverse transcriptase and proliferation of leukemia cells." http://www.ncbi.nlm.nih.gov/entrez/query.fcgi?cmd=Retrieve&db=pubmed&dopt=Abstract&list_uids=14572878

- "Inhibition of human colon carcinoma development by lentinan from shiitake mushrooms (Lentinus edodes)." http://www.ncbi.nlm.nih.gov/pubmed/12470439

- *Medicinal Mushrooms: An Exploration of Tradition, Healing, & Culture (Herbs and Health Series)* by Christopher Hobbs and Harriet Beinfield (2003)

- *The Cancer Prevention Diet: Michio Kushi's Macrobiotic Blueprint for the Prevention and Relief of Disease* by Michio Kushi and Alex Jack (1994)

- Memorial Sloan-Kettering Cancer Center: Shiitake Mushroom, http://www.mskcc.org/mskcc/html/69377.cfm

- Shiitake Mushroom, http://www.cancer.org/Treatment/TreatmentsandSideEffects/ComplementaryandAlternativeMedicine/DietandNutrition/shiitake-mushroom

- Medicinal Mushrooms II, http://www.christopherhobbs.com/website/library/articles/article_files/mushrooms_med_02.html

- "The potential of fungi used in traditional Chinese medicine: shiitake (*Lentinula edodes*)," by Dawn Soo (2002) http://www.world-of-fungi.org/Mostly_Medical/Dawn_Soo/Dawn_Soo_SSM.htm

## Suehirotake - Schizophyllum commune

Suehirotake mushrooms have been used for medicinal purposes for thousands of years. It is said these mushrooms are successful in treating cervical cancer, though little evidence can be found.

### Further Reading & References

- Mushroom Harvest, http://www.mushroomharvest.com/catalog/product_info.php?products_id=163 (Note: not an endorsement; for informational purposes only)

- Memorial Sloan-Kettering Cancer Center: MGN-3, http://www.mskcc.org/mskcc/html/69301.cfm

# The Beer's Yeast Cure

Yeasts are eukaryotic micro-organisms classified in the kingdom Fungi, with the 1,500 species currently described estimated to be only 1% of all yeast species. Living cells of beer's yeast in a cellular fluid form is a beneficial drug that has been administered for thousands of years by cultures like the Sumerians, the Babylonians, and the Egyptians.

In 1930, the Italian Professor Dr. Giocondo Protti, head of the Research and Treatment Centre of Tumors in Busto Arsizio undertook extensive research into beer's yeast. He discovered that beer's yeast selectively attacks and destroys the morbid growth of cancer tissue. His discovery of selective oncolytic characteristics - about which he reported in Munich - aroused considerable scientific interest. Protti's collaborator, the German physician Professor Dr. Gottschalk from Munich, pointed out that beer's yeast is capable of turning cell respiration of (pathological) fermentation into oxygen respiration.

In experiments with rats, Dr. Triebel (Klinik für Geschwulst Krankheiten Braunschweig), ascertained this extraordinary phenomenon: rats with cancer instinctively pounced only on food rich in beer's yeast, and experienced a prompt improvement of their condition. The beer's yeast-treated rats survived 2 to 3 months longer than the untreated control group. At the beginning of the experiment, the rats had tumor masses weighing as much as, or even exceeding, their total body weight. In comparison with a life expectancy of three years, 2 to 3 months represented a significant life extension.

Other experiments by Jochle (Main Laboratory of Schering AG, Berlin) were conducted on mice. Even for the so-called incurable adenocarcinoma, Jochle could increase the survival time of mice by 30% with the intratumorous administration of beer's yeast. In addition to its oncolytic action, beer's yeast seems to have a beneficial effect on irradiation therapy.

It was observed that simultaneous therapy by means of beer's yeast and radiation significantly improved the general condition of beer's yeast-treated patients compared to patients who only received radiation. Beer's yeast stimulated appetite, sleep, and intestinal peristalsis.

Beer's yeast protects the mucous membranes, which is especially important in throat and gullet cancers. It is remarkable that beer's yeast-treated patients apparently hardly ever suffer from swallowing problems or inflammations of the mouth. It also inhibits hair loss. Finally, it has proved very useful to commence the beer's yeast therapy (1 litre per week) before starting with radiation.

Not only internal radiation damage is positively influenced by the beer's yeast cure, hyperkeratoses, skin atrophies, formation of rhagades with infections, nail deformation, and nail bed inflammations are also avoided significantly by means of preliminary and simultaneous beer's yeast therapy.

Thus, Professor Dr. Ries, Bayerische Krebsgesellschaft (Bavarian Cancer Association) could establish in his radiation therapeutic department in Munich, that, "...Radium damage was improved in a substantial way, inflammations disappeared, as well as skin atrophies, which were replaced by normal epithelium. Furthermore, hyperkeratotically thickened skin became tender and smooth again. Until today, none of the other conservative treatment methods has ever obtained such results."

In its written stipulations for cancer patients, the Bavarian Cancer Association consequently advises the use of beer's yeast preparations against the disease - in addition to other 'alternative' treatments such as metabolic active alimentation, vitamin and enzyme therapy, regeneration of the bowels, and mesenchyma activating organ preparations.

With regard to composition, the cellular fluid beer's yeast preparation called Metz Panaktiv, is a broad spectrum active agent; the action of its numerous components is described below.

First, beer's yeast contains a powerful antitoxic capacity due to its sulfurous content. Sulfurous components within the human body are always combined with protein complexes, and precisely this protein characteristic inactivates the sulphurous components quite easily by warmth, oxygen and dehydration.

Beer's yeast has a high content (100 g. contains 0.12 g.) of the sulphurous glutathione which has been long known for its antitoxic and antioxidant capacity.

A second aspect of the anti-tumorous action of beer's yeast, according to Professor Dr. Gottschalk, must be sought in its connective-tissue-stimulating characteristic. He ascertained that when beer's yeast is administered, an 'explosion' of connective tissue takes place in the peritumorous area and that the newly formed connective tissue grows into the disintegrating tumor mass.

Furthermore, beer's yeast is reportedly a purifying agent for the liver. This purification is caused by the B-group vitamin (amply contained in beer's yeast) and by liver regenerating agents such as oric acid and choline.

### Further Reading & References

- The Beer's Yeast Cure, http://www.karlloren.com/biopsy/book/p6.htm

# Thiazolidine-4-Carboxylic Acid (TAC)

Thiazolidine-4-carboxylic acid (TAC) is an anti-cancer agent found in the shiitake mushroom. This mushroom is one of the very few foods which naturally contain TAC.

TAC is especially hydrophobic (water-repellent), and it is believed that when cancer cells absorb it they lose their ability to absorb water; thus they die. Normal cells are not affected similarly.

TAC is somewhat toxic; however, vitamin C supposedly neutralizes or apparently eliminates the toxicity of TAC. See in References below.

Professor Andrew Victor Schally, a Nobel Laureate, and his colleagues have been exploring the anti-cancer possibilities of compounds which include this acid in their composition. This acid has other names: '4-Thiazolidine-carboxylic acid', 'Timonacic' and 'Thioproline'.

### Further Reading & References

- *Nutrients and Cancer Prevention (Experimental Biology and Medicine)* by Kedar N. Prasad and Frank L. Meyskens Jr. (Jul 30, 1990)

- "Marked formation of thiazolidine-4-carboxylic acid, an effective nitrite trapping agent in vivo, on boiling of dried shiitake mushroom (Lentinus edodes)," http://pubs.acs.org/doi/abs/10.1021/jf00100a015

# Tricholoma Matsutake

Matsutake, also known as Tricholoma matsutake, is the common name for a highly sought after mycorrhizal mushroom that grows in Asia, Europe, and North America. Matsutake has a symbiotic relationship with the roots of several tree species; it grows under trees.

The odor and taste of the matsutake are quite distinctive. Considered spicy and complex, it is unlike any other related mushrooms. It's considered an excellent source of protein, vitamins, including vitamins A, B6, and C, as well as thiamine, niacin, and riboflavin, and minerals such as potassium, sodium, iron, copper, phosphorous, and calcium. These mushrooms have no cholesterol and only traces of fat.

Matsutake mushrooms are believed to have natural anti-cancer properties with no side-effects. Some of the anti-cancer components include glycans, polysaccharides AB-P and AB-FP, various steroids, uronyde, and some nucleic acid elements. These are considered the carcinostatic (i.e. cancer-growth-inhibiting) properties of the mushroom and have been proven helpful in research on animal subjects at a rate exceeding 85%. It appears these mushrooms prevent the metastasis of carcinoma cells because of the strong effect they have on the immune system.

In a 2003 study of a number of different fungus-derived substances, the Matsutake extract performed well. The antitumor effects of biological response modifiers (BRMs) were examined in an experimental mouse model using a double grafted tumor system*:

"Some BRMs prevented metastases by utilizing the anti-tumor immunological cascade reactions, which activate macrophages in the body. The following BRMs were analyzed: PSK was a hot water extract of cultured mycelia from Coriolus versicolor and a protein bound beta-glucan. Lentinan was purified from fruit bodies of Lentinus erodes and is a beta-glucan. The agaricus preparation was extracted from fruit bodies of Agaricus blazei and a protein-bound alpha-, beta-glucan.

The M2 fraction prepared from Matsutake inhibited the growth of both primary and metastatic tumors. The M1 fraction did not inhibit either primary or metastatic tumors. Immunosuppressive acidic protein (IAP) is produced by activated macrophages. The PSK, Agaricus preparation and M2 fraction of the Matsutake preparation induced IAP but the lentinan and M1 fraction did not."

### Further Reading & References

- *"Activation of antitumor immunity by intratumor injection of biological preparations." http://www.ncbi.nlm.nih.gov/entrez/query.fcgi?cmd=Retrieve&db=pubmed&dopt=Abstract&list_uids=14619462

- Matsutake, http://en.wikipedia.org/wiki/Matsutake

- The American Matsutake: Tricholoma magnivelare, http://www.mushroomexpert.com/tricholoma_magnivelare.html

- "Matsutake mushrooms - health benefits. SteadyHealth.com, "http://www.steadyhealth.com/about/matsutake_mushrooms_health_benefits.html

# Marine Treatments

## Bengamides/Marine Sponges

Sponges are probably the simplest form of animal. Found throughout the oceans and in fresh water, a sponge is a creature with no mouth, gut, muscles, nerve cells, or sensory organs. However, sponges come in a wide variety of shapes and colors.

Sponges have amazing regeneration capabilities, as a chopped up sponge can re-grow from as little as a single cell. Other surprising complexities beyond the obvious simplicity of sponges have caught the attention of organic chemists. Sponges have existed for longer than 500 million years and, some believe, may have even been the ancestors of all animal life, according to recent genetic evidence.

Despite being stationary, soft-bodied creatures, sponges have evolved a diverse line of chemical defenses. As a primary defense, they make themselves unappealing or toxic to predators by creating potent chemicals. It is the creation of these chemicals that has won the interest of both medical researchers and pharmaceutical companies, all with an eye on new drug development.

Dr. Phillip Crews, a long-time chemistry professor at the University of California Santa Cruz, has developed a Marine Natural Products Laboratory with nearly 800 pure compounds. Each of these compounds consists of complex chemicals that have been isolated from sponges and other marine organisms. Dr. Crews has also accumulated thousands of extracts with chemical mixtures they have not yet had time to separate and analyze.

Dr. Crews has funded many research expeditions with money from the National Institutes of Health, among other sources. Over the years, he has concentrated his expeditions around the South Pacific islands, including Fiji, the Solomon Islands, and Papua New Guinea. These areas in particular have wide variety within their coral reef habitats along with extensive biological and chemical diversity when it comes to sponges.

The extract of each sponge is made up of hundreds of chemicals. It is the hope of Dr. Crews and other scientists that one such compound will provide a new treatment for diseases like cancer or arthritis.

The most promising drug lead to come out of the program so far is a group of compounds called bengamides, which Crews first isolated from sponges collected in the Benga Lagoon in the Fiji Islands. The bengamides have shown potent antitumor activity, and the pharmaceutical company Novartis has been investigating them for clinical use. A bengamide-derived drug is currently in clinical trials to test its safety and effectiveness as a treatment for breast cancer.

Several patents have been registered or are pending to add bengamide derivatives to medicaments to be used in the treatment of cancer.

### Further Reading & References

- Adventures in Organic Chemistry, http://review.ucsc.edu/winter-03/chemistry.html

- Bengamide Derivatives, Method For The Production Thereof And Use Thereof For The Treatment Of Cancer, http://www.patsnap.com/patents/view/EP1680405A1.html.

# Bryostatins

Bryostatins are a unique family of chemicals suspected to have anticancer properties. From a scientific standpoint, bryostatins are a group of macrolide lactones that were first isolated in the 1960s from extracts of moss animals (aquatic invertebrate animals) called Bugula neritina.

Bryostatins are potent modulators of PKC, or protein kinase C. The effects of bryostatins on different forms of PKC vary, showing that Bryostatin 1 can inhibit cell growth under certain circumstances while exciting cell differentiation and apoptosis under other circumstances. Bryostatin 1 was also shown to act synergistically when combined with other anti-cancer drugs. This could potentially make drug combinations more effective against a large variety of tumor cells.

Bryostatin 1 as a drug on its own has not shown significant activity in tumor patients. It also has the potential for severe side-effects when administered on its own. Because of this, most researchers are focusing on a combination therapy that includes Bryostatin 1 and other chemotherapeutic antitumor agents.

As of today, at least 20 different bryostatins have been isolated and further studies regarding their effects on cancer treatment are planned.

### Further Reading & References

- Bryostatin 1 affects P-glycoprotein phosphorylation but not function in multidrug-resistant human breast cancer cells, http://www.ncbi.nlm.nih.gov/pubmed/9815959

- A phase II trial of bryostatin 1 in patients with non-Hodgkin's lymphoma, http://www.ncbi.nlm.nih.gov/pmc/articles/PMC2363763/

# Shark Cartilage/Cartilate/Cartilade/Benefin/AE-941/Neovastat

In China, shark cartilage has been a delicacy for centuries. The Chinese consume it in the form of Shark Fin Soup. They consider it a rejuvenator and aphrodisiac. Unfortunately, heavy fishing of sharks in Chinese waters will likely lead to the extinction of certain shark species.

Though it is widely believed that sharks don't get cancer, that is a myth. Malignant tumors are indeed rare in sharks, but they have been found. Regardless, there are substances in the cartilage of sharks that may inhibit the formation of new blood vessels used by tumors to grow (this process is also known as angiogenesis).

The cartilage of sharks has been studied as a potential treatment for cancer for over 30 years. Shark cartilage was first thought to contain a substance that blocks blood vessel growth following studies that came out in the 1980s. Then again in 1998 and 2005, published reports came out that showed clinical trials of shark cartilage as a possible cancer treatment.

Among the theories as to why shark cartilage is useful in treating cancer, the most likely is that the cartilage actually makes substances that block the growth of new blood vessels that feed a tumor and help it grow.

Shark cartilage is administered in a variety of ways. Patients can take it by mouth in pill or powder form, or intravenously in the vein or abdomen. Another option is to have slow-release plastic pellets surgically implanted in the body.

Other administration methods include the use of skin patches. Some believe that retention enemas or absorption through the vaginal cavity are more efficient ways of getting the compounds into the body, as they are then absorbed without the presence of the digestive enzymes.

In addition, oral administration is an option, though some have questioned whether oral ingestion of shark cartilage could have a clinically meaningful effect on cancer because cartilage is broken down in the digestive tract. What is absorbed gets broken down by the liver, meaning very little can reach the cancer site to have any appreciable effect.

Professor Henry Brem of the Johns Hopkins School of Medicine refuted research done by William Lane, PhD for Rutgers and author of a popular book on the subject, *Sharks Don't Get Cancer.* Brem concluded that Lane's research never produced conclusive evidence showing the oral form of cartilage has any benefit. Brem's criticism is credible because he worked with Dr. Judah Folkman in the 1980s. Dr. Folkman was one of the first to publish a study on the manner in which cartilage could shut down angiogenesis in lab-cultured tumors.

Many of the shark cartilage products sold in pill or powder form have not been tested for safety or efficacy. Reportedly, many of these products were created by unreliable parties. Advocates of shark cartilage also claim it can prevent as well as treat cancer. Little or no evidence seems to exist for its prevention benefits.

Despite the questions and problems about shark cartilage therapy, some laboratory studies seem to support its ability to slow the growth of new blood vessels.

In 1983, Dr. Robert Langer and Dr. Anne Lee at M.I.T. published research* in the prestigious journal *Science* which showed that cartilage stopped new blood vessel development and stopped tumor growth. They reported that for the first 14 days, while a tumor was developing its network of blood vessels, there was no tumor growth either in untreated control animals or in animals treated with cartilage.

However, after 14 days, once the blood vessel network was in place, without the shark cartilage the tumor growth went up almost 400%. With shark cartilage, there was no growth at all. Their research also showed that shark cartilage is 1,000 times more potent as an inhibitor than any other type of cartilage.

Research on mice with melanoma had the same results. For the first two weeks, there was no tumor growth. After two weeks, the tumor growth was very active without shark cartilage, but there was almost no tumor growth at all in the animals given shark cartilage.

In a study in Mexico, seven out of eight patients responded dramatically to cartilage treatment. The only therapy was shark cartilage. After eleven weeks of therapy, five patients were tumor-free and two had tumors reduced by 85%.

Other research, this time in Cuba, received a great deal of publicity on *60 Minutes*, the popular news program. It involved patients with cancer of the prostate, breast, brain, stomach, liver, ovarian, uterus, esophagus, tonsils, and urinary bladder. All were very advanced terminal cancer patients, not expected to live more than three or four months. At the beginning all these patients were completely bedridden. At the end, those who survived were running, walking, playing, and doing normal activities.

The dosage level is one gram per kilo of body weight. So a man who weighs 80 kilos (176 pounds) would be taking 80 grams of shark cartilage per day.

There's no definitive answer to whether shark cartilage offers hope to patients who have not responded to conventional treatments.

*Further Reading & References*

- *Lee, Anne, and Robert Langer. Shark Cartilage Contains Inhibitors of Tumor Angiogenesis. Science 221:1185-1187, 1983.

- *Sharks Don't Get Cancer: How Shark Cartilage Could Save Your Life,* by I. William Lane, Linda Comac (1992)

- Folkman, Judah. Tumor Angiogenesis: Therapeutic Implications. The New England Journal of Medicine 285:1182-1186, 1971.

- Folkman, Judah and Michael Klagsbrun. Angiogenic Factors. Science 235:442-447, 1987.

- Shark Cartilage, http://www.cancer.org/Treatment/TreatmentsandSideEffects/ComplementaryandAlternativeMedicine/PharmacologicalandBiologicalTreatment/shark-cartilage

- Cartilage (Bovine and Shark) (PDQ®), http://www.cancer.gov/cancertopics/pdq/cam/cartilage/HealthProfessional/page5

- "Shark Cartilage Therapy Evaluated," by I. William Lane, PhD, http://www.dynamicchiropractic.com/mpacms/dc/article.php?id=41108

- Langer, R. et al., Science., p. 70, July 1976

# Shark Liver Oil/Alkylglycerols/Squalamine

In addition to the cartilage, the shark's liver is believed to contain health maintaining substances. It is a rich source of vitamin A and contains substances that promote both healing and the production of white blood cells.

Shark liver oil has been studied in Sweden for many years. It was found to contain alkylglycerols, chemicals found in a mother's milk as well as the immune system organs, including the liver, spleen, bone marrow, lymphatic tissues, and, importantly, in the blood.

A 2003 study reported on the cytostatic (inhibiting cell growth) and cytotoxic (having a toxic effect on cells) effects of alkylglycerols:

"BACKGROUND: Shark liver oil, with a standardized concentration of alkylglycerols and their methoxy derivates, has been widely used in Scandinavian countries as complementary medicine in the treatment of different forms of cancer. The aim of our study was to verify the hypothesized antiproliferative effect of alkylglycerols in different human cancer cell lines. …. RESULTS: The prostate cells from DU-145, PC-3 and PCa-2B showed a dramatic reduction in the colony number even after relatively small doses of 0.5 and 0.1 mg/ml medium. Flow cytomery showed an increased percentage of apoptotic cells of ovarian and prostate carcinoma, while mammary carcinoma cells showed predominantly necrotic cells after exposure to Ecomer. CONCLUSIONS: The alkylglycerols and their methoxy derivates present in Ecomer shark liver oil showed a clear apoptotic/necrotic effect on human prostate and mammary carcinoma cell lines."*

One chemical found in shark liver oil is squalamine, which appears to shut down a tumor's ability to connect to and develop its own blood supply (angiogenesis).

Consider an excerpt from the book *Shark Liver Oil: Nature's Amazing Healer* by Neil Solomon, M.D., Ph.D., Richard Passwater, Ph.D., and Ingemar Joelsson, M.D., Ph.D.:

"The Brohults of Sweden - Astrid, Sven, and their son Johan - together with Dr. Ingemar Joelsson and others, have studied the effects of AKGs (Alkylglycerols) on patients with varying forms and manifestations of cancer.

"In the course of their work, they have witnessed reduced mortality rates, protection against radiation damage, stimulation and formation of white and red blood cells and platelets, the slowing of cancer growth, accelerated wound healing, and strengthening of the immune system."

One compound found within shark liver oil, called squalamine, shows particular promise. According to researchers, animal trials demonstrated that squalamine effectively shut down a tumor's ability to connect to and develop its own blood supply. Once tumors are isolated from the nourishment they need, the hope is that the immune system will cause the tumor to shrink. Some researchers even believe squalamine could represent a powerful new weapon in the anticancer arsenal.

### *Further Reading & References*

- *Cytostatic and cytotoxic effects of alkylglycerols (Ecomer). http://www.ncbi.nlm.nih.gov/pubmed/14586289?dopt=Abstract

- *Shark Liver Oil: Nature's Amazing Healer* by Neil Solomon, et al (1997)

- "Shark Liver Oil: Health Benefits and Side Effects," http://www.steadyhealth.com/articles/Shark_Liver_Oil___Health_Benefits_and_Side_Effects_a988.html

- Shark Liver Oil, http://www.cancer.org/Treatment/TreatmentsandSideEffects/ComplementaryandAlternativeMedicine/PharmacologicalandBiologicalTreatment/shark-liver-oil

# Animal and Insect-Based Treatments

## Antistasin/Mexican Leech

Antistasin is an anticoagulant derived from the salivary glands of the Mexican leech. It inhibits blood coagulation and metastasis. See **Anticoagulants**.

### Further Reading & References

- "Antistasin, an inhibitor of coagulation and metastasis, binds to sulfatide (Gal(3-SO4) beta 1-1Cer) and has a sequence homology with other proteins that bind sulfated glycoconjugates." http://www.jbc.org/content/264/21/12138.abstract

- "Antistasin, a leech-derived inhibitor of factor Xa. Kinetic analysis of enzyme inhibition and identification of the reactive site." http://www.jbc.org/content/264/28/16694.short

## Bee Pollen

Bee pollen is produced by bees through a combination of flower pollen and nectar. It has a high nutritional content and is believed to have an anti-carcinogenic principle that could be added to food.

Bee pollen is made up of a blend of minerals, carbohydrates, lipids, protein, polysaccharides, and essential fatty acids.

Most clinical data show benefits from bee pollen are limited and somewhat benign. Regardless, it is said to help with many ailments, including cancer prevention, allergies, asthma, diabetes, GI disorders, and alcoholism.

William Robinson of the US Bureau of Entomology at the Agricultural Research Administration conducted a study where a particular strain of mice was bred to develop and eventually die from cancer tumors. Tumors would appear in the mice when they were between 18 and 57 weeks of age, followed quickly by death. Bee pollen mixed in with food was administered to one group of mice while another group received food only.

Dr. Robinson reported that the mice not given bee pollen developed tumors at an average of 31 weeks and died shortly after. For mice that received bee pollen, tumor development didn't occur till an average of 41 weeks. After 62 weeks, seven mice in the bee pollen group had still not developed tumors. At that point, the study was terminated.

Dr. Robinson's conclusion was that bee pollen or some extract from it could help prevent or treat cancer if added to food.

Patients who are allergic to bee stings, honey, ragweed, or chrysanthemum are advised to not take bee pollen.

*Further Reading & References*

- Memorial Sloan-Kettering Cancer Center: Bee Pollen, http://www.mskcc.org/mskcc/html/69132.cfm

- *User's Guide to Propolis, Royal Jelly, Honey, & Bee Pollen (Basic Health Publications User's Guide) - Paperback* by Leigh Broadhurst (2005)

- Health Benefits of Bee Pollen, http://www.bee-pollen-health.com/health-benefits-bee-pollen.html

- Robinson, William. "Delay in the Appearance of Palpable Mammary Tumors in C3H Mice Following the ingestion of Pollenized Food." Journal of the National Cancer Institute, 1948.

# Bee Propolis

Propolis is a resinous mixture that honey bees collect from tree buds and other botanical sources. It is used as a sealant for unwanted open spaces in the hive. Propolis is used for small gaps while larger spaces are usually filled with beeswax.

Propolis is believed to protect bees from disease and parasites. Its composition varies, but it is most often dark brown in color. Some alternative doctors recommend it as an anti-bacterial and anti-viral.

Propolis is believed to offer support for the pulmonary system, tissue regeneration, strengthening of capillaries, and anti-rheumatic inhibition of melanoma and carcinoma tumor cells.

*Further Reading & References*

- *Bee Propolis: Natural Healing from the Hive (Nature's Remedies)* by James Fearnley (2001)

- *User's Guide to Propolis, Royal Jelly, Honey, & Bee Pollen (Basic Health Publications User's Guide)* by C. Leigh Broadhurst (2005)

- *The Bee's Propolis - Nature's Miracle Cure* by Dr. Karkar (2008)

- Bee Propolis and its Medicinal Uses, http://www.pharmainfo.net/reviews/bee-propolis-and-its-medicinal-uses

- Health from the Hive: Honey...Bee Pollen...Bee Propolis...Royal Jelly by Carlson Wade (1992)

# Bee Royal Jelly

Royal jelly is a honey bee secretion that is used in the nutrition of larvae, as well as adult queens. It is secreted from the glands in the hypopharynx of worker bees, and fed to all larvae in the colony. Feeding the larvae of developing bees extensive amounts of royal jelly insures the development of a queen with fully formed ovaries.

A research team in Canada found that mice that were fed Royal jelly were fully protected from the developments of leukemia or other tumors. Control mice died from ascitic tumors in less than 14 days, while mice receiving appropriate mixtures of cells and royal jelly all failed to develop tumors.

It is believed royal jelly can help generate new cells as well as assist the immune system in the healing process. Royal jelly can be obtained as a supplement from nutritional outlets.

### Further Reading & References

- Super Royal Jelly, http://www.enerex.ca/products/super_royal_jelly.htm (Note: not an endorsement; for informational purposes only)

- *User's Guide to Propolis, Royal Jelly, Honey, & Bee Pollen (Basic Health Publications User's Guide)* by C. Leigh Broadhurst (2005)

- Health from the Hive: Honey...Bee Pollen...Bee Propolis...Royal Jelly by Carlson Wade (1992)

- Royal Jelly and Fighting Cancer, http://www.beeroyaljelly.net/royal-jelly-and-fighting-cancer

- The Buzz on Bee Products, http://www.bee-pollen-health.com/bee-products.html

# Bee Venom/Melittin

Melittin is the active component of bee venom. Percentage level of its contents in bee venom is 50-60%. Melittin provides very strong anti-inflammatory and anti-bacterial effect. Scientists at Australia's Commonwealth Scientific and Industrial Research Organization of Molecular Science use melittin to develop cancer treatments that should have fewer side effects than other drugs used to fight the disease.

The sting of a bee may eventually hold the secret to killing cancer cells. The venom's mellitin is a molecule that kills cells by slicing through the cell walls, destroying the cells. Australian researchers have altered the structure of the mellitin molecule to remove the part that causes the allergic reaction while still maintaining its ability to kill cells.

The next step is to target the killing activity of mellitin to cancer cells only, without harm to healthy cells. Researchers hope to achieve this by attaching the modified mellitin to an antibody molecule that specifically recognizes cancer cells. This combination of a toxin and an antibody is known as an Immunotoxin.

Chemotherapy drugs are not specific; they attack normal cells thereby causing unwanted side effects such as hair loss, vomiting and weight loss. Such symptoms limit the amount of drug that can be administered and hence its effectiveness. Immunotoxins will generate a new class of cancer drugs that can attack a wide range of cancer cells. This approach, if successful, could overcome the major drawbacks of chemotherapy treatment. Mellitin appears to be far less toxic than the plant and bacterial toxins used in earlier work. New immunotoxin drugs may reduce potential side effects while still retaining the specific killing of target cancers.

A team of researchers from the University of Technology, Sydney (Australia) and CSIRO Division of Molecular Engineering is working on putting the two types of molecules together in the hope of producing an effective and highly specific anti-cancer drug. Such a drug would have big advantages over traditional chemotherapy, which is much less specific and results in the death of many healthy cells as well as cancerous ones. In preliminary experiments, researchers were able to chemically couple bee venom with an antibody specific for myeloma cells (a type of cancer found in bone marrow). However, the process of sticking onto the antibody is difficult and can lead to unwanted chemical changes. Thus, researchers are turning to genetic engineering to create a single synthetic gene that will code for the antibody and the bee toxin, if successful.

In 1999, a research team led by Dr. Samuel Wickline at the Siteman center of Cancer Nanotechnology Excellence at Washington University in St. Louis published a study about a material they discovered that easily adheres to melittin and is able to protect the body from its effects. The nanoparticles they worked with, which they called "nanobees," were tiny spheres made from a mixture of an oily substance known as perfluorocarbon, plus lipids (fatty substances) and lecithin (found in egg yolks).

Mice in the experiment received one hundred trillion nanobees per dose, thanks to the nanoparticles. Normally, this amount of melittin would have caused massive death of red blood cells and eventually killed all the mice, but with the coatings this was avoided.

Nanobees also appear to protect the melittin itself from the body's defense system, which makes it possible to circulate longer and thus locate more tumors. In the test mice, there was a decrease in both tumors and precancerous lesions.

The scientists hope that this treatment will go into clinical trials and be available to people soon. Nanoparticles are already being used to encapsulate approved cancer drugs, as in one study with docetaxel, a prostate cancer drug, which uses the nanoparticle to deliver the drug directly to the tumor rather than having it circulate in the body and potentially harm other cells.

### *Further Reading & References*

- "Purity control of different bee venom melittin preparations by capillary zone electrophoresis," http://www.sciencedirect.com/science?_ob=ArticleURL&_udi=B6TG9-457CV9F-P4&_user=10&_coverDate=08%2F19%2F1994&_rdoc=1&_fmt=high&_orig=search&_origin=search&_sort=d&_docanchor=&view=c&_searchStrId=1595382434&_rerunOrigin=google&_acct=C000050221&_version=1&_urlVersion=0&_userid=10&md5=dcc6f1fad519f5881631a9e05759475a&searchtype=a

- Succinyl bee venom melittin is a leukocyte chemotactic factor, http://www.nature.com/nature/journal/v267/n5613/abs/267713a0.html

- "Sweeter than Honey," Triple Helix Online, http://triplehelixblog.com/2009/12/sweeter-than-honey/

# Bovine Cartilage/BovineTracheal Cartilage (BTC)

Bovine cartilage was developed by a Harvard-trained physician named John F. Prudden. Dr. Prudden used it to treat cancer as early as the 1980s and published multiple records on how bovine cartilage prompted remissions in a variety of intractable malignancies from cancers such as pancreatic, metastatic breast, and glioblastoma multiforme.

Therapeutic bovine cartilage itself is taken from the tracheal cartilage of cows. It is administered orally and through parenteral routes and appears to have antitumor and immune-regulatory effects. Bovine cartilage is also believed to have at least one angiogenesis inhibitor (angiogenesis is the formation of new blood vessels).

At least three mechanisms of action have been proposed to explain the anticancer potential of cartilage. One is that it is toxic to cells, another is that it stimulates the immune system, and the third, as mentioned, is that it inhibits angiogenesis. Cartilage also appears to be relatively resistant to invasion by tumor cells.

A variety of names have been used for Processed Bovine Cartilage, including VitaCarte, CATRIX, and BTC. There is evidence that that BTC does work some of the time, and that remissions achieved through the use of BTC are often sustained for extremely long periods of time.

BTC therapy consists of ingesting capsules, three grams three times per day.

BTC may make particular sense for patients with pancreatic cancer, since the prognosis of this cancer has been so poor with conventional therapy, and since there have been a few spectacular successes with BTC.

Compared to shark cartilage, BTC is said to be better documented, less expensive, and easier to take. Nausea and vomiting appear to be possible side effects, along with changes in the patient's taste perception, fatigue, and dizziness. The U.S. Food and Drug Administration has not approved cartilage as a cancer treatment.

### Further Reading & References

- American Cancer Society: Bovine Cartilage, http://www.cancer.org/Treatment/ TreatmentsandSideEffects/ComplementaryandAlternativeMedicine/ PharmacologicalandBiologicalTreatment/bovine-cartilage

- WebMD: Bovine Cartilage, http://www.webmd.com/vitamins-supplements/ingredientmono-155-BOVINE%20CARTILAGE.aspx?activeIngredientId=155&activeIngredientName=BOVIN E%20CARTILAGE

- National Cancer Institute: Cartilage (Bovine and Shark), http://www.cancer.gov/cancertopics/ pdq/cam/cartilage/Patient

- Memorial Sloan-Kettering Cancer Center: Bovine Cartilage, http://www.mskcc.org/mskcc/ html/69150.cfm

- Boost Your Health With Bovine Cartilage by Sally Eauclaire Osborne (1999)

- The Successful Use of Bovine Tracheal Cartilage in the treatment of cancer by D.C. David Kirchhof and N.D. Elisabeth Kirchhof (1995)

- Bovine Cartilage, http://cancerguide.org/btc.html

- Bovine and Shark PDQ, National Cancer Institute, http://www.cancer.gov/cancertopics/pdq/cam/ cartilage/HealthProfessional/page3

# Butyric Acid/Butyrate

There is evidence to suggest that milk fat contains a number of components with anticarcinogenic properties, including butyric acid. Butyric acid may play a role in the inhibition of breast and colon tumors:

"A study published in the January 2000 issue of *Carcinogenesis* shows that human colorectal cancer cells can be made more sensitive to butyrate (a European cancer therapy) when the butyrate is combined with a COX-2-inhibiting drug. Butyrate helps to induce the differentiation and death (apoptosis) of colorectal tumor cells, but is not readily available in the United States. The doctors conducting this study stated that dietary modification (using therapies such as butyrate) along with COX-2-inhibiting drugs could be considered in the treatment of colon cancer."

### Further Reading & References

- Parodi-PW 1997 Butyric acid from the diet: actions at the level of gene expression. Journal-of-Nutrition; 127 (6) 1055-1060

- Parodi-PW 1996 Milk fat components: possible chemopreventive agents for cancer and other diseases. Australian-Journal-of-Dairy-Technology; 51 (1) 24-32. Also see Parodi 1997.

- Smith-JG; German-JB 1995 Milk fat components: possible chemopreventive agents for cancer and other diseases. Food-Technology; 49 (11) 87-90

- "The histone deacetylase inhibitor sodium butyrate induces breast cancer cell apoptosis through diverse cytotoxic actions including glutathione depletion and oxidative stress." http://www.ncbi.nlm.nih.gov/entrez/query.fcgi?cmd=Retrieve&db=pubmed&dopt=Abstract&list_uids=15547708

# Contortrostatin

Contortrostatin is a protein extracted from the venom of the southern copperhead, a poisonous snake. It does not kill cancer cells, but stops their growth by inhibiting angiogenesis, as well as preventing metastases (the spread of cancer). A compound in this protein appears to inhibit cancer cell migration. It is not cytotoxic, i.e., cell-killing in the way of conventional chemotherapy drugs.

Contortrostatin is unique from all other disintegrins described to date in that it is a homodimer, which means it has two identical peptide chains held together by covalent disulfide bonds. Findings indicate that contortrostatin blocks several critical steps in tumor metastasis, and is, therefore, more potent than other agents which only block a single step.

In addition, contortrostatin significantly inhibits invasion of breast cancer cells through an artificial barrier similar to the tissue surrounding blood vessels. This action is most likely due to the ability of contortrostatin to inhibit cell motility.

At the University of Southern California, a study showed that it slowed the growth of tumors in mice implanted with human breast cancer cells by up to 70%. Dr. Francis Markland found that contortrostatin reduced breast tumor metastasis by 60-70%, and lung tumor metastasis by 90%, in mice implanted with human breast cancer cells. Contortrostatin slows metastasis by interrupting the adhesion and invasion of tumor cells into surrounding healthy cells. Side effects are reported to be milder than those of chemotherapy drugs.

In another study, Contortrostatin was injected daily into tumors in one group of mice while a saline solution was injected into the tumors of a control group. It was found that the size of the tumor masses in the contortrostatin-treated mice were significantly smaller than those in saline-treated mice. Even more promising, the contortrostatin-treated group showed 65% to 85% inhibition of lung metastasis, as compared to the saline-treated group.

### Further Reading & References

- Snake Venom Protein Paralyzes Cancer Cells, http://jnci.oxfordjournals.org/content/93/4/261.full

- "Contortrostatin, a dimeric disintegrin from Agkistrodon contortrix contortrix, inhibits breast cancer

THE COMPLETE GUIDE TO ALTERNATIVE CANCER TREATMENTS

progression," http://www.ncbi.nlm.nih.gov/pubmed/10966001

- Contortrostatin, http://www.cancure.org/choice_of_therapies_continued.htm

- *Snake venom metalloproteases - structure and function of catalytic and disintegrin domains [An article from: Comparative Biochemistry and Physiology, Part C]* by O.H.P. Ramos and H.S. Selistre-de-Araujo

# DGS1

The suppliers of this product, available in honey or capsule form, state on their website:

"… we have arranged nearly 40,000 pounds of quartz (rock crystal) with specific geometric orientation which allows them to capture energy frequencies. In this enclosed space containing quartz, 1,000 rose bushes and some wild flower plants, judiciously selected for their therapeutic properties, permit thousands of bees to produce energizing honey that is truly remarkable. By this apiculture process that is unique in the world, we produce honey which, once blended with certain essential oils, has exceptional effects for the well-being of humans."

In describing the stated ingredients, the site says:

"DGS Honey, Pure Honey, the Essential Oils of Vervain, Pine, and Cedar products have numerous therapeutic properties that have been known and used for thousands of years."

Its immune system enhancing claims are:

"Through regular and daily use, the natural product DGS1 revitalizes the immune system, provides you energy, and contributes tremendously to improve quality of life."

A number of testimonials at the supplier's website illustrate its helpful effects with prostate cancer, metastatic cancer in both lungs and cancerous tumor of the colon, and numerous metastases of the liver.

### Further Reading & References

- All Natural Health Remedies: DGS1, http://www.allnaturalremedies.net/product/product.html (Note: not an endorsement; for informational purposes only)

# Glandular Therapy/Live Cell Therapy/Thymus Extracts

The thymus is one of our major immune system glands. It is composed of two soft pinkish gray lobes lying in bib-like fashion just below the thyroid gland and above the heart. To a large extent, the health of the thymus determines the health of the immune system. The thymus is responsible for many immune system functions, including the production of T lymphocytes, a type of white blood cell that protects against the development of cancer. The thymus gland also releases several hormones that regulate many immune functions.

In 1931, Dr. Paul Niehans (1882-1971), a Swiss physician, initiated live cell therapy. After a surgical accident by a colleague, Niehans attempted to replace a patient's severely damaged parathyroid glands with those of a steer. When the patient began to rapidly deteriorate before the transplant could take place, Niehans decided to dice the steer's parathyroid gland into fine pieces, mix the pieces in a saline solution, and inject them into the dying patient. Immediately, the patient began to improve and, in fact, lived for another 30 years.

The idea that "like cures like" is the guiding principle of homeopathy and a tenet of glandular therapy, also called live cell therapy, tissue therapy and organotherapy. Glandular therapy – the use of animal glands or extracts to stimulate diseased human glands – is a healing technique that reportedly dates back to hunter/gatherer times.

Thymus extracts are extracts derived from the thymus glands. Typically, they come from the thymus gland of young calves. In one notable study published in the *New England Journal of Medicine* involving calf thymus extract, glandulars (as they're sometimes called) were tested on humans. Seventeen patients with lymphocytic abnormalities (tumorous growths and organ lesions) received daily injections of thymus peptide extract. A separate control group of 20 people with the same illness underwent chemotherapy. Of the 17 patients in the test group, ten responded to the thymic extract and experienced full remission after one year.

### Further Reading & References

- The Thymus Therapy, http://www.karlloren.com/biopsy/book/p8.htm

- Thymus Extracts, http://www.ritecare.com/nutritional/natcell_thymus.html ((Note: not an endorsement; for informational purposes only)

- Glandulars: An Old Therapy Back In Vogue, http://www.vitamintrader.com/articles/1997_02_Gland.html

- Osband, M., Lipton, J., et al. "Histiocytosis-X: Demonstration of abnormal immunity T-cell histamine

- H2 receptor deficiency, and successful treatment with thymic extract," N Engl J Med, 304: 146-53,1981.

- *Immunological Aspects of Neoplasia - The Role of the Thymus (Cancer Growth and Progression)* by Bela Bodey, Stuart E. Siegel, and Hans E. Kaiser (2004)

- Osband, M., Lipton, J., et al. "Histiocytosis-X: Demonstration of abnormal immunity T-cell histamine H2 receptor deficiency, and successful treatment with thymic extract," N Engl J Med, 304: 146-53, 1981.

# Immune Therapies

## Bacillus Calmette-Guerin (BCG)

BCG is a type of bacteria used in the treatment of cancer, usually to stimulate the immune system. It is a form of biological therapy used by both conventional and progressive oncologists, and is reported to be especially effective against malignant melanoma. BCG is used for superficial bladder cancer following surgery to remove the tumor/s. A catheter is used to place the BCG solution into the bladder. The solution contains live, weakened bacteria that activate the immune system.

The BCG solution used for bladder cancer is different from the BCG vaccine that is a vaccine for tuberculosis. Doctors are not quite sure how BCG works for bladder cancer. It seems to encourage cells of the immune system to grow and become very active in the lining of the bladder. These cells probably kill off any cancer cells that might grow back or have been left behind in the bladder lining. The treatment apparently does help to keep bladder cancers from coming back.

Thomas Keane, MD, professor and chairman of urology at the Medical University of South Carolina in Charleston, S.C. remarks on a 2002 study: "This is a good study that supports use of maintenance BCG therapy in patients with high risk superficial bladder cancer," But Keane said the study had fewer patients and a shorter follow-up time than most of the other studies the authors compared it to, which makes valid comparisons difficult, since there is less likelihood that problems — such as recurrence of the cancer — will show up when fewer patients are followed for less time. And giving BCG as often as every month could suppress the immune response to it, killing fewer cancer cells, he added.

Since BCG produces some serious side effects, researchers will continue to try to find the lowest dose of BCG that will prove effective, said Keane.

### Further Reading & References

- National Cancer Institute: Bacillus Calmette-Guerin, http://www.cancer.gov/dictionary/?CdrID=44581

- Cancer Resources: BCG, http://www.oncolink.org/resources/glossary_terms.cfm

## Bestatin

Bestatin is an immunomodulating agent with low toxicity that has a significant effect on the immune system. Bestatin displays immunostimulant and antitumor activity, along with being a potent aminopeptidase inhibitor. The hypothesis is that it inhibits aminopeptidase by stimulating apoptosis (natural cell death) in malignant cells.

In a randomized, double-blind, placebo-controlled study reported in 2003, bestatin increased survival rates for Stage-1 lung cancer patients receiving surgery. Researchers were looking at whether adjuvant treatment with bestatin could prolong survival rates of patients with Stage-1 squamous-cell lung carcinoma. Study participants were divided into a bestatin group and a placebo group.

The 5-year survival rate for the bestatin group was 81%, while the placebo group had a rate of 74%. The 5-year cancer-free survival rate was 71% for the bestatin group and 62% for the placebo group. The results were deemed statistically significant.

Few negative side effects were observed in either group. Researchers concluded that patients treated with bestatin as a postoperative adjuvant therapy showed statistically significant improved survival results compared to those who received a placebo.

### Further Reading & References

- *"Randomized double-blind placebo-controlled trial of bestatin in patients with resected stage I

- squamous-cell lung carcinoma." http://www.ncbi.nlm.nih.gov/entrez/query.fcgi?cmd=Retrieve&db=PubMed&list_uids=12697853&dopt=Abstract

- Clinical trials of bestatin for leukemia and solid tumors, http://www.springerlink.com/content/x7I7881331382572/

- Bestatin Reduces Recurrences in Patients with Stage I Squamous Cell Lung Cancer, http://professional.cancerconsultants.com/news.aspx?id=29512

# Colostrum

Colostrum is the first breast secretion that a mammal provides for its newborn during the first 24-48 hours of that newborn's life. It contains numerous immune system and growth factors as well as essential nutrients, trypsin, and protease inhibitors that protect it from destruction in the GI tract. It is estimated that colostrum triggers at least fifty processes in the newborn.

Bovine (cow) colostrum is biologically transferable to all mammals, including humans, and is apparently much higher in immune factors than human mother's colostrum. Laboratory analyses of immune and growth factors from bovine colostrum are identical to those found in human colostrum except for the fact that the levels of these factors are significantly higher in the bovine version. Dr. John Maras says: "For example, human colostrum contains 2% of IgG while cow colostrum contains 86% of IgG, the most important of the immunoglobulins found in the body".

Bovine colostrum contains a blocking hormone to prevent the calf from becoming sensitized to its own mother's immune factors. Studies indicate that all species, including man, benefit from the immune boosting properties of bovine colostrum with no reports of allergic or anaphylactic reactions to date. It is in a very limited supply because colostrum is only available for a day or two after calving.

The needs of the newborn calf must be met first and only high quality colostrum is taken from cows that have been certified free of antibiotics, pesticides, and synthetic hormones. Colostrum must be processed at low temperatures so that the immune and growth factors remain biologically viable. The past 20 years has also witnessed the publication of over 2003 research papers supportive of both colostrum and its numerous components.

In *Colostrum, Life's First Food*, Dr. Daniel G. Clark's basic message, as printed on the back cover of his book, is that "bovine colostrum rebuilds the immune system, destroys viruses, bacteria, and fungi, accelerates healing of all body tissue, helps lose weight, burn fat, increase bone and lean muscle mass and slows down and even reverses aging."

According to Clark and the well-known naturopathic physician, Dr. Bernard Jensen, colostrum has a therapeutic role to play in AIDS, cancer, heart disease, diabetes, autoimmune diseases, allergies, herpes, bacterial, viral and parasitic infections, gingivitis, colds, flu and much more. Colostrum has antioxidant properties, is anti-inflammatory, and is a source of many vitamins, minerals, enzymes, and amino acids.

Ayurvedic physicians have used bovine colostrum therapeutically in India for thousands of years. The most important components of colostrum can be broken down into two major categories: immune system factors and growth factors.

**Immune system factors:**

- *Immunoglobulins* (A, D, E, G, and M) are the most abundant of the immune factors found in colostrum; IgG neutralizes toxins and microbes in the lymph and circulatory system; IgM destroys bacteria while IgE and IgD are highly antiviral.

- *Lactoferrin* - an antiviral, anti-bacterial, anti-inflammatory, iron-binding protein with therapeutic effects in cancer, HIV, cytomegalovirus, herpes, chronic fatigue syndrome, Candida albicans, and other infections. Lactoferrin helps deprive bacteria of the iron they require to reproduce and releases iron into the red blood cells, enhancing oxygenation of tissues. Lactoferrin modulates cytokine release and its receptors have been found on most immune cells including lymphocytes, monocytes, macrophages, and platelets.

- *Proline-Rich Polypeptide* (PRP) - a hormone that regulates the thymus gland, stimulating an underactive immune system or down-regulating an overactive immune system as seen in autoimmune disease (MS, rheumatoid arthritis, lupus, scleroderma, chronic fatigue syndrome, allergies, etc.).

**Growth Factors:**

- Epithelial growth factor (EgF)

- Insulin-like growth factor-I and II (IGF-1 and IGF-II)

- Fibroblast growth factor (FgF)

- Platelet-derived growth factor (PDGF)

- Transforming growth factors A & B (TgA and B)

- Growth hormone (GH)

These all help stimulate cell and tissue growth by stimulating DNA formation.

Genetically engineered versions of IGF-1 and GH are now marketed as anti-aging and AIDS drugs. They are found naturally and in high concentrations in colostrum. Several studies show that these growth factors are capable of increasing T-cell production, accelerate healing, balance blood glucose, reduce insulin need, increase muscle and bone growth and repair while metabolizing fat for fuel.

It is generally safe for children to take colostrum, though they require proportionately lower doses. Flu-like symptoms (also known as Herxheimer reactions, resulting from the sudden release and elimination of toxins in the body) may occur in as many as 40% of cases, but symptoms are usually mild and disappear with consistent supplementation at a consistent dosage.

Throughout hundreds of years of use and over 1,000 clinical studies, colostrum has proven itself to be completely safe and without side effects or drug interactions. There is no known toxicity from ingesting colostrum at any dose.

### *Further Reading & References*

- *Colostrum: Nature's Gift to the Immune System (Health Learning Handbook)* by Beth M. Ley (2000) *Immune System Control: Colostrum & Lactoferrin* by Beth M. Ley (2000)

- *Colostrum: Nature's Healing Miracle (Volume 1)* by M.D., M.P.H. Donald R. Henderson and Deborah Mitchell (2002)

- *Colostrum: Life's First Food the White Gold (Dr. Jensen's Health Handbooks Series)* by Bernard Jensen (1993)

- *Colostrum: Amazing Immune System Enhancer* by C. M. Hawken (1999)

- *The Colostrum Miracle: The Anti-Aging Super Food That Can Boost Immunity and Prevent Premature Aging by The Editors at the Doctors' Prescription for Healthy Living Magazine* (2004)

- Memorial Sloan-Kettering Cancer Center: Bovine Colostrum, http://www.mskcc.org/mskcc/html/69151.cfm

- National Cancer Institute: hyperimmune bovine colostrums, http://www.cancer.gov/drugdictionary/?CdrID=600855

# Dr Coley/Coley's Toxins

The grandfather of bacterial treatments is Coley's toxins. Dr. William B. Coley (1862-1936), Harvard Medical School graduate, eminent New York City surgeon, and Sloan-Kettering researcher was an early US cancer pioneer who used a special vaccine to induce fever and inflammation in cancer patients.

Here is an excerpt on the history of Coley's Toxins:*

Dr. Coley was prompted by frustration after losing his first patient at Memorial Hospital, a 19-year-old female bone cancer patient, despite an early detection followed by prompt amputation of her arm and a good prognosis.

He examined records of all bone cancer patients that ended in failure and death. Coley discovered that one patient, who had been given up by his doctors, had walked out of the hospital in apparently perfect health. On his deathbed, this patient had suffered two attacks of erysipelas, a severe skin infection caused by bacteria Streptococcus pyogenes.

Coley's first attempts to produce reaction in cancer patients by injecting streptococcus cultures into them ended in failure. He then managed to get a particularly virulent culture from a famous German bacteriologist, Robert Koch, through a friend. The patient who received this culture developed a severe case of erysipelas with high fever. Within a few days, the tumors on his tonsils and neck completely disappeared. In 1893, Coley published his first paper on the new method.

Because using live bacteria was dangerous and caused an ordeal for the patient, Coley later tried to and succeeded in improving his method. Instead of using bacteria, he mixed the toxins of the strep with those of another germ, Bacillus prodigiosus, which today is called Serratia marcescens. This seemed to work similarly to the live culture.

Best results were obtained when Dr. Coley or his colleague supervised the production of toxins. Parke-Davis, the pharmaceutical company, also produced the toxins commercially for many years, but they heated the formula, which reduced its effectiveness. Despite that, even these weakened toxins, Parke-Davis formula # IX, showed a 37% cure rate for inoperable patients.

In 1943 NCI researcher M.J. Shears discovered that the biologically active substance in Coley's toxins is lipopolysaccharide (LPS), which occurs in the cell walls of gram-negative bacteria.

By 1953, however, all the production of the toxins in the United States stopped.

For over 30 years starting in the late 50s or early 60s, Dr. Frances Havas, professor emeritus of the Department of Microbiology and Immunology at Temple University School of Medicine, Philadelphia, studied the effects of Coley's toxins in mice and humans. The results of her studies were generally favorable, even in advanced patients.

In 1976, randomized trials of mixed bacterial vaccines (MBV) - as Coley's toxins are now called - began at Memorial Sloan-Kettering.

In 1991, K.F. Kolmel and colleagues in Gottingen, Germany reported favorable results obtained on treatment of advanced melanoma with Coley's toxins.

This highly successful method of curing cancer has remained more or less sidelined for over a century. The method was added to the list of unproven treatments by the American Cancer Society, generally seen as a "blacklist" of forbidden cancer treatments. Coley's toxins are not used in conventional cancer treatment today, not because they are judged ineffective or experimental, but mostly because they are inexpensive and cannot be patented.

In 1962, Dr. Barbara Johnston, M.D. published a double blind study on Coley's toxins. This study was conducted at New York University-Bellevue Hospital. The results were clear-cut. In the control group treated with a fever inducing placebo, only one patient of 37 showed any signs of improvement. Of the 34 patients treated with Coley's toxins, 18 showed no improvement, 7 noted decreased pain, while 9 showed such benefits as tumor necrosis, apparent inhibition of metastases, shrinkage of lymph nodes, and disappearance of tumors.

Coley's toxins have been researched and used in China. Zhao and others published 1991 preliminary results of these trials. China is so enthusiastic it established a special hospital in Beijing where cancer patients can be treated with Coley's toxins.

One of the few centers where Coley's toxins treatment is currently available is at the Issels

Treatment Center in Tijuana, Mexico (http://www.isselstreatmentcenter.com/). At this clinic, Coley's toxins are used in combination with the Gerson diet and other forms of immunotherapy.

Dr. Coley's daughter, Helen Coley Nauts, D.Sc. and former executive director of the Cancer Research Institute, Inc., in New York City charted Coley's results with help from her medical colleagues. Together, they documented 894 cases treated with Coley's vaccine.

Mrs. Nauts gathered promising results showing the following 5-year survival rates:

- Giant cell bone tumor: 79%

- Breast cancer: 65%

- Bone cancer: 90%

- Inoperable breast cancer: 65%

- Hodgkin's disease: 67%

- Inoperable ovarian cancer: 69%

- Inoperable malignant melanoma: 60%

Overall, patients with inoperable tumors of various kinds had 45% 5-year survival, while those with operable tumors had 50%.

Mrs. Nauts reported the first results of randomized trials of MBV (Coley's toxins) at a 1982 conference held in Cologne, Germany. The trials began in 1976 at Memorial Sloan-Kettering. First results showed advanced non-Hodgkin's lymphoma patients receiving MBV had a 93% remission rate as opposed to 29% for controls who received chemotherapy alone.

### *Further Reading & References*

- *Coley's Toxins/Issel's Fever Therapy, http://www.cancerguide.org/coley.html

- Coley, William B. A Preliminary Note on the Treatment of Inoperable Sarcoma by the Toxic Product of Erysipelas, Post-graduate 8:278-86, 1893.

- Coley, William B. The Cancer Symposium at Lake Mohonk, American Journal of Surgery (New

- Series) 1:222-25, October 1926.

- Nauts, Helen Coley. Immunotherapy of Cancer by Bacterial Vaccines. Paper read at International

- Symposium on Detection and Prevention of Cancer. New York, April 25 - May 1, 1976.

- Johnston, Barbara, "Clinical Effects of Coley's Toxin. 1. Controlled Study. 2. A Seven-Year Study." Cancer Chemotherapy Reports 21:19-68, August 1962.

- Nauts, Helen Coley, Bacterial Products in the Treatment of Cancer: Past, Present, and Future. Paper read at the International Colloquium on Bacteriology and Cancer, Cologne, Federal Republic of Germany, March 16-18, 1982.

- *Third Opinion: An International Resource Guide to Alternative Therapy Centers for Treating and Preventing Cancer, Arthritis, Diabetes, HIV/AIDS, MS, CFS, and Other Diseases* by John M. Fink (Aug 15, 2004)

# Immuno-Augmentative Therapy (IAT)/Lawrence Burton

Immunoaugmentative therapy (IAT) consists of injections of blood proteins into a patient from a healthy human donor. This therapy has not been proven to be effective, but proponents believe it helps restore the body's natural immune ability, particularly when fighting cancer.

IAT was developed by Lawrence Burton, whose doctoral work was in experimental zoology. He served as the senior investigator and senior oncologist in the cancer research unit of the pathology department of St. Vincent's Hospital in New York, a post he held until 1973.

His cancer research was based in a pathology unit. He worked with real tumors, not cell lines, and with real patients and not laboratory rats. Burton's work led to the development of a serum that would, he argued, inhibit the growth of cancer tumors. This serum was derived from certain proteins found in blood: a tumor antibody, a tumor complement that activated the antibody, an antibody blocking protein and 'de-blocker' that neutralizes the blocker. Burton, with an associate Frank Friedman, isolated these blood fractions.

Burton's theory was that when these four elements were in a balanced ratio in the blood cancer, cells would be routinely destroyed. His serum therefore was a way of bringing about this balance. He called this method of dealing with cancer 'Immuno-augmentative therapy'.

The patient's blood was analyzed every day for the ratio of these four proteins. Following that, a personalized serum was developed to correct any deficiencies. Gradually, Burton's work came to the attention of Pat McGrady who, at the time, was an editor working for the American Cancer Society. McGrady later reported seeing Burton inject some mice with his tumor-inhibiting factor. "They injected the mice and the lumps went down before your eyes - something I never believed possible."

In 1966, Burton repeated this demonstration in front of a group of science writers. The result was a story in the Los Angeles Times with a headline that read, "15-minute cancer cure for mice." Oncologists attending the seminar deemed Burton and Friedman frauds. Friedman eventually gave up in disgust while Burton fled to the Bahamas. The Bahamian government allowed him to set up a clinic in Freeport despite political interference.

Patients who could afford it made their way to the Bahamas to be treated. There were frequent demands from establishment medical bodies that he conduct clinical trials - a request he spurned on the grounds that, when dealing with the terminally ill, this is tantamount to murder.

Burton's clinic was abruptly closed down in 1985. The NCI and other bodies had convinced the Bahamian government that Burton's serum products were a source of hepatitis B and AIDS (so were blood transfusions in the United States, at the time). They had extremely weak evidence that Burton's clinic deserved to be singled out for this alleged offense. Outraged patients lobbied Congress and the result was that Congress ordered a study of alternative cancer treatments. Dr Burton was allowed to reopen his clinic, which continues the work today under the direction of Dr. R. J. Clement. Burton himself died of heart disease in 1993 at age 67.

One patient, Curry Hutchinson, diagnosed as having metastasized malignant melanoma of the lung, told the authors of a *Penthouse* article:

"When I came here I was in a wheelchair. My mother had to care for me constantly. Two months later, she was able to go home. I'm walking, jogging, swimming - alive...My improvements are unbelievable... Burton's critics claim there's no proof his therapy works. I disagree. I'm proof."

*Further Reading & References*

- Null G, Steinman, L. The politics of cancer: suppression of new cancer therapies: Dr. Lawrence Burton. Penthouse 1977:75-76,188-197.

- *The Cancer Industry: The Classic Expose on the Cancer Establishment, Updated Edition* by Ralph W. Moss (1996)

- *Cancer Action Plan: Useful, Innovative, Alternative Cancer Therapies,* by Simon James Kelly and Enrida Kelly (2003)

- Immunoaugmentative therapy (IAT), http://www.wellness.com/reference/allergies/immunoaugmentative-therapy-iat/

- American Cancer Society: Immuno-Augmentative Therapy, http://www.cancer.org/Treatment/TreatmentsandSideEffects/ComplementaryandAlternativeMedicine/PharmacologicalandBiologicalTreatment/immuno-augmentive-therapy

- IAT — Immune Augmentation Therapy, http://immunemedicine.com/

# Lactoferrin

Lactoferrin exists naturally in the breast milk of most mammals, and is found throughout the human body. It occurs in all secretions that bathe mucous membranes, such as saliva, tears, bronchial and nasal secretions, hepatic bile, and pancreatic fluids. It is an essential factor in the immune response. The lactoferrin in mother's milk provides powerful immune protection to the newborn.

Lactoferrin binds iron in the blood, keeping it away from cancerous cells, bacteria, viruses and other pathogens that require iron to grow. Thus it inhibits angiogenesis and decreases tumor growth.

Research also suggests that the lactoferrin protein activates specific strands of DNA that turn on the genes that launch the immune response. It has also been shown to have anti-viral activity. Lactoferrin can also kill H. pylori bacterium, the bacteria that cause ulcers.

Lactoferrin is concentrated in oral cavities where it will come in direct contact with pathogens (i.e. viruses, bacteria, etc.) and kills or greatly suppresses these pathogens through a variety of different mechanisms. In fact, there are specific receptors for lactoferrin found on many key immune cells, such as lymphocytes, monocytes and macrophages, and it is known to be directly involved in the upregulation of the immune system's natural killer (NK) cell activity.

Lactoferrin appears to play a key role as a host defense (protector) at the mucosal surface in the gut. Based on research observations, it is thought that lactoferrins are not absorbed via traditional routes in the gut, but instead may act directly on intestinal epithelial cells and the gut-associated lymphoid tissue (GALT) cells, probably through a receptor-mediated mechanism.

Lactoferrin has been shown to improve inflammatory diseases in animals. Its release during inflammation suggests it is involved with phagocytosis. Suppression of intestinal overgrowth and bacterial translocation of enterobacteria as well as a protective effect against infection caused by methicillin-resistant Staphylococcus aureus (MRSA) and Candida albicans has been reported in mice. In a rat model of colon cancer, lactoferrin taken orally suppressed the formation of precancerous lesions in the large intestine and the incidence of carcinoma was reduced significantly.

Multiple studies using both rats and mice exposed to a toxic chemical (azoxymethane) known to cause tumors throughout the gastrointestinal tract, administered concomitantly with lactoferrin, showed a large reduction in intestinal polyp development. Just as important, there were no toxic effects to intestinal epithelial tissues.

Another animal study found that the addition of lactoferrin to cancer-prone mice subjected to cancer-causing chemicals reduced the number of tumors and suppressed angiogenesis (the production of new blood vessels), which tumors need to survive. This study also found lactoferrin "significantly inhibited" liver and lung metastasis of cancer cells in these animals. In addition to what appears to be direct cancer inhibiting properties of lactoferrin, additional studies have found it increased natural killer (NK) cell toxicity to several cancer cell lines at low concentrations. This shows lactoferrin plays a systemic role in improving immune cell effectiveness to cancer cells, as well as a direct effect through mechanisms that are not fully clear at this time.

Intriguing human research supports functional uses for lactoferrin. In the guts of human babies, increases in bifidobacteria (beneficial intestinal flora) were reported in those fed lactoferrin-enriched infant formula. In adults with skin fungal infections, symptoms improved with oral consumption of lactoferrin.

Yet another study found lactoferrin to be very effective at suppressing the growth of human pancreatic cancer cells. So much so, the researchers concluded that lactoferrin: "…might become one of the new drugs of choice for the adjuvant therapy against pancreatic cancer." Several studies suggest lactoferrin reduces oxidative stress. Diseases such as cancer, heart disease and AIDS are all closely related to oxidative stress either as a causative factor or as a factor in progression of the disease. One study that examined the role of whey proteins, multifermented whey proteins and lactoferrin in oxidative stress made this statement:

"We can conclude that whey protein, lactoferrin and multifermented whey are good candidates as dietary inhibitors of oxidative stress and should be considered as potential medicinal foods in various pathologies as HIV infection and cancer."


### Further Reading & References

- "Expression and prognostic value of lactoferrin mRNA isoforms in human breast cancer," http://www.ncbi.nlm.nih.gov/entrez/query.fcgi?cmd=Retrieve&db=pubmed&dopt=Abstract&list_uids=15543612NatureTreatments

- *Immune System Control: Colostrum & Lactoferrin* by Beth M. Ley (2000)

- *Lactoferrin: Interactions and Biological Functions (Experimental Biology and Medicine)* by T. William Hutchens and Bo Lönnerdal (1997)


# Whey/Immunocal™/HMS-90™

Whey or milk plasma is the liquid remaining after milk has been curdled and strained. It has significant anti-cancer properties. In vitro research has shown that the growth of breast cancer cells is strongly inhibited when exposed to low concentrations of whey protein.

In an attempt to determine what protein possesses the best cancer fighting abilities, female rats were fed a diet containing either soy protein isolate, whey, or casein while the scientists attempted to induce tumors using the chemical 7,12-dimethylbenzanthracene.

Also, the rats were mated with others fed the same protein to see if these protective effects could be passed on to the next generation. All rats grew well on these proteins. However, as the months went by, tumors developed in the casein and soy-fed rodents. The whey protein rats, on the other hand, were virtually all cancer-free.

The whey and soy proved to be better than casein, while whey protein proved to be at least twice as effective as soy in reducing both tumor incidence and multiplicity. In many instances, this protective effect of whey protein was passed on to the second generation.

Another clinical study showed a regression in some cancerous tumors when patients were administered 30 grams per day of whey protein powder. Likewise, animals fed whey protein before being subjected to dimethylhydrazine (DMH), a strong cancer-causing agent, mounted a much more vigorous immune response than animals fed any other type of protein. More importantly, any resulting tumors were smaller and far fewer in number in the animals fed whey protein.

This study was confirmed by additional research showing that rats subjected to DMH and fed whey protein showed fewer tumors and a reduced pooled area of tumors. The researchers concluded that whey protein offered "considerable protection to the host," compared with other proteins, including soy.

It is interesting to note that the concentration of glutathione in tumor cells is often much higher than in surrounding normal cells, meaning that cancer cells will respond differently to nutrients and drugs that alter glutathione status. This discrepancy in glutathione status between normal cells and cancer cells also makes it harder to kill cancer cells with chemotherapy. Because the surrounding cells have lower levels of glutathione to begin with, anything that further suppresses glutathione puts normal healthy cells in danger long before cancer cells are affected.

Instead, cancer patients need a compound that can target cancer cells and deplete only their glutathione. Whey protein appears to be just such a compound. When introduced in studies, cancer cells responded to whey protein by losing glutathione, while normal cells actually increased in glutathione and cellular growth. No other protein was reported to show the same effect. Even the mechanism by which whey protein acts is not fully understood.

Whey protein is effective because of its abnormally high biological value, which is a measure of the nitrogen retained for growth or maintenance, expressed as a percentage of the nitrogen absorbed. Whey, with the highest biological value of any protein, is absorbed, utilized and retained in the body better than other proteins. This has caused athletes to make whey protein concentrate a best-seller. In fact, one recent pilot study found whey protein isolate corrected the immune suppression often seen in athletes suffering from over-training syndrome.

Proteins with a high biological value are more tissue-sparing, making whey protein concentrate a good choice for people suffering from wasting diseases such as cancer, AIDS, and/or aging-related muscle losses.

Whey also appears to have a direct in vitro effect on bone cell growth. It was found to stimulate protein synthesis, DNA content, and increased hydroxyproline content of bone cells. When these results were added to the observation that animals fed whey protein powder had stronger bones, researchers concluded, "These findings suggest that whey protein contains active components that can activate osteoblast cell proliferation and differentiation. Also these active components can probably permeate or be absorbed by the intestines. We propose the possibility that the active component in the whey protein plays an important role in bone formation by activating osteoblasts."

In addition, whey is a highly complex protein made up of many sub-fractions, including beta-lactoglobulin, immuno-globulins, bovine serum albumin (BSA), lactoperoxidases, lysozyme, lactoferrin and others. Each of these subfractions has its own unique biological properties and benefits.

One sub-fraction, lactoferrin, is found in tiny amounts in the human body, yet appears to be a first-line immune system defense. It binds to iron so strongly that it inhibits the growth of iron-dependent bacteria and can block the growth of many pathogenic bacteria and yeast. Its antimicrobial action may even improve effectiveness of antibiotics.

In the digestive tract, lactoferrin may help by stimulating intestinal cell growth and enhancing the growth of "good" intestinal microflora. A strong antioxidant, lactoferrin has positive immunomodulatory effects and scavenges free iron, which prevents uncontrolled iron-based free radical reactions and protects certain cells from lipid peroxidation.

In another study, lactoferrin was shown to inhibit colon carcinogenesis in male rats treated with another carcinogenic chemical, azoxymethane. See **Lactoferrin**.

Most importantly, these protective effects were demonstrated with easy to achieve, realistic amounts of lactoferrin; about the same as contained in high quality whey oligopeptide formulations.

Immunocal/HMS 90, a patented concentrated whey protein isolate has been shown to raise glutathione (GSH) levels by 35%. By maintaining high intracellular GSH levels, oxidative damage is minimized. See **Antioxidants**.

Immunocal/HMS 90 contains three bioactive proteins: the thermobiles — serus albumin, alpha lactalbumin and lactoferrin. Alpha lactalbumin increases the following neurotransmitters and amino acid tryptophan:

- Serotonin

- Melatonin

- Pinoline

- 5-MeO-DMT (5-methoxy-dimethyltryptamine)

- DMT (dimethyltryptamine)


*Further Reading & References*

- "Diets containing whey proteins or soy protein isolate protect against 7,12-dimethylbenz(a) anthracene-induced mammary tumors in female rats." http://www.ncbi.nlm.nih.gov/entrez/query.f cgi?cmd=Retrieve&db=pubmed&dopt=Abstract&list_uids=10667471

- Lands LC, Grey VL, Smountas AA. Effect of supplementation with a cysteine donor on muscular

- performance. 1: J Appl Physiol. 1999 Oct;87(4):1381-5.

- "Effect of supplementation with a cysteine donor on muscular performance." http://www.ncbi.nlm. nih.gov/entrez/query.fcgi?cmd=Retrieve&db=PubMed&list_uids=10517767&dopt=Abstract

- Whey Beats Rat Breast Cancer.(Brief Article): An article from: Food Ingredient News (2005)

- Modified whey protein may offer anticancer benefits.: An article from: Emerging Food R&D Report (2005)

- USDA Agricultural Research Service: A New Whey To Prevent Cancer? http://www.ars.usda.gov/ is/ar/archive/oct00/whey1000.htm

# Inositol/Inositol Hexaphosphate (IP-6)

Dr. AbulKalam M. Shamsuddin MD, PhD, is Professor of Pathology at the University of Maryland School of Medicine in Baltimore. Since 1975, he has been researching the processes of cancer formation, cancer prevention and cancer treatment. Inventor of a rapid, simple and inexpensive screening test for colorectal cancer, he is also the pioneering scientist who demonstrated the immune-enhancing and anti-cancer actions of IP-6 & Inositol, for which he was awarded the US patent #5,082,833.

Inositol hexaphosphate (IP-6) is an extract from rice bran that improves natural killer cell activity and is absorbed by cancer cells, where it stops cell proliferation and restores normal function. Various studies show that IP6 has potential for cancer treatment and prevention.

Dr. Shamsuddin's theory is that, since all cancers, irrespective of their type and origin, have a common defect of uncontrolled cell proliferation, IP-3 is a key regulator of cell growth, and IP-6 & Inositol yield IP-3. Therefore, IP-6 and Inositol should be effective against many different types of cancers, and across species.

Dr. Shamsuddin wrote about these studies in *IP-6: Nature's Revolutionary Cancer- Fighter*. His research has shown that IP-6 can slow or stop the growth of cancer cells in the laboratory and in mice. Dr. Shamsuddin has reported that while IP-6 doesn't actually kill cancer cells, it makes them behave like normal cells, thus eliminating the danger they pose. A number of laboratory studies have confirmed his findings. Research suggests that IP-6 can boost immune function, help lower cholesterol, prevent formation of kidney stones, reduce the risk of heart disease and stroke, and prevent the complications of diabetes.

Some alternative doctors perform chelation intravenously with a mild mineral chelator called EDTA. But this approach is said to be time-consuming and costly, and the tumor grows in between treatments. Alternatively, IP-6 is sometimes recommended to be taken orally to perform chelation therapy at home. It is recommended that IP-6 should be consumed in between meals so as not to interfere with mineral absorption from foods. It should only be taken with water, as vitamin C in juices interferes with its action. Anemic individuals will feel weak after taking IP-6.

Nearly two decades of research with animals reveals that IP-6 shrinks all types of tumors (brain, lung, prostate, breast, liver, colon) when given to animals in drinking water. Study results show a 60% reduction in the number of lung tumors in mice by the use of inositol compared to an untreated control group. The authors conclude: "among the compounds tested, myo-inositol is most effective after carcinogen treatment."

IP-6 has also reproducibly inhibited the growth of human prostate cancer cells in the laboratory, and demonstrated its effectiveness in the prevention of colon cancer.

### Further Reading & References

- *IP-6: Nature's Revolutionary Cancer-Fighter* by AbulKalam M. Shamsuddin, MD, PhD. (1998)

- *Nature's Ultimate Anti-Cancer Pill: The IP-6 with Inositol Question and Answer Book* - by Coles Stephen (1999)

- "Anti-angiogenic activity of inositol hexaphosphate (IP6)." http://www.ncbi.nlm.nih.gov/entrez/query.fcgi?cmd=Retrieve&db=pubmed&dopt=Abstract&list_uids=15297368

- "Inositol hexaphosphate (IP6) enhances the anti-proliferative effects of adriamycin and tamoxifen in breast cancer." http://www.ncbi.nlm.nih.gov/entrez/query.fcgi?cmd=Retrieve&db=pubmed&do

pt=Abstract&list_uids=12846414

- Inositol Phosphates Have Novel Anticancer Function Authors: Shamsuddin AM Source: J. Nutr. 1995;125:725S-732S.

- Inositol-Phosphate-Induced Enhancement of Natural Killer Cell Activity Correlates with Tumor

- Suppression Authors: Baten A, Ullah A, Tomazic VJ, Shamsuddin AM Source: Carcinogenesis. 1989; IP6 in Treatment of Liver Cancer. I. IP6 Inhibits Growth and Reverses Transformed Phenotype in HepG2 Human Liver Cancer Cell Line. Authors: Vucenik I, Tantivejkul K, Zhang ZS, Cole KE, Saied I, Shamsuddin AM Source: Anticancer Res. 1998; 18(16A):4083-4090.

- IP6 in Treatment of Liver Cancer II. Intra-Tumoral Injection of IP6 Regresses Pre-Existing Human

- Liver Cancer Xenotransplanted in Nude Mice. Authors: Vucenik I, Zhang ZS, Shamsuddin AM Source: Anticancer Res. 1998; 18(6A):4091-4096.

- IP6-Induced Growth Inhibition and Differentiation of HT-29 Human Colon Cancer Cells: Involvement of Intracellular Inositol Phosphates Authors: Yang G, Shamsuddin AM Source: Anticancer Research. 1995; 15:2479-2488.

- IP6: A Novel Anti-Cancer Agent Authors: Shamsuddin AM, Vucenik I, Cole KE Source: Life Sciences. 1997; 61(4):343-354.

- Novel Anti-Cancer Functions of IP6: Growth Inhibition and Differentiation of Human Mammary Cancer Cell Lines in Vitro Authors: Shamsuddin AM, Yang GY, Vucenik I Source: Anticancer Research. 1996; 16:3287-3292.

- Up-Regulation of the Tumor Suppressor Gene p53 and WAF1 gene expression by IP6 in HT-29 Human Colon Carcinoma Cell Line Authors: Saied IT, Shamsuddin AM Source: Anticancer Res. 1998; 18(3A):1479-1484.

# Iscador/Mistletoe/Iscar/Viscumalbum/Plenosol/Helixor/Iscucin/ Anthroposophical Cancer Treatment

Mistletoe treatment is available in Germany, where it is the most commonly used biologic therapy for cancer. It is also frequently used in Switzerland, the Netherlands, the United Kingdom, Austria and Sweden. Physicians in these countries can legally prescribe commercial preparations of mistletoe. Although condemned by the American Cancer Society, it is approved for use in Germany and Switzerland.

Iscador is the trade name for a number of preparations made with different types of mistletoe that grow on different kinds of trees and therefore exhibit different properties. These are further combined with homeopathic (extremely small) doses of such metals as silver, copper, and mercury.

The Lukas Clinic in Arlesheim, Switzerland is a major center where this therapy is carried out. However, any doctor can procure the capsules.

As a leader of the Anthroposophical movement, Rudolph Steiner, PhD popularized the use of mistletoe in the early 20th century. A certain lectin in mistletoe has been found to inhibit the growth of proliferating cells. By the 1980s, about 40,000 patients worldwide were receiving Iscador, a fermented form of mistletoe that is administered by injection.

The Anthroposophical Cancer treatment includes:

- Vegetarian diet

- Regular physical activity

- Bowel cleansing

- Yarrow liver compress

- Social engagement

- Hepatodoron, Formica, Stibium

- Therapeutic Eurythmy

- Artistic therapy

- Standard therapy (chemo, radiation, hormonal treatment) when indicated and requested

- Mistletoe therapy, such as with Iscar®, Iscucin®, or Helixor®

Multiple published studies show that mistletoe extracts can inhibit metastasis, and reduce the size of and cause necrosis of induced tumors in rodents by stimulating the immune system.

Steiner's proposal in the early 1920s that mistletoe might be therapeutic for cancer was based on the process he called "spiritual science" in which he combined spiritual and scientific thought as "complementary" modes of insight.

Steiner believed that cancer resulted from imbalances in forces affecting the human body and that the "lower organizing forces" were responsible for cell division, growth and expansion, while the "higher organizing forces" were responsible for limiting and organizing that growth, for controlling cell differentiation and producing overall body form. These forces were in balance in a healthy person, while in people with cancer, the higher organizing forces were weak. The resulting imbalance, he theorized, could lead to an excess proliferation of cells, loss of form and, eventually, to tumor formation.

It was Steiner's belief that cancer involved not only physical disorder in the body, but also disruptions among "different levels of matter, life, soul, and spirit."

Steiner's ideas about mistletoe's potential effectiveness for cancer arose from his analysis of the semiparasitic plant's characteristics. The form of the plant is spherical rather than vertical, the force of gravity does not influence its growth, and it grows on different species of host trees, taking water and minerals from the sap and supplying the tree with sugars. As it avoids contact with the earth, the plant does not have roots. It produces berries all year long and flowers in the winter.

Steiner concluded that mistletoe grew independently from earth forces and seasonal cycles, opposite to the way he believed tumors developed.

From these characteristics, Steiner concluded that mistletoe would be a valuable therapeutic agent, stimulating the "higher organizing" forces which he felt were inadequate in people with cancer. He also believed that mistletoe might be combined with certain metals in high dilution to enhance its activity.

Steiner also developed specific artistic activities that he felt would contribute to recovery from cancer, such as clay modeling, movement therapy (eurythmy), and speech formation that he believed would strengthen patients' "formative forces."

The Iscador extract of mistletoe is given by subcutaneous injection at a site close to the tumor, starting with low doses and gradually increasing them until the patient reacts by showing a clear objective or subjective improvement in general health, the tumor slows down, or the patient experiences a fever reaction. This is seen as a good sign.

One of its most obvious effects is that it increases the size of the thymus gland substantially (by nearly 100% in some animal studies) and the thymus becomes much more active. This is a significant finding as the thymus is an important immune system gland.

Not all cancers respond well to Iscador. Leukemia, apparently, does not. Iscador reportedly works best with carcinomas and melanomas.

The best results with Iscador are claimed for its use with solid tumors both before and after surgery and radiation. Given 10 to 14 days before surgery, it is thought to help prevent metastatic spread due to surgery and to promote recovery. It is thought by proponents to improve survival rates for cancers of the cervix, ovaries, breast, stomach, colon, and lung.

A second use of Iscador is for advanced stage, inoperable solid tumors. At this time, proponents claim patients might experience improvements in their general condition, alleviation of side effects of conventional therapies, less pain, cessation of tumor growth and, occasionally, regression of tumors.

Proponents also claim that the use of Iscador in these cases sometimes results in a better demarcation between the tumor and surrounding tissue that then makes surgery possible. The best results for inoperable tumors are thought to be with cancers of the bladder, stomach, intestine, genital organs, and skin. It is also claimed that bone metastases are retarded in some cases. Results are thought to be less promising for inoperable cancers of the breast, lungs and esophagus.

Although mistletoe is poisonous, Iscador is relatively non-toxic. It is suggested that it can accompany any other anti-cancer treatment as no negative interactions with other medications have been reported. However, people with heart problems, pregnant women and people taking a prescription drug containing a monoamine oxidase inhibitor should not take it.

In addition to fighting cancer, it has the effect of aiding sleep, providing pain relief and stimulating weight gain. Many patients report being reinvigorated. A study reported in 2004 evaluating its use in primary, non-metastatic breast cancer patients receiving conventional therapy, showed it considerably reduced the side effects of conventional therapy.

In a study reported in 2004 evaluating its use in primary, non-metastatic breast cancer patients receiving conventional therapy, the researchers found it considerably reduced the side-effect of conventional therapy. See References below.

Despite the treatment's semi-mystical origins, it has since been scientifically validated. Extracts of mistletoe have been shown to kill cancer cells in the laboratory and to stimulate the immune system, according to a report by the National Cancer Institute that summarizes the anticancer effects of mistletoe.

ISCADOR is available under the brand name ISCAR® in the US.


### Further Reading & References

- *Iscador: Mistletoe in Cancer Therapy* by Christine Murphy (2001)

- "Efficacy and safety of long-term complementary treatment with standardized European mistletoe

- extract (Viscum album L.)." http://www.ncbi.nlm.nih.gov/entrez/query.fcgi?cmd=Retrieve&db=pubmed&dopt=Abstract&list_uids=15460213

- Herbal Therapies for Cancer, http://www.commonwealhealth.org/herbs.html

- "Suzanne Somers's Use of Mistletoe," Annie Apple Seed Project, http://www.annieappleseedproject.org/suzsomuseofm.html

# Lactobacilli/Probiotics/Prebiotics

Lactobacillus is a genus of bacteria also called lactic acid bacteria. Probiotics are defined as live microorganisms that, when administered in adequate amounts, confer a health benefit on the host. The ingestion of probiotic bacteria is intended to support and supplement the billions of bacteria that normally exist in a healthy human colon. These so-called intestinal flora are vital to good health.

There is mounting evidence that selected probiotic strains can provide health benefits to their human hosts, including significant anti-cancer benefits. Prebiotics are the foods that contain nutrients that nourish these healthy bacteria.

Lactobacillus acidophilus and Lactobacillus bulgaricus are well-known yogurt culture bacteria. A myriad of healthful effects have been attributed to the probiotic lactic acid bacteria. There is a wealth of evidence of the anticancer effect of consumption of lactic cultures in fermented or unfermented dairy products. For example, Lactobacillus casei and Bifidobacterium longum were shown to suppress the proliferation of tumor cells and prolong survival.

The immunomodulatory and antitumor effects of lactic acid bacteria have been shown in studies to have a direct antiproliferative effects on tumor cell lines in vitro as well as effects on immune cells in vivo, and antitumor effects on tumor-bearing mice with prolonged survival periods. See References below.

In another study, Lactobacillus rhamnosus was shown to be more cytotoxic to human bladder cancer cells than Mycobacterium Bovis (bacillus Calmette-Guerin), which is used by both conventional and alternative cancer physicians. See **BCG**.

Because intestinal bacteria play an extremely important role in the digestion of otherwise incompletely-digested proteins and other food substances, these beneficial bacteria are an important part of the detoxification of the body. Lactobacillus plantarum is believed to be especially productive of proteolytic enzymes (enzymes that act on protein and clear protein wastes from the system). This form of bacteria it noted for its ability to eliminate or reduce most other bad bacteria and fungi. In addition, Lactobacillus plantarum has a beneficial effect on the immune system, as it changes the immune cells and influences the production of cytokines. One consequence of this is the normalization of the colon pH.

PRObiotic Foods include:

- Yogurt

- Kefir

- Tempeh

- Miso

- Kim Chi

- Sauerkraut

- Other 'fermented' foods


PREbiotic foods include:

- Oatmeal

- Flax

- Barley

- Other whole grains

- Greens (especially dandelion greens, but also spinach, collard greens, chard, kale, mustard greens, etc.)

- Berries and other fruit

- Legumes (lentils, kidney beans, chickpeas, navy beans, white beans, black beans, etc.

Many alternative and integrative cancer doctors consider colon health to be essential to recovery from cancer and poor colon health to be one of the principal causes of cancer. As a well-established therapy for restoring and maintaining colon health, probiotic "friendly bacteria" supplements are a highly reasonable and well-supported therapy not only for the prevention and treatment of cancer but for general good health.

### *Further Reading & References*

- Beating Cancer With Nutrition by Patrick Quillin (2005)

- User's Guide to Probiotics: Learn How "Healthy Bacteria" Can Help You Fight Infections and Restore Your Health by Earl Mindell (2010)

- Health Benefits of Probiotics (Latest Research Showing Benefits for Digestion, Cholesterol, Yeast Infection, Immune System, Colon Cancer, Ulcers, etc) by Beth Ley-Jacobs (2000)

- The Probiotic Solution by Mark Brudnak (2003)

- *"Immunomodulatory and antitumor effects in vivo by the cytoplasmic fraction of Lactobacillus casei and Bifidobacterium longum." http://www.ncbi.nlm.nih.gov/entrez/query.fcgi?cmd=Retrieve&db=pubmed&dopt=Abstract&list_uids=15028884

- "Lactobacillus species is more cytotoxic to human bladder cancer cells than Mycobacterium Bovis (bacillus Calmette-Guerin)." http://www.ncbi.nlm.nih.gov/entrez/query.fcgi?cmd=Retrieve&db=pubmed&dopt=Abstract&list_uids=12394766

# Maruyama Vaccine/Specific Substance Maruyama (SSM)

Maruyama Vaccine was developed by the late Dr. Chisato Maruyama, Professor Emeritus at Nippon Medical School, Japan. When treating Hansen's Disease and Tuberculosis patients with a vaccine he had developed, Dr. Maruyama noticed that the number of Cancer patients was extremely small among these patients. In 1965, Maruyama Vaccine was injected twice a week to a patient with terminal cancer with only two or three months to live. The patient recovered his strength, and the tumor almost disappeared.

Maruyama Vaccine has no effect to directly kill cancer cells. It causes interferon to be produced which activates macrophages which in turn, inhibit an increase of cancer cells.

### Further Reading & References

- What is Maruyama Vaccine? http://www.tim.hi-ho.ne.jp/keisaku/index1.html

# MGN-3/BioBran/Peakimmune4

Dr. Mamdooh Ghoneum of Drew University of Medicine and Science developed MGN-3/ BioBran from breaking down rice bran with enzymes from the Shiitake mushroom. The product, which is a functional food, is called BioBran in the United Kingdom and Europe. In the US it is called MGN-3 and was manufactured by Lane Labs. It is no longer available from Lane Labs according to an FDA ruling on July 9th, 2004 due to medicinal claims made by the manufacturer — not because it doesn't work. MGN-3/ BioBran has been clinically proven to help powerfully enhance depleted immune systems. It is now manufactured and sold under the name Peakimmune4.

In general, manufacturers of supplements are not permitted to make claims regarding the treatment and cure of diseases. Violations of this regulation sometimes result in a supplement's removal from the market, although the claims may be perfectly true.

While MGN-3/BioBran/Peakimmune4 has acquired a remarkable reputation, it is just one of a wide selection of immune system supplements that have been proven highly effective.

The cellular picture of this treatment is as follows: The human immune system is comprised of more than 130 subsets of white blood cells. About 15% of them are called Natural Killer (NK) cells. These provide the first line of defense for dealing with any form of invasion to the body. Each cell contains several small granules, which act as 'ammunition.' When an NK cell recognizes a cancer cell, for instance, it attaches itself to the cell's outer membrane and injects these granules directly into the interior of the cell. The granules then 'explode,' destroying the cancer cell within five minutes. The killer cell then moves on to other cancer cells and repeats the process. As long as NK cells remain active, the body is able to keep disease under control. In its lifetime, a single NK cell can kill as many as 27 cancer cells, sticking to them and then injecting lethal chemical granules that can destroy the abnormal cell in less than five minutes.

MGN-3/BioBran is reported to not only stimulate NK cell activity by more than 300%, but also T-cell and B-cell activity by 250% and 200% respectively. It can do this without any toxicity or other adverse side effects, unlike synthetic cytokines currently used by oncologists, such as interleukin-2, which can be extremely toxic.

It appears to be able to do this by increasing the body's production of natural cytokines (substances such as interferons, interleukins, and tumor necrosis factors), which not only help destroy rogue cells and viruses directly, but kick-start the immune system by increasing the activity of the lymphocytes (B-cells, T-cells and especially NK-cells). B-cells focus on producing antibodies whilst the T-cells and NK cells circulate through the body directly destroying virally or bacterially infected cells as well as cells that have turned cancerous.

Cancers of the blood, such as leukemia and multiple myeloma, show the greatest response, while good results have been seen in other cancers like lymphoma, ovarian, prostate, and breast cancer. When the body is stressed or in a diseased state, the immune system can become overloaded and the activity of these protector cells becomes sluggish. This is often compounded by medical treatment (such as chemotherapy in the case of cancer) that further depresses the immune system. A weak immune system is less able to prevent cancer cells and infections from taking hold and spreading in the body.

Dr. David G. Williams stated in his health newsletter, **Alternatives**, "If MGN-3 were a drug, it would be front-page news, the top story of every newscast in the country. But MGN-3 isn't a drug, it probably won't even make the news, and it could even threaten the multi-billion dollar profits of the U.S. drug industry."

Dr. Ghoneum's findings have been demonstrated in test-tube experiments as well as seven published studies involving 72 patients. In a study presented to the American Association for Cancer Research, he reported on five patients with breast cancer. Each patient was treated with the same dosage of three grams a day of MGN-3/ BioBran from a Japanese manufacturer. NK cell activity increased within two weeks and continued to do so as the study progressed. At the end of the six- to eight-month study, two of the patients were in complete remission. In a study reported the following year, 27 patients with various types of cancers including breast, cervical, prostate, leukemia and multiple myeloma were tested for NK cell activity by 51 Chromium- release assay before and after only two weeks treatment with MGN-3/ BioBran.

### Further Reading & References

- NetNutri.com, www.natura.org.uk/biobran.htm (Note: not an endorsement; for informational purposes only)

- MGN-3 Research Data Index, http://www.research-data.com/Latest-Findings/MGN3-Index.htm

- Biobran MGN-3 Immunomodulator, http://www.biobran.org/

- Biobran MGN-3 - An Overview, http://www.biobran.org/overview/

# Dr. Hasumi

In Japan, Dr. Hasumi claims outstanding success in curing cancer with a vaccine made from the patient's own urine; however, it works only if the immune system is still sufficiently strong.

The Electro-Chemical & Cancer Institute developed a cancer vaccine in 1946, the Hasumi Vaccine, and started its clinical application in 1948. The Hasumi Vaccine has been in clinical use since. At first, the concept of this vaccine was based on the simple premise and a methodological question: "How we can let the body's immune system distinguish cancer cells from normal cells?"

In those days, the research was based on the theory of virus-induced cancer propagation, an idea totally rejected by the then reigning medical circle of Japan.

Since 1988, the present organization has made efforts to extract membrane antigen from cancer cells. In 2000, through joint research with the University of Maryland (USA), the physiological activity of the Hasumi Vaccine was demonstrated and has paved the way for the cancer vaccine to steadily prevail. In 1999, through joint research with the Jefferson Medical College of Thomas Jefferson University (USA), the clinical research of dendritic cell vaccine, a new type of cancer vaccine, was started.

The product's website states, "To date, more than 130,000 people have been treated with the Hasumi Vaccine and today approximately 16,000 people in Japan and 6,000 people overseas are continuing treatment with the vaccine. The therapeutic advantage of the Hasumi Vaccine has been demonstrated to prevent recurrence after cancer surgery."

Approximately one-third of the patients who take the vaccine do so against a secondary cancer. Some terminal, grown tumors have been reported to vanish in rare cases.

### Further Reading & References

- Shukokai Clinic, http://www.shukokai.org/index3e.html

# Dr. Virginia Livingston/Livingston Approach

Dr. Virginia Livingston, like Roy Rife and Gaston Naessens, took as her starting point the belief that a microbe —one that could change shapes —was the cause of cancer. This ability of a microorganism to "shape-shift" is called pleomorphism and the organisms are referred to as pleomorphs. It's important to add that this theory of cancer causation is controversial and only weakly supported by evidence pro or con, due to the scientific establishment's hostility.

Dr. Livingston reportedly saw such a microbe in 1947 and from then on directed all her work to combating it. She named the microbe Progenitor cryptocides (meaning 'hidden, ancestral killer'). She claimed to find this microbe everywhere she looked - even in sperm.

She believed that everyone has this microbe but that it is held in check by the immune system until stress, diet, or even surgery or other traumatic events weaken or damage the immune system. Then the microbe multiplies in overwhelming numbers, becoming invasive and promoting the growth of cancer tumors.

She and her researchers demonstrated that solutions containing P. cryptocides but free of bacteria, sealed off from external contamination, subsequently become populated by bacteria, proving that the microbe changes forms. Such organisms have also been associated with arthritis and multiple sclerosis. She discovered that the microbe secreted a growth hormone that was identical to that which coats the placenta surrounding a fetus. She believes that this hormone, human chorionic gonadotrophin (HCG), also coats tumor cells.

The purpose of the hormone is to alert the immune system not to interfere with the contents of the HCG coated bundle. Clearly, some biochemical signal is needed to prevent the body's immune system from attacking a new fetus. According to Livingston, this is the mechanism. Others have since claimed they confirmed it. HCG has to be kept in check by antibodies or it will grow out of control. One substance that does neutralize it is abscisic acid.

Dr. Livingston's regime is to rebuild the immune system with a vegetarian raw food diet, vitamin and mineral supplements, gamma globulin injections and - the key differentiating element of the therapy - an autogenous vaccine [a vaccine cultured from the patient's own blood] given in conjunction with a BCG vaccination (an attenuated bovine tuberculosis bacillus vaccine that Livingston describes as "a close relative of Progenitor cryptocides"). See **BCG**.

She claimed an 80% remission rate.

In 1965, a friend convinced Livingston to try to help her husband, a physician with a malignant lymphoma of the thymus gland. She "treated him with an autogenous vaccine as a nonspecific immune stimulation, mild antibiotics, and diet. He died of a heart attack, after living almost twenty additional years."

In 1968, she founded what was to become the Livingston-Wheeler Medical Clinic. Over the 22 years from 1968 until Dr. Livingston's death in 1990, the Livingston-Wheeler Clinic became one of the landmark alternative therapy clinics in the United States and one of the treatment centers of choice for many cancer patients seeking other options. It is still in operation, essentially providing the same treatment originally designed by Livingston. The clinic employs a wide range of other cancer therapies in addition to those described here.

### Further Reading & References

- *Conquest of Cancer: Vaccines and Diet* by Virginia Livingston-Wheeler, Edmond G. Addeo

- *Cancer: A New Breakthrough* by Virginia Livingston (1993)

- *Physician's Handbook* by Virginia Livingston-Wheeler (San Diego: Livingston-Wheeler Medical Clinic)

- UCSD Medical Center: Livingston Wheeler Therapy, http://cancer.ucsd.edu/outreach/PublicEducation/CAMs/livingston.asp

- Memorial Sloan-Kettering Cancer Center: Livingston-Wheeler Therapy, http://www.mskcc.org/mskcc/html/69283.cfm

- The Healing Journal: A tribute to Dr. Virginia C. Livingston, http://www.thehealingjournal.com/node/96

# VG-1000/Dr. Govallo/Immuno Placental Therapy (IPT)

Dr. Valentine Govallo, a Russian immunologist developed a vaccine from the human placenta after a live birth, which appears to wake up the immune system of cancer patients to the invading cancer.

Dr. Govallo, believed the immune system itself was hindering the activity of the immune system, emitting certain "blocking factors". Since some of these blocking factors seem to bear a striking resemblance to those emitted by an embryo during pregnancy, Govallo had the brilliant idea of using placental extracts to immunize the patient against the fetus-like behavior of the cancer cells. He found that an extract of human chorionic villi effectively blocks all reactions of cell immunity when added to a test tube of white blood cells.

Records of Govallo's first trial with 45 patients and IPT in 1974 show 29 (64.4%) still alive after more than 20 years. Side effects are those typical of many vaccinations: fever, malaise, flulike symptoms for 1 to 2 days. Due to the strong possibility of "tumor lysis syndrome" (i.e., disintegration of the tumor) because of the newly mounted immune attack, it is critical that detoxification and full nutritional strategies, including the use of coffee enemas, be in place before a course of IPT.

In cancer patients, Govallo found a quantitative reduction of the tumor mass after immunization with placental extract, and decreased production of blocking factors, just as a decrease in the production of blocking factors reduces tumor mass.

Govallo has stated it is not yet exactly clear how the placental extract effect works. The statistics in his book show a 77.1% 5-year survival rate. He published his results in *Immunology of Pregnancy and Cancer.*

His first "prototype" placental anticancer extracts were crude, natural compounds which had to be shipped in dry ice. Since 1999, however, there is a second generation extract, VG-1000, which has all the advantages of a modern product. It is lyophilized, standardized, and manufactured under strict quality control rules. Due to its amino acid content, it is accepted as a food supplement in a (drink) ampoule.

VG-1000 is most beneficial in the kind of cancer known as carcinoma, for example breast cancer, prostate cancer, lung cancer, etc. VG-1000 is also helpful in melanomas, a type of skin cancer. It is also indicated for some sarcomas (cancers of muscle, bone, and connective tissue) and in leukemia.

"Patients recently subjected to chemotherapy or radiation respond more slowly to VG-1000 as they have a depressed immune system. However, patients who have had neither radiation nor chemotherapy respond very favorably. Thus, VG-1000 is clearly indicated as first-line treatment for persons with recently diagnosed cancers, as well as to help prevent recurrence."

Beginning in 1975, Dr. Govallo treated over one hundred patients, most with cancers that were considered incurable. More than 60% of his earliest patients have reportedly survived ten (10) years or longer with healthy immune systems.

### Further Reading & References

- CHIPSA's - Center for Integrative Medicine in Tijuana, Baja California, Mexico http://chipsa.com/

- San Diego Clinic, Tijuana, Mexico http://www.cancure.org/san_diego_clinic.htm

- *Immunology of Pregnancy and Cancer* by Valentin I. Govallo, M.D. (1993)

- VG-1000 Cancer Vaccine, http://www.cancure.org/VG1000_cancer_vaccines.htm

# Transfer Factor/Transfer Factor Plus

Dr. H. Sherwood Lawrence made a discovery in 1949 that an immune response could be transferred from a donor to a recipient by injecting an extract of leukocytes. According to records, "He found that this extract contained a factor capable of transferring immunity. He named the substance transfer factor. In the fifty years since Lawrence's pioneering work, an estimated $40,000,000 has been spent on research, resulting in over 3,000 scientific papers documenting the benefits of transfer factors. The world's leading scientists and physicians have established the safety and remarkable immune system benefits of transfer factor."*

These transfer factors are small peptides of approximately 44 amino acids that have the ability to express cell-mediated immunity from immune donors to non-immune recipients.

Transfer Factor Plus is a patented blend of proven immune system builders such as Inositol Hexaphosphate, Cordyceps, Beta Glucans, Maitake and Shiitake Mushrooms. These ingredients work together to trigger and enhance the various immune protective mechanisms of the body.

"Clinical studies show that Transfer Factor Plus can increase Natural Killer cell activity up to 248% above baseline."

With Transfer Factor Plus as part of an aggressive nutraceutical regime with Stage IV endstage cancer, a clinical study showed that survival was extended and quality of life increased.

### Further Reading & References

- *Dr. H. Sherwood Lawrence, http://www.int-a1.com/4life/company/people/Dr_H.Sherwood_Lawrence.htm

- Transfer Factor Molecules And The Immune System, http://tf4health.com

- "Increased tumor necrosis factor alpha (TNF-alpha) and natural killer cell (NK) function using an integrative approach in late stage cancers" http://www.ncbi.nlm.nih.gov/entrez/query.fcgi?cmd=Retrieve&db=pubmed&dopt=Abstract&list_uids=12148949

# TVZ-7 Lymphocyte Treatment/Zwitterionic Piperazine

TVZ-7 [zwitterionic piperazine] is an extract of cytokines – immune system hormones – and other immune activating chemicals, taken from cultured B lymphocytes. Mature B lymphocytes are white cells that live in the spleen, lymph glands and peripheral lymphoid tissue.

TVZ-7 can independently [recognize] "antigens", anything foreign to the body, and mount an attack by creating antibodies. Though the scientists behind TVZ-7 are not yet quite sure how exactly it works, it has induced dramatic responses in cases of pancreatic, liver and brain cancer, as well as having an impact on pain control.

### Further Reading & References

- *Complementary/Holistic Medicine for Brain Cancer - It's Your Life, Live It!* by Michael Braham (2010)

- Non-Toxic Complementary Therapies: TVZ-7 Lymphocyte Treatment, http://www.canceraction.org.gg/therapies-and-recipes/non-toxic-complementary-therapies

# Vitamins And Other Natural Substances

## Antioxidants

While oxygen is necessary to maintain life, the by-products created when cells use oxygen can be harmful to cells. These by-products, called 'free radicals' occur naturally when oxygen in the bloodstream combines with any of a diverse group of chemicals. Substances that give rise to free radicals can be found in polluted air, cigarette smoke, chemical toxins such as benzene, food additives and re-heated cooking oil, high energy radiation, heavy sun burning, radiation in cancer therapy and radioactivity, heavy physical training, long lasting inflammations, some drugs, alcohol, smoking, and heavy metals.

The mercury from tooth fillings is thought to be the main chronic generator of free radicals.* In this case, the antioxidant melatonin is believed to protect against the effects of mercury, which is implicated in many diseases.

Free radicals together with 'non-radicals', e.g., hydrogen peroxide, are known as "reactive oxygen species" (ROS). Scientists know today that free radicals carry out much of the actual destructive work in disease, infection, stress, and aging. Further, free radicals are known to cause defects in normal RNA as well as in life perpetuating DNA, the genetic information of the cells. The damage by ROS to DNA, though thought to be a frequent event in the normal human cell, is also regarded as the fundamental molecular event leading to cancer.

Antioxidants are organic substances that include vitamins C, E, and A, the mineral selenium, carotenoids including beta-carotene, and melatonin. Antioxidants can be found in foods, or in enzymes made in cells. Glutathione peroxidase and superoxide dismutase (SOD) are body enzymes that function as antioxidants. Many antioxidants are also available in supplement form.

A great many foods are rich in antioxidants including citrus fruits, tomatoes, peppers, strawberries, broccoli, peaches, and cabbage. Even coffee and beer are reportedly rich in antioxidants, although they contain other substances that are less desirable. Vitamins A, C, E, beta carotene, and the mineral selenium have been investigated for possible protective abilities against cancer.

Normally, ROS and antioxidants are in balance. ROS are a normal part of our metabolism, and they are active when fighting bacteria and vira. However a large permanent excess of ROS leads to oxidative stress, cell damage and in the long run, chronic diseases. To become stable, free radicals need to steal electrons from other molecules, so they constantly seek out healthy cells and attack their vulnerable outer membranes, eventually causing cellular degeneration and death. Antioxidants come to the rescue by binding with free radicals, transforming them into non-dangerous compounds.

"If free radicals are left to their own devices, they may cause heart damage, cancer, cataracts, and weaken your immune system," says Nicole Nisly, M.D., UI Health Care specialist in alternative medicine at the UI Family Care Center.

There is considerable evidence that antioxidants slow or possibly prevent the development of cancer. It is estimated that 30 to 35 percent of all cancers may be associated with poor nutritional habits. Research on certain vitamins and minerals indicates that diets high in foods containing antioxidants lead to lower rates of cancer.

The study of antioxidant use in cancer treatment is a rapidly evolving area.** A number of reports show a reduction in adverse effects of chemotherapy when given concurrently with antioxidants. The combination of antioxidants and chemotherapy agents needs more investigation, because published research indicates the cautious and judicious use of a number of antioxidants can be helpful in the treatment of cancer, alone and in combination with conventional cancer treatments such as radiation and chemotherapy. The majority of alternative cancer doctors recommend antioxidant-rich foods and supplements as an essential part of cancer treatment.

Numerous animal studies have been published demonstrating decreased tumor size and/or increased longevity with the combination of chemotherapy and antioxidants. A study was conducted on small-cell lung cancer in humans using combination chemotherapy of cyclophosphamide, Adriamycin (doxorubicin), and vincristine with radiation and a combination of antioxidants, vitamins, trace elements, and fatty acids. The conclusion was, "…antioxidant treatment, in combination with chemotherapy and irradiation, prolonged the survival time of patients".

Human studies found melatonin plus chemotherapy to induce greater tumor response than chemotherapy alone. Additionally, physicians need to remain aware of the large body of evidence showing a positive effect of antioxidants in the period following chemotherapy administration. The general protocol with conventional treatment is to follow a watch-and-wait strategy after treatment is concluded.

This is a period when supplemental therapies are highly indicated and have been demonstrated to result in a higher percentage of successful outcomes. A recent review article by Prasad** summarizes the need for a nutritional protocol involving multiple dietary antioxidants to enhance the efficacy of standard and experimental cancer therapies and decrease their toxicity, and to prevent the recurrence of cancer.


### Further Reading & References

- *"Mercury induces cell cytotoxicity and oxidative stress and increases beta-amyloid secretion and tau phosphorylation in SHSY5Y neuroblastoma cells." J Neurochem. 2000 Jan;74(1):231-6, http://www.ncbi.nlm.nih.gov/entrez/query.fcgi?cmd=Retrieve&db=pubmed&dopt=Abstract&list_uids=10617124

- **Prasad KN, Kumar A, Kochupillai V, Cole WC. "High doses of multiple antioxidant vitamins: essential ingredients in improving the efficacy of standard cancer therapy. J Am Coll Nutr 1999;18:13-25." http://www.ncbi.nlm.nih.gov/entrez/query.fcgi?cmd=Retrieve&db=PubMed&list_uids=10067654&opt=Abstract

- "The SU.VI.MAX Study: A Randomized, Placebo-Controlled Trial of the Health Effects of Antioxidant Vitamins and Minerals." Arch Intern Med. 2004 Nov 22;164(21):2335-2342, http://www.ncbi.nlm.nih.gov/entrez/query.fcgi?cmd=Retrieve&db=pubmed&dopt=Abstract&list_uids=15557412

- "Inhibition of Cancer Cell Proliferation in Vitro by Fruit and Berry Extracts and Correlations with Antioxidant Levels II Proliferation in Vitro by Fruit and Berry Extracts and Correlations with Antioxidant Levels." J Agric Food Chem. 2004 Dec 1;52(24):7264-7271, http://www.ncbi.nlm.nih.gov/entrez/query.fcgi?cmd=Retrieve&db=pubmed&dopt=Abstract&list_uids=15563205

- VandeCreek L, Rogers E, Lester J. Use of alternative therapies among breast cancer outpatients compared with the general population. Altern Ther Health Med 1999;5:71-76.

- Singh DK, Lippman SM. Cancer chemoprevention part 1: retinoids and carotenoids and other classic antioxidants. Oncology 1998;12:1643-1660.

- Weijl NI, Cleton FJ, Osanto S. Free radicals and antioxidants in chemotherapy induced toxicity. Cancer Treat Rev 1997;23:209-240.

- Labriola D, Livingston R. Possible interactions between dietary antioxidants and chemotherapy. Oncology 1999;13:1003-1012.

- Schmitt CA, Lowe SW. Apoptosis and therapy. J Pathol 1999;187:127-137.

- Chinery R, Brockman JA, Peeler MO, et al. Antioxidants enhance the cytotoxicity of chemotherapeutic agents in colorectal cancer: a p53-independent induction of p21 via C/EBP-beta. Nat Med 1997;3:1233-1241.

- Mediavilla MD, Cos S, Sanchez-Barcelo EJ. Melatonin increases p53 and p21WAF1 expression in MCF-7 human breast cancer cells in vitro. Life Sci 1999;65:415-420.

- Seifter E, Rettura G, Padawer J. Vitamin A and beta-carotene as adjunctive therapy to tumor excision, radiation therapy and chemotherapy. In Prasad K, ed. Vitamins Nutrition and Cancer. New York: Karger Press; 1984:2-19.

- Thatcher N, Blackledge G, Crowther D. Advanced recurrent squamous cell carcinoma of the head and neck. Cancer 1980;46:1324-1328.

- Shimpo K, Nagatsu T, Yamada K, et al. Ascorbic acid and adriamycin toxicity. Am J Clin Nutr 1991;54:1298S-1301S.

- Taper HS, de Gerlache J, Lans M, et al. Non-toxic potentiation of cancer chemotherapy by combined C and K3 vitamin pre-treatment. Int J Cancer 1987;40:575-579.

- Sue K, Nakagawara A, Okuzono SI, et al. Combined effects of vitamin E (alpha-tocopherol) and cisplatin on the growth of murine neuroblastoma in vivo. Eur J Cancer Clin Oncol 1988;24:1751-1758.

- Myers CE, McGuire WP, Liss RH, et al. Adriamycin: the role of lipid peroxidation in cardiac toxicity and tumor response. Science 1977;197:165-167.

- Naganuma A, Satoh M, Imura N. Effect of selenite on renal toxicity and antitumor activity of cis-diamminedichloroplatinum (II) in mice inoculated with Ehrlich ascites tumor cell. J Pharm Dyn 1984;7:217-220.

- Berry JP, Pauwells C, Touzeau S, et al. Effect of selenium in combination with cis-diamminedichloroplatinum (II) in the treatment of murine fibrosarcoma. Cancer Res 1984; 44:2864-2868.

- "Multiple dietary antioxidants enhance the efficacy of standard and experimental cancer therapies and decrease their toxicity." Integr Cancer Ther. 2004 Dec;3(4):310-22. Prasad KN, http://www.ncbi.nlm.nih.gov/entrez/query.fcgi?cmd=Retrieve&db=pubmed&dopt=Abstract&list_uids=15523102

- Antioxidants in Cancer Therapy: Their Actions and Interactions With Oncologic Therapies, http://www.chiro.org/nutrition/ABSTRACTS/Antioxidants_in_Cancer_Therapy_Part_1.shtml

# Alpha Lipoic Acid (ALA)/Lipoic Acid

Alpha-lipoic acid is an antioxidant that is produced naturally in the body. It functions as a co-factor for a number of important enzymes responsible for the conversion of food to energy (ATP). However, most lipoic acid arises from diet or from supplements. In nature, lipoic acid is found in the leaves of some plants and in red meat. Unlike other antioxidants, lipoic acid is both fat and water-soluble and is easily absorbed and transported across cell membranes. This unique quality offers protection against free radicals both inside and outside the cell while other antioxidants only provide extracellular protection.

Research has shown alpha-lipoic acid to be an efficient free radical scavenger, effective in numerous neurodegenerative disorders, and an agent that prevents deficits in nerve blood flow, oxidative stress and distal sensory conduction. With its capabilities as a precursor to glutathione (GSH-a major antioxidant in the body), alpha-lipoic acid has been shown to be a potential therapeutic agent fighting against cancer and HIV.

Lipoic acid has the ability to regenerate other antioxidants like vitamin E, vitamin C and GSH for further use, after they have eradicated free radicals. Numerous clinical trials have shown the benefits of supplementing with lipoic acid for medical problems such as moderating blood sugar concentrations, symptoms of cardiovascular ailments, blurred vision, memory loss, and liver complication.

Alpha lipoic acid has been shown to help chelate (bind with and remove) iron, copper, and cadmium which are metals that can give rise to increased free radical activity in the body. It is therefore a useful detoxifying agent. If chelating heavy metals like mercury, another moving agent like DMSA should be used, as lipoic acid only forms weak bonds with mercury and could merely move this toxin elsewhere in the body.

Alpha lipoic acid has been found to have a number of positive impacts in relation to cancer. In its antioxidant capacity, it protects a complex called NF kappa B. NF Kappa B is involved in controlling cell division and is often damaged in cancer cells (by free radicals). When this damage happens, oncogenes (genes that have the potential to cause cancer) can take over the cell cycle leading to uncontrolled cell division and cancer. ALA in conjunction with N-Acetyl Cysteine has been found to repair functional defects in the immune systems of cancer patients as well.

See **Antioxidants**.

## *Further Reading & References*

- *Alpha Lipoic Acid Breakthrough: The Superb Antioxidant That May Slow Aging, Repair Liver Damage,*

- *and Reduce the Risk of Cancer, Heart Disease, and Diabetes* by Burt Berkson (1998)

- *Alpha Lipoic Acid: Nature's Ultimate Antioxidant* by Allan E. Sosin, et al (1998)

- *The Antioxidant Miracle: Put Lipoic Acid, Pycnogenol, and Vitamins E and C to Work for You* by Lester Packer and Carol Colman (1999)

# Arginine/L-arginine/Tumorex/Jimmy Keller

The terms L-arginine and arginine are frequently used interchangeably. Arginine is an amino acid that can both inhibit cancer and help it grow, depending on how it is converted. It is converted in two different ways: it can become L-ornithine, or it can become nitric oxide. Each has different actions with regard to cancer. If it's converted to nitric oxide, it helps the type of immune cells that attack cancer. If it's converted to L-ornithine, it can help cancer grow.

In a Japanese study on rats implanted with sarcoma, 50% of the animals receiving arginine had metastases to the liver versus 100% for those not receiving it. Similarly, 75% had lung metastases versus 100%.

In 1992, University of Pennsylvania researchers reported that arginine has a beneficial effect on the immunity of cancer patients. People who underwent surgery for upper gastrointestinal malignancies would recover crucial aspects of their immunity only if given arginine, RNA and omega-3 fatty acids; otherwise, certain immune responses would stay depressed. They concluded that the three supplements "significantly improved immunologic, metabolic, and clinical outcomes in patients with upper gastrointestinal malignancies who were undergoing major elective surgery."

In a different study on patients with colorectal cancer, 30 grams of L-arginine a day for 3 days before surgery caused the tumors to have more antigens (for immune cells to home in on).

Breast cancer patients undergoing chemotherapy have also benefitted from arginine. In a study from the University of Aberdeen, women who took 30 grams/day for 3 days prior to each chemo treatment had stronger immunity.

In other studies, the growth of human breast cancer cells in vitro has been slowed with supplemental arginine. Arginine can also block the growth of mammary tumors in rodents. Arginine can have the opposite effect on some cancers – for example, at least one pancreatic cancer cell line is arginine-dependent.

An arginine preparation called Tumorex was used by the healer, Jimmy Keller, who claimed it healed his melanoma. He reportedly treated many people successfully but was eventually imprisoned. The defense kept copies of more than 350 letters and affidavits sent to the U.S. District Court in Brownsville in support of Jimmy Keller and his clinic. Many of the letters can be read at http://www.karlloren.com/Jimmy_Keller/page6.htm.

### Further Reading & References

- Brittenden J, et al. 1994. Dietary supplementation with L-arginine in patients with breast cancer (>4 cm) receiving multimodality treatment: report of a feasibility study. Br J Cancer 69:918-21.

- Brittenden J, et al. 1994. Natural cytotoxicity in breast cancer patients receiving neoadjuvant chemotherapy: effects of L-arginine supplementation. Eur J Surg Oncol 20:467-72.

- Cho-Chung YS, et al. 1980. Arrest of mammary tumor growth in vivo by L-arginine: stimulation of NAD-dependent activation of adenylate cyclase. Biochem Biophys Res Commun 95:1306-13.

- Daly JM, et al. 1992. Enteral nutrition with supplemental arginine, RNA, and omega-3 fatty acids in patients after operation: immunologic, metabolic, and clinical outcome [see comments]. Surgery 112:56-67.

- Heys SD, et al. 1997. Dietary supplementation with L-arginine: modulation of tumor-infiltrating lymphocytes in patients with colorectal cancer. Br J Surg 84:238-41.

- Levy HM, et al. 1954. Effect of arginine on tumor growth in rats. Cancer Res 14:198-200.

- Singh R, et al. 2000. Arginase activity in human breast cancer cell lines: NT-Hydroxy-L-arginine selectively inhibits cell proliferation and induces apoptosis in MDA-MB-468 cells. Cancer Res 60:3305-12.

- Swaffar DS, et al. 1994. Inhibition of the growth of human pancreatic cancer cells by the arginine antimetabolite L-canavanine [see comments]. Cancer Res 54:6045-48.

- Tachibana K, et al. 1985. Evaluation of the effect of arginine-enriched amino acid solution on tumor growth. J Parenteral Ent Nutr 9:428-34.

# Beta-Carotene/Alpha-Carotene

$\beta$-Carotene, more familiarly spelled beta-carotene, is an organic compound and classified as a terpenoid. It is a deeply colored red-orange pigment abundant in plants and fruits. The appetizing colors of fresh fruits and vegetables often derive from the presence of special groups of antioxidants, including beta-carotene. Carotenoids in general are fat-soluble compounds which range in hue from light yellow to deep orange. The flagship carotenoid is beta-carotene, the orange pigment evident in carrots and cantaloupe.

The body converts beta-carotene to vitamin A. As a dietary supplement, some research suggests beta-carotene appears to be ineffective in preventing cancer or heart disease. However, whole foods that are high in beta-carotene and other carotenoids do appear to offer health benefits and protection. The whole foods should therefore be preferred to supplements.

Carrot juice is considered an excellent cancer-fighting juice because of its high levels of beta-carotene and alpha-carotene. Some research suggests that beta-carotene is actually carcinogenic in habitual cigarette smokers although beneficial to non-smokers.

See **Antioxidants**.

### *Further Reading & References*

- "Dietary carotenoids, connexins and cancer: what is the connection?" http://www.ncbi.nlm.nih.gov/entrez/query.fcgi?cmd=Retrieve&db=pubmed&dopt=Abstract&list_uids=15506943

- Nutrition—A Cancer Battle Plan, http://www.torontoadvisors.com/Kefir/cancerbattle.htm

- Foods That Heal, http://www.annieappleseedproject.org/foodsthatheal.html

# Bioflavonoids

Bioflavanoids include hesperetin, hesperedin, eriodictyol, quercetin, quercitrin, and rutin. The human body cannot produce bioflavanoids, so they must be supplied in the diet.

The darker colors of fruits and vegetables are often supplied by a group of compounds called bioflavonoids, which typically range from bright yellow to deep purple hue. There are over four hundred bioflavonoids in the human diet. They are widely distributed in fruits, vegetables, beverages, and spices. A typical North American consumes about one gram of bioflavonoids per day. Asians may consume over five grams per day, much of it coming from herbs and spices.

Bioflavonoids are potent antioxidants that not only contribute to the health benefits of fruits and vegetables but also to the therapeutic effects of many traditional Chinese and Indian herbal remedies. The bioflavonoids which give grapes their purple color are believed responsible for the protection against heart disease attributed to red wine.

Epigallocatechin gallate (EGCG), the bioflavonoid that is the main constituent of green tea, is credited with the protection against cancer that results from drinking it. Bioflavonoids found in soy beans have weak estrogen-like activity. The low frequency of breast cancer in East Asia, where soy is a major source of protein, has been attributed to the mild estrogen-blocking effect of soy flavonoids. This theory is unproven. Preliminary research indicates that soy flavonoids can block the estrogenic effects of dioxin.

Bioflavonoids, including those found in apples, onions, tea, and red wine, are now being studied for possible cancer-fighting properties. In one 24-year study, people who ate bioflavonoid-rich foods had a 20% lower risk for cancer.

Laboratory and animal studies have even indicated that some of the compounds in green tea might have the capacity to selectively destroy cancer cells (black tea does not appear to do the same).

Ubiquinone, more familiar as Coenzyme Q10 or CoQ10, is a fat-soluble vitamin-like compound that assists in generating energy within our cells. It's been demonstrated to be a highly effective anti-oxidant. Although it exists naturally in the body, it can also be supplemented by eating beef, pork, mackerel, salmon, sardines, anchovies, and nuts.

Bioflavanoids enhance the absorption of Vitamin C and it is often advised that the two should be taken together. Bioflavanoids act synergistically with Vitamin C to preserve the structure of the capillaries. Sources of bioflavanoids are the white skin beneath the peel of citrus fruits, peppers, buckwheat, black currents, apricots, cherries, grapefruit, grapes, lemons, oranges, prunes, and rose hips.

Herbs that contain bioflavanoids are chervil, elderberries, hawthorn berry, horsetail, rose hips, and shepherd's purse.

Quercetin is known as "king of the flavonoids" because of its preventive and curative abilities. It is considered one of the best antihistamines for relieving hay fever and allergies. Plus, it is an anti-inflammatory for ailments such as rheumatoid arthritis.

Some consider quercetin more effective than vitamin E when it comes to lowering cholesterol and the risk of heart disease and stroke. It safeguards LDL (the bad cholesterol) from oxidation, helping to prevent it from clogging arteries.

High-dose quercetin therapy is said to be especially beneficial as it slows the advance of many different types of cancer. It is known to stop the growth of leukemia cells and halt the progress of breast cancer. Recommended human dosage is about a thousand milligrams. For aggressive therapy, the recommended dose is two thousand milligrams. It should be taken on an empty stomach, divided throughout the day.

In a recent study in which it was used with cisplatin on lung tumor cells, quercetin was found to amplify the growth and apoptosis (cell death) of tumor cells:

"Experience over several years has indicated that chemotherapy, even if widely used, does not always remain effective in the therapy of lung tumors and, in addition, is linked to serious side effects. In parallel, some plant polyphenols are known to exert a proapoptotic action on tumor cells while, in contrast, representing anti-cancerogenic antioxidants in living organisms. Our studies were aimed at comparing the effects of a polyphenol, quercetin, and cisplatin on cells of various types of lung cancer in in vitro conditions. In these studies we also attempted to define the relationship between the dose and the duration of the activity of the compounds. Cisplatin alone was found to induce only a small reaction in the cells, while in combination with quercetin its antiproliferative and pro-apoptotic effects were amplified, depending upon the type of tumor, the dose and the duration of the drug's action."**

### Further Reading & References

- *Anti-proliferative properties of prenylated flavonoids from hops (Humulus lupulus L.) in human prostate cancer cell lines* by L. Delmulle, A. Bellahcene, W. Dhooge, and F. Comhaire (2007)

- *Bioflavonoids* by Earl Mindell (1998)

- *All About Bioflavonoids* by Daniel Gastelu (2002)

- **Borska S, Gebarowska E, Wysocka T, Drag-Zalesinska M, Zabel M. Folia Morphol (Warsz). 2004

- Feb;63(1):103-5. "The effects of quercetin vs cisplatin on proliferation and the apoptotic process in A549 and SW1271 cell lines in in vitro conditions." http://www.ncbi.nlm.nih.gov/entrez/query.fcgi ?cmd=Retrieve&db=pubmed&dopt=Abstract&list_uids=15039912

- Bioflavonoids, http://www.holisticbird.org/pages/nbiflavonoids.htm

# Carnitine/Levocarnitine

Carnitine is a naturally occurring amino acid, also known as a quaternary ammonium compound. It is biosynthesized from lysine and methionine (both amino acids). This process occurs in the liver and kidneys. Carnitine is a necessary component of heart and skeletal muscle tissue.

Carnitine functions to transport fatty acids across the inner mitochondrial membranes. Mitochondria are tiny organelles within cells, sometimes called "cellular power plants." This amino acid is essential for brain cells and healthy neurological function, and it promotes longevity by helping to provide cells with the necessary energy to function. Carnitine deficiencies are common.

Low levels of carnitine have been noted in patients with cancer, diabetes, certain types of heart disease, and alcoholism. There are different types of carnitine. Elemental (active) L-carnitine fumarate has an extra molecule of fumaric acid that helps maintain Krebs' Cycle function, and acetyl-carnitine crosses the blood brain barrier quickly and aids in neurological function. Carnitine supplementation results in increased plasma and tissue levels of carnitine.

In healthy heart tissue, carnitine is present in adequate amounts to provide sufficient fatty acids, which are the principal energy substrate of the heart.

Levocarnitine (another name for carnitine) has been shown to assist patient recovery from the effects of chemotherapy treatment. A specially designed energy drink each day could boost cancer patients left exhausted by chemotherapy, according to research published in the *British Journal of Cancer*. Fatigue is one of the most common side effects of treatment for cancer, robbing patients of the energy to perform everyday tasks and severely impairing their quality of life.

Scientists believe many cases of fatigue, which affects 80% of chemotherapy patients, occur when treatment disrupts a patient's metabolism. This depletes levels of carnitine, which is vital for providing energy to our muscles.

But Italian scientists have found that giving people a substance called levocarnitine, which is taken in a pineapple-flavored drink, help them recover from the effects of treatment. In their study, 90% of those who received the supplement recovered from their fatigue within a week.

Lead researcher Dr. Francesco Graziano, of Urbino Hospital in Italy, comments: "After chemotherapy, many patients have low levels of carnitine in their blood and we think that's one of the reasons they feel so exhausted. It seemed logical that boosting carnitine levels with a dietary supplement might restore that lost energy. Our study was the first to take this new approach to treating fatigue and the results, although preliminary, were very encouraging."

Dr. Graziano and his colleagues studied 50 patients who had reported feeling fatigue during the course of their chemotherapy. Researchers used detailed questionnaires to assess each patient's degree of fatigue and took blood samples to measure carnitine levels. Then they gave patients an energy drink containing levocarnitine, which is converted to carnitine in the body. After a week of treatment, their progress was assessed. On average, blood carnitine levels increased by 50% over the course of the week. And the questionnaires revealed that 45 of the 50 patients (90%) no longer felt fatigued.

Prof Gordon McVie of Cancer Research UK, owners of the *British Journal of Cancer*, says, "Treating patients more effectively doesn't just mean keeping them alive for longer; it also means preserving their quality of life.

"We are getting better at reducing the side effects associated with modern drugs, but chemotherapy still robs many patients of the energy they need to live their life to the full. A simple dietary supplement to restore a patient's zip would be a valuable step forward and these initial results are certainly encouraging."

### Further Reading & References

- *The Carnitine Miracle: The Supernutrient Program That Promotes High Energy, Fat Burning, Heart Health, Brain Wellness and Longevity* by Robert Crayhon (2001)

- L-Carnitine by Brian Leibovitz (1999)

- *British Journal of Cancer*, June 17, 2002; 86(12):1854

- L-Carnitine: Lipid Metabolism and Weight Management, http://www.healingedge.net/pdf/l_carnitine.pdf

# Conjugated Linoleic Acid (CLA)

Conjugated linoleic acid (CLA), a fatty acid, has promising anti-cancer effects. The effect of CLA is reportedly more powerful than any other fatty acid in modulating tumor development.

Numerous studies have been published on CLA's powerful anti-cancer effects. Even more significant is the fact that only relatively small amounts of CLA are required to achieve its effects. The studies showed that to produce healthful benefits, only 3 to 4 grams of CLA daily are required.

Studies show CLA may help protect against many diseases including atherosclerosis and cancer. In a paper in the 'Journal of Nutrition' (1999 December), evidence of significant cancer prevention was shown when CLA was added to the diet. This study revealed CLA to be a "potent cancer preventative agent in animal models." Specifically, it was determined that feeding CLA to female rats while they were young and still developing conferred life-long protection against breast cancer. This astounding preventative action was achieved by adding CLA at the dose of 0.8% of the animal's total diet. This corresponds to 3-4 g for a human (1% of diet).

Meat and milk from grass-fed cattle and sheep have been found to be good sources of CLA, containing from three to five times more CLA than products from grain-fed animals. Eggs are also rich in CLA. CLA is available in supplement form.

### Further Reading & References

- *Advances in Conjugated Linoleic Acid Research* by Jean-Louis Sebedio, et al (2003)

- *Advances in Conjugated Linoleic Acid Research* by Martin P. Yurawecz (2006)

- Alternative Cancer Treatments: http://www.cancertutor.com/

# Co-enzyme Q10/Coenzyme Q/CoQ10/Ubiquinone/Stockholm Protocol Cancer Treatment/Q-Gel®

Coenzyme Q10 is an oil-soluble, vitamin-like substance that can be found in most eukaryotic cells and mitochondria in particular. It aids in aerobic cellular respiration and generates ATP (cell energy). CoQ10 also helps stimulate heart muscles and the immune system in several different ways, mainly through higher antibody levels, and greater numbers and/or activities of the cancer fighting macrophages and Tcells. There may be other ways Co-Q10 aids in the fight against cancer that have not yet been isolated. It is best known as an antioxidant. Antioxidants help the body use oxygen more efficiently.

Coenzyme Q10 has also demonstrated potent anti-cancer properties. CoQ10 may be able to halt cancer.

Dr. William Campbell Douglass reported research findings and case histories in his newsletter *Second Opinion* that showed a correlation between CoQ10 and breast cancer. Low levels of CoQ10 were found in women with breast cancer. Increased levels were associated with regression and remission.

Dr. Douglass points out that CoQ10 dissolves in fat and that it is therefore most absorbable in either a special wafer form (to which some oil has been added) or taken with a tablespoon of olive oil. Some authorities recommend coconut oil. Since CoQ10 has many health benefits, a minimum dose of 50 mg daily is appropriate for prevention of degenerative diseases, for improved energy, and for general health. Cancer patients may want to increase that dosage dramatically to 400-600 mg daily. They are advised to discuss large doses with a doctor.

Among other Co10 researchers, Dr. Karl Folkers of the University of Texas, Austin reports regression of breast cancer, not only at the original site, but even of cancer that had spread (metastasized) to the liver—usually a sign of terminal illness. Unlike conventional treatment, CoQ10 is completely non-toxic and stimulates the immune system, rather than depressing it. In several studies, CoQ10 worked wonders with patients who had chosen to take chemotherapy, reducing the toxicity of such treatment. In one study, patients who were given CoQ10 had little or no toxicity, even though they were given much larger doses of the toxic chemotherapy agent than were given to the control group. This inverse correlation is significant.

According to Ralph Moss, who wrote *Antioxidants Against Cancer*, Dr. Folkers held the first clinical trial of Co Q10 at a clinic in Copenhagen, Denmark in 1993. He writes, "Doctors treated 32 patients with advanced, 'high risk' breast cancer. In addition to appropriate surgery and conventional treatment, each patient was given 90 mg of CoQ10 per day. They also received other vitamins, minerals, antioxidants, and essential fatty acids. On this regimen, 6 of the 32 patients showed partial tumor regressions, significant in 'advanced' patients."

Moss goes on to tell the story of how one of the six women independently increased her dosage from 90 to 390 mg per day. The following month, her doctors reported that the tumor was no longer palpable. A mammogram the following month confirmed that the tumor had disappeared.

This pattern was repeated by another woman in the group who also upped her dosage to 300 mg and saw her own tumor disappear. A clinical exam not only confirmed the tumor was gone but also showed no evidence that a tumor had been there in the first place. There was also no evidence of distant metastases.

Dr. Folkers's study was significant for two reasons. For one, all the patients involved received chemotherapy along with Co-Q10. It is impossible to know what the results would have been without the toxic and immune-system-destroying chemotherapy. Second, the dosages of Co-Q10 given by the doctors were much too low to make a difference (90 mg). Instead, the patients themselves made the most impressive discoveries.

Where the dosage was only 90 mg, results were sporadic. However, when dosages were in the range of 400-600 mg, and perhaps higher, results were substantial. (Note: A person should gradually build up to dosages above 100 mg.)

The most bioavailable form of CoQ10 is called ubiquinol. However, this substance is extremely unstable. The most common form of CoQ10 found in commercial food supplements is ubiquinone, a more stable form, which the body must convert to ubiquinol. Supplement manufacturers now report that a more stable, albeit more expensive, ubiquinol supplement can now be manufactured that reportedly has more nutritional value than the less expensive ubiquinone supplements.

### Further Reading & References

- Coenzyme Q10 / Co Q10 / Stockholm Protocol, http://www.cancertutor.com/Cancer/Q10.html

- Q-gel, http://www.qgel.com/

- *Natural Strategies For Cancer Patients* by Russell L. Blaylock (2003)

- *The Coenzyme Q10 Phenomenon* by Stephen T. Sinatra, M.D., F.A.C.C. (1998)

- *Antioxidants Against Cancer*, Ralph Moss (1999)

# DHEA (Dehydroepiandrosterone)

As a natural sterone (steroid hormone) produced by the adrenal gland, DHEA is the most common sterone in human blood. Secretions are highest in a person's early twenties and begin to decline at around age 25. By age 70, DHEA production is only a fraction of what it was 50 years earlier.

Research has shown a correlation between low DHEA levels and a declining immune system. Alzheimer patients have low DHEA levels, when compared to their healthy counterparts. In view of its potential to boost immune function, DHEA is being used in the fight against HIV, dementia, and cancer. It has also been clinically shown to help brain neurons establish contact. A small amount of sulphate DHEA and micronized DHEA can convert into testosterone and then be used as a treatment for prostate cancer.

In vitro studies have also found DHEA to have both anti-proliferatives and apoptotic (cell killing) effects on cancer cell lines, though the significance of this finding is yet to be determined.

Elevated levels of DHEA in conjunction with higher endogenous sex hormones are associated with an increased risk of breast cancer for both pre- and postmenopausal women.

An interesting article has been published in *Steroids* 2003 Jan;68(1):73-83 that correlates endogenous DHEA to anti-proliferative action on human cancer cell lines under the title "Anti-proliferative action of endogenous dehydroepiandrosterone metabolites on human cancer cell lines." by S. Yoshida et al. at Department of Gastroenterology and Hepatology, Institute of Clinical Medicine, University of Tsukuba, 1-1-1 Tennodai, Tsukuba, 305-8575, Ibaraki, Japan.

DHEA is commonly sold in supplement form.

### Further Reading & References

- DHEA (Dehydroepiandrosterone): http://newagecities.com/neighborhoods/mindworks/content/DHEA.asp

- Yoshida S., et al. "Anti-proliferative action of endogenous dehydroepiandrosterone metabolites on human cancer cell lines." *Steroids*. 2003 Jan;68(1):73-83. http://www.ncbi.nlm.nih.gov/entrez/query.fcgi?cmd=Retrieve&db=PubMed&list_uids=12475725&dopt=Abstract

- Key, T.; Appleby, P.; Barnes, I.; Reeves, G. (2002). "Endogenous sex hormones and breast cancer in postmenopausal women: reanalysis of nine prospective studies." *J. Natl. Cancer Inst.* 94 (8): 606–16.

- Yang, N. C.; Jeng, K. C.; Ho, W. M.; Hu, M. L. (2002). "ATP depletion is an important factor in DHEA-induced growth inhibition and apoptosis in BV-2 cells". *Life Sci.* 70 (17): 1979–88.

- Loria, R. M. (2002). "Immune up-regulation and tumor apoptosis by androstene steroids." *Steroids* 67 (12): 953–66.

# Gamma Linolenic Acid (GLA)/Borage Oil/Evening Primrose Oil/ Eurasian Black Currant Oil

Studies have shown that Gamma-Linolenic Acid (GLA), an omega-6 fatty acid, is effective in killing cancer cells.

GLA is an inflammation-fighter found in the oils of various plants. Particularly good sources are the seeds of the hardy borage plant (Borago officinalis), the yellow-blossomed evening primrose (Oenothera biennis), and the deciduous Eurasian black currant shrub (Ribes nigrum).

In one study, terminally ill patients suffering from pancreatic cancer tripled their life expectancy after taking extensive doses of GLA. It is also believed that tumor growth and metastasis can be quelled with GLA-especially in melanoma and colon or breast cancer.

GLA is not found in fish oils and must be obtained from the plant sources mentioned above.

### Further Reading & References

- Gamma-Linolenic Acid: What You Need to Know by C.W. Newman, et al

- "On theophylline and evening primrose oil in the treatment of cancer" - Letters to the Editor, http://www.findarticles.com/p/articles/mi_m0ISW/is_2002_June/ai_86387594

- American Cancer Society: Gamma Linolenic Acid, http://www.cancer.org/Treatment/TreatmentsandSideEffects/ComplementaryandAlternativeMedicine/PharmacologicalandBiologicalTreatment/gamma-linolenic-acid

# Glutathione

Glutathione is glutathione sulfhydryl (GSH), a peptide (very small protein or protein fragment) that occurs naturally within the body, where it is assembled by individual cells from its three components— the amino acids glycine, glutamate (glutamic acid), and the all important cysteine. Because it contains three amino acids it is referred to as a tripeptide.

Of these amino acids, cysteine is the rarest. It is a sulfur-containing amino acid that contributes the sulfhydryl group to the molecule, making it also the most important of the raw ingredients. When cells have cysteine they can efficiently manufacture GSH. Cysteine is missing or deficient in many diets. And unfortunately it has difficulty surviving the trip from the mouth to the cells unless it's part of a larger protein, making supplementation with oral cysteine, or L-cysteine, impractical. Although it may raise GSH levels to some extent, L-cysteine is oxidized in the digestive tract and enters the bloodstream only with difficulty. Its toxicity also makes it a poor candidate for oral supplementation.

Doctors have been using pharmaceuticals like NAC (N-acetyl-cysteine) for years to raise glutathione levels in their patients. In fact, most traditional glutathione studies on humans have been conducted with NAC. However, drugs like NAC must be swallowed or injected repeatedly to maintain elevated GSH levels. They also produce side effects such as rash, wheezing, nausea, vomiting, cramps and diarrhea, making them unsuitable for longterm or supplemental use.

Whey proteins, derived from milk, can contain GSH precursors. They are easily digested, passed into the bloodstream and taken to individual cells where they penetrate the cell wall and are metabolized into glutathione. They are also fragile and easily 'denatured' (broken down), so that by the time they are processed, although they retain their nutritional value, they are no longer bioactive.

Studies have shown that tumor cells have elevated levels of glutathione which makes them resistant to chemotherapy drugs. Depleting glutathione in these cells makes them more vulnerable to the effects of the drugs and to the gene that promotes apoptosis. Undenatured whey protein isolate is known to deplete cancer cells of their glutathione. Supplementation of carnitine and lipoic acid has also been shown to improve glutathione levels.

See **Antioxidants and Whey**.

### *Further Reading & References*

- Kumaran S, Savitha S, Anusuya Devi M, Panneerselvam C. Mech Ageing Dev. 2004 Jul;125(7):507-

- 12. "L-carnitine and DL-alpha-lipoic acid reverse the age-related deficit in glutathione redox state in

- skeletal muscle and heart tissues." http://www.ncbi.nlm.nih.gov/entrez/query.fcgi?cmd=Retriev e&db=pubmed&dopt=Abstract&list_uids=15246746

- *Glutathione: The Ultimate Antioxidant* by Alan H. Pressman and Sheila Buff (1998)

- *New Hope for Serious Diseases: The Healing Power of Glutathione* by Howard Peiper (2008)

# Glyconutrients, Glycoproteins, Glycobiology

Glyconutrients are a blend of sugars manufactured by Mannatech, Incorporated, a multinational firm that specializes in distribution of the supplement. They claim glyconutrients support the process individual tissue cells use to recognize and communicate with each other.

More specifically, they state that glyconutrients provide the body with the necessary nutrients for biochemical functions. The company's message is that a steady supply of glyconutrients is needed to provide the body with the nutrients necessary to make glycoforms to cover the surface of all cells (every cell in the human body is covered with glycoforms). If the balance of glycoforms is off, a cell becomes dysfunctional and may not recognize a cancer cell. This leads to the rapid growth of more cancer cells because the immune system does not kick in to recognize the foreign invaders.

According to Ray Sahelian, M.D. the term "glyconutrients" is ambiguous as it was "…created by a company that sells through multilevel marketing channels." Dr. Sahelian states there is no mention of glyconutrients in the medical literature, though several websites promote the products.

Proponents feel there is a large potential for using glyconutrients in alternative cancer treatments. Dr. Ben Carson, a world-renowned professor of neurosurgery, oncology, plastic surgery, and pediatrics at John Hopkins University had a very aggressive type of cancer that reversed itself with the use of high dosages of glyconutrients. It is important to remember that glyconutrients do not actually cure cancer. Rather, they improve the immune system by supplying the nutrients necessary to make the essential glycoforms for the surface of each cell.

In 2007, the owner of Mannatech, Inc., was charged with promoting an illegal marketing scheme that encourages consumers to believe glyconutrients are an effective way to combat serious disease.

*Glycoprotein,* on the other hand, is an accepted term and is mentioned in the nutrition textbook *Modern Nutrition in Health and Disease.* And, according to a 2008 article on glycobiology, "The discipline of glycobiology contributes to our understanding of human health and disease through research, most of which is published in peer-reviewed scientific journals. Recently, legitimate discoveries in glycobiology have been used as marketing tools to help sell plant extracts termed 'glyconutrients.' The glyconutrient industry has a worldwide sales force of over half a million people and sells nearly half a billion dollars (USD) of products annually."

Glycoproteins have shown promise as potential biomarkers for cancer detection. In a 2010 issue of the journal *Cancer Research,* scientists found that cancer patients produce antibodies that target abnormal glycoproteins. These are proteins with sugar molecules attached which are made by their tumors. This suggests the possibility that antitumor antibodies in the blood could potentially provide a source of biomarkers for early cancer detection.

### Further Reading & References

- Frequently Asked Questions about Glyconutrients, http://glycoinformation.com/nobel.html

- *Sugars That Heal: The New Healing Science of Glyconutrients* by Emil I. Mondoa and Mindy Kitei (2002)

- *Miracle Sugars: The Glyconutrient Link to Disease Prevention and Improved Health* by Rita Elkins MH (2003)

- Over 200 Alternative Cancer Treatments: http://www.cancertutor.com/Other/Big_List.htm

- Alternative to Traditional Cancer Treatment, http://www.diseaseeducation.com/diseases/Cancer.php

- "Glyconutrients, an honest review," by Ray Sahelian, MD, http://www.raysahelian.com/glyconutrients.html

- Antibodies Against Abnormal Glycoproteins Identified as Possible Biomarkers for Cancer Detection," National Cancer Institute, http://www.cancer.gov/newscenter/pressreleases/2010/autoantibodysignatures

# Melatonin

Melatonin is a naturally-produced hormone from the pineal gland but is also available as a manufactured supplement. Research shows this hormone plays a significant role in sleep-waking patterns.

Research has shown that individuals who work night shifts are potentially at greater risk for cancer, and it is postulated that this is linked to melatonin levels. The body's melatonin levels normally rise during the hours of darkness, but this process is suppressed by exposure to artificial light. The higher levels of cancer that have been observed in long-term night shift workers may be explained by their underexposure to normal night-time darkness and resulting depressed melatonin levels. In any case, it's been amply demonstrated that melatonin supplements are an effective cancer treatment.

It has been shown in experiments with rodents that melatonin may counteract chemotherapy-induced immune suppression, as a major drawback to chemotherapy is the destruction of many important immune system functions and various blood cells.

Dr. Lissoni and colleagues, from the Division of Radiation Oncology, S. Gerardo Hospital, in Milan, Italy, evaluated the role of melatonin given with chemotherapy to test whether the same positive effect could be replicated in humans. In his trial, eighty patients were randomized to receive either chemotherapy alone, or chemotherapy with melatonin.

The patients had a range of cancer types. Thirty-five had lung cancer and were receiving cisplatin, 31 had breast cancer and were receiving mitoxantrone, and 14 had gastrointestinal tract tumors and were receiving 5-fluorouracil. Patients in the study group received evening melatonin doses of 20 mg.

Results of the study showed patients given the melatonin had a higher number of platelets. They also felt less weakness and had less nerve damage. Loss of hair and nausea did not appear to be influenced by the melatonin.

The study authors say, "This pilot study seems to suggest that the concomitant administration of the pineal hormone melatonin during chemotherapy may prevent some chemotherapy-induced side-effects, particularly myelosuppression and neuropathy."

In a separate study on non-small cell lung cancer, the tumors of patients who received added melatonin responded to the treatment at nearly double the rate (11 out of 34) when compared to those who did not receive melatonin (6 out of 35). In addition, the percentage of one-year survival rates was significantly higher in patients who received melatonin in conjunction with chemotherapy as opposed to those who received chemotherapy alone (15 out of 34 vs. 7 out of 36).

Over the years, a number of studies have shown that melatonin plays a positive role in the therapy of cancer patients. At this point, the ideal dose of melatonin to use with various types of cancers is not known. However, there is enough evidence to at least consider the nighttime use of a small amount of melatonin, perhaps in the 0.5 to 3 mg range, in anyone who has cancer.

For those with breast cancer, melatonin is recommended if DHEA, Premarin, or any other estrogen-related drug is also being administered. Melatonin blocks estrogen receptors on breast cells, stopping them from proliferating in response to estrogen and other factors that promote tumor growth. Melatonin also protects breast cells against chemical carcinogens, free radical damage, cortisol-induced damage, and non-estrogen dependent cellular changes that lead to breast cancer.

For seven years, researchers assayed the effects of melatonin treatment on leukemia and cancer patients. They reported that leukemia and cancer are nearly impossible to eradicate without melatonin treatment. However, though melatonin appears to be necessary as part of a treatment arsenal, it is not believed to be able to stand on its own as a cancer cure. Leukemic strains vary in their response to melatonin; myeloid acute or chronic leukemia has to be cured with significantly lower dosages.

In addition, excellent results have been observed in epithelial or connective tissue tumors as melatonin assists in reaching a balanced equilibrium which allows a normal or almost usual existence for a patient.

Treatment with melatonin seldom requires hospitalization, though periodic blood analysis is recommended.

Melatonin has excellent antioxidant properties and is able to enter cells and subcellular compartments with ease. In contrast, most antioxidant nutrients have difficulty penetrating cell membranes. Entry into cell membranes is crucial in protecting intracellular molecules from oxidative damage. An antioxidant molecule must have access to subcellular compartments (i.e. the mitochondria) in order to quench the hydroxyl radicals, considered by some to be the most damaging of all free radicals. See **Antioxidants** for the definition of free radicals.

Melatonin induces drowsiness and improves sleep quality. As such, it should be taken in the evening. Melatonin is inexpensive and readily available to Americans.

Note: Do not attempt melatonin treatment except under the care of a qualified physician. Pregnant women and women seeking to become pregnant should avoid melatonin because of its ability to act as a contraceptive.

### Further Reading & References

- *The Melatonin Hypothesis: Breast Cancer and Use of Electric Power* by Richard G. Stevens, Bary W. Wilson, and Larry E. Anderson (1997)

- *The miracle of melatonin: The amazing pill that slows aging, fights memory loss & Alzheimer's, eases symptoms of PMS, protects against cancer & heart disease, ... night's sleep, and more!* by James O'Brien (1996)

- *Melatonin: From Contraception to Breast Cancer Prevention* by Michael Cohen (1996)

- *The Melatonin Miracle: Nature's Age-Reversing, Disease-Fighting, Sex-Enhancing Hormone* by Walter Pierpaoli (1996)

- *Melatonin* by Russel J. Reiter, Jo Robinson (1996)

- *Melatonin: The Anti-Aging Hormone* by Suzanne Le Vert (1995)

- Lissoni P, Tancini G, Barni S, Paolorossi F, Ardizzoia A, Conti A, Maestroni G. Treatment of cancer chemotherapy-induced toxicity with the pineal hormone melatonin. Support Care Cancer, March, 5:126-9, 1997, http://www.ncbi.nlm.nih.gov/pubmed/9069612

- Memorial Sloan-Kettering Cancer Center: Melatonin, http://www.mskcc.org/mskcc/html/69298.cfm

- American Cancer Society: Melatonin, http://www.cancer.org/Treatment/TreatmentsandSideEffects/ComplementaryandAlternativeMedicine/PharmacologicalandBiologicalTreatment/melatonin

- NCI Office of Cancer Complementary and Alternative Medicine: "Melatonin, Chronobiology, and Cancer." http://www.cancer.gov/cam/attachments/MelatoninSummary.pdf

## Monoterpenes

Monoterpenes are a class of terpenes with a unique molecular structure. Biochemical processes such as oxidation relate to actions performed by monoterpenoids. Monoterpenes are found in several essential oils located in fruits, vegetables, and herbs.

Monoterpenes appear to be effective in treating both early and late-stage cancers by preventing carcinogenesis during both the initiation and growth stages.

### Further Reading & References

- Cancer chemoprevention and therapy by monoterpenes, http://www.ncbi.nlm.nih.gov/pmc/articles/PMC1470060/

# Theanine

Theanine is an amino acid in green tea. Theanine appears to work with cancer medications, making them more effective against the disease. Research on mice found that an injection of the chemotherapy drug Doxorubicin (Adriamycin) alone failed to slow tumor growth. However, the combination of theanine and Adriamycin significantly reduced the tumor weight by 62% on average. Other studies have confirmed that theanine found in green tea can suppress tumor growth and proliferation, especially when used in combination with Doxorubicin.

It was found that patients who added theanine to their diets while undergoing Doxorubicin chemotherapy experienced fewer and less severe side effects.

### Further Reading & References

- *Theanine, The Relaxation Amino Acid Latest Research on Green Tea and Theanine, An Amazing*

- *New Amino Acid* by Dr. Billie Sahley (2004)

- Memorial Sloan-Kettering Cancer Center: L-Theanine, http://www.mskcc.org/mskcc/html/69285. cfm

- WebMD: Theanine, http://www.webmd.com/vitamins-supplements/ingredientmono-1053-THEANINE.aspx?activeIngredientId=1053&activeIngredientName=THEANINE

# Tocotrienols (a class of Vitamin E compounds)

Tocotrienols are part of the vitamin E family and are an essential nutrient for the body. They help protect cell membranes, active enzyme sites, and DNA from experiencing radical damage. They're found in certain vegetable oils, barley, wheat germ, saw palmetto, and certain grains.

Several research studies show that tocotrienols are able to delay tumor growth and initiate death within cancer cells.

Human studies have shown that daily doses of up to 240 mg. of tocotrienols for 16 months produce no adverse side effects. This finding does not address possible long-term effects of such high doses.

See **Vitamin E**.

### Further Reading & References

- "Tocotrienols Kill Cancer Cells," http://www.wellnessresources.com/health/articles/tocotrienols_ kill_cancer_cells/

- "Tocotrienols show promise against cancer growth," http://www.nutraingredients.com/Research/ Tocotrienols-show-promise-against-cancer-growth

- "Tocotrienols are good adjuvants for developing cancer vaccines," http://www.biomedcentral. com/1471-2407/10/5

# The B Vitamins

B vitamin supplementation should be approached with care. Vitamin $B_{12}$ can act both as a tumor promoter and a tumor-inhibitor; its tumor-enhancing activities are partially controlled by methionine. Vitamin $B_6$ (pyridoxine) is deficient in many cancer patients and has been used to enhance the outcome of radiotherapy in a controlled prospective trial.

Hans Ladner and Richard Salkeld, a team of German and Swiss researchers, reported an important controlled clinical trial in which 300 mg of pyridoxine (vitamin $B_6$) was given throughout a 7-week course of radiotherapy to half of a group of 210 patients aged 45 to 65 with endometrial cancer. They found a 15% improvement in 5-year survival compared to patients who did not receive the supplement, and found no side effects from the supplementation. The theoretical basis for the study was animal experiments showing that healthy animals subjected to whole body radiation, or animals carrying tumors, developed tryptophan metabolism disorders that resembled those created by vitamin $B_6$ deficiency states.

In humans, these metabolic disorders resembling vitamin $B_6$ deficiency states are found in Hodgkin's disease, and bladder and breast cancer. One study suggested that vitamin $B_6$ supplementation to correct the metabolic abnormality might prevent recurrence of bladder cancer.

Ladner and Salkeld confirmed "the beneficial effects of pyridoxine administration on radiation-induced symptoms — nausea, vomiting, and diarrhea — in gynecological patients treated with high-energy radiation." They also observed that impairment of the vitamin $B_6$ status could be remedied by ingesting 300 mg of pyridoxine on a daily basis.

The researchers went on to study vitamin $B_6$ status in 6,300 gynecological cancer patients with cervical, uterine, endometrial, ovarian, and breast cancers. Prior to radiotherapy, patients with uterine, ovarian, and breast cancer showed pronounced impairment of vitamin $B_6$, $B_1$ and $B_2$ status. This was especially true with advanced tumor progression. Following irradiation, the vitamin B status became progressively more impaired.

Ladner and Salkeld concluded that quality of life and survival improved in conjunction with $B_6$ supplementation. They also found that chemotherapy (doxorubicin, cisplatin, and cyclophosphamide) generated no obvious deterioration of vitamin B6 status in women with metastatic endometrial or breast cancer who received $B_6$ supplementation.

This study on the improved quality of life for women with gynecological and breast cancer who take vitamin $B_6$ supplements in conjunction with radiotherapy is particularly provoking considering similar results with vitamin C. See **Vitamin C**.

## Further Reading & References

- *Diabetes, new therapies: Clinically proven usage of vitamin $B_6$* by John Marion Ellis (1995)

- *Free of pain: $B_6$ deficiency U.S.A. : the cause of soft tissue rheumatism* by John Marion Ellis (1988)

- Prog Clin Biol Res. 1988; 259:273-81.Vitamin B6 status in cancer patients: effect of tumor site, irradiation, hormones and chemotherapy. Ladner HA, Salkeld RM. Department of Radiology, University Gynecology Clinic, Freiburg, West Germany. http://www.ncbi.nlm.nih.gov/pubmed/3283751

# Ursodeoxycholic Acid (UDCA)

Ursodeoxycholic Acid is a type of bile acid and is a metabolic byproduct of intestinal bacteria.

Studies* in both humans and experimental models of colon cancer indicate that secondary bile acids promote tumor development. UDCA, in contrast, was found to inhibit colon cancer in rats.

### Further Reading & References

- *"Ursodeoxycholic acid inhibits the initiation and postinitiation phases of azoxymethane-induced colonic tumor development." http://www.ncbi.nlm.nih.gov/entrez/query.fcgi?cmd=Retrieve&db=PubMed&list_uids=12433708&dopt=Abstract

# Vitamin A/Emulsified Vitamin A/Vitamin A Palmitate/Retinoids/Retinol/Accutane

Vitamin A has repeatedly been shown to enhance the immune response to tumor cells and assist in the fight against cancer. The association of vitamin A and cancer was initially reported in 1926 when rats, fed a vitamin A-deficient diet, developed gastric carcinomas. The first investigation showing a relationship between vitamin A and human cancer was performed in 1941 by Abels and colleagues who found low plasma vitamin A levels in patients with gastrointestinal cancer.

Since then there have been several studies to prove that this treatment needs to be taken seriously - Proponents claim that vitamin A has the potential to reverse precancerous lesions.

Vitamin A cannot be synthesized in the body and must therefore be taken in with food as either vitamin A alcohol (retinol) or its esters, or as beta-carotene (a pro vitamin split in the intestine to form vitamin A). Natural, pre-formed vitamin A is found only in foods from animal sources while beta-carotene is found in plant sources.

Unlike beta-carotene, vitamin A is not an antioxidant, so its benefits relate to its possible roles in reversing tumor development and boosting immune function. Preformed vitamin A is found in natural sources such as milk, cheese, yogurt, fish liver oils, liver, egg yolk, butter, and cream.

At Stockholm's Karolinska Hospital, scientists gave healthy subjects vitamin A pills. After a few years, they found that vitamin A decreased the risk of cancer: the higher the dose, the less likely that cancer developed.

Scientists at the NCI scientists followed nearly 2,500 men over the age of 50, for ten years. It was found that the lower their blood serum level of vitamin A, the greater their risk of developing prostate cancer. In another NCI study in 1974, blood was obtained from over 25,000 people. Over 100 of these developed prostate cancer during the next 13 years. Once again, the less vitamin A (retinol) they had in their blood, the greater their odds of developing prostate cancer.

Six hospitals in southwestern France provided 106 cases of lung cancer for a dietary study. As with prostate cancer, it was found that the lower the consumption of vitamin A and its pro-vitamin, beta-carotene, the greater the chances of developing lung cancer. French scientists confirmed the protective value of beta-carotene and provided new evidence that vitamin A also has a protective effect. In experimental animals, cancer forms in two phases: Initiation and promotion. This vitamin seemed to inhibit the tumor promotion phase, while beta-carotene complemented this action by inhibiting tumor initiation.

Dutch scientists studied the blood levels of vitamin A in 86 patients with cancers of the head and neck. Some of these patients had tumors at other sites as well. 31% of the patients with just head and neck cancers had low serum levels of vitamin A. But 60% of those also with other cancers had low levels of Vitamin A. About two-thirds of all these cancer patients had low beta-carotene levels.

The scientists also concluded that it was possible that low vitamin A levels play a role in causing a second tumor of the head or neck. They recommended that patients with head and neck tumors be given vitamin supplements in order to prevent a second tumor from forming.

According to Peter Greenwald, Director of the Division of Cancer Prevention and Control at the National Cancer Institute (NCI), retinoids have the capacity to modify the cancer cell, in some cases actually causing the differentiation, or return to a normal state, of cancer cells. ("Retinoids" refer to Vitamin A (retinol) and its isomers, derivatives (retinal, retinoic acid), and synthetic analogues.)

"Retinoids are of special interest for use in clinical prevention because they can exert their antineoplastic activity in cells that are already dedifferentiated or initiated into a malignant state."

This means retinoids can sometimes stop the cellular process of loss of differentiation that characterizes the progression of cancer. This is of critical interest to people with cancer.

For example, researchers have found that vitamin A can suppress abnormal differentiation of prostate epithelial cells in laboratory tests after a potentially malignant state has been induced by chemical exposure or radiation. According to Greenwald, when the vitamin A was removed from the culture medium, "full expression of the malignant phenotype occurred." And with human promyelocytic leukemia cells, retinoids returned malignant cells to full differentiation with the shape and biochemical characteristics of a healthy granulocyte.

Other retinoids have "consistently arrested malignant progression in three different rodent bladder cancer systems" and have inhibited the development of cancer in chemically induced breast and skin cancer models.

### Further Reading & References

- *Cancer Therapy* by Ralph W. Moss, Ph.D.

- Greenwald, P., "Principles of Cancer Prevention: Diet and Nutrition," Cancer. Principles and Practice of Oncology, 3rd ed., V.T. DeVita, Jr., S. Hellman, and S.A. Rosenberg (eds.) (Philadelphia, PA: J.B. Lippincott, 1989).

- de Vries N, Snow GB. "Relationships of vitamins A and E and beta-carotene serum levels to head and neck cancer patients with and without second primary tumors." http://www.ncbi.nlm.nih.gov/entrez/query.fcgi?cmd=Retrieve&db=pubmed&dopt=Abstract&list_uids=2278703

# Vitamin B17

See **Laetrile/Amygdalin/VitaminB17/Sarcarcinase/Nitriloside/Mandelonitrile**.

# Vitamin B17 Metabolic Therapy/Harold Manner

It has been proposed that cancer is a nutritional and toxicity problem featuring low levels of certain important enzymes in the body as well as a deficiency in the dietary element Vitamin B17.

Professor John Beard surmised that cancer was partly caused by a deficiency of the pancreatic enzymes trypsin and chymotrypsin. People on diets rich in animal meat were losing the preventative effects of these enzymes because the enzymes were being constantly employed to break down the animal proteins in their diet. These pancreatic enzymes were shown by Beard to strip down and digest the protein coating of cancer cells. It was this life-saving action that was described by the Edinburgh embryologist in his *Unitarian or Trophoblastic Thesis of Cancer*.

Later, biochemist Ernst T. Krebs and others added further pieces to the cancer puzzle, reporting that while these pancreatic enzymes were doubtless the first line of defense against malignant attack, those people with a marked lack of hydrocyanic acid (Vitamin B17) in their diet were also prone to cancer. Krebs had determined that hydrocyanic acid's active component, laevo-mandelonitrile ('laetrile'), reacted with cancer cells to produce hydrogen cyanide and benzaldehyde, which were selectively released at the cancer site, killing the malignant cells. Krebs further found out that excess quantities of laetrile were broken down by the enzyme rhodanese, which was available in plentiful supply throughout the body, but not at cancer sites.

But it was Harold Manner, Ph.D., who publicly put the picture together and developed what has come to be known as Vitamin B17 Metabolic Therapy. Harold Manner was a fairly orthodox biology professor at Loyola University in Chicago. He decided to study the controversial chemical "laetrile," or amygdalin. He admits in his book *Death of Cancer* that his late 1970s studies would either elevate or damn the anti-cancer substance. His research was some of the most pro-laetrile research ever conducted, which "dropped a bombshell" on medical orthodoxy.

Manner showed with trials that it was a combination of dietary changes involving raw, whole foods, vitamin B17, pancreatic enzymes, emulsified Vitamin A, and full nutritional supplementation that proved most effective against cancer.

Manner also recognized that our bodies are often damaged by environmental toxins and behavioral lifestyles that cause the body to initiate a healing process. Usually pancreatic enzymes terminate this healing process upon completion of the task. In the event, though, that there are insufficient enzyme levels, due to high animal protein diets or general malnutrition, that healing process may not terminate but go on to form a site-specific tumor. In his trials, he obtained a 76%-plus regression rate with breast cancer and, more importantly, showed a high level of protection against primary cancers metastasizing to the deadly secondary state.

Today, some of Dr. Manner's assumptions about digestive enzymes are being confirmed by new human and animal research (by Dr. Nicholas Gonzalez, among others).

*Death of Cancer* chronicles Dr. Manner's research on laetrile, enzymes, vitamin C, and vitamin A against cancer. This combination caused complete cancer regression in 90% of the breast cancer-ridden rats tested.

See **Hydrocyanic Acid**.

### Further Reading & References

- *Death of Cancer* by Harold Manner (1979)

- *The Unitarian Or Trophoblastic Thesis Of Cancer* by Ernst T. Krebs, Jr., Ernst T. Krebs, Sr., and Howard H. Beard (Reprinted From the Medical Record, 163:149-174, July 1950) http://www.navi.net/~rsc/unitari1.htm

- *The Cancer Syndrome* by Ralph W. Moss (1982)

- *World Without Cancer: The Story of Vitamin B17* by G. Edward Griffin

- *Alive and Well: One Doctors Experience With Nutrition in the Treatment of Cancer Patients* by Philip E. Binzel Jr.

- *Laetrile Control for Cancer* by Glenn D. Kittler

- Some scientific information about Laetrile and cancer by Richard H Bolt

- *Laetrile, nutritional control for cancer with vitamin B-17* by Glenn D Kittler

- *Politics, Science and Cancer: The Laetrile Phenomenon* by Markle

- *The Little Cyanide Cookbook; Delicious Recipes Rich in Vitamin B17* by June De Spain

- *Vitamin B-17--forbidden weapon against cancer;: The fight for Laetrile* by Michael L Culbert

- *Laetrile Control for Cancer* by H. Knaus

- *Too Young to Die: Dramatic Use of Laetrile to Conquer Terminal Cancer* by Rick Hill

# Vitamin B3/Niacin

Niacin is a water-soluble vitamin, also known as Vitamin B3. The term niacin refers to nicotinic acid and nicotinamide, which are both used by the body to form the coenzymes, nicotinamide adenine dinucleotide (NAD) and nicotinamide adenine dinucleotide phosphate (NADP) which are required by more than 150 enzymes involved in respiration and the transfer of electrons. Without these enzymatic reactions, the body's energy production would shut down.

Dr. Max Gerson successfully treated many cancer patients with a regime that included 50 mg of niacin 8-10 times per day.

Niacin supplements in animals were shown to be able to reduce the cardiotoxicity of Adriamycin, a chemotherapy drug, while not interfering with its tumor killing capacity. Niacin combined with aspirin in 106 bladder cancer patients receiving surgery and radiation therapy provided for a substantial improvement in 5-year survival (72% vs. 27%) over the control group. Niacin seems to make radiation therapy more effective at killing hypoxic cancer cells. Loading radiation patients with 500 mg to 6,000 mg of niacin has been shown to be safe and one of the most effective agents known to eliminate acute hypoxia in solid malignancies.

### Further Reading & References

- *Beating Cancer with Nutrition* by Patrick Quillin (2005)

- Cancer Solutions: Niacin and Cancer, http://www.cancersolutions.org/2008/02/niacin-and-cancer_06.html

- National Cancer Institute: Niacin, http://www.cancer.gov/drugdictionary/?CdrID=38351

# Vitamin C/Ascorbic Acid/Ascorbate

Vitamin C has many properties which makes it an excellent cancer fighter. It is a detoxifying agent, an antioxidant, and helps to produce antibodies. It is also very important in preventing growing tumors from invading adjacent tissue.

Linus Pauling Ph.D., who won the Nobel Prize for Chemistry in 1954 and for Peace in 1962, partnered with Ewan Cameron, M.B., Ch.B., F.R.C.S. (Edinburgh and Glasgow), who was Medical Director of the Linus Pauling Institute of Science and Medicine, on several cancer patient studies involving vitamin C.

Cameron and Pauling treated a large series of terminally ill cancer patients with extensive doses of vitamin C. As Linus Pauling stated during an interview in 1996, "I became interested in vitamin C and cancer in 1971 and began working with Ewan Cameron, M.B., Ch.B., chief surgeon at Vale of Leven Hospital in Scotland. Cameron gave 10 grams of vitamin C a day to patients with untreatable, terminal cancer. These patients were then compared by Cameron and me to patients with the same kind of cancer at the same terminal stage who were being treated in the same hospital but by other doctors — doctors who didn't give vitamin C, but instead just gave conventional treatments.

They gave a later group of terminally ill patients a broad spectrum of other vitamins and minerals with their vitamin C. These patients had even larger increases in life expectancy. Results were best with cancers of the reproductive system.

"Cameron's terminal cancer patients lived far longer compared to the ones who didn't get 10 grams a day of vitamin C. The other patients lived an average of six months after they were pronounced terminal, while Cameron's patients lived an average of about six years."

This "megadose" vitamin therapy involves the intravenous injection of large amounts of vitamins. This treatment has been extensively evaluated at the Vale of Leven Hospital in Scotland under the supervision of Dr. Cameron. The experiments found that terminal cancer patients who received large, daily doses of vitamin C along with their regular treatment lived much longer than patients who did not receive vitamin C; they also had less pain and in general, a much improved quality of life. There were also some complete remissions.

A Mayo Clinic study did not confirm the Cameron and Pauling results for Vitamin C, and each side accused the other of methodological errors.

Dr. Hoffer of Victoria, Canada later expanded on the Pauling/Cameron treatment protocol by adding large amounts of vitamin E, vitamin B-3, other B vitamins, beta-carotene, and some minerals. Those of Dr. Hoffer's cancer patients who followed this regimen lived, on the average, about 16 times longer than those who did not.

In January 1994, Dr. Donald Lamm and his colleagues at the West Virginia University School of Medicine reported that daily megadose vitamin therapy significantly lessens the risk of recurrence in bladder cancer patients. Patients who received the therapy, on the average, had less than half the tumor recurrence rate than did patients who did not receive it. Dr. Lamm's vitamin combination included multivitamins (RDA dosages) plus 40,000 IU vitamin A, 100 mg vitamin $B_6$, 2,000 mg vitamin C, 400 IU vitamin E, and 90 mg zinc(32). Vitamin C is involved in the maintenance of a healthy immune system as well as protecting against a variety of cancers. It has also been shown to demonstrate an inhibitory effect on tumor growth. It is found in citrus fruits, broccoli, green peppers, and many other fruits and vegetables.

There is solid evidence that this vitamin is essential for optimal functioning of the immune system.

Natural killer (NK) cells are among the immune components involved in fighting cancer, and these are only active if they contain relatively large amounts of Vitamin C. Vitamin C also boosts the body's production of interferon which has anti-cancer activity.

In 1989, Belgian researchers reported in *Cancer* that sodium ascorbate (vitamin C) and vitamin K3 were administered separately and in combination to human breast, oral, and endometrial cancer cell lines. When combined, both vitamins displayed a synergistic inhibition of cell growth at much lower concentrations. When administered separately, each was found to have an inhibiting effect on cancer cell growth at high concentrations,

The presumed mechanism of the synergistic effect of these vitamins C and K3 is hydrogen peroxide production. Hydrogen peroxide has long been a chemical of interest among some practitioners of alternative cancer therapies. (See **Hydrogen Peroxide**.) The observed effect on cancer cells was connected to the formation of hydrogen peroxide, suggested by the suppression of the inhibitory effect the addition of catalase to the culture.

Two different hospitals in Japan conducted uncontrolled trials in the 1970s that confirmed the increase in survival time of terminal cancer patients supplemented with ascorbate. The highest increase in survival time was recorded in relation to uterine cancer, while the smallest increases were with lung and stomach cancer. The best results came from ingesting 30-60 grams daily.

Stress has been shown to have a link to cancer in that it reduces plasma levels of vitamin C. This was demonstrated in patients with uterine, cervical, and ovarian cancer, and in leukemia and lymphoma, as well as in experimental animals.* This provides additional justification for increasing vitamin C supplement intake in cancer patients, since stress from cancer lowers vitamin C levels and it is known that low vitamin C levels reduce immune function.

The potential effects of vitamin C are closely related to dietary iron. According to Swiss researcher Alfred Hanck, "Iron deficiency is an aggravating factor in cancer patients. Only ferrous iron is absorbed and ascorbic acid converts food ferric iron to bioavailable ferrous iron. Vitamin C improves hemoglobin status and thus oxygen supply of tissue, with an increase in oxidative energy production. ... The cytotoxic effect of ascorbic acid against malignant cells is significantly increased by chelation with ferrous iron. ... This increased efficacy is attributed to the longer half-life of the ascorbate iron complex during cell contact compared to ascorbic acid."

Vitamin C is helpful when used in conjunction with radiotherapy. Hanck reviewed the literature and describes the study:

Decreases of multiple vitamin levels, including vitamins E, $B_{12}$, folic acid, and C were observed during radiotherapy. The lethal effect of radiation against tumor cells along with potentiation or augmentation was also demonstrated when ascorbic acid was co-administered. The effects of radiation therapy with adjunct ascorbic acid treatment were investigated in cancer patients in a prospective clinical trial.

The patients were randomly divided into two groups. Cancer diagnoses included cancer of the tongue, tonsil, cervix, esophagus, neck, skin, lip, and cheek, and Ewing's sarcoma. Progressive disease was seen after one month in 5% of the control group and 3% of the study group. These values increased to 20% of the control group after 4 months and 7% in the study group.

Based on 20 cases, Hanck reported that 45% of the control group survived without disease while 50% were with disease at 6 months. Compare that to 67% of the vitamin C group surviving without disease while only 33% were with disease at 6 months. He also found that patients suffered less anemia, less pain, and less loss of appetite and weight if they were given vitamin C. Side effects of radiotherapy also tended to be reduced. He urged further clinical investigations of the effects of high doses of vitamin C.

In a related study, Paul Okunieff of Massachusetts General Hospital also found vitamin C to protect both the skin and bone marrow against the effects of radiation. It was not found to be toxic to the tumor itself, nor did it protect the tumor from radiation.

Another potentially significant finding for cancer patients is the protective effect vitamin C has demonstrated against potential damage to the heart by Adriamycin (ADR, doxorubicin) in animal studies.

Experimental studies by Kedar N. Prasad of the University of Colorado Health Science Center have demonstrated that two forms of vitamin C, sodium L-ascorbate and sodium D-ascorbate, enhanced the effectiveness of radiotherapy and the chemotherapeutic agents 5-fluorouracil (5-FU) and bleomycin when used on mouse neuroblastoma cells but not on rat glioma cells.

An indirect association has been demonstrated between high vitamin C intake and a lowered risk of cancer. This is especially true for cancer of the esophagus and stomach. The association is indirect because foods known to contain high levels of vitamin C were analyzed rather than vitamin C itself. High consumption of fresh fruit specifically has been shown to protect against gastric cancer.

Experimental evidence demonstrates that vitamin C can also inhibit the formation of carcinogenic nitrosamines, which are found in tobacco smoke, marijuana, some cosmetics, corrosion inhibitors, rubber products, rubber nipples for baby bottles, and cured meats.

Precursors of nitrosamines are found in many foods: they react with sodium nitrite, a food preservative, to form carcinogenic nitrosamines in the acidic environment of the human stomach. Since vitamin C can inhibit the formation of nitrosamines in the stomach, this is widely assumed to be the basis for its protective effect against gastric cancers specifically.

This capacity of vitamin C to reduce nitrosamine levels in the stomach was demonstrated with esophageal cancer patients in a study performed in northern China's Lin-Xian province, an area where esophageal cancer is common. A positive correlation was found when researchers measured levels of nitrosamines in the stomach and lesions in the esophageal epithelium: the higher the nitrosamine levels, the more lesions were found. They then gave experimental subjects 100-mg of vitamin C supplements three times a day, an hour after meals. They found a marked decrease in urinary nitrosamine products, which became comparable to those in people in areas with low esophageal cancer risk.

Gladys Block, Ph.D., of the NCI showed significant protective effects of vitamin C after surveying 33 of 46 epidemiological studies. In terms of vitamin C consumption, those in the top fourth of vitamin C intake demonstrated approximately half the cancer risk of the lowest fourth. But 21 of the 29 studies assessing fruit intake demonstrated a protective effect, especially when it came to cancers of the esophagus, larynx, oral cavity, pancreas, stomach, rectum, and cervix.

Block concluded, "While it is likely that ascorbic acid, carotenoids, folate, and other factors in fruit and vegetables act jointly, an increasingly important role for ascorbic acid in cancer prevention would appear to be emerging."

In the premalignant condition uterine cervical dysplasia, a case-controlled study of vitamin C consumption showed a protective role. However, a case-controlled study of colon cancer did not demonstrate the same effect.

The protective effect of vitamin C may be due to its ability to inhibit the oncogenic transformation of cells. Richard Schwarz of the University of California at Berkeley demonstrated that the presence of vitamin C in a culture of primary avian tendon cells and oncogenic Rous sarcoma virus "stabilizes the normal state [of the cells] by reducing virus production and promoting the synthesis of differentiated proteins."

Another protective aspect of vitamin C is its antioxidant activity.

Free radicals are potentially carcinogenic compounds created by both healthy and diseased cells in the course of cell respiration and intermediary metabolism. According to Carmia Borek of the departments of pathology and radiology at Columbia University College of Physicians and Surgeons, "The cellular oxidant state is of the utmost importance also in cellular protection against the oncogenic potential of radiation and chemicals. Inherent cellular factors comprised of enzymes, vitamins, micronutrients and low molecular weight substances are protectors."

These include superoxide dismutase and catalase, peroxidase and thiols, vitamin A, vitamin C, vitamin E, and selenium. These antioxidants serve to defend the cells against elevated levels of free radicals produced by radiation, chemical carcinogens, and tumor promoters. The free radicals damage cells to varying degrees.

Borek goes on to summarize the field as follows, "Free radicals are continuously produced by living cells. ... Under optimal cellular metabolic conditions, cellular antioxidants are sufficient to impart protection against oxidant stress. However, under conditions of exposure to carcinogens or to unfavorable metabolic stress, which enhances free radical levels, inherent protection may prove to be inadequate leading eventually to neoplastic [cancerous] transformation. ... Under stressful conditions, cells require the external addition of antioxidants to enable them to cope with the excess load of free radicals and to minimize the oxidative damage and oncogenic transformation."

Some nutrient antioxidants act directly; other agents such as selenium will impart their protection by inducing high levels of inherent protective enzyme systems, which destroy peroxides. This enables the cell itself to increase its scavenging powers and to cope with the "overload" of free radicals and their toxic products thus preventing the onset and progression of malignant transformation.

The role of vitamin C as one of the primary defenses against oxygen free radicals is described by Etsuo Niki at the University of Tokyo:

"Free radicals attack lipids, proteins, enzymes, and DNA to eventually cause a variety of pathological events and cancer. ... When aqueous radicals were generated in the whole blood, ascorbic acid [vitamin C] scavenged them faster than any other antioxidants and protected lipids and proteins more effectively than bilirubin, uric acid, or tocopherol (vitamin E)."

Similarly, Balz Frei and Bruce Ames at the University of California at Berkeley investigated the effectiveness of selected antioxidants in human blood plasma. Ascorbic acid proved to be the most effective of all the antioxidants they tested and the only one that could prevent the initiation of lipid peroxidation [the "spoilage" of fats], rather than simply lowering the rate at which the process occurs. They also found that the effect increased with the plasma concentration of ascorbic acid.

Another pathway for the protective effects of vitamin C was proposed by Joachim Liehr at the University of Texas Medical Branch who found in animal studies that vitamin C may also play a role in inhibiting estrogen-induced carcinogenesis by reducing concentrations of metabolic byproducts of estrogen.

Swiss researcher Alfred Hanck commented on the potential effects of vitamin C:

"Iron deficiency is an aggravating factor in cancer patients. Only ferrous iron is absorbed and ascorbic acid converts food ferric iron to bioavailable ferrous iron. Vitamin C improved hemoglobin status and thus oxygen supply of tissue, with an increase in oxidative energy production. . .The cytotoxic effect of ascorbic acid against malignant cells is significantly increased by chelation with ferrous iron. . ."

Dr. Kedar Prasad, Director of the Center for Vitamins and Cancer Research at the University of Colorado School of Medicine, states on using vitamin C to treat cancer: "Most people associate antioxidants with their ability to eliminate free radicals, which helps prevent cancer."

Research in 2004 shows that how ascorbic acid is delivered has a big impact on the amount that actually becomes physiologically available. A study by NIH scientists showed that much more vitamin C gets taken up when it is given via the intravenous route than when the vitamin is taken orally. The blood concentration of vitamin C when given intravenously was nearly 7 times greater than when the same amount was given orally. And the maximum tolerated dose was nearly 20 times higher.

A new trial utilizing intravenous vitamin C was announced in 2003 by Dr. Jeanne A. Drisko of the University of Kansas Medical Center.

"At this plasma level, vitamin C is chemotoxic to the cancer cells and appears to be nontoxic to healthy cells. But we are following white cell and platelet counts and other markers for possible toxicity from the vitamin C. Most patients need between 75 and 100 grams infused to get to that plasma level."

Intravenous vitamin C is a common therapy employed by many alternative and integrative doctors and clinics in the treatment of cancer.

### *Further Reading & References*

- *Hanck, "Vitamin C and Cancer." In Tryfiates and Prasad, eds., Nutrition, Growth and Cancer, 312.

- *Cancer and Vitamin C: A Discussion of the Nature, Causes, Prevention, and Treatment of Cancer With Special Reference to the Value of Vitamin C* by Ewan Cameron, Linus Pauling (1993)

- *Vitamin C and Cancer: Medicine or Politics?* by Evelleen Richards

- Evaluation of publicly available scientific evidence regarding certain nutrient-disease relationships: 8B.

- *Vitamin C and cancer* by Howerde E Sauberlich

- *Vitamin C & Cancer: Discovery, Recovery, Controversy* by Abram, Md. Hoffer, et al

- *Fight Cancer with Vitamins and Supplements* by Kedar N. Prasad, Ph.D., and K. Che Prasad, M.D.

- *Vitamin C Against Cancer* by H.L. Newbold

- *Vitamin C : The Future Is Now* by Jeffrey S. Bland

- *Challenge Cancer and Win! Step-By-Step Nutrition Action Plans for Your Specific Cancer* by Kim Dalzell, et al

- *World Without Cancer: The Story of Vitamin B17* by G. Edward Griffin

- Murata A, Morishige F and Yamaguchi H. Prolongation of survival times of terminal cancer patients by administration of large doses of ascorbate. International Journal for Vitamin and Nutrition Research. 23(Supp): 101-13. 1982.

- Pauling L et al. Effect of dietary ascorbic acid on the incidence of spontaneous mammary tumors in RIII mice. Proceeding of the National Academy of Sciences. 82(15): 5185-89. August 1985.

- Riordan N, Riordan H and Casiari J. Clinical and experimental experiences with intravenous vitamin C. Journal of Orthomolecular Medicine, Special Issue: Proceedings from Vitamin C as Cancer Therapy Workshop, Montreal. 15(4): 201-13. 1999.

- Campbell A, Jack T and Cameron E. Reticulum cell carcinoma: two complete spontaneous regressions, in response to high-dose ascorbic acid therapy. A report on subsequent progress. Oncology. 48(6): 495-97. 1991.

- Karunanithy R Saha N, Ng SE. Serum and red blood cell magnesium, copper, and zinc content in G6PD deficiency. Am J Hematol. 35(2): 136-8. Oct1990.

- Riordan N et al. Intravenous ascorbate as a tumor cytotoxic chemotherapeutic agent. Medical Hypothesis. 9(2): 207-13. 1994.

- Lesperance ML, Olivotto LSA, Forde N, et al. Mega-dose vitamins and minerals in the treatment of non-metastatic breast cancer: an historical cohort study. Breast Cancer Res Treat. 2002;76: 137-143.

- Hoffer A, Pauling L. Hardin Jones biostatistical analysis of mortality data for cohorts of cancer patients with a large fraction surviving at the termination of the study and a comparison of survival times of cancer patients receiving large regular oral doses of vitamin C and other nutrients with similar patients not receiving those doses. J. Orthomol Med. 1990;5: 143-154 .Reprinted in Cancer and Vitamin C, E. Cameron, L. Pauling, Camino Books. P.O. Box 59026, Philadelphia, PA 19102; 1993.

- "Chapter 3: Case Study of Scientific Corruption," Cancer Tutor, http://www.cancertutor.com/WarBetween/War_Pauling.html

- *Vitamin C and Cancer: Discovery, Recovery, Controversy* by A. Hoffer

- *Antioxidants Against Cancer* by Ralph W. Moss Ph.D.

- Nitrosamines, NaturalPedia, http://www.naturalpedia.com/Nitrosamines-2.html

- Deficiency, NaturalPedia, http://www.naturalpedia.com/Deficiency-49.html

- *Choices In Healing: Integrating The Best of Conventional and Complementary Approaches to Cancer* by Michael Lerner, http://www.commonweal.org/pubs/choices/12.html

- "The Dr. Ewan Cameron, M.D. and Linus Pauling, PhD Vitamin C Experiment," Cancer Tutor, http://www.cancertutor.com/WarBetween/War_Pauling.html

# Vitamin D/Cholecalciferol/Calcitriol

Few vitamins can provide such an array of health benefits as vitamin D. Vitamin D is formed in the skin of animals and humans by the action of short-wave ultraviolet light, the so-called fast-tanning sun rays. Precursors of vitamin D in the skin are converted into cholecalciferol, a weak form of vitamin D3, which is then transported to the liver and kidneys where enzymes convert it to 1,25-dihydroxycholecalciferol, the more potent form of vitamin D3.

Fat-soluble vitamin D supplements are available in two forms. Vitamin D3 is believed to exhibit the most potent cancer- inhibiting properties and is the preferred form of the vitamin. More than 10 substances belong to a group of steroid compounds that exhibit vitamin D activity. Vitamin D2 (ergocalciferol), derived from plants and yeast, is a form of the vitamin commonly added to milk and some nutritional supplements. The first vitamin D to be discovered was a crude mixture called vitamin D1; it is not available as a supplement. Although the list of vitamin-D-rich foods is limited, it is acquired from foods such as egg yolks, butter, cod liver oil, and from cold-water fish such as salmon, herring and mackerel.

Vitamin D is not prevalent in foods. A study conducted at the Bone Research Laboratory at Boston University School of Medicine revealed that fortified milk may not be a reliable source of vitamin D. Only 29% of commercial milk samples tested were within 80-120% of the amount stated on the label.

Most milk products were overfortified, and a few milk cartons contained no vitamin D at all. Vitamin D milk fortification procedures vary widely. Some dairies place their vitamin D preparations in refrigerated storage, and others do not, which may affect the vitamin D content of the final product. Sunshine is still the most economical and beneficial way to improve circulating vitamin D levels. The skin synthesizes vitamin D when exposed to sunlight. In addition, the lack of sunlight exposure could lead to thinning bones and an increased risk for cancer.

Evidence of vitamin D's protective effect against cancer is compelling. For more than 50 years, medical literature suggests regular sun exposure is associated with substantial decreases in death rates from certain cancers and a decrease in overall cancer death rates. Recent research suggests this is a causal relationship that acts through the body's vitamin D metabolic pathways. For instance, some evidence points to a prostate, breast and colon cancer belt in the United States, which lies in northern latitudes under more cloud cover than other regions during the year. Rates for these cancers are apparently two to three times higher than in sunnier regions.

Vitamin D may also go beyond cancer prevention and provide tumor therapy. Laboratory tests have shown vitamin D to be a potent angiogenesis inhibitor – these are agents that help inhibit the growth of new, undesirable blood vessels that tumors require for nutrient supply and growth.

Laboratory tests have shown that vitamin D can kill cancer cells. In clinical use, vitamin D was administered to seven patients who had experienced recurrent cancer after radical prostatectomy (surgical removal of the prostate). Six patients showed reduced PSA's. However, vitamin D in the form offered by most supplements tends to be ineffective. More work is needed to find a form of vitamin D that is more active and easily assimilated. Calcitriol, obtainable by prescription, can be useful as a source of assimilable vitamin D.

Vitamin D also works at another stage of cancer development. Tumor cells are young, immortal cells that never grow up, mature, and die off. Because vitamin D derivatives have been shown to promote normal cell growth and maturation, drug companies today are attempting to engineer patentable forms of vitamin D for anti-cancer therapy.

Johns Hopkins researchers designed vitamin D analogs called deltanoids that delay the onset and reduce the frequency of skin cancers in mice but do not cause significant bone-calcium loss or growth inhibition. Drug companies have tried to do this in the past.

"What we did was to take some of the best structural changes that large pharmaceutical companies have made public and incorporated those changes with a structural change that we discovered here eight years ago in a different portion of the molecule," said one researcher. The researchers hope eventually to put a deltanoid into human clinical trials.

Dark-skinned people require more sun exposure to make vitamin D. The thickness of the skin layer called the stratum corneum affects the absorption of UV radiation. Black human skin is thicker than white skin and thus transmits only about 40% of the UV rays for vitamin D production. Darkly pigmented individuals who live in sunny equatorial climates experience a higher mortality rate (not incidence) from breast and prostate cancer when they move to geographic areas that are deprived of sunlight exposure in winter months.

The rate of increase varies, and researchers hesitate to quote figures because many migrant black populations also have poor nutrition and deficient health care that confound statistics somewhat. Although excessive sun exposure may give rise to skin cancer, researchers as early as 1936 were aware that skin cancer patients have reduced rates of other cancers. One researcher estimates moderate sunning would prevent 30,000 annual cancer deaths in the United States.

Sunning before 10 a.m. and after 3 p.m. avoids the sun's harshest UV radiation that can cause skin damage. People who live in areas of winter cloud cover, are homebound, or don't get enough sun should consider naturally compounded vitamin D3 (cholecalciferol) supplements.

### Further Reading & References

- *Vitamin D Analogs in Cancer Prevention and Therapy (Recent Results in Cancer Research)* by J.

- Reichrath, W. Tilgen (2003)

- *Naked at Noon: Understanding Sunlight and Vitamin D* by Krispin Sullivan

- *Vitamin D* by R. Bouillon, et al

- *Vitamin D* by Feldman, David, et al

- *Vitamin D: Physiology, Molecular Biology, and Clinical Applications* by M. F. Holick, et al (1999)

- Studzinski GP, Moore DC. Sunlight--can it prevent as well as cause cancer? Can Res 1995;55:4014- 22.

- Angwafo FF. Migration and prostate cancer: an international perspective. J Natl Med Assoc 1998 Nov; 90 (11 suppl):S720-3.

- Ansleigh HG. Beneficial effects of sun exposure on cancer mortality. Prev Med 1993;22:132-40.

- Shokravi MT, et al. Vitamin D inhibits angiogenesis in transgenic murine retinoblastoma. Inv Oph 1995;36:83-7.

- Studzinski GP, Moore DC. Vitamin D and the retardation of tumor progression. In Watson RR, Mufti SI, editors, Nutrition and cancer. Boca Raton: CRC Press, 1996. p 257-82.

- Neer RM. Environmental light: effects on vitamin D synthesis and calcium metabolism in humans. Ann NY Acad Sci 1985;453:14-20.

- Heaney RP. Lessons for nutritional science from vitamin D. Am J Clin Nut 1999;69:825-6.

- Holick MF, et al. The vitamin D content of fortified milk and infant formula, New Eng J Med

- 1992;326:1178-81.

- Hicks T, et al. Procedures used by North Carolina dairies for vitamin A and D fortification of milk. JDairy Sci 1996;79:329-33.

- Grimes DS, et al. Sunlight, cholesterol and coronary heart disease. Q J Med 1996;89:579-89.

- "Vitamin D and breast cancer: insights from animal models." Welsh J. http://www.ncbi.nlm.nih. gov/entrez/query.fcgi?cmd=Retrieve&db=pubmed&dopt=Abstract&list_uids=15585794

# Vitamin E/Alpha Tocopheryl Succinate/Gamma Tocopherol

The evidence is not clear-cut when it comes to cancer and commercially available alpha-tocopherol acetate vitamin E supplements. It appears that other forms of vitamin E found in food (such as gamma tocopherol and tocotrienols) may also be responsible for providing the protective effect against breast cancer shown in some surveys which evaluated total vitamin E intake.

Many types of cancer are believed to result from oxidative damage to DNA caused by free radicals. Antioxidants such as vitamin E help protect against the damaging effects of free radicals, which may contribute to the development of chronic diseases such as cancer.

Vitamin E also may block the formation of nitrosamines, which are carcinogens formed in the stomach from nitrites consumed in the diet. Vitamin E may also protect against the development of cancers by enhancing immune function. Human trials and surveys examining the association of vitamin E with incidence of cancer have included study findings released in early 2005 that suggest a diet rich in vitamin E could help ward off bladder cancer, the fourth leading cancer killer among men. The study suggests getting plenty of vitamin E by eating foods like nuts and olive oil. It appears to cut in half people's risk of bladder cancer, which kills about 12,500 Americans annually.

Vitamin E enhances the effect of ionizing radiation on tumor cells in culture without affecting the radiation response of normal tissues. Vitamin E also enhances the effects of hyperthermia on tumor cells in culture, and inhibits the production of prostaglandin E series, which are known to suppress the host's immune system. Finally, vitamin E reduces the toxic effects of some chemotherapeutic agents. These studies suggest that vitamin E may be one of the important anticancer agents, which could play a very significant role in the prevention and treatment of cancer.

The Nurse's Health Study followed 83,234 women at baseline (at the inception of the study) and sought to assess the incidence of breast cancer during a 14-year follow-up. The study showed that premenopausal women with a family history of breast cancer who consumed the highest quantity of vitamin E enjoyed a 43% reduction in breast cancer incidence compared to only a 16% risk reduction for women without a family history of breast cancer. Based on this study, vitamin E appears to protect against genetic-predisposed breast cancer better than environmentally induced breast cancer.

However, other studies which have reviewed the effects of standard vitamin E supplements (alpha-tocopherol acetate) taken by themselves have failed to decisively show a protective benefit for cancer. As stated above, it is possible that other forms of vitamin E found in food (such as gamma tocopherol and tocotrienols) may be responsible for providing the protective effect against breast cancer shown in some surveys which evaluated total vitamin E intake. This is why vitamin E supplements that contain other tocopherols and tocotrienols, not just alpha-tocopherol, are often recommended.

In 2002, a researcher at Wake Forest University School of Medicine compiled and analyzed the large volume of published data about vitamin E and breast cancer. Her comprehensive work was published in the *Journal of Nutritional Biochemistry*. The results confirmed that certain vitamin E compounds found in food confer a significant protective effect, but that commercial alpha-tocopherol acetate supplements fail to reduce the incidence of breast cancer for most women.

The data indicates that some other vitamin E compounds in food may account for the dramatic reductions in breast cancer incidence when dietary intake levels of vitamin E are measured. As discussed above studies have indicated that the form of vitamin E used in most commercial preparations (alpha-tocopherol acetate) has not been shown to protect against breast cancer. It is the tocotrienols, one of the 8 members of the vitamin E family, however, which have demonstrated the most significant potential to not only reduce breast cancer incidence, but also to inhibit the propagation of existing breast cancer cells. Tocotrienols have been shown to inhibit the growth of estrogen receptor positive breast cancer cells by as much as 50% in culture.

Gamma-tocopherol, a form of vitamin E found in many plant seeds but not widely available in nutritional supplements, might halt the growth of prostate and lung cancer cells, stated US researchers in December 2004. Their findings lend weight to the growing support for supplements containing a mixture of vitamin E forms, in preference to those containing only alpha-tocopherol.

In the December 2004 online edition of the *Proceedings of the National Academy of Sciences*, a team from Purdue University reported that Gamma-tocopherol, found naturally in walnuts, sesame seeds and corn, was found to slow down the proliferation of lab-cultured human prostate and lung cancer cells.

Previous research by the same team found that gamma-tocopherol inhibits inflammation, which had already been implicated in cancer development. The researchers theorized that it might retard the progress of cancer and cardiovascular disease, and to test their hypothesis they exposed cultures of cancerous prostate and lung cells to the vitamin. Normal prostate epithelial cells were used as a control group.

Lead researcher Qing Jiang said, "We discovered that as we increased the quantity of gamma-tocopherol, the cancer cells grew more slowly. But the normal prostate cells were not affected and grew normally. This could indicate that the vitamin could be used to target lung and prostate cancer cells without the damaging side effects of chemotherapy."

The study also revealed that gamma-tocopherol caused cell death by interrupting synthesis of fatty acid molecules called sphingolipids. Jiang stated, ""This is also a novel discovery. Although there have been prior indications that some form of vitamin E may cause cell death in some mouse cell lines, we are the first to provide a mechanism for such an effect."

Scientists have been studying vitamin E for more than three-quarters of a century, but most efforts have focused largely on alpha-tocopherol, one of eight known forms in the vitamin's family.

Alpha-tocopherol was found early on to have the most beneficial effects on laboratory animals fed diets deficient in vitamin E, and also is the major form found in body tissues. For these reasons, it has been nearly the only form of the vitamin to be included in most manufactured nutritional supplements.

Specialist supplement manufacturers in the US are beginning to offer 'full spectrum' or 'complete complex' vitamin E products in order to provide all eight forms of the vitamin in a supplement.

Some evidence associates higher intake of vitamin E with a decreased incidence of prostate cancer, although the evidence is not overwhelming.

The objective of any cancer therapy is to induce the cancer cells to differentiate in a way which promotes programmed cell death (apoptosis). Several studies indicate that tocotrienols induce breast cancer cell apoptosis.

K.N. Prasad, an authority on vitamin E, has demonstrated that, among the several forms of vitamin E, vitamin E succinate appears to be the most effective in reducing growth and enhancing differentiation of mammalian cancer cell lines in laboratory experiments. This may be so because "tumor cells pick up this form of vitamin E more readily than they do other forms." High-dose alpha-tocopherol has reduced growth of human neuroblastoma cells in living cancer patients, and has reduced benign mastitis (inflammation) of the breast. Vitamin E enhances the effectiveness of some chemotherapies, radiation, and hyperthermia on cancer cell lines.

Alpha-Tocopheryl succinate has been shown to cause efficient apoptosis in breast cancer cells, in a study published in 2005.

With respect to protecting against chemotherapy side-effects, Prasad states: "In animal studies, vitamin E has been shown to reduce cardiac and skin toxicity from doxorubicin, and lung fibrosis related to bleomycin--two very widely used chemotherapies. In addition to protecting the heart against damage from doxorubicin in animal studies, vitamin E has been reported to have a possible protective effect in humans against hair loss from doxorubicin therapy."

Werbach summarizes a study by Wood in the New England Journal of Medicine: "69% of patients on doxorubicin [Adriamycin] receiving 1600 IU dl-alpha-tocopherol acetate [vitamin E] daily did not develop alopecia [hair loss]. Those who did develop alopecia were believed to have received the vitamin E too late before chemotherapy, as it should be started 7 days prior to commencement."

These vitamin E studies represent stunning examples of the underutilization of scientific nutrition in cancer. Each year, hundreds of thousands of women around the world take doxorubicin at the same time they undergo breast surgery. They not only undergo the personal loss of part or all of their breast, they also lose their hair.

In addition, many end up with heart damage, a known side effect of doxorubicin in many situations. Vitamin E in an admittedly preliminary study was shown to protect against hair loss with doxorubicin. Further, animal studies show that it may protect against heart damage. Both results argue strongly for further research.

If some oncologists maintain that there is not yet enough evidence to recommend to patients undergoing doxorubicin treatment that they take vitamin E, then getting that evidence should be a national research priority. If others answer that there is already sufficient evidence to recommend taking vitamin E with doxorubicin, that raises the equally troubling question of why most patients are not told they should take vitamin E when undergoing this therapy. For the biomedical cancer researcher, perhaps protecting women against hair loss when fighting for their lives with breast cancer may seem trivial.

But for the patient-centered medical practitioner, protecting women with breast cancer against hair loss is not at all trivial. Hair loss makes a profound difference in the suffering that women undergo. Therefore, if this is a preventable problem, it should be a vital matter to conduct the inexpensive and innocuous research that would settle the matter of hair loss and vitamin E and make the outcome a standard element in doxorubicin protocols. But even for the strictly biomedical researcher, unconcerned with hair loss, the issue of preventing heart damage with vitamin E should be a real priority. Again, the studies would be inexpensive and potentially lifesaving.

It should be noted that many of the salutary effects of the antioxidant vitamins A, C, and E on cancer, according to Prasad, are achieved best by their synergistic interactions. Thus, studies of the individual nutrients may understate their potential for suppressing cancer cell growth, encouraging cell differentiation toward normality, enhancing immune function, potentiating the effects of existing anticancer therapies, and protecting the body from the harmful side effects of some of these therapies.

The best therapeutic results will undoubtedly follow inclusion of a full range of nutrients, not the isolated study of one nutrient that's found in whole foods in conjunction with many others.

See also **Tocotrienols**.

### *Further Reading & References*

- *Vitamins Against Cancer; Fact and Fiction*, K.N. Prasad.

- *The Vitamin E Factor : The Miraculous Antioxidant for the Prevention and Treatment of Heart Disease, Cancer, and Aging* by Andreas Papas (1999)

- *The Antioxidant Miracle: Put Lipoic Acid, Pycnogenol, and Vitamins E and C to Work for You* by Lester Packer, Carol Colman

- *The Vitamin E Factor : The Miraculous Antioxidant for the Prevention and Treatment of Heart Disease, Cancer, and Aging* by Andreas Papas

- *Dr. Wilfrid E. Shute's complete updated vitamin E book* by Wilfrid E Shute

- *DRI Dietary Reference Intakes for Vitamin C, Vitamin E, Selenium, and Carotenoids* by Institute Of Medicine

- *Vitamin E: For a Healthy Heart and a Longer Life* by Herbert Bailey

- *Fight Cancer with Vitamins and Supplements: A Guide to Prevention and Treatment* by Kedar N. Prasad Ph.D., et al

- Vitamins and Cancer: Human Cancer Prevention by Vitamins and Micronutrients by Frank L., Jr.

- Meyskens, Kedar N. Prasad

- *Vitamins in Cancer Prevention and Treatment: A Practical Guide* by Kedar N. Prasad

- *Modulation and Mediation of Cancer* by Vitamins by F.L. Meyskens, K.N. Prasad

- *Prevention's Healing with Vitamins : The Most Effective Vitamin And Mineral Treatments For Everyday Health Problems And Serious Disease* by Alice Feinstein (Editor)

- *Nutrients in Cancer Prevention and Treatment (Experimental Biology and Medicine)* by Kedar N. Prasad, et al

- *Cancer and Nutrition* by K. N. Prasad

- Jiang, Qing, et al. "Gamma-Tocopherol or Combinations of Vitamin E Forms Induce Cell Death in Human Prostate Cancer Cells by Interrupting Sphingolipid Synthesis." 2004 December online edition of the *Proceedings of the National Academy of Sciences*, Purdue University.

- Sigournas G., et al. dl-alpha-tocopherol induces apoptosis in erythroleukemia, prostate, and breast cancer cells. Nutr. Cancer 28 (1997) 30-35.

- National Academy of Sciences, Diet, Nutrition and Cancer, 9-p;10.Ibid.

- Kedar N. Prasad, "Summary and Overview." In Poirier et al., eds., Essential Nutrients in Carcinogenesis, 543-p;7.

- K.N. Prasad, "Mechanisms of Action of Vitamin E on Mammalian Tumor Cells in Culture." In Tryfiates and Prasad, eds., Nutrition, Growth and Cancer, 363-p;75. Ibid., 364.

- K.N. Prasad, "Modification of the Effect of Pharmacological Agents, Ionizing Radiation and Hyperthermia on Tumor Cells by Vitamin E." In Prasad, ed., Vitamins, Nutrition and Cancer, 76-p;104.

- K.N. Prasad et al., "Vitamin E Enhances the Growth Inhibitory and Differentiating Effects of Tumor Therapeutic Agents on Neuroblastoma and Glioma Cells in Culture," Proceeds of the Society for Experimental Biological Medicine 164(2):158-p;63 (1980). Abstracted in Werbach, Nutritional Influences on Illness, 109-p;10.

- L. Wood, "Possible Prevention of Adriamycin-Induced Alopecia by Tocopherol," New England Journal of Medicine 312:1060 (1985). Abstract cited in Werbach, ibid.

- Wang XF, Witting PK, Salvatore BA, Neuzil J. "Vitamin E analogs trigger apoptosis in HER2/erbB2-overexpressing breast cancer cells by signaling via the mitochondrial pathway (2005)." http://www.ncbi.nlm.nih.gov/entrez/query.fcgi?cmd=Retrieve&db=pubmed&dopt=Abstract&list_uids=15582575

- "Gamma-tocopherol halts cancer cells in lab study," Bone & Joint Health http://www. nutraingredients.com/Research/Gamma-tocopherol-halts-cancer-cells-in-lab-study

# Vitamin F/Omega 3 Fatty Acids

Another vitamin critical to the prevention of cancer that has never been recognized by the FDA is omega-3 fatty acid or vitamin F. Only recently has the FDA approved one particular brand of this nutrient, permitting the manufacturer to claim specific health benefits (and to charge far higher prices than consumers pay for identical nonpatented omega-3 oils). Vitamin F is an essential fatty acid, with "essential" meaning the body cannot manufacture it from other nutrients. Vitamin F is required for the production of hemoglobin which is used by red blood cells to transport oxygen.

Dr. Johanna Budwig spent her life investigating fatty acids and found that without exception, the blood of unhealthy people always has very low levels of essential fatty acids. This directly impacts the ability of blood to carry oxygen to tissues.

Essential fatty acid deficiency is probably more common than any other nutrient deficiency, and is aggravated by the consumption of hydrogenated and partially hydrogenated oils. These manufactured oils, not found in nature, actively interfere with the metabolism of healthy fatty acids in the body.

In addition, preservatives in prepared foods generally interfere with the oxidation of fats, and become poisons when consumed.

Fats quickly become rancid when exposed to light, heat, or air. Good sources of essential fatty acids include flaxseed, walnuts, pumpkin seeds, sesame seeds, sunflower seeds, and the germ of wheat and corn. (Fish oils are also good, provided they have not been heated to get rid of the fishy taste and extend the shelf life). The whole seeds can be eaten fresh or sprouted.

Seeds containing Omega 3 fatty acid can also be cooked without damaging the oil provided the temperature remains relatively low. Cancer experts unanimously agree that the oils are better consumed uncooked — in salad dressings or mixed with milk or juice.

Health food stores may have non-rancid flaxseed oil in refrigerated dark glass bottles.

Dr. Szent-Gyorgy won the Nobel Prize in 1937 for discovering that essential fatty acids combined with sulphur-rich proteins (such as those found in dairy products) increase oxygenation of the body. Dr. Budwig applied this discovery in clinical trials by feeding cancer patients a mixture of 3-6 Tbsps. flaxseed oil and 4 oz. (1/2 cup) low-fat cottage cheese daily. She reported very high levels of success at reversing cancer, and the Budwig Protocol remains one of the most popular alternative cancer treatments.

The mixture is most effective if the flaxseed oil and low-fat cottage are thoroughly mixed or blended. Pineapple or other fruit can be added to improve the taste. After about three months, improvements should be seen in the blood of cancer patients, and the malignant tumors begin to shrink. When used for prevention by people who are cancer-free, the maintenance dose is 1 Tbsp. flaxseed oil daily per hundred pounds of body weight, blended with organic cottage cheese or quark, provided the patient can tolerate milk products. According to some sources, patients who are milk intolerant can substitute tofu.

See **Dr. Johanna Budwig**.

*Further Reading & References*

- *Flax Oil As a True Aid Against Arthritis Heart Infarction Cancer and Other Diseases* by Dr Johanna Budwig (1994)

- *The Oil Protein Diet Cookbook* by Dr Johanna Budwig (2003)

- *Healthy Fats for Life : Preventing and Treating Common Health Problems with Essential Fatty Acids* by Lorna R. Vanderhaeghe, Karlene Karst (2004)

- *Understanding Fats & Oils: Your Guide to Healing With Essential Fatty Acids* by Michael Murray and Jade Beutler (1996)


# Vitamin K/Vitamin KK2/Vitamin K3

Vitamin K is a fat-soluble vitamin that is most well-known for the important role it plays in blood clotting. However, vitamin K is also absolutely essential to build strong bones and prevent heart disease, and it plays a crucial role in other bodily functions besides blood clotting. It is so important that it is recommended as a supplement because many people do not get enough of it on a daily basis through foods. In fact, vitamin K is sometimes referred to as "the forgotten vitamin" because its major benefits are often overlooked. Studies have shown that vitamins $K_1$ and $K_2$ are effective against cancer.

There are three types of Vitamin K:

- Vitamin $K_1$ (phylloquinone) is found naturally in plants. Vitamin K (vitamin $K_1$) is natural and nontoxic at even 500 times the RDA.

- Vitamin $K_2$ (menaquinone) is made by the bacteria that line the gastrointestinal tract. Vitamin $K_2$, which is made in the human body and also produced by fermented foods, is also a superior form of vitamin K.

- Vitamin $K_3$ (menadione) is a synthetic form that is man-made, and is not recommended. In infants given synthetic vitamin $K_3$ by injection, toxicity has been reported.


A study published in the September 2003 *International Journal of Oncology* found that treating lung cancer patients with vitamin K2 slowed the growth of cancer cells, and previous studies have shown benefit in treating leukemia.

The anticancer effects of vitamin $K_1$ have been demonstrated in a number of human trials. In a study published in the August 2003 issue of *Alternative Medicine Review*, 30 patients with hepatocellular carcinoma, a type of liver cancer, took oral vitamin $K_1$. In six patients, the disease stabilized. Seven patients had a partial response, and seven others had improved liver function. For 15 patients, abnormal levels of prothrombin normalized.

Research suggests that vitamin K may help to keep calcium out of artery linings and other body tissues, where it can be damaging. Vitamin K also helps to prevent hardening of the arteries which is a common factor in coronary artery disease and heart failure.

Vitamin K is also one of the most important nutritional interventions for improving bone density. It helps to keep calcium locked into the bone matrix.

As published in the March 2004 *Life Extension* magazine, researchers have found many other beneficial effects of vitamin K including:

- Vitamin K deficiency may be a contributing factor to Alzheimer's disease, and vitamin K supplementation may help to fight this disease

- Topical vitamin K may help to reduce bruising

- Vitamin K deficiency may interfere with insulin release and blood sugar regulation in ways similar to diabetes

- Vitamin K may have antioxidant properties

Being a fat-soluble vitamin is important because dietary fat is necessary for its absorption. This means that in order for your body to absorb it effectively, you need to eat some fat along with it.

### *Further Reading & References*

- Vitamin K - A Medical Dictionary, Bibliography, and Annotated Research Guide to Internet References (2004) September 2003 International Journal of Oncology

- American Cancer Society: Vitamin K, http://www.cancer.org/Treatment/ TreatmentsandSideEffects/ComplementaryandAlternativeMedicine/ HerbsVitaminsandMinerals/vitamin-k

- Reuters: Higher vitamin K intake tied to lower cancer risks, http://www.reuters.com/article/ idUSTRE62U4VO20100331

- *Fight Cancer with Vitamins and Supplements: A Guide to Prevention and Treatment* by Kedar N. Prasad Ph.D. and K. Che Prasad M.D. (2001)

- *Health Benefits of Vitamin K2: A Revolutionary Natural Treatment for Heart Disease And Bone Loss* by Larry M. Howard and Anthony G. Payne (2006)

# Minerals

## Arsenic/Arsenic trioxide/Arsenic trisulfide

A form of arsenic, once used as insect poison, has won U.S. FDA approval as a leukemia and cancer treatment after studies found that small doses helped patients with a rare but deadly form of the disease.

Two years ago, Chinese researchers reported that low doses of arsenic trioxide induced remission in patients with acute promyelocytic leukemia (APL).

Researchers at Memorial Sloan-Kettering Cancer Center have now become the first investigators in the Western world to show that arsenic effectively induces remission in-patients who have relapsed with APL, a potentially fatal type of cancer that affects the blood and bone marrow. The findings were reported in a 1998 issue of the *New England Journal of Medicine*:

"We now know that arsenic can safely bring patients with APL into remission, which may ultimately give them a second chance at life," stated Dr. Raymond P. Warrell, Jr., the senior author of the study and a leukemia specialist at Memorial Sloan-Kettering Cancer Center.

In the pilot study, 12 patients who had relapsed from conventional therapy were treated with low doses of arsenic trioxide. Eleven of the 12 patients achieved remission anywhere from 12 to 39 days after treatment started, with mild side effects. One patient died from a cancer complication five days after arsenic treatment began, and could not be evaluated in the study. Once remission was achieved, each patient received a brief treatment break, followed with repeated courses of arsenic trioxide therapy every three to six weeks thereafter. After two cycles of therapy, the investigators conducted additional tests to determine whether any molecular evidence of leukemia remained. Three patients tested positive and later relapsed with APL, while eight patients tested negative for molecular evidence of APL and remained in remission as long as 10 months. Several patients received up to six courses of arsenic treatment without experiencing cumulative side effects.

Dr. Steven Soignet, the lead author of the study stated: "Based on these highly sensitive molecular results, treatment with arsenic trioxide appears to exceed the effectiveness of any single drug to treat APL. Still, this is not a cure. More studies will tell us how truly effective arsenic trioxide will be over the long term."

Arsenic trioxide works by killing the cancerous cells that cause APL, including those that have become resistant to the most successful form of treatment - a drug called all-trans retinoic acid that was also pioneered by Dr. Warrell.

"This finding shows that arsenic trioxide does not discriminate between APL that is resistant or not resistant to retinoic acid, which may mean that we can use it at the outset of treatment for patients with APL," said Dr. Soignet.

Arsenic trioxide has also been shown to target multiple myeloma cells. Interestingly, arsenic trisulfide has always been a component of Hoxsey's yellow powder, a well-known alternative cancer treatment. Forms of arsenic and stibnite are found in many of the most highly studied pastes. Both Hoxsey treatment and Mohs microsurgery methods, as well as some Ayurvedic practitioners, claim that arsenic can be rendered nontoxic.

It should obviously only be used under careful supervision. Patients need to take great care as several studies state that arsenic in drinking water has led to sarcoma. In fact, arsenic is one of the most common carcinogens in U.S. drinking water, found most often in the western half of the country.

### Further Reading & References

- "Multiple myeloma." http://www.ncbi.nlm.nih.gov/entrez/query.fcgi?cmd=Retrieve&db=pubmed &dopt=Abstract&list_uids=15561686

- "Arsenic Shows Promise as Cancer Treatment, Study Finds," http://www.sciencedaily.com/ releases/2010/07/100712154428.htm

- "Arsenic Treats Cancer?" http://www.ivanhoe.com/channels/p_channelstory. cfm?storyid=24794

## Beres Drops Plus (Dr. Jozsef Beres)

"In Hungary he carried out tests on 235 patients who had 'no chance of recovery.' After giving them the drops nearly one-third found their tumors had subsided."*

The formula is said to include EDTA and succinic acid plus minute amounts of cobalt, vanadium, magnesium, manganese, iron, glycine, nickel, boron, zinc, sodium, copper, chlorine, and fluorine.

### Further Reading & References

- *Miracle Drops? "Wendy cancels cancer op after tumour shrinks." http://www.whale.to/cancer/ beres.html

## Calcium

Calcium is a chemical element essential for living organisms due to its ability to move in and out of the cytoplasm, acting as a biochemical signal for multiple cell processes. Calcium is a major material in bones as well as an important part of a healthy diet. Though 99% of the body's calcium is stored in the bones and teeth, calcium serves other important functions in the body such as aiding in muscle contraction, depolarizing cells, and proliferating the action potential of cells.

Dr. Carl Reich, M.D., considered by many to be the father of preventive medicine, was the first North American doctor to prescribe mega doses of minerals and vitamins to his patients. He reported back in the 1950s that his patients were able to cure themselves of almost all degenerative diseases by consuming several times the RDA of calcium, magnesium, vitamin D, and other nutrients. By the 1980s, Dr. Reich had reportedly cured thousands. Yet, his medical license was revoked for expounding the idea that the consumption of mineral nutrients such as calcium could prevent cancer and a host of other diseases. Conventional medicine rejected this thesis and continues to do so. However, by the late 1990s, other medical professionals were also discovering that calcium supplements could indeed help reverse cancer.

Adequate mineral consumption is necessary in order to supply the blood with the crucial minerals required to maintain an alkaline pH of 7.4. When a person's diet lacks minerals, the body removes crucial minerals, such as calcium, from the saliva, spinal fluids, bones, kidneys, liver, etc., in order to maintain the blood at pH 7.4. This causes the de-mineralized fluids and organs to become acidic and therefore anaerobic, thus inducing not only cancer, but a host of other degenerative diseases, such as heart disease, diabetes, arthritis, lupus, etc.

Harvard researchers analyzed data on 87,998 women from the Nurse's Health Study and 47,344 men from the Health Professionals Follow-up Study. Both were long-term longitudinal studies that generated landmark research over the past several decades. Out of the more than 135,000 eligible participants in the cohorts, there were 626 cases of colon cancer among the women and 399 cases among the men. The researchers compared data from the participants' food frequency questionnaires with the incidence of colon cancer.

Colon cancer cases were classified as distal (occurring on the left side, or in the descending colon) or proximal (occurring on the right side, or in the ascending colon). The researchers found that people who consumed between 701 and 800 mg of calcium each day were half as likely to develop distal colon cancer as those who consumed 500 mg a day of calcium or less. However, no association was seen between calcium intake and proximal colon cancers.

An interesting point is that the beneficial calcium intake levels in this study are considerably below those often recommended by nutrition experts; most sources recommend that women and men over 50 get 1,200 mg of calcium each day. And the authors note: "calcium intake beyond moderate levels may not be associated with further risk reduction." The current RDA of calcium is 1000 to 1500 mg.

Many people promote the benefits of coral calcium, which is a salt of calcium that comes from fossilized coral reefs and is composed of both calcium carbonate and trace minerals. Proponents of coral calcium claim it is an ideal treatment and cure for cancer, though there is no medical evidence that supports these claims. In 2004, the National Center for Complementary and Alternative Medicine issued a consumer advisory warning about false and misleading marketing claims promoting the benefits of calcium supplements.

In contrast, calcium carbonate is by far the most common and least expensive type of calcium supplement. Some studies suggest absorption of calcium carbonate is as effective as absorption of calcium from milk. Calcium supplements can be obtained from retailers.

Milk and soymilk are both plentiful sources of dietary calcium because they contain high calcium concentrations that are easily absorbed. In addition, several juices have high calcium levels.

### Further Reading & References

- *The Calcium Factor* by Robert Barefoot (2006)

- *Death By Diet* by Robert Barefoot (2002)

- *The Calcium Bomb: The Nanobacteria Link to Heart Disease & Cancer* by Douglas Mulhall, et al (2004)

- *Calcium Signalling in Cancer* by G. V. Sherbet (2000)

- *Evaluation of the scientific evidence for a relationship between colorectal cancer risk and calcium, vitamin D or dairy intake* by Bonny Specker

- *Calcium in Cell Cycles and Cancer* by James F., Ph.D. Whitfield (1995)

- *The Calcium Connection: A Revolutionary Diet and Health Program to Reduce Hypertension, Prevent Osteoporosis, and Lower the Risk of Cancer* by Cedric Garland, Frank Garland (1989)

- *Calcium, Vitamin D, and Prevention of Colon Cancer* by Martin S. Newmark, et al (1991)

- Calcium, http://en.wikipedia.org/wiki/Calcium

# Cesium

Over seventy-five years ago, Dr. Otto Warburg published a Nobel Prize winning paper describing the environment of the cancer cell. A normal cell undergoes an adverse change when it can no longer take up oxygen. In the absence of oxygen, the cell reverts to a primitive nutritional program to sustain itself, converting glucose, by fermentation. The lactic acid produced by fermentation lowers the cell pH (acid/alkaline balance) and destroys the ability of DNA and RNA to control cell division. The cancer cells begin to multiply unchecked.

Cesium, a naturally occurring alkaline element, has been shown to affect the cancer cell in two ways. Firstly, cesium limits the cellular uptake of the nutrient glucose, starving the cancer cell and diminishing fermentation. Secondly, cesium raises the cell pH to the range of 8.0, neutralizing the weak lactic acid and stopping pain within 12 to 24 hours. A highly alkaline pH range of 8.0 is a deadly environment for the cancer cell; the cancer cell dies within a few days and is absorbed and eliminated by the body.

By the late 1970's mass spectrographic and isotope studies had shown that tumor cells exhibit a preference for certain alkaline minerals: potassium, rubidium, and especially cesium. Further, specific antioxidants, including vitamin C, and zinc were shown to enhance the uptake of these alkaline minerals by the cancer cell.

In preliminary research, Sartori (1984) found no response when cesium was given alone to 50 patients over a period of three years. When cesium was given along with minerals such as magnesium, potassium, and selenium and some vitamins and chelating agents, the patients experienced a 50% recovery from primary breast, colon, prostate, pancreas, lung, and liver cancer and lymphoma, Ewing sarcoma of the pelvis, and adenocancer of the gallbladder.

Sartori indicated that the typical dosage is 6-9 g divided into three doses daily. High exposure to cesium can result in burns to body tissue and death (Environmental Protection Agency, 2002). Side effects include nausea, diarrhea, anorexia, and tingling of the lips, hands, and feet (Neulieb, 1984). Cesium therapy should be undertaken only under the care of a doctor.

Physicist and cancer researcher A. Keith Brewer said cesium defeats cancer cells by doing one of two things. The first method is to change the pH of cancer cells when taken orally, meaning cesium raises the pH levels of cancer cells while leaving the pH of normal cells unaffected. When the pH of a cancer cell goes above 7.5, it dies.

The second method by which cesium can defeat a cancer cell is to starve it by limiting the uptake of glucose. Cancer cells that can no longer use oxygen sustain themselves on glucose. According to Dr. Rogers writing in *Pain Free in Six Weeks*, "Sugar and alcohol are like fertilizer for cancer."

Brewer said animal studies at the University of Wisconsin in Platteville confirmed his theories about how cancer cells take in cesium. Tests on mice given the minerals cesium and rubidium showed notable shrinkage in the tumor masses within two weeks as well as none of the side effects of cancer.

In areas of the world where there is a high cesium content in the soil, cancer is virtually unknown: Hopi Indians of Arizona, the Hunza of North Pakistan, and the Indians of Central and South America.

Evaluation of the nutrient content of certain diets in regions with low incidence of cancer has advanced the use of certain alkaline metals, i.e., rubidium and cesium, as natural chemotherapeutic agents. The rationale for this approach, termed "high pH" therapy, resides in using cesium to change the acidic pH range of the cancer cell towards weak alkalinity that endangers the cancer cell's survival. According to the therapy's proponents, the formation of acidic and toxic materials, normally formed in cancer cells, is neutralized and eliminated.

See also **High pH Therapy/Dr Brewer/Cesium Chloride**.

### Further Reading & References

- *Nutrients and Cancer: An Introduction to Cesium Therapy* H. E. Sartori, M.D. Life Science Universal Medical Center, Suite 306, 4501 Connecticut Avenue, Washington, DC 20008

- *The High pH Therapy for Cancer - Tests on Mice and Humans* was published in Pharmacology Biochemistry & Behavior, v.21, Suppl., 1, pp. 1-5.

- *The High pH Therapy for Cancer Tests on Mice and Humans* http://www.mwt.net/~drbrewer/highpH.htm

- *Swimming In A Deadly Sea: Awash In Radiation* http://www.cancer-coverup.com/default.htm

- Brewer, A.K. 1984. *The High pH Therapy for Cancer*. Retrieved April 17, 2010 from http://www.cancer-coverup.com/brewer/printbrewerreport.htm.
  5 Rogers, S. 2001. *Pain Free in Six Weeks*. Quoted by Henderson, B. in *Cancer Free*, p. 204.

# Colloidal Silver

Colloidal silver is a form of silver sometimes promoted by alternative medicine, though its use is contentious. It has disinfectant properties and is used by some physicians for wound dressings, particularly as a result of the rise in antibiotic-resistant bacteria.

Silver has a toxic effect on bacteria, algae, and fungi in vitro (i.e. in lab cultures). Among elements that have this effect, silver is the least toxic for humans to use.

Since the 1990s, colloidal silver has been marketed as an essential mineral supplement with the ability to prevent or treat many diseases, cancer included. However, silver is not an essential mineral in humans and support for colloidal silver's effectiveness as a disease treatment is unproven.

This is a comment on one of several colloidal mineral drinks that advocates believe shows promise for cancer treatments:

"Naturopathic Medicine regards Cancer as a viral and fungal [candida septicemia] process. Microorganisms depend on a specific enzyme to breathe. Colloidal Silver is a catalyst that disables these enzymes, and as a result they die. To this day, there has been no recorded case of adverse effects from it when it is properly prepared. There also has been no recorded case of drug interaction with any other medication. Unlike pharmaceutical antibiotics which destroy beneficial enzymes, Colloidal Silver leaves the tissue-cell enzymes intact."

Conventional medicine maintains colloidal silver may pose some dangers if taken internally, though it is widely considered acceptable when used externally.

### *Further Reading & References*

- Naturopathic Protocol for Cancer, http://www.doctorajadams.com/cancer.html

- *Colloidal Silver Today: The All Natural, Wide-Spectrum Germ Kill*er by Warren Jefferson (2003)

- *Colloidal Silver : Making the Safest and Most Powerful Medicine on Earth for the Price of Water* by Mark Metcalf (20010

- *The Wonders of Colloidal Silver* by Dhyana L Coburn, et al 1997)

- Medical Uses of Silver, http://en.wikipedia.org/wiki/Medical_uses_of_silver

# Copper

Copper is one of the colloidal minerals that may have great potential for treating cancer.

"In 1930, work in France indicated that injections of colloidal copper mobilized and expelled tumor tissue. Recent work with mice in the U.S. has shown that treatment of solid tumors with non-toxic doses of various organic complexes of copper markedly decreased tumor growth and metastasis and thus increased survival rate. These copper complexes did not kill cancer cells but caused them to revert to normal cells. Based on work in the treatment of cancers using copper complexes, researchers have found that these same complexes may prevent or retard the development of cancers in mice under conditions where cancers are expected to be induced."

Copper supplementation is somewhat controversial, even among alternative doctors, in anything higher than minimal doses.

### *Further Reading & References*

- "A Brief History of The Health Support Uses of Copper'" http://www.purestcolloids.com/history-copper.htm

# Germanium (Ge-132)

Germanium is a trace element that enhances the availability of oxygen to both healthy cells and cancer cells. Since Otto Warburg's work, it is known that cancer cells cannot thrive in an oxygen-rich environment. They cannot survive. Dozens of scientific studies have shown that germanium appears to have a wide range of health benefits, including the ability to boost the immune system, normalize high blood pressure and cholesterol, protect the body against harmful cellular aberrations and abuse, provide some pain relief, alleviate rheumatoid arthritis symptoms and generally normalize physiological functions.

Germanium exhibits a remarkable ability to stimulate the immune system in cancer patients as well as healthy individuals. In many experiments, Japanese and American scientists found evidence which suggests that germanium activates the body's own defenses.

A number of prominent researchers such as Dr. Parris Kidd and Dr. Frank Summerfield have stated that germanium is the ideal immunostimulant.

U.S. doctors have used the inorganic form of germanium on patients with anemia since 1922. In 1967, Japanese scientist Dr. Kazuhiko Asai was the first to synthesize an organically bound compound, germanium sesquioxide (Ge-132).

Even the healing miracles at the French Catholic shrine of Lourdes have been attributed to germanium because of its prevalence in the local water. In the Pyrenees on the French Spanish border, Lourdes is a small city with a population of about 10,000. Numerous hotels, boarding houses, and inns are clustered all over town and around its famous cathedral, accommodating guests from all over the world, mostly the ailing who seek a cure with the help of the healing waters gushing out of the rock on which the cathedral is built.

The August 9, 1971 issue of *Newsweek* carried the following story.

"A three year old girl contracted kidney cancer. One of the kidneys was excised, but the cancer spread to the cranial bone. She became emaciated, her hair had fallen out, and her skin had turned yellow. Her whole system was affected by cancer and the doctors had given up her case as hopeless.

"As a last resort, the parents sat her in a wheelchair and went to Lourdes, where the cancer-stricken girl was dipped in the sacred water of which she also drank. No sign of improvement appeared, and the discouraged parents brought their daughter back to Glasgow, Scotland, to let her die at home.

"On the morning of the third day after their return, the girl suddenly sat up in bed and asking for an orange, she began eating it. From then on her condition began to improve and several days later, the tumor disappeared and she was once a gain a healthy girl."

This story was accompanied by a photograph showing the girl in good spirits. The case created a major sensation in the medical circles of Scotland, and the fame of the miraculous water of Lourdes spread further.

Several studies have shown GE-132, a laboratory version of the naturally occurring compound from Japan, has excellent anti-tumor activities and helps the patient in strength and quality of life. It is thought to do this by strengthening the immune system. Germanium also seems to stimulate interferon production.

Dr. Asai of Japan's Coal Research Institute noted the high concentrations of germanium in coal and theorized that germanium must be present in plants since coal is composed of fossilized plants.

He went on to prove that the highest concentrations of germanium were found in plants commonly used for medicinal purposes such as ginseng, shitake mushrooms, aloe, comfrey, and garlic. Shelf fungus, a substance highly regarded by the Russians for centuries in the treatment of cancer, had the highest levels. An analysis of the healing waters of Lourdes, France also revealed significant quantities of germanium.

The major energizing feature of germanium appears to be that it works at the cellular lever, which is also the most basic level of the body. Cumulative evidence suggests that germanium raises the cell's oxygen supply, thus enhancing the cell's ability to generate energy.

At the 1987 meeting of the Orthomolecular Medical Society, researchers told the symposium that germanium appears to work by increasing tissue oxygenation. *The Townsend Letter for Doctors and Patients* says: "Its oxygenation phenomenon allows greater organism function with reduced oxygen intake. It creates an oxygen economy with extremely fast-acting effects. Those with Raynaud's syndrome, for example, will feel warmth in the affected fingers and toes one half hour after taking germanium. Healthy people will feel the warmth in a couple of minutes."

Jeff Rinehardt, Ph.D. and nutritional biochemist with the Marin Clinic of Preventative Medicine in

California, has found that germanium's antiviral powers were particularly potent in one patient suffering from the Epstein Barr virus, a very debilitating infection related to herpes, which, like herpes, has no known cure. Dr. Rinehardt believes germanium will someday be viewed in the same light as selenium, though it may take 10 to 20 years.

As Dr. Rinehardt says, many diseases are typified by hypoxia, which is an insufficient supply of oxygen to cells and tissues within the body. He goes on to say, "Many diseases can be looked upon as a chemical imbalance in the body, an imbalance of electrons and protons. With germanium, you have a compound that can get to these sites and begin to modify and reestablish homeostasis, a healthy biochemical balance in the cells. Many researchers believe germanium helps the cell metabolize oxygen more efficiently, which would account for its energizing effects."

Germanium's ability to increase tissue oxygenation may explain why it offers measurable effects on maintaining healthy cells and organs.

According to Dr. Kidd, germanium normalizes many physiological functions such as lowering high blood pressure in humans and rats. It also restores deviant blood characteristics to their normal range including pH, glucose, the minerals sodium, potassium, calcium and chlorides, triglycerides, cholesterol, uric acid, hemoglobin and leucocytes (white blood cells).

All of these clinical studies illustrate germanium's role as an adaptogen, a nontoxic substance that normalizes body functions indirectly.

If the immune system is depressed, ingestion of germanium may be one way to help the body defend itself. Researchers Dr. Kidd and Dr. Summerfield believe that germanium's ability to stimulate the body's natural defense mechanisms makes it an ideal candidate for combating viruses, funguses, bacteria, and especially candida albicans, a yeast infection.

It should be noted that germanium does not directly kill viruses and bacteria. Some researchers believe germanium plays an active role in returning the body's defenses to normal, enabling the body to fight off the invading germs. This is the prime reason why the International AIDS Treatment Conference approved germanium's use for clinical testing on AIDS patients.

Germanium appears to significantly enhance the body's production of interferon. In animal experiments, germanium has reduced the harmful effects of influenza.

Research suggests germanium may exhibit an ability to help normalize the body's defenses in cancer patients. This is a huge benefit, as many cancer patients are immuno-deficient. This theory is backed by a report by Fujio Suzuki and Richard Pollard in *The Journal of Interferon Research* (1984) which states that studies in immune-suppressed animals and patients with malignancies (cancer) or rheumatoid arthritis may be restored to normal T-cells, B lymphocytes and antibody-forming cell function when given Ge-132.

Japanese doctors also observed that Ge-132 normalized activity in immune cells such as T lymphocytes and NK cells and increased interferon production in seven cancer patients, according to a report given at the International Symposium at Osaka in July of 1981. The doctors concluded that Ge-132 had increased the patients' resistance in both malignancies and rheumatic disorders. According to this study, one patient's abdominal cancer disappeared after 16 months of Ge-132 treatment and intermittent therapy with a chemotherapy agent. Another patient's post-operative condition was controlled well on Ge-132 alone.

When free radicals abound, tissue injury and disease states such as cancer can occur based on their tendency to be highly reactive molecules, thus reducing the cell's oxygen supply. While aerobic (oxygen-using) cells exhibit regular controlled growth patterns, anaerobic (oxygen-deprived) cells show abnormal growth. Based on this, a number of researchers, including Otto Warburg, believe the prime cause of cancer is oxygen deprivation in the cell.

According to Dutch researcher, Dr. Schuitemaker, "It [germanium] is involved as a catalyst in the supply of oxygen to oxygen-poor tissue, such as cancerous growths … It lessens the peroxidation of fatty acids, thus establishing the role of germanium in free radical pathology."

As a preventative aid, this treatment's advocates suggest 25 to 100 mg per day. In treating chronic conditions such as ongoing viral symptoms, yeast infections, and food allergies, Dr. Jeff Anderson, a practitioner from Corte Madera, California, has recommended that his patients take between 300 and 500 mg a day. Dr. Asai often treated seriously ill people with daily doses of one or two grams.

In substances high in germanium such as garlic, ginseng, and aloe, the amount of Ge-132 is extremely small. For this reason, germanium supplements are often more expensive than some nutritional compounds. Naturally-synthesized germanium sesquioxide seems to be the best source of this vital element.

### *Further Reading & References*

- Asai, Germanium Research Institute, *Ge-132: Outline*, Tokyo, Japan. 1984.

- Asai, Kazuhiko, Ph.D.; Norihiro, Kakimoto, Pharmacist; and Saito, Michael T., M.D., Ph.D.; 1976 International Medical Convention of Surgeons, *Germanium Research of Surgical Patients*.

- Fujio, Suzuki, R. R. Bruthiewicz and R. B. Pollard, *Ability of Sera From Mice Treated with Ge-132, an Organic Germanium Compound, To Inhibit Experimental Murine Ascites Tumors*. BR.. Journal Cancer 52: 757-763.1985.

- Fujio Suzuki and Richard B. Pollard, *Prevention of Suppressed Interferon Gamma Production in Thermally Injured Mice* by Goodman, Sandra, *Therapeutic Effects of Organic Germanium*. Medical Hypothesis 26:207, 1988.

- Hisashi, Aso, Fujio, Suzuki, Ct. al., *Introduction of Interferon and Activation of NK Cells and Macrophages in Mice by Oral Ad-ministration of Ge-132, an Organic Germanium Compound*. Microbiology Immunology, Volume 29 (1), 65-74, 1985.

- Isao Sato, Bao Ding Yuan, Toshio Nishimura and Nobuo Tanaka, *Inhibition of Tumor Growth and Metastasis in Association with modification of Immune Response by Novel Organic Germanium Compounds,* Journal of Biological Response Modifiers 4:159-168.1985.

- Kamen, Betty, Ph.D., *Germanium-A New Approach to Immunity*, Nutrition Encounter, Inc., Larkspur, CA 1987

- Kidd, Parris M., *Germanium-I 32 (Ge-I 32): Homeostatic Normalizer and Immunostimulant. A Review of its Preventive Efficacy. International Clinical Nutrition Review* 7:11, 1987.

- Miller, Dana and Stephen A. Levine, Ph.D., *Doctors Report on Germanium Benefits*, Let's Live Magazine, December 1987.

- Mitsugu, Hachisu, HirokoTakahashi, Takemi Doeda and Yashuham Sekizawa, *Analgesic Effect of Novel Organogermanium Compound, Ce-132.* Journal of Pharm. Dyn. 6:814-820; 1983.

- Nobuko Kumano and Yushi Nakai, et. al., *Inhibition of Lewis Lung Carcinoma with the Organogermanium Compound Ge-I32.* Current Chemotherapy and Immunotherapy. Proceedings of the 12th International Congress of Chemotherapy. July 19-24, 1981.

- *Organic Germanium*, American Institute for Biosocial Research, Life Sciences Division, Botanical Medial Series, Number 7, 1987.

- Schuitemaker, Dr. G. E., *Germanium: A Mineral of Great Promise*, Orthomolecular, Number 3, 1987

- Walker, Morton, D.P.M., *Germanium Oxygenation/Immune Enhancing Effects Sparks Excitement*, Townsend Letter for Doctors. #528611.

- Y. Mizushima, Y. Shoji and K. Kaneko: *Restoration of Impaired Immunoresponse by Germanium in Mice*, International Archives of Allergy and Applied Immunology, 63: 338-339. 1980.

- *Cytostatic and cytotoxic effects of alkylglycerols (Ecomer)*. http://www.ncbi.nlm.nih.gov/entrez/ query.fcgi?cmd=Retrieve&db=pubmed&dopt=Abstract&list_uids=14586289

- Germanium: The Missing Element, http://www.stopcancer.com/germaniumstor2.htm

- Alternative Cancer Therapies, cont., The Cancer Cure Foundation, http://www.cancure.org/ choice_of_therapies_continued.htm


# Lithium and Iodine

Iodine is regarded in some circles as a major cancer treatment/preventative. Its compounds are a staple in nutrition for most biological functions and it contributes to the production of acetic acid and polymers.

When breast tissue cells lack in iodine, they are more likely to be abnormal, precancerous, or cancerous. Deficiency in this mineral is also related to child mortality. In addition, lack of this mineral can be a factor in chronic fatigue and fibromyalgia, ADD/ADHD, and even chronic headaches. Many also believe lack of iodine is a cause of breast cancer, breast cysts, prostate cancer, and other types of cancer.

As a treatment, iodine is reported to kill breast cancer cells without killing normal cells in the process. This makes it unusually ideal as both a treatment and preventive tool for breast cancer.

Scientists who have studied iodine and the doctors who use it in their practice believe we need 83 times as much as the government's recommended daily allowance (RDA).

A Michigan M.D., David Brownstein, has reported promising clinical results when supplementing his patients with high levels of this vital mineral. He reports that a 45-year-old woman came to him with a 15-year history of breast cysts. After receiving iodine therapy, she commented on the healthy state of her breasts, saying "The two rocks I had are now soft and normal-feeling. All of the cysts are gone and all of the pain is gone."

Another patient of Dr. Brownstein's, a 55-year-old man, suffered from depression and loss of vision for three years. After careful review, his problem appeared to be low thyroid function caused by extreme iodine deficiency. After starting a supplement protocol that included iodine, he reported the difference was like "night and day … I feel like I am 20 years old."

Dr. Brownstein also reports treating a woman with late-stage breast cancer by prescribing high doses of iodine for 26 days. Soon after, she was cured. Similarly, Dr. Brownstein treated another woman with breast cancer who also tested very low for iodine levels. She had a history of breast cysts, typical of women with iodine deficiency. With the help of iodine supplements she was able to stop the progress of her tumors without resorting to surgery, radiation, or chemotherapy.

Lithium and Iodine-131 (I-131) are also reported to work together in the body to treat thyroid cancer.

Lithium may also be a useful adjuvant for I-131 radiation therapy of thyroid cancer, augmenting both the accumulation and retention of I-131 in lesions.


### Further Reading & References

- "Lithium as a Potential Adjuvant to 131I Therapy of Metastatic, Well Differentiated Thyroid Carcinoma1." Sung-Soo Koong, James C. Reynolds, Edward G. Movius, Andrew M. Keenan, Kenneth B. Ain, Mark C. Lakshmanan and Jacob Robbins http://jcem.endojournals.org/cgi/content/full/84/3/912

- *Iodine: Why You Need It, Why You Can't Live Without It* by David Brownstein, M.D. (2005, 4th edition)

- "Cancer-Fighting Mineral is Almost Totally Ignored," *Cancer Defeated*, http://cancerdefeatednewsletter.com/10/021010.html


# Magnesium/Magnesium Chloride/Magnesium Chloride Hexahydrate Therapy

Magnesium has an impressive healing effect on a wide range of diseases as well as in its ability to rejuvenate the aging body. It is essential for many enzyme reactions, especially in regard to cellular energy production, for the health of the brain and nervous system and also for healthy teeth and bones. Many studies have shown an increased cancer rate in regions with low magnesium levels in soil and drinking water. In Egypt the cancer rate was only about 10% of that in Europe and America. In the rural areas, it was practically non-existent. The main difference was an extremely high magnesium intake of 2.5 to 3g (2,500 to 3000 mg) in these cancer-free populations, ten times more than in most Western countries.

It may come as a surprise that in the form of magnesium chloride, magnesium is also an impressive infection fighter.

The first prominent researcher to investigate and promote the antibiotic effects of magnesium was a French surgeon, Prof. Pierre Delbet MD. In 1915, he was looking for a solution to cleanse wounds of soldiers because he found that traditional antiseptics actually damaged tissues and encouraged infections instead of preventing them. In all his tests magnesium chloride solution was by far the best. Not only was it harmless for tissues, but it also greatly increased leukocyte activity and phagocytosis, the destruction of microbes.

Later, Prof. Delbet performed experiments with the internal application of magnesium chloride and found it to be a powerful immune-stimulant. In his experiments, phagocytosis increased by up to 333%. This means that after magnesium chloride intake the same number of white blood cells destroyed up to three times more microbes than before.

Gradually, Prof. Delbet found magnesium chloride to be beneficial in a wide range of diseases. He also found a very good preventative effect on cancer and cured precancerous conditions such as leukoplakia, hyperkeratosis, and chronic mastitis. He was also surprised that many of these patients experienced euphoria and bursts of energy. Epidemiological studies confirmed that regions with magnesium-rich soil had lower cancer rates than did regions with low magnesium levels.

Another French doctor, A. Neveu, cured several diphtheria patients with magnesium chloride within two days. He also published 15 cases of poliomyelitis that were cured within days if treatment was started immediately, or within months if paralysis had already progressed. Neveu also found magnesium chloride effective with asthma, bronchitis, pneumonia and emphysema, and several other health problems.

In more recent years, Dr. Raul Vergini and others have confirmed these earlier results and have added more diseases to the list of successful uses: acute asthma attacks, shock, tetanus, herpes zoster, and several more including beneficial effects in cancer therapy. In all of these cases, magnesium chloride had been used and gave much better results than did other magnesium compounds.

A healthy cell has high magnesium and low calcium levels. Up to 30% of the energy of cells is used to pump calcium out of the cells. The higher the calcium level and the lower the magnesium level in the extra-cellular fluid, the harder is it for cells to pump the calcium out. The result is that with low magnesium levels the mitochondria (a cell's energy source) gradually calcify and energy production decreases. It may be fair to say that our biochemical age is determined by the ratio of magnesium to calcium within our cells.

Those with low blood pressure and a tendency towards inflammation should also greatly reduce their intake of phosphorus and high-phosphorus foods. Sodas are perhaps the highest source of phosphorus in the American diet. A high level of phosphorus in the blood tends to cause magnesium and calcium levels to be low. This is the insight that enabled Percy Weston to develop his mix of alkalizing powders to combat cancer supposedly caused by the high levels of phosphorus in the food chain from the overuse of superphosphate fertilizer (See **Percy's Powder**).

Finally, Indian scientists demonstrated how breast tumor incidence in rats could be reduced from 100% to between 46-57% by single applications of magnesium chloride, selenium, Vitamin C or Vitamin A. In combinations of two, tumor incidences were further reduced to between 25.9-31.8%. When all four nutrients were given, tumor incidence was reduced by 88% -- all the way down to only 12%.

Hydrated magnesium chloride contains about 120 mg of magnesium per gram or 600 mg per rounded teaspoon. It has a mild laxative effect. As a good maintenance intake to remain healthy, it is suggested to take a teaspoon daily in divided doses with meals. It may be used instead of table salt, as it has a somewhat salty taste.

Caution: Magnesium supplementation should be avoided with severe kidney problems (severe renal insufficiency), and with myasthenia gravis. Patients with severe adrenal weakness or with very low blood pressure are advised to take care. Too much magnesium can cause muscle weakness. If this happens it is often advised to temporarily use more calcium.


*Further Reading & References*

- *Supplement to The Art of Getting Well: Magnesium Chloride HexahydrateTherapy*, Pierre Delbet, M.D., A. Neveu, M.D., Raul Vergini, M.D. Responsible editor/writer Anthony di Fabio.

- Ramesha A et al. Chemoprevention of 7, 12-dimethylbenz[a]anthracene- induced mammary carcinogenesis in rat by the combined actions of selenium, magnesium, ascorbic acid and retinyl acetate. Jpn J Cancer Res; 81(12): 1239-46. 1990.

- *The Cure For All Advanced Cancers* by Hulda Regehr Clark (1999)

# Molybdenum

Molybdenum is necessary for the metabolism of dietary fats. It has been used in many forms of arthritis with success. It is necessary for the formation of tooth enamel and hence helps prevent tooth decay. It is needed for the following enzymes xanthine oxidase, aldehyde oxidase, nitrate reductase and sulphite oxidase.

The average human body contains about 9,000 mg (nine grams) of Molybdenum. Molybdenum is an antioxidant and is important in the defense against cancer and carcinogens. It has a defense role within the gastrointestinal tract by detoxifying compounds that cause cancer. Molybdenum is important for kidney function and helps excrete heavy metals like mercury.

Molybdenum is often found with iron in relation to energy cycles. The brain and nervous system rely on molybdenum to stay in balance. This is why molybdenum deficiency can cause anxiety and irritability.

Molybdenum helps aldehyde oxidase break down formaldehyde and many other aldehydes which we absorb from the clothes we wear, furniture we own, chipboard, carpets, glues, perfumes, etc. These are inhaled and need to be eliminated, but aldehydes can also be produced internally by bacteria, parasites, fungi, yeast, etc.

The most important function of molybdenum appears to be to keep copper in check. When copper becomes too plentiful, it ceases to be a nutrient and starts becoming a toxin. Molybdenum appears to moderate excess copper.

Molybdenum has been shown to prevent breast and gastrointestinal cancers and to protect the body from the carcinogenic effects of dietary nitrosamines. Some studies conducted in Japan and China have linked low levels of molybdenum with an increased risk of stomach and esophageal cancers.

In animal studies, molybdenum has had an inhibitory effect on the appearance of breast cancers. A derivative of molybdenum, has been observed to achieve a "100% tumor inhibition until day 30."

Molybdenum deficiency is said to be virtually nonexistent in the U.S. and is usually seen only in people who have been on prolonged tube or intravenous feeding or have a genetic inability to metabolize molybdenum. Symptoms of deficiency include rapid heartbeat and breathing, headaches, night blindness, anemia, mental disturbances, nausea and vomiting.

The recommended daily allowance (RDA) of molybdenum for adults is 75 - 250 mcg per day. It's unlikely the average person needs to supplement with higher doses. According to some authorities, additional molybdenum is advisable with cancer of the throat and esophagus.

Tetrathiomolybdate, a molybdenum compound which antagonizes copper, is now in clinical trial to determine if copper depletion therapy via molybdenum is a viable approach for the treatment of cancer.

"A new anticopper drug, tetrathiomolybdate (TM), developed for Wilson's disease, is a very promising antiangiogenic agent. Copper levels lowered into an antiangiogenic window by TM have shown efficacy against cancer in a variety of animal models as well as in patients. The only significant toxicity so far results from overtreatment and excessive bone marrow depletion of copper. The resulting anemia and/ or leukopenia is easily treatable by dose reduction or drug holiday. The underlying concept for TM efficacy as an anticancer agent is that when the body's copper status is in the window, cellular copper needs are met and toxicity is avoided. Copper status is relatively easily monitored by following serum ceruloplasmin, a copper-containing protein secreted by the liver at a rate dependent upon the amount of copper in the liver available to incorporate into the protein. The authors speculate that the copper level is a primitive angiogenesis and growth-signaling regulator that has been retained throughout evolution."

*Further Reading & References*

- "Cancer therapy with tetrathiomolybdate: antiangiogenesis by lowering body copper--a review. Brewer GJ, Merajver SD." http://www.ncbi.nlm.nih.gov/entrez/query.fcgi?cmd=Retrieve&db=pubmed&dopt=Abstract&list_uids=14664727

- Kopf-Maier P, Leitner M, Voigtlander R, Kopf H. "Molybdocene dichloride as an antitumor agent." http://www.ncbi.nlm.nih.gov/entrez/query.fcgi?cmd=Retrieve&db=PubMed&list_uids=161840&dopt=Abstract

# Selenium/Selenomax

There are many studies of large human populations that demonstrate the powerful anticancer benefits of this important essential trace mineral. Selenium is considered a non-accumulating trace nutrient

Dr. E. J. Crary of Smyrna, Georgia, stated that "Selenium is the most potent broad-spectrum anticarcinogenic agent that has yet been discovered." The scientific and medical literature is filled with studies that demonstrate selenium's anticancer effects in humans. A review published in 1986 reported that at least fifty-five published studies confirm selenium's cancer-protective effect. The epidemiologic studies showed that low blood levels of selenium correlate with increased incidence of almost all kinds of cancer.

In an epidemiological study, Dr. Raymond Shamberger demonstrated an inverse association between selenium availability and age-adjusted mortality for all types of cancer after categorizing the states and cities in the United States according to selenium availability in the diet (classified as low, medium, and high). He concluded that the more selenium an area had available, the lower the levels of cancer in that area.

Dr. Gerhard Schrauzer of the University of California in San Diego studied, circa late 1970s, the relationship between selenium and breast cancer induced in female mice. With trace amounts of selenium added to their diets, over a 70% reduction in breast cancer was realized. Dr. Schrauzer went on to say that if women would take 200-300 mcg of selenium daily, the majority of breast cancers could be eliminated within a relatively short period of time.

In a worldwide study, Dr. Schrauzer analyzed the blood-bank data from seventeen countries around the world. He reported that areas with low levels of selenium in the diet had higher levels of leukemia and cancers of the breast, colon, rectum, prostate, ovary, and lung. For example, he found that the blood levels of selenium in Japan, Taiwan, Thailand, the Philippines, Puerto Rico, and Costa Rica were over three times as high as samples from the United States and European countries. The corresponding breast cancer mortality rates in Europe and the U.S. were from two to five times greater than in Asian and Latin American countries with higher selenium levels in the soil.

In another study with mice, Dr. Schrauzer was able to show that for maximum protective effect, selenium supplementation must be introduced as early in life as possible. This is because malignant transformation may occur even at a very young age, and selenium exerts its protective effects only prior to this event. This study also showed that dietary selenium prevents and impedes tumor development only as long as it is supplied in adequate amounts.

The same study showed a rapid increase in tumors if selenium supplementation ceased in mid-life. Dr. Schrauzer's conclusion was that selenium supplementation was most effective when maintained throughout the entire life span.

In another important study, selenium's anticarcinogenic activity was demonstrated during both the initiation and the promotion phases of carcinogenesis. In addition, the same research demonstrated that supplementary selenium impedes the reappearance of tumors in animals whose tumors had regressed following ovariectomy. The study's authors state, "The data suggest that selenium is not only effective in prevention but can also be used as an adjuvant chemotherapeutic agent."

A case control study conducted in Finland by J.T. Salonen et al. (published in the *American Journal of Epidemiology* in 1984) followed a random sample of over 8,100 people for six years. At the conclusion of the study, low serum levels of selenium appeared to correlate with increased total cancer mortality. The risk of low selenium was greatest in individuals who were also low in plasma levels of vitamins A and E. This finding suggests that other factors influence the anticarcinogenic effects of selenium.

Cancer mortality rates throughout the United States, following a county-by-county analysis, confirmed a significant inverse association between selenium availability and total cancer mortality in both men and women, i.e. the higher the naturally-occurring selenium level in a county, the lower the cancer death rate. In a study of skin cancers, lower plasma selenium levels were associated with higher levels of basal cell and squamous cell carcinoma.

Dr. Robert C. Donaldson, an oncologist at the Veterans Administration Hospital in Saint Louis, Missouri found that his cancer patients had very low blood selenium levels, which agreed with the scientific literature linking low levels of selenium with increased rates of cancer. Deciding to study this problem, he enlisted the help of Nutrition 21, a company that produces standardized organically bound high-selenium yeast. Nutrition 21 agreed to supply him with selenium-rich yeast for his cancer patients.

Dr. Donaldson discovered that in most of his patients, normal doses of selenium did not produce much of an increase in the blood levels of selenium. In fact, very high oral doses of selenium were required to bring up the blood levels of selenium in his cancer patients. In a letter to *Nutrition* dated May 11, 1979, he indicated:

"We are now able, with nearly 100% regularity, to increase the blood levels by several fold by giving 1,000 to 2,000 micrograms of selenium daily and then dropping back to a maintenance dose."

In one case, a dosage level of 2,700 mcg/day for two months followed by six weeks of 5,000 mcg/day was required to bring up the patient's selenium blood levels. Take note that the doses used by Dr. Donaldson were potentially toxic as selenium is a trace mineral, i.e. selenium is found in tiny amounts in a healthy individual. Dosages from 2,700 mcg to 5,000 mcg per day could produce symptoms of selenium toxicity in a normal person.

Dr. Donaldson also found that many cancer patients apparently don't absorb selenium well. Potentially toxic levels of oral selenium had to be administered in order to achieve normal blood selenium levels. When normal blood selenium levels were reached, Dr. Donaldson documented marked improvement in his patients and, in some cases, remission of advanced cancers.

Some patients with relatively low levels of selenium (.223 parts per million or ppm) experienced dramatic tumor regressions when supplemental selenium raised their blood levels to normal. For other patients, tumor regression was not evident until the levels reached .40 ppm to .50 ppm, while still others required reaching blood levels of .80 ppm.

An additional benefit of selenium is that it can counteract the effects of cadmium in the human prostate. Cadmium is believed to play a major role in the increase in prostate cancer incidence in men exposed to high levels. Selenium has been shown to inhibit the growth stimulation induced by cadmium.

A study in China reported that a daily dose of 500 mcg of selenium over a period of several years is safe for healthy humans. Dr. Schrauzer reports that dosages of 2,000 to 5,000 mcg per day will produce toxicity symptoms after several months. However, since the early symptoms of selenium toxicity such as nausea, weakness, and discoloration of the fingernails are obvious, high doses have apparently not been reported to have caused any fatalities.

According to animal studies, selenium-enriched onions, broccoli, garlic, and Brazil nuts are particularly effective in the inhibition of tumors. A fresh, unshelled Brazil nut contains about 80 mcg of selenium. This level supposedly declines to 20 mcg in shelled nuts that have been exposed to air. Selenium supplements, many derived from selenium-enriched yeast, are commercially available. In the yeast-derived products, the selenium is present in an organic form. Supplements with inorganic selenium have been introduced commercially, but the experimental data indicate that inorganic forms of selenium are less effective than organic ones.

Some advocates recommend between 300 and 400 mcg of organic selenium orally each day for cancer patients, but this dosage should be combined with regular laboratory assessment of blood selenium levels to prevent toxicity when selenium is used to treat cancer. 200 mcg of selenium daily is deemed completely safe.

### Further Reading & References

- *Selenium: Are You Getting Enough to Reduce Your Risk of Cancer* by Edgar Drake (2001)

- *Selenium Against Cancer and Aids* by Richard A. Passwater (1999)

- *Selenium and Cancer: Larry C. Clark Memorial Issue* by Leonard A. Cohen (2010)

- "Alternatives In Cancer Therapy" by Ross, R.Ph. Pelton, Lee Overholser, http://curezone.com/diseases/cancer/selenium.asp

- Nutrition classics. *Journal of the National Cancer Institute*, April 1970, Vol. 44, No. 4: Relationship of selenium to cancer.

- Inhibitory effect of selenium on carcinogenesis. By 4. Raymond J. Shamberger. Nutr Rev. 1985 Nov;43(11):342-4. No abstract available. PMID: 3935987 [PubMed - indexed for MEDLINE]

# Tellurium/AS-101

Tellurium is a chemical element that looks very much like tin. It is a brittle, mildly toxic, silvery metalloid. Some consider it useful against cancer.

AS-101 is a synthetic organic tellurium compound that boosts the immune system by increasing cytokine production.

### Further Reading & References

- Cancer Therapy by Ralph W. Moss, PhD (20050

- "Use Of Tellurium Compounds For Treatment Of Basal Cell Carcinoma And/Or Actinic Keratosis." http://www.freepatentsonline.com/y2010/0150869.html

# Vanadium

Vanadium is a soft, gray ductile transition metal that occurs naturally in about 65 different minerals and fossil fuel.

The minerals vanadium and sulfur were used to create 24 new drugs to combat cancer in a study done at the Parker Hughes Institute. The same study found vanadium could destroy 14 different cancer cell lines. This was true both in the laboratory and for human cell lines.

It appears vanadium compounds have preventive effects against chemical carcinogenesis. Further study is needed.

### Further Reading & References

- "Vanadium in cancer treatment." http://www.ncbi.nlm.nih.gov/pubmed/12050018

# Zinc

Zinc can both enhance and retard tumor growth. In epidemiological studies, the National Academy of Sciences report described a study in England and Wales where gastric cancer was higher in people whose gardens had high zinc levels in the soil. Schrauzer and his colleagues examined food intake in 27 countries and reported a direct correlation between higher zinc intake and a higher incidence of leukemia and cancers of the intestine, breast, prostate, and skin.

They concluded that zinc increases cancer risk by its known antagonism to selenium (that is, an excess of zinc can cause a deficiency of selenium). Schrauzer also found that high zinc in blood samples collected from healthy donors across the United States correlated directly with mortality rates from large bowel, breast, ovary, lung, bladder, and oral cancer in the different areas where the blood was collected. Zinc and selenium levels in the blood were inversely related. On the other hand, two studies of esophageal cancer found zinc levels to be lower in the diet of countries where that cancer is common and lower in the blood of patients with esophageal cancer than in normal controls. Clearly, in the latter studies, "the altered zinc levels may have followed, rather than preceded, the onset of cancer."

The experimental evidence collected in the National Academy of Sciences report supports the epidemiological evidence, showing both the enhancing and retarding effects of zinc on tumor growth.

Zinc deficiency appears to retard the growth of transplanted tumors, whereas it enhances the incidence of some chemically induced cancers. In some experiments, dietary zinc exceeding nutritional requirements has been shown to suppress chemically induced tumors in rats and hamsters, but when given in drinking water it counteracts the protective effect of selenium in mice. These data are insufficient to explain the effects of zinc and of interactions between zinc and other minerals on tumorigenesis.

Zinc has become a popular supplement especially for the treatment of enlarged or infected prostates; however, a study from the National Cancer Institute shows that taking more than 100 mg of zinc supplements a day doubles a man's chances of developing advanced prostate cancer. The safe dose for healthy individuals is generally thought to be 30 to 50 mg per day.

A deficiency of zinc can lead to depressed activity of NK cells and other white blood cells.

Using high amounts of zinc reportedly causes a deficiency of copper and thereby prevents the formation of new blood vessels, (angiogenesis) and stops tumor growth, especially if the zinc therapy is combined with shark or bovine cartilage therapy and a protocol aimed at alkalizing the body.

### Further Reading & References

- Boik J. Cancer & Natural Medicine: *A Textbook of Basic Science and Clinical Research.* Princeton, Minn: Oregon Medical Press; 1996: 28, 29, 76, 182, 183, 251.

- Linus Pauling Institute: Zinc and Prostate Cancer, http://lpi.oregonstate.edu/ss05/zinc.html

- "Zinc in Cancer Prevention." http://www.springerlink.com/content/l244170308126307/

# Treatment Programs

## 714-X/Gaston Naessens/Immunostim

714-X is a chemical compound that contains camphor, a natural substance that comes from the wood and bark of the camphor tree. Nitrogen, water, and salts are added to camphor to make 714-X. It was developed in the 1960s in Canada, based on the theory that there are somatids in the blood, which are tiny living things. The number of somatids a person has in his or her blood indicates whether cancer has the likelihood of forming. Mainstream science has not accepted the existence of somatids.

In the blood of healthy people, the somatid cycle has but three phases after their formation in the red blood cells: somatid, spore, and double-spore.

But in people who have cancer or other degenerative diseases, the somatid unfolds 13 additional phases, for a total of 16 phases of the complete macrocycle. That is why the existence of any of phases 4 to 16 in the blood is a sign of a weakened natural defense system. In its additional phases, the somatid morphs into different types of bacteria, yeasts, and other microorganisms, according to Naessens. For this reason, advocates of the theory dub the somatid a pleomorph or "shape-changing" organism that actually changes its fundamental nature during its life cycle.

Naessens considers the elucidation of this cycle one of the high points of his long career. Over the years, others have also seen phases of this cycle including ten scientists who wrote about them between 1840 and 1900. Since 1900 and the present, over 50 scientists have observe and written about these particles.

Most related scientific writings address the bacterial phase. Researchers believed they were working with an externally generated "cancer microbe." Naessens, however, claimed to have defined a sequence of changes of the pleomorphism – the changes from one type of organism to another -- of a microbe normally resident in the human body. At the different stages of the cycle, the form of the somatids may resemble bacteria, yeasts, or fungi.

This means it could be possible to track and monitor cancer by observing the number and forms of somatids in the blood. If the somatids are exposed to a type of trauma such as pollution or radiation, they enter an uncontrolled growth cycle that leads to cancer. Naessens theorized that cancer cells are deficient in nitrogen, and that injecting 714-X into the lymph system would cause them to convert to normal cells.

Advocates claim the 714-X treatment returns the somatids to a normal state, thereby inhibiting and slowing down the growth of cancer. 714-X has been used by thousands of patients and hundreds of doctors across Canada, the United States and Europe. In spite of this demand, 714-X is only legally available in Canada for patients who are considered to be in the terminal stages of a degenerative disease.

Naessens's ideas are so far-reaching that since the early 1960s, Naessens was pursued with fury by medical authorities. Is 714-X just a worthless nostrum, with possibly dangerous side effects? Or is it an ingeniously designed and unique product, which has the ability to stabilize or even reverse symptoms in people with cancer, AIDS, and other chronic illnesses?

Clearly a great deal is at stake. If true, Naessens's ideas could yield an entirely revolutionary way of viewing the origin of cancer and other chronic illnesses. His pleomorph theory has gained considerable acceptance among advocates of alternative cancer treatments, even those who don't view 714-X as a first-line treatment. It has to be said that most advocates of the pleomorph theory are self-taught cancer experts rather than those who have received medical training.

As he developed 714-X, Dr. Naessens selected camphor as a carrier because he believes it has special affinity for cancer cells. He included ammonium salts because he believed they improve the circulation of lymph in cancer patients. He also believed that the ammonium salts activate certain kinins that inhibit abnormal cell growth and enhance the healthy functioning of the immune system.

Dr. Naessens discovered that tumor cells produce a substance, cocancerogenic K factor, that paralyzes the immune system. 714-X seems to neutralize CKF, thereby enabling the immune system to more readily identify and destroy cancer cells.

714-X acts to strengthen, or unblock, the dysfunctional immune system. If a patient is seriously affected by lung or oral cancer, and is unable to take the treatment orally, it can be administered through the nose using a nebulizer. The nasal route has been recommended for patients with lung or oral cancers. Advocates claim a long-term remission rate of 75% for 714-X.

The Cancer Cure Foundation states, "714-X is a homeopathic combination of ammonium compounds, camphor, phosphors and salts of silicate. A similar product is Immunostim. Recently NCI has agreed to study 714-X."

CERBE Distribution Inc. is the private company in charge of the popularization of the scientific knowledge brought by Gaston Naessens' Somatidian Orthobiology. See http://www.cerbe.com/

- Further information on the NCI review of 714-X is at http://www.cancer.gov/cam/attachments/714-X_follow.pdf and http://www.annieappleseedproject.org/drugdevgroup.html

CERBE Distribution Inc. describes its product and recommended protocol below:

"It is important to be aware that our product does not require any special monitoring. Our clients remain under their attending physician's care, using conventional tests to monitor their health, as they would if not using 714-X.

"In most cases of autoimmune or degenerative diseases, we recommend using 714-X by injection only, basic treatment. When there is cancer in the right breast, the lungs, the esophagus, or anywhere else in the head, we recommend adding a second use of our product from the second 21 days cycle on. We appreciate receiving a complete description of the diagnosis (when it was given, where the disease is located in the body, the treatments to date (conventional and/or alternative), name of the person who will be using our product, date of birth...) in order to recommend the proper protocol.

"Here is the protocol we recommend when there is cancer in the right upper quadrant of one's body (including left lung, joined organs...): one would do a first 21 day cycle using only the injection, basic treatment, and take the mandatory 2 day break. From Day 1 of the second cycle and all following cycles, one would do the injection in the morning and 12 hours later would also breathe the product in using a nebulizer. One would use both methods daily, always taking a 2 day break between cycles.

"We recommend using 714-X for a minimum of 6 to 8 cycles. Once the minimum number of cycles is completed, we recommend to keep on using it until conventional tests show there is no sign of disease.

"One learns to do the injection by watching a video, "714-X: How does it work?" We also send written instructions and are here to coach, if needed. We use a 26G 3/8" 1cc (0,45mm x 10 mm, 1ml) Tuberculin syringe. We can provide them ($10US/tray of 25), if unable to purchase them locally.

"We recommend avoiding these products while using 714-X: vitamins E & B12, supplementally. In a regular diet they do not cause any problem. Flaxseed oil, bee pollen and royal jelly can be used as sources for those vitamins while using 714-X. We also recommend avoiding all antiangiogenic products (shrinking blood vessels, cutting off the blood supply) such as shark or bovine cartilage, thalidomide, certain chemos or others. When one is currently receiving or considering receiving chemo, please check how that particular chemo kills cancerous cells. If it does so by cutting off the blood supply, by shrinking blood vessels, it is antiangiogenic and 714-X cannot be used at the same time as such products. It would be asking one's body to do two opposing actions at the same time. Once antiangiogenic treatments are over, we recommend waiting for at least a week, preferably two, before starting on 714-X.

"An important fact to understand about our product is: to 714-X all diseases, as long as autoimmune or degenerative, are the same: an imbalance our product will assist the body in correcting by revitalizing the immune system, by supporting the body's natural defenses thus enabling the body to fight back at disease. 714-X does not work directly on diseased cells, does not work on a specific disease but works on an imbalance. The theory behind the product says that when an immune system is balanced, we stay healthy: our immune system recognizes foreign cells and eliminates them.

"The goal of 714-X is to get the immune system back on track (it is an immunomodulator; if an immune system is overworking, it brings it back to balance, if not working, 714-X will stimulate it into working again); in doing so it enables the body to fight back at disease...The least benefit one would obtain by using our product is by enjoying a better quality of life.....It is difficult to predict how much cleansing and repairing will go on in one's body ...Many factors are involved in the process: treatments, of course, conventional and/or alternative, but one's willingness to make lifestyle adjustments such as diet corrections, stress management, environment (emotional, physical), core beliefs, ...many factors will influence the pace at which one's body will cleanse and repair itself.

"Possible side effects are flu like symptoms: slight fever, nausea, aching muscles, tiredness....they usually subside within a few days. Our product is nontoxic. It cannot hurt nor harm in any way. The results vary from one person to the other, depending on many factors such as diet, stress management, environment (physical, emotional, etc...), core beliefs... all those factors and many others will influence the pace at which one will cleanse and repair one's body.

"714-X is designed to improve natural defenses, and to stimulate the immune system. The 714-X product does not necessarily eliminate abnormal cells. 714-X has been integrated in the Canadian Emergency Drug Program since January 1990 (Now called Special Access Program). 714-X has therefore been applied for various degenerative diseases, with some interesting results; unfortunately, in Canada, access to the program is only for advanced terminal cases. . .

"We can summarize the action of 714-X by saying that first 714-X activates deep cellular cleansing, and then it stimulates cellular repair mostly for damaged cells caused either by disease and/or some conventional treatments.

"714-X has a unique mode of intromission. It has to be injected in the lymphatic system according to a specific protocol (injection technique available on videocassette). The reason for this special and unusual route is simple; patients with degenerative disease have lymph fluid which is clogged up, inducing stagnation and promoting intoxication. 714-X liquefies the lymph system allowing the toxins to be removed from the body."

### Further Reading & References

- *The Galileo of the Microscope* concerning the trial of Gaston Naessens was written in 1991 by Christopher Bird

- Videotape: *Introduction to the Somatidian Orthobiology* - 1998 (91 min). Including: *Basics of Gaston*

*Naessens' Biological Theory*, Interview with Jacinte Levesque-Naessens and a host.

- Bird C. Gaston Naessens vs. scientific medicine. *Townsend Letter for Doctors* 1991 May; 94:313-320.

- Diamond WJ, et al. *An alternative medicine definitive guide to cancer.* Tiburon: Future Medicine Publishing, Inc., 1997:32,871.

- Kaegi E, on behalf of the *Task Force on Alternative Therapies of the Canadian Breast Cancer Research Initiative.* Unconventional therapies to cancer: 6. 714-X. Canadian Medical Association 1998;158:1621-1624.

- 714-X. BC Cancer Agency Cancer Information Centre. (BCCA Cancer Information Centre search file 2400)

- 714-X Alternative Cancer Treatment Comparison, http://alternativecancer.us/714-X.htm

- National Cancer Institute: Questions and Answers About 714-X, http://www.cancer.gov/cancertopics/pdq/cam/714-X/Patient/page2

# 21 Day Curing Program

The 21 Day Curing Program is described in the book *The Cure for All Advanced Cancers* by Hulda Clark, Ph.D., N.D.

The book description reads: "Cancer can now be cured, not only the early stages, but also advanced cancer, stages four and five, including imminent death. We are not accustomed to thinking about a cure. We think of remission as the only possibility. But this book is not about remission. It is about a cure … The Cause of the malignancy is explained in the earlier book, *The Cure For All Cancers.* But removing the malignancy left behind the tumors as they were, prior to the malignant development. So, eliminating tumors became the focus of additional research, and is the subject of this book.

"The success rate for advanced cancer is about 95% … It is a total approach that not only shrinks tumors, but also normalizes your blood chemistry, lowers your cancer markers, and returns your health. The small failure rate (5%) is due to clinical emergencies that beset the advanced cancer sufferer. However, if you combine the advice in this book with access to hospital care, even "hopeless" patients can gain the time necessary to become well again."

Dr. Clark's 21 Day Program for Advanced Cancers was introduced for severely ill patients in cancer stage 4, the most advanced stage of cancer, often implying imminent death. Dr. Clark identifies three tasks:

- Kill clostridium bacteria. (Clostridium is a tumor-making strain of bacteria, which supplies the DNA, the toxic amines and also isopropyl alcohol which will eventually contribute to malignancy).

- Kill all other parasites.

- Remove metals, malonic acid (which comes from some common foods, tapeworm larvae and plastic teeth), and other carcinogens from the body.

Dr. Clark's organization is reported to have been built from the grassroots up by her former patients, and relatives of patients. They have seen that her therapy works; many are alive today because of her.

Information on the Dr. Clark Research Association can be found on the web-site http://www.drclark.net

As Cathy Kopasek, Manager, New Century Press stated, "95% success rate! So you can count on this method, not merely hope it will work for you."

Videos are also available describing the 21 day program:

- *The Cure* is the most popular video documentary about the research of Hulda Clark, Ph.D., N.D. The video features testimonials from prominent figures from around the world, including an interview with the physician to Pope John Paul II, who claims to have successfully applied the Hulda Clark programs. The video has an interview with Dr. Clark, and goes over the herbal cleanses, liver cleanse, zapping protocol, and dental clean-up.

- The video, *Cure Yourself*, is much more technical than the video *The Cure*. *Cure Yourself* goes into detail on the 21 day program and would be suitable for health providers who are interested in the technical and medical information underpinning Dr. Clark's 21 day program.

Hulda Clark's videos can be accessed at http://www.drclarkbooks.com/.

Thousands of testimonials exist acclaiming her methods and the success people have achieved through using them. A booklet of a thousand testimonials is available for $10 from the Dr. Clark Information Center, located at http://www.drclark.net/.

See **Dr. Hulda Clark/ Dr. Clark's Treatment**.

### Further Reading & References

- *The Cure for All Diseases* by Hulda Regehr Clark (1995)

- *The Cure For All Advanced Cancers* by Hulda Regehr Clark (1999)

- *The Cure for All Cancers: Including over 100 Case Histories of Persons Cured* by Hulda Regehr Clark (1993)

- *The Cure and Prevention of all Cancers* by Hulda Regehr Clark (2008)

- *The Cure For HIV / AIDS* by Hulda Regehr Clark (2002)

- *Syncrometer Science Laboratory Manual* by Hulda Regehr Clark (2000)

- University of Washington study shows the Dr. Clark zapper inhibits the growth of leukemia cells

- Dr. Clark Information Center, http://www.drclark.net/news/lairesearch.htm

# Controlled Amino Acid Treatment (CAAT)

Angelo P. John, a cancer theorist for more than 40 years, developed an extremely interesting and promising nutritional approach to help cancer patients. CAAT - Controlled Amino Acid Treatment -- is a novel approach to cancer treatment. The treatment has been used since 1994 in very advanced-cancer patients combined with or without conventional treatment of radiation and/or chemotherapy. Angelo

John develops these nutritional programs for cancer patients with the cooperation of the patient's oncologist or with nutritionally oriented complementary and alternative physicians who work with cancer patients.

CAAT is an amino acid and carbohydrate deprivation protocol that uses scientifically formulated amino acids. Based on the fact that the needs of normal cells and cancer cells are quite different, the diet of the cancer patient is manipulated to include a blend of amino acids (protein building blocks in the body). Cancer cells are literally starved to death.

The program consists of:

- A strict diet

- A special amino acid blend — the exact blend depends to some extent on the type of cancer being treated

- Certain nutritional supplements, and the avoidance of others


The treatment attacks cancer cells in four ways:

- Helps to prevent new blood vessel formation (angiogenesis), which is necessary for the growth of solid cancers.

- Interferes with the cancer cell's ability to produce energy by blocking a process called glycolysis in cancer cells.

- Reduces the ability of the body to produce factors that stimulate growth of cancers.

- Interferes with the production of specific amino acids that are necessary for DNA replication in cancer cells.


The diet is quite strict and is low in both carbohydrates and protein. Fat intake is moderate and involves specific fats. The amino acid blend reduces certain amino acids (such as glycine, valine, leucine, and isoleucine) and increases others, resulting in reduced production of the protein elastin, which is necessary for angiogenesis.

In contrast to normal cells, which produce energy primarily through the use of oxygen, cancer cells produce energy by a process known as glycolysis because their mitochondria (energy producing structures in cells that utilize oxygen) are damaged and not capable of utilizing oxygen the way normal cells do. The theory is that the strict diet and the blend of amino acids attack the glycolysis process in cancer cells, thus helping to prevent the production of energy in cancer cells.

Certain growth factors produced in the body, such as human growth hormone and insulin growth factor 1 (IGF1) tend to stimulate cancer growth. This program with its reduced calorie and protein diet tends to reduce the production of these growth factors. The growth of cancer cells requires certain amino acids (like glycine) and nutrients (like vitamin B6) for replication of the cancer cells' DNA. The reduction of these nutrients in this CAAT protocol helps to inhibit DNA replication in cancer cells.

A number of nutritional supplements are part of the program. These may include, but are not limited to:

- Vitamins A, C and D

- D-Limonene

- N-Acetylcysteine (NAC)

- Grape Seed Extract

- Lycopene and others

On the other hand, most of the B vitamins, especially vitamin B6, are avoided because they enhance the glycolysis process or DNA replication.

Regardless of the cancer type, all cancer cells survive through the same biochemical processes. CAAT interferes with these processes and causes the cancer cells to die, significantly increasing the patients' chance of recovery. However, because each patient is unique, CAAT is designed for one's specific needs, taking into account the patient profile and medical history. A personalized amino acid deprivation formula and food plan is designed for each patient's individual requirements.

### Further Reading & References

- *Controlled Amino Acid Treatment (CAAT)-A Novel Nutritional Approach to Cancer Treatment* by Michael B. Schachter, MD, CNS, FACAM

- A.P. John Institute for Cancer Research http://www.apjohncancerinstitute.org/

## Cancell/Cantron/Entelev/Entele/Protocel/Protoc/Sheridan's formula/Jim's Juice/Crocinic Acid/JS-114/ JS-101/126-F

Cancell is a nontoxic treatment for cancer developed in the 1930's by Jim Sheridan, an analytical chemist for the Dow Chemical Company. It is now more commonly known by the name Protocel. There is a great deal of mystery surrounding Cancell. Apparently the idea for this drug came to Sheridan in a dream on an afternoon in September, 1936. He saw a multilayered rainbow made up of the various respiratory enzymes of the oxidation-reduction ('redox') system. The dream suggested to the young chemist a cure for cancer.

Cancell is described by advocates as an assembly of synthetic chemicals that react with the body electrically rather than chemically. Sheridan says cancer is a protein disease and that there are three types of cells: normal, primitive, and cancerous. He stated that Cancell causes cancer cells to become primitive and to self-destruct.

Advocates claim that human and animal studies proving Cancell's worth have been done, but are being suppressed by the establishment. The FDA conducted a secret study that resulted in 80-85% cure rates, but the FDA denies that any such study was ever conducted. Unlike many such stories, convincing evidence exists that the study indeed took place.

In Sheridan's view, the cancer cell exists at a "critical point" between a truly primitive cell (like yeast) and a normal human cell. The goal of Cancell is to push the cancer cell into the primitive state. "Cancell tries to take away the last vestiges of normality" from cancer cells, Sheridan said, "So, they are no longer on the boundary line." He added, "Once the cancer cell is definitely into the primitive stage, the body deals with it as the body does any other foreign object. It gets rid of it."

Cancell contains a chemical that can inhibit respiration. Sheridan claims that by 1942, he was already getting between 70 and 80% anti-tumor responses in mice. In 1953, just as human clinical tests were about to begin, representatives of the American Cancer Society blocked them. Around this time, Sheridan began giving Cancell away to patients who asked for it.

In the 1980s, Sheridan met foundry owner Ed Sopcak who took up where he left off, giving 20,000 bottles of Cancell away, even paying for the postage. All of it was made in their homes. Sopcak advised patients to go off all other medications before taking Cancell or at least not to take megadoses of vitamins C and E while on this medication. Clinical results can take up to 3 months. Cancell "does not actually kill the cancer cell in the usual meaning of the word kill" Sheridan stated. In 1989, the FDA obtained a permanent injunction against the distribution of Cancell in interstate commerce.

By 1990, the NCI finally agreed to test Sheridan's formula with its stringent laboratory procedures, using a variety of cancer cell lines in Petri dishes ("in vitro"). The results were impressive and showed that the formula worked on all cancer cell lines tested. These cancer cell lines included leukemia, non-small cell lung cancer, small cell lung cancer, colon cancer, central nervous system cancer, melanoma, ovarian cancer, and renal cell (kidney) cancer. (People who have used it have reportedly found it to work on virtually every other type of cancer as well.)

The mystique and lack of transparency as to its contents helped the FDA to discredit Cancell, though thousands of people have used it. The only evidence Sheridan and Sopcak were able to offer was a file of letters testifying that Cancell works.

Between the 1930s and the early 1950s, Sheridan developed another product called Entelev as a treatment for cancer. There is a long history of how the ACS, FDA, and NIH reportedly tried to destroy this product, too. Currently, the original Entelev formula is held by two different companies. The products of these two companies are Protocel and Cantron. There are testimonials on the Internet for each of these products. Nevertheless, "Today, the Sheridan family endorses Protocel as THE Cancell formula."

"According to a 1989 FDA evaluation, Cancell [now called Protocel and Cantron] consists of nitric acid, sodium sulfite, potassium hydroxide, sulfuric acid, inositol, and catechol."

Here is another description of its formulation:

"Cantron is a unique nutritional formulation containing vitamins, minerals and a proprietary blend of organic compounds:

- Vitamins: trace amounts of the B vitamin Inositol.

- Minerals: Copper, Sodium, and Potassium.

- Proprietary blend of organic compounds: Catechol (from Pyrocatechol) and the following Hydroxyquinones; Tetrahydroxyquinone, Rhodizonic Acid, Croconic Acid, Triquinol, Leuconic Acid.

"The ingredients in Cantron are used for their bioelectrical properties (not their chemical properties), for their roles in cellular respiration, and for their anti-oxidant properties."

Advocates advise that certain other treatments and supplements should not be used in conjunction with Protocel or Cantron. These include:

- Vitamin C (limited to 100 mg)

- Vitamin E (limited to 32 IU)

- Co-Q10 (limited to 60 mg)

- Selenium (limited to 60 mg)

- Essiac Tea

- Burdock Root

- Refined sugar

- Ozone, acupuncture, homeopathic, hydrogen peroxide

- 714-X

- Colloidal Silver

- Refined grain (or anything refined)

- Alcohol

Because the Protocel/Cantron patient can't use antioxidants such as vitamins C and E -- normally considered essential in other cancer therapy programs -- the patient's cancer markers should be closely monitored and the therapy abandoned within a few months if clear progress isn't being made.

### Further Reading & References

- Paul Winter's excellent site at http://www.alternativecancer.us is recommended.

- *The Cancell Controversy: Why Is A Possible Cure For Cancer Being Suppressed?* by Louise B. Trull

# CellFood

CellFood is a supplement that delivers oxygen, minerals, enzymes, and amino acids at the cellular level. It is a proprietary formulation developed by Everett Storey — who was reportedly proclaimed a 'genius' by his colleague Albert Einstein — and it has been on sale in the US since 1969. It is also available in the UK and over 40 countries worldwide.

CellFood is intended to enhance nutrient absorption and increase metabolism. Contained in this formula are "aerobic" proteins, 17 amino acids, 34 enzymes, 78 major and trace elements, deuterons, electrolytes and dissolved 'nascent' oxygen. It promotes greater availability of vitamins, minerals, herbs and other nutrients.

CellFood increases oxygen in the body at a cellular level. When CellFood is ingested, according to its advocates, vital oxygen and hydrogen are released into the body, increasing oxygen at a cellular level. Because CellFood's nutrients are in an ionic state, they are absorbed very quickly and efficiently into the body. The body uses this additional oxygen to diminish bacteria, viruses, parasites, fungi, yeast, pathogens, and free radical scavengers. In addition to supporting the body's immune system, it reportedly combats degenerative diseases and rebuilds tissue, slowing down the aging process, and even reversing it.

By oxidizing toxins and waste, the body expels them through normal channels of elimination, such as respiration, perspiration, urination and defecation.

The nutrients in CellFood are in colloidal form, meaning they are minute and negatively charged. Most body fluids (like blood and lymph) are colloidal and negatively charged. The body perceives CellFood as a normal, healthy bodily fluid and allows the nutrients in CellFood to pass immediately through the sensitive membranes of the mouth, throat, and esophagus directly into the bloodstream creating an up to 95% absorption rate.

CellFood increases cellular respiration. According to proponents, when it is mixed into water an exothermic reaction takes place, providing oxygen and hydrogen to the individual cells of the body. The steady flow of oxygen and hydrogen to all parts of the body allows for simultaneous oxygenation and reduction within the cells. CellFood users report recovering from respiratory and allergy related conditions such as asthma, sinus, and upper respiratory infections.

Increased levels of oxygen combine with the other important nutrients to enable the cells and organs to function properly, allowing the body to function at its best. By providing the body with required building blocks, CellFood strengthens the immune system, as has been shown by research at Immunosciences Laboratories in the US. This is one of the most frequently reported benefits and substantiated by research at the University of Pretoria in South Africa, which showed that athletes taking CellFood had increased vitality and better performance.

Once the energy potential in the body is increased due to the additional supply of oxygen, the natural mechanism in the body increases metabolism of waste material and eliminates toxins more effectively. The enzymes and amino acids improve metabolism so that the body can derive greater nutritional value from food and other supplements.

The increase in oxygenation of cells has been perceived valuable in combating cancer since Dr. Otto Warburg stated that cancer cannot survive in an oxygen rich environment.

### Further Reading & References

- *CellFood: Vital Cellular Nutrition for the New Millennium* by Dr. David S. Dyer (2000)

# Deuterium-Depleted Water

The deuterium depletion therapy is a completely original approach to inhibit the growth of cancer cells in the body. The core of the invention is a new therapeutic modality using deuterium-depleted water, a novel tool of sub-molecular medicine, for treatment and prevention of cancer.

Deuterium is a hydrogen isotope that plays a role in cell division. Deuterium surplus or depletion knocks out the system controlling division. Some biologists think that without deuterium, cancer cells receive some kind of shock. While healthy cells adapt very fast to the new environment, tumorous ones cannot, so they die.

"Dr. Gabor Somlyai and his colleagues at the National Institute of Oncology discovered that the alive cells can feel if the amount of hydrogen isotope changes. Plant cells stop their photosynthesis and on the contrary, they take up oxygen as they breathe. Research with mice in which human tumor was transplanted proved the same thing. While they were drinking deuterium-depleted water, the tumor became smaller or even disappeared. The mice in the control group died. Experimental data suggests that deuterium atoms modify biochemical reactions in a concentration-dependent manner."

The basic principle of the technology is the reduction of deuterium from the water and thus from all the diseased cells of the body. This procedure has been found to inhibit the growth of cancer in laboratory animals and to affect various biological processes.

It was discovered, in the early 1990s, that decreasing the deuterium concentration of the body below normal physiological levels delays the progression of several types of cancer in mice and prolongs their survival.

Depletion of body deuterium can simply be achieved by consumption or prolonged administration of deuterium depleted water and nutrients deficient in deuterium. It was therefore postulated that deuterium depletion would have therapeutic use in patients with cancer and other neoplastic diseases.

A human phase II double blind clinical trial was started in Hungary in August of 1995. The intermediate evaluation was completed in May of 1997 resulting in a 68% decrease in prostate cancer.

The proportion of patients with improving efficacy was statistically significantly greater in the treated group. The size of the prostate decreased significantly in the treated group, while in the control group it was regarded as unchanged. The patients in the treated group had more positive changes in their symptoms, along with a significantly longer survival period.

These examples provide some evidence for the anti-tumor effect of deuterium depleted water (dd-water); connections are evident, and improvement and survival rates exceed statistical values that could be attributed to "spontaneous" improvement.

In the case of tumors of the central nervous system, deuterium depleted water can play a role at least as great in the preparation for surgery as is possible later in post-treatment. With brain surgery, the doctor is often faced with the problem that although he knows that because of the tumor he should remove more tissue, this would endanger the patient's life or cause significant and permanent disability.

If the results to date can be confirmed, it might be advantageous if patients consumed deuterium depleted water 2-3 months prior to surgery. This would enable the surgeon to remove a more compact tumor isolated from its surroundings, with less damage to adjacent healthy tissue. Post-treatment with deuterium depleted water after surgery would in the optimal case destroy remaining tumor cells.

### Further Reading & References

- *Defeating Cancer: The Biological Effect of Deuterium Depletion* by Gabor Somlyai (Includes case descriptions) (2002)

# DMSO and MSM

Dimethyl sulphoxide (DMSO) is a clear, colorless, and largely odorless liquid that has demonstrated clear anti-tumor qualities. Over 6,000 articles in the scientific literature establish a solid claim for it to be recognized as an anti-cancer weapon. Veterinarians use it freely when treating cancer in animals.

DMSO is derived from lignin, the natural material that bonds together the cells of trees. It is actually a by-product of paper manufacturing, extracted during the manufacturing of pulp, and was first synthesized in 1866. As medication, DMSO was used initially in the 1960's.

Following FDA approval for experimental use, it was applied in topical form to relieve pain, reduce swelling, heal injuries such as muscle strains and sprains, and treat arthritis. It remains widely popular among laypeople for these applications.

It was accidentally discovered that DMSO acts as a catalyst for conventional chemotherapy and plays a major role in slowing down the development of cancerous tumors. When given to a patient undergoing chemotherapy, it may support a reduction in the dosage needed of the chemotherapeutic agent.

DMSO has been used by several alternative and integrative clinics to treat cancers of the bladder, ovary, breast, and skin. When administered to humans, DMSO is absorbed rapidly and produces a garlic-like taste and odor on the breath and skin that can last as long as three days. It can be given orally, by injection or by enema. Treatments usually last approximately four weeks.

DMSO stimulates various parts of the immune system and scavenges hydroxyl radicals, the most potent of free radicals. Since free radicals promote tumor growth this may be one of the mechanisms by which DMSO interferes with the development of cancer. It may also explain why patients who receive DMSO while undergoing either chemotherapy or radiation (both of which generate free radicals in order to kill cancer cells) are far less prone to such side effects as hair loss, nausea, and dry mouth.

DMSO has a wide range of biological activities because it creates very powerful bonds with water molecules. This allows it to penetrate membranes and to pass from one organ or tissue to another with great ease. It is thought to have a wider range of biochemical actions than any other known chemical agent.

A Chilean study showed that DMSO used with low doses of a chemotherapeutic drug was able to obtain remissions in 44 out of 65 cancer patients. This result was even more impressive because these patients had all previously been treated with chemotherapy without success. Twenty-six of the cases involved women with metastatic breast cancer. Twenty-three obtained remission.

There is a theory, rejected by mainstream science, that a kind of bacteria, known as dwarf bacteria, can be implicated in some cancers. It is believed that these bacteria have the ability to change their shape and size and to become as small as a virus. There is experimental support for this suggestion. Several other alternative physicians have also observed the "pleomorphism" phenomenon.

Some advocates of this theory claim that DMSO in very low concentrations has the ability to kill these bacteria, which are otherwise extremely drug resistant. DMSO, in a 12.5% solution, shows long-term inhibitory action on cancer tumors in laboratory settings.

One dramatic and very well known case of a DMSO-implicated cancer cure occurred in 1970, when the mother of 3-year old Clyde Robert Lindsey of Pasadena, Texas took her son to see Dr. Eli Tucker of Houston. Clyde had a very deadly cancer known as Letterer-Siwe disease. The cancer had spread throughout his body and orthodox doctors considered the case to be hopeless. Dr. Tucker gave the boy a dilute mixture of DMSO mixed with haematoxylon, a chemical normally used as a dye to trace the location of pathological animal cells. The haematoxylon-DMSO combination therefore had a special affinity for tumor cells.

Inside the cells, the haematoxylon oxidizes and this has the effect of inactivating the substance that surrounds the cancer cells, which then starve to death. Five drops of this substance in a glass of distilled water every morning daily eliminated all signs of Clyde's cancer.

Side effects to taking DMSO are a garlicky taste in the mouth and smelly breath, headaches, dizziness, mild nausea, localized skin rashes or a burning feeling on the skin.

DMSO is a powerful solvent that penetrates "through skin and meat all the way to the bone", and the nutritional sulfur in DMSO, Methylsulfonylmethane (MSM), is the main ingredient that allows this penetration.

This breakdown product of DMSO was discovered in 1963 by Dr. Stanley Jacobs at Oregon Health Sciences University. Studies by Dr. Jacobs show that MSM significantly slows the development of both mammary and colon tumors and may reduce pain and inflammation.

Dr. Jacobs was granted a patent for its use as a nasal spray that prevents snoring, and several other patents for health benefits. MSM allows cell walls to be more permeable and flexible so that they take in nutrients and give off toxins more easily. Along with water and salt, MSM is the most plentiful chemical compound in the body. It is absolutely essential to body growth and self-healing.

When old cells die and are replaced by new cells, the new ones will be shriveled, wrinkled, and leathery if insufficient MSM is present in the body. MSM is best aided by vitamin C in doing its work, according to advocates of this protocol.

It is thought there is widespread MSM deficiency because of our diets. The best natural sources of MSM are fresh rainwater, milk, and very fresh fruits and vegetables. MSM is the first thing to evaporate out of fruits and vegetables when they are harvested, boiled, pasteurized, or allowed to sit. MSM is reported to be non-toxic in quantities of up to 10 grams per 100 pounds of body weight.

MSM has been proven in laboratory tests to cure snoring and lupus, to relieve arthritis, and to significantly lengthen the lives of cancer victims. It has been shown to "melt away" scar tissue in burn victims, to improve breathing in emphysema victims, to strengthen hair and nails dramatically, to rejuvenate wrinkled skin, to ward off allergies and to heal bee stings. It has been used by athletes for years because it eases the pain of sore muscles. It is essential in rebuilding the body's connective tissue and collagen, a quality of obvious benefit to cancer victims.


See **Dimethyl Sulfoxide (DMSO)**.


*Further Reading & References*

- *DMSO: Nature's Healer* by Dr. Morton Walker (1993)

- *The Miracle of MSM: The Natural Solution for Pain* by Stanley W. Jacob MD, et al (1999)

- *The Persecuted Drug: The Story of DMSO* by Sr. Pat McGrady (1982)

- *DMSO: The complete up-to-date guide-book: a practical step-by-step guide providing a wealth of information to anyone interested in the use of DMSO* by David G Williams

- *DMSO: The New Healing Power* by Morton, D.P.M. Walker

- *DMSO* by Kurt W Donsbach

- *DMSO Pain Killer* by Barry Tarshis

- *DMSO: The True Story of a Remarkable Pain Killing Drug* by Barry Tarshis

- *DMSO Handbook a Complete Guide to the History and Use of DMSO* by Bruce Halstead

- *The Miracle of MSM: The Natural Solution for Pain* by Stanley W. Jacob MD, et al

- *The MSM Miracle* by Earl Mindell

- *MSM the Definitive Guide: The Nutritional Breakthrough for Arthritis, Allergies and More* by Stanley W. Jacob, Jeremy Appleton (2002)

- *Dr. Earl Mindell's The Power of MSM* by Earl Mindell, et al

- *The Miracle of MSM: The Natural Solution for Pain* by MD Stanley W. Jacob et al

- *MSM: The Natural Pain Relief Remedy* by Deborah Mitchell

- *MSM (Methylsulfonylmethane): Your Natural Repair Kit* by Deanne Tenney

- *All About MSM* by Margaret Dennison (1999)


# Dr. Burzynski/Antineoplastons

Dr. Stanislaw Burzynski is both a doctor and a biochemist who works in Houston, Texas. His groundbreaking discovery was a group of peptides and amino acid derivatives occurring naturally in our bodies that have the effect of inhibiting the growth of cancer cells. Burzynski calls these peptides 'antineoplastons'. They have the effect of "reprogramming" cancer cells to die like normal cells.

Dr. Burzynski theorized that certain anti-neoplastons, or naturally occurring peptides, could inhibit the growth of tumor cells without interrupting normal cell growth. Burzynski first isolated his antineoplastons from human urine and later synthesized these compounds in the laboratory. He uses about 10 types of antineoplastons in both oral and intravenous fashion.

In Burzynski's view, there is a biochemical defense system, completely different from the immune system, that allows defective cells to be corrected through biochemical means. Antineoplastons are at the heart of this defense system. Blood samples from cancer patients show that they have only 2-3% of the amount typically found in a healthy person.

Burzynski's method requires the injection of antineoplastons into the bloodstream. The result is tumor shrinkage and even remission. Often this occurs in a matter of a few weeks. In an interview, Burzynski stated that excellent results are obtained for prostate cancer and brain cancers, specifically childhood gliomas.

When interviewed, Burzynski reported excellent results for prostate and brain cancers and childhood gliomas in particular. He also said he was impressed with sustained-response results for non-Hodgkin's lymphomas (80% of tumors reduced by 50%) and pancreatic cancers (70% of tumors reduced by 50%).

The treatment also achieves significant (although lesser) success with breast cancer, lung cancer and colon cancer.

These rates of success do not represent cures, but "responses" to the treatment, generally meaning tumor shrinkage. There was a chance the cancers could recur.

In humans, normal cells die off after 20 to 60 divisions. They enter a terminal differentiation at that point and die. In animals, they can sometimes revert, but not in humans.

According to Burzynski, cancer cells do not die as long as cell division continues. Tumors grow as long as cells remain, in a sense, immortal. When cells are highly malignant, between 20 and 60 divisions can happen very quickly. Since the goal is to have them quickly die while seeing the tumor reduce in size, it is important to force differentiation.

He believes this is the reason behind the positive results he achieved with glioblastomas and pancreatic cancers. They're particularly fast-moving cancers. In breast cancer, where one finds slower tumor growth, it takes much longer to see results unless chemotherapy or interferon are also administered.

Burzynski has only been able to explore a small corner of the research that antineoplastons open up. At present, antineoplastons bring benefit to only a portion of patients seeking help at the Burzynski Clinic, most of whom are suffering not only from advanced disease but also from the toxic side effects of previous cancer treatment. Burzynski's frank advice to one patient with metastatic ovarian cancer was that she probably would not benefit from his therapy. Other people have been urged not to come, and this honest approach to accepting patients is greatly to his credit. This is in marked contrast to conventional medicine, where hundreds of thousands of dollars are expended on inefficacious treatments of terminal patients.

In one study of 20 patients with astrocytoma, mostly in an advanced stage, four went into early remission, two showed partial remission, and ten showed stabilization i.e. tumor regression of less than 50%. Some of these subsequently went on to complete remission. Burzynski holds more than twenty patents and has had more than 150 papers published.

Nevertheless, the FDA and the American Cancer Society consider him a quack. Some insurance companies refuse to cover his treatments. Antineoplaston was placed in the ACS's Unproven Therapies list in 1983. This is equivalent to being blacklisted in the conventional medicine community. Yet even official reports show that Burzynski's treatment has resulted in objective improvements in 86% of advanced cancer patients.

The FDA took him to court in 1983. He was allowed to continue his work, but only in the State of Texas - and none of his drugs could be shipped across state lines. In 1985, the FDA raided his Institute armed with illegal search warrants and seized 200,000 confidential documents. They have never been returned. The doctor was acquitted by a jury of all charges.

### Further Reading & References

- The Burzynski Clinic http://www.cancermed.com/

- *The Burzynski Breakthrough: The Most Promising Cancer Treatment ... and the Government's Campaign to Squelch It* by Thomas D. Elias (2000)

- *The Cancer Industry* by Ralph W. Moss Ph.D.

# Dr. Hulda Clark/Dr. Clark's Treatment

Dr. Hulda Clark Ph.D.,N.D., was an independent research scientist specializing in biology, biophysics and cell physiology. In 1979, Dr. Clark left government research to begin private consulting full-time and in 1985 developed a radio electronic technique for scanning the human body, the Syncrometer, which tests for viruses, bacteria, fungi, parasites, solvents and toxins. This gave her clues to the cause of cancer, HIV and other diseases. Her health books are best sellers – at one time they were in the top 3% of books sold on Amazon.com.

Her theories are based on the simple idea that the human body heals itself if kept in good condition. No matter how many symptoms a person has, she attributes them to only two causes of health problems:

- Pollutants (toxins which make it difficult for organs to do their work– especially isopropyl alcohol)

- Parasites (protozoa, amoeba, worms that utilize our food and leave us with their wastes).

Her solution to good health is as follows:

- Parasites - electronic and herbal treatment

• Pollution - avoidance

Her strategy to return to health is:

• Kill all parasites, bacteria, viruses, and fungi.

• Remove toxic molds, metals and chemicals from food and body products.

• Clear and wash away gallstones, secretions and debris already formed that hinder healing.

• Use herbs and special food factors to hasten healing, being careful to use only unpolluted products.

Hulda Clark is more concerned with the food that's free from parasites, bacteria and chemicals rather than with the style of nutrition or lack thereof in dealing with cancer. Her approach is different from those who specialize in cancer-controlling foods and nutrition.

Flatworms, roundworms, protozoa, bacteria, and viruses are killed using a combination of an electronic device called a 'zapper' and an herbal parasite killing program. Dr. Clark has found that this can benefit almost every illness. The zapper is a handheld battery operated (9V) frequency generator that uses a positively offset square wave to electrocute parasites. Its effectiveness is believed to be because it regenerates the white blood cells by building a positive magnetic field in the body. It is a recognized medical device, but should not be used by people with pacemakers or by pregnant women. (See **Zappers**.)

The herbal program kills remaining parasites throughout the body which cannot be reached by the electric current. It consists of black walnut hull tincture, wormwood capsules, and cloves taken over 3 weeks. A weekly maintenance program is then recommended to prevent reinfection from the home, pets, undercooked dairy products and undercooked meat. She believed uncooked meat is the main source of intestinal flukes.

She contended that isopropyl alcohol is a key pollutant. Foods and products polluted with isopropyl alcohol include shampoo, hair spray and mousse, cold cereals, cosmetics, mouthwash, decaffeinated coffee, vitamins, minerals and supplements, bottled water (polluted with antiseptics from the bottling procedure), rubbing alcohol, white sugar, shaving supplies, carbonated beverages and store-bought fruit juice. Dr. Clark recommends homemade products, unprocessed foods and a limited number of tested supplements. Once you stop using isopropyl alcohol, it disappears from your body within three days.

When isopropyl alcohol is present in the body, the intestinal fluke uses another organ as a secondary host and that organ becomes cancerous. Other solvents in the body produce other diseases. For example, benzene causes the intestinal fluke to use the thymus for its secondary host, ruins the immune system and AIDS develops. Wood alcohol invites pancreatic flukes to use the pancreas as a secondary host and diabetes develops. Dr. Clark states that cancer could be eliminated if laws required testing for solvents in animal feeds and human foods. A significant reason for isopropyl alcohol pollution is the chemicals used by manufacturers to sterilize food-handling equipment.

After cancer is stopped, the patient can get well if the toxins that invited parasites, bacterial, and viral invaders are removed. Removing toxins from the affected organs lets them heal. For example, lung lesions will not heal unless cigarette smoking, Freon, asbestos, and fiberglass exposure is stopped. Carcinogens draw the cancer to the organ: nickel draws cancer to the prostate, barium draws cancer to the breast. Dr. Clark considers the most serious threats to be: Freon (CFCs or refrigerant), copper from water pipes, fiberglass or asbestos, mercury from amalgam tooth fillings, lead from joints in copper plumbing, formaldehyde in foam bedding and new clothing, and nickel, usually from dental metal.

Dental, diet, body, and home clean-ups aim to remove parasites and pollutants at their source. The body constantly fights to remove pollutants, but if you are being "re-supplied" with them, the body cannot heal. See **Dr. Clark Cleanups**.

The dental clean up has been found crucial in shrinking tumors and restoring health. This is subject on which many alternative cancer experts agree. Dr. Clark advises:

- Remove all metals and large plastic fillings from the mouth.

- Remove all infected teeth and clean cavitations.


Silver or amalgam fillings contain 48-55% mercury, 33-35% silver, and various amounts of copper, tin, zinc, and other metals that corrode and seep into the body. Mercury is continually released from mercury fillings in the form of mercury vapor and abraded particles, which can be increased 15-fold by chewing, brushing, and hot liquids. Research has shown that mercury, even in small amounts, damages the brain, heart, lungs, liver, kidneys, thyroid, pituitary and adrenal glands, blood cells, enzymes, and hormones, and suppresses the body's immune system.

At the beginning of the 20th century Dr. Weston Price, head of the American Dental Association, found that root canal therapy, often used to save a tooth that has become infected or dead, had serious side effects. He showed thousands of instances of disease created from devitalized (i.e. dead) teeth, from head and neck pain to rheumatism and cancer. Most patients with devitalized teeth had thyroid dysfunction. The dental establishment, heavily committed to mercury amalgam fillings and root canals, ignored his findings. Safe treatment requires extracting the dead tooth rather than filling the root, and removing any infected tissue from around the tooth. Later the space can be filled with a bridge or partial denture.

Personal care products -- particularly petroleum products, alcohol, asbestos, colorings, dyes, formaldehyde, and perfume – are often toxic. These chemicals were not in use fifty or sixty years ago. Likewise for many other substances that have found their way into the human body. The tested ingredients in 99% of perfumes are labeled as toxic hazards and are not allowed in the agriculture industry. So, apart from avoidance of processed foods, Dr. Clark warns against commercial salves, ointments, lotions, colognes, perfumes, deodorants, toothpaste, soaps, washing powders etc. and gives recipes for homemade substitutes, e.g. borax powder for cleaning.

Cleaning up the home environment to make it safe includes:

- Removing paints, varnishes, thinners, cleaners, and chemicals from the house.

- Sealing cracks around pipes.

- Changing CFC-cooled refrigerators for non CFC ones (Dr. Clark found Freon concentrated in cancerous organs, where it facilitates the accumulation of other toxins).

- Checking air conditioners for leaks.

- Sealing or removing uncovered fiberglass.

- Removing clothes dryers, hair dryers containing asbestos and old radiators and electric heaters which give off asbestos.

- Changing copper plumbing to PVC plastic.

She suggests if you have been quite ill to move to a warm climate where you can avoid heating and cooling, and spend more time outdoors.

Clark recommended the Syncrometer, a device that makes it possible to test exactly which toxins and parasites cause a patient's cancer. The Syncrometer can be used for diagnosing and monitoring progress until cured. It consists of an audio oscillator circuit, which includes the body as part of the circuit. Dr. Clark maintained that every living and non-living entity produced certain specific frequencies which can be heard with the audio oscillator. Every living creature broadcasts its presence like a radio station.

The Syncrometer tests for parasites or pollutants in any product or body tissue by using samples of those parasites or pollutants. Cancerous tumors grow in the body for at least three years before they are big enough to be detected by medical imaging techniques, but according to advocates, the Syncrometer can detect them long before that.

For detoxifying the body, Dr. Clark recommends vitamins, minerals, and herbs from safe sources. Apart from parasite and dental cleanses, she gives detailed instructions for liver, kidney, and bowel cleanses. She recommends that the liver cleanse should not be done if the liver contains living parasites, and is best carried out after a parasite cleanse and then a kidney cleanse. The liver cleanse is reportedly the single most important thing you can do for your health. Medical herbalists, naturopaths and other natural healers speak highly of her cleanses.

Thousands of testimonials exist acclaiming her methods and the success people have achieved through using them. A booklet of a thousand testimonials is available for $10 from the Dr. Clark Information Center, located at http://www.drclark.net/.

See **Dr. Clark Cleanups**.

### *Further Reading & References*

- *The Cure for All Diseases* by Hulda Regehr Clark (1995)

- *The Cure For All Advanced Cancers* by Hulda Regehr Clark (1999)

- *The Cure for All Cancers: Including over 100 Case Histories of Persons Cured* by Hulda Regehr Clark (1993)

- *The Cure and Prevention of all Cancers* by Hulda Regehr Clark (2008)

- *The Cure For HIV / AIDS* by Hulda Regehr Clark (2002)

- *Syncrometer Science Laboratory Manual* by Hulda Regehr Clark (2000)

- "University of Washington study shows the Dr. Clark zapper inhibits the growth of leukemia cells'"

- Dr. Clark Information Center, http://www.drclark.net/news/lairesearch.htm

# Dr. Josef Issels

Dr Josef Issels (1907-1998) of Germany was a pioneer in alternative cancer treatment who established what he called a whole-body therapy to deal with the whole-body problem of cancer. The therapy combined ozone-oxygen treatments, diet, fever therapy and even low dose chemotherapy and radiation.

His theoretical basis is as follows. The body has four interrelated defense systems. First, there are the lymphocytes and antibodies that are normally considered to be the entire immune system. Secondly, there are the eliminating and detoxifying organs: liver, kidneys, skin, and intestine.

Third, there are friendly bacteria in the epithelial tissues of the body and lastly there is the connective tissue where organic salts are stored and toxins are digested or bound chemically to make them inert.

Dr. Issels made a big point of insisting that infected teeth and tonsils should be removed - including all teeth filled with mercury amalgam and teeth whose pulp has been removed through root canal treatment. He believed that these impair the immune system.

Dr. Issels achieved remarkable remissions, even in advanced cases, through a combination of therapies designed to shrink the tumor and repair the body's defense mechanisms. His "whole body" approach included anticancer vaccines, an anticancer diet emphasizing organic raw foods, and fever therapy to stimulate immune function. He also used a variety of methods to rebuild the immune system and change the body's biochemistry to eliminate an environment favorable for the development of cancer.

Occasionally he also used very low-dose chemotherapy, surgery, radiation, and ozone therapy in combination with immunotherapy. He prescribed organ extracts to repair damage to organs and improve their functioning. He also administered organ-specific RNA and DNA, proteolytic enzymes to destroy the protein coat surrounding tumors, as well as vitamins and minerals to strengthen the body's enzyme activity.

His program also includes psychotherapy to deal with the emotional factors that he felt could hinder recovery.

Dr. Issels gave patients a "fever shot" once a month to raise the body temperature as high as 105 F. He induced active fever with the ethical drug Pyrifer, made from specially treated coli bacteria. He induced passive fever by means of hyperthermia - the patient was placed inside a cylinder containing electrodes that bombarded his or her body with ultra short waves.

He tried to motivate cancer patients to wage a fulltime struggle against cancer. As one example, his cancer patients were routed out of their beds to do light mountain climbing in the Bavarian Alps. The patients also participated in a daily exercise regime that included jogging.

Two independent studies - one at King's College Hospital in London, the other at the University of Leyden in Holland - confirmed that about 17% of Issel's incurable, terminal patients led normal, cancer-free lives for at least five years. Their life expectancy upon admission had been less than one year. Comparable five-year survival figures for conventional chemotherapy and radiation treatment are less than 2-3%.

Here are 5-year survival statistics as depicted at http://www.issels.com/:

- For incurable patients:

  - 2% survived with conventional treatment

  - 17% survived with Issels's treatment (these "incurable" cancer patients went on to lead full cancer-free lives, some for up to 45 years.)

- Of 370 patients with various cancers who received the Issels treatment as a follow-on to conventional cancer treatments, only 13% suffered a recurrence of their cancer compared to an expected recurrence rate of 50%

Dr. Issels with his Whole Body Therapy achieved, as published in the *Clinical Trials Journal*:

- 87% five-year survival with non-metastasized cancer patients, in a study published in *Clinical Trials Journal* (London), 1970, 7, No. 3

- 16.6% five-year survival with late-stage cancer patients, in a study published in *Die Medizinische* 1959, No. 40

- 17% five-year survival with late-stage cancer patients, in a study published in *General Practitioner*, March 1971

These are good survival figures for late-stage cancer patients.

In the 1950's and 60's, the German medical establishment boycotted and isolated Dr. Issels. Finally, the German medical authorities leveled trumped-up charges of fraud and manslaughter against him, and in 1960, he was imprisoned. Eventually, however, he was acquitted of all charges.

Dr. Josef Issels died in California on 11 February 1998, a few weeks after his 90th birthday.

### *Further Reading & References*

- *Issels Hypothesis of the Pathogenesis of Cancer* by Dr. Josef Issels

- *Dr. Issel's textbook - Cancer, A Second Opinion* by Dr. Josef Issels

- Issels, J. Immunotherapy in Progressive Metastatic Cancer - A Fifteen-Year Follow-up. Clinical Trials

- Journal, August 1970: 357-365 - editorial by Phillips S. Dr Joseph Issels and the Ringberg Klinik.

- *Cancer - Whole-body Approach and Immunotherapy, lecture given in New York*, 1980, by Dr. Josef Issels.

- Cancer Cure Foundation: The Issels Cancer Treatment, http://www.cancure.org/issels_therapy.htm

- *The Cancer Industry* by Ralph W. Moss Ph.D.

- *Cancer Therapy* by Ralph W. Moss Ph.D. (1992)

- Richard Walters: *Options. The Alternative Cancer Therapy Book.*

- *Third Opinion* (Fourth Edition) by John M. Fink (2010)

# Dr. Matthias Rath

Matthias Rath was born in 1955 in Stuttgart, Germany. He studied Medicine in Germany and subsequently worked as a scientist at the University Hospital in Hamburg and the German Cardiac Center in Berlin, and served as head of Cardiovascular Research at the Linus Pauling Institute in Palo Alto, USA. Matthias Rath has made a place for himself in alternative therapy with his belief and research that vitamins, some in high dosages, and other nutritional supplements, protect against cancer. He states that the preparations made in his laboratories are able to cure cancer.

According to Rath, diseases appear when the balance between mechanisms breaking down and building the connective tissue shifts towards breakdown. If disease organisms or cancer cells can dissolve the surrounding connective tissue, a disease may spread in the body.

Rath claims that the plasminogen activator/plasmin system plays a critical role in this process: the reaction chain results in the activation of collagenase, which breaks down collagen. By gaining access to the blood vessels, cancer cells can then spread in the circulatory system.

Rath proposes that the body can normally block enzymes that destroy connective tissue by means of two mechanisms: with the intrinsic enzymatic block, or with the help of nutritional supplements. According to Rath, almost all people suffer from a chronic vitamin deficiency and almost all diseases are caused by a lack of lysine and vitamin C. Lysine can allegedly suppress the plasmin-induced proteolysis by occupying the binding sites on plasminogen.

In diseases, the body's production of proline becomes insufficient, which is why this amino acid also has to be consumed. The brand name 'Cellular Health' was chosen for the supplements because they target the body's cells as their active site.

Matthias Rath believes the mechanism of 'cancer spread' that he has identified is both the decisive breakthrough in blocking cancer as well as a breakthrough in the struggle against infectious diseases (including AIDS), and virtually all other diseases.

Hundreds of studies to date have shown that high dosages of vitamin C, vitamin E, beta-carotene, and other nutritional supplements can prevent some types of cancer. With the publication of the results of Rath's research in 1992, the significance of lysine was recognized as a medical breakthrough.

According to Rath, the foundation of modern cancer therapy is high dosages of vitamins. Only lysine in high doses combined with vitamin C can slow down or even stop the connective tissue destruction process.

Vitamin C, proline, lysine, and polyphenol from green tea are able to stem the invasion of cancer cells. (Research at Rath's research institute demonstrates that the combination of nutritional supplements recommended by Rath **can completely stop the spread of cancer cells**. In experiments, the spread of cancer cells was blocked - skin and breast cancer completely, colon cancer by 91%.

According to his information, cases of lung, breast, liver, esophageal, bladder, and testicular cancer, as well as lymphomas, have been successfully treated using Cellular Health. Rath repeatedly refers to his own research. Rath notes that sometimes, especially in cases of advanced illness, even Cellular Health cannot fully restore health.

If taken for cancer prevention, Rath recommends three or five preparations, depending on whether risk factors (more advanced age, greater risk of illness in the family) are present or not. If taken as natural therapy against cancer, Rath recommends six preparations.

The staged program recommended by the supplier calls for beginning with one preparation, "Vitacor Plus," and adding a new one every month.

The pharmaceuticals (Vitacor Plus, Epican Forte, Vita C Forte, Arteriforte, Lysine C Drink, Prolysin C) contain vitamins, trace elements, amino acids, flavonoids, and other nutritional supplements in differing compositions.

## Epican Forte™

Rath claims that laboratory research confirms that maximum inhibition of enzymatic activity is best achieved, not by nutrient megadoses, but by specific nutrient combinations and levels. The Epican Forte formula was developed using the principles of nutrient synergy, and contains a combination of Vitamin C, L-Lysine, L-Proline, Epigallocatechin from Green Tea, and other critical nutrients in precise levels for maximum effectiveness.

Several studies document an anticoagulating effect of vitamin C. Therefore, patients with coagulation disorders and patients that are about to be operated on should not take high doses of vitamin C (more than about 2g/d).

### Further Reading & References

- Rath, M.: Cellular Health Series - Cancer. 2/2001, MR Publishing, Sta. Clara, CA 95054

- http://www.natuerlich-gegen-krebs.de/de/index.html, 23.9.2002

- Brown, J. et al., American Cancer Society Workgroup on Nutrition and Physical Activity for Cancer

- Survivors: Nutrition during and after Treatment: A Guide for Informed Choices by Cancer Survivors.

- In: CA A Cancer Journal für Clinicians. A Nutritional Guide for Cancer Survivors. May/June 2001, Bd.

- 51/3, 153 ff.

- Key, T. et al., The effect of diet on risk of cancer. The Lancet, Bd. 360, 861

# Dr. Robert Jones DIY Cancer Treatment/Phenergan

According to Dr. Robert Jones, the successful treatment of cancer requires the total elimination of malignant cells in the body. The aim of his therapy is to procure necrosis (tumor death) by disrupting energy metabolism in both primary and secondary (metastatic) growths. In marked contrast with conventional treatments, the procedure is highly selective; both side effects and associated risks are negligible. Patients are asked to be realistic and not to allow hopes to rise too high; it is impossible to provide any guarantee of the desired outcome. Careful adherence to the advice provided is necessary.

According to Jones, certain drugs acting on the central nervous system possess the additional property of causing injury to tumors by interfering with energy production. Some belong to the large group of drugs known as phenothiazines, many of which have been in use for half a century. Their diverse uses include the treatment of schizophrenia, nausea, and pain.

The active drug in this form of cancer treatment is the phenothiazine Phenergan (promethazine), currently used as an antihistamine, as a pediatric sedative, and to quell travel sickness. Introduced in 1947, its effects on the central nervous system are much less marked than those of most other phenothiazines. In most countries, Phenergan can be purchased over the counter in the form of 10mg and 25mg tablets; other phenothiazines are available only on prescription. Formulations in which the drug is provided in conjunction with other drugs are not recommended.

This novel and unconventional therapy has several unusual features. First, a new chemotherapeutic target is selected within the cancer cell. The majority of anticancer drugs currently in use are supposed to react with DNA located mostly in the nuclei. In marked contrast, phenothiazines trigger a cytotoxic mechanism within the cancer cell itself. The production of chemical energy in its powerhouses (mitochondria) is disrupted initially by intensifying their natural state of partial disability, and then by destroying them.

Second, in order to produce its anti-cancer action, Phenergan has to be taken according to a specific schedule. The maintenance of continuous destructive pressure against malignant growths constitutes an essential feature of the treatment. Despite Dr. Jones's claim of supportive scientific evidence and in spite of several requests, no cancer charity or pharmaceutical firm has agreed to conduct any kind of clinical trial. Patent protection for Phenergan has long ago run out. In consequence, the potential profits are too modest to attract commercial interest.

For the detailed protocol for treating cancer with Phenergan, including dosages and frequency, see the references below. The protocol involves taking certain supplements, including vitamins, certain minerals, and omega-3 fatty acids.

According to its advocates, the treatment is gentle and humane. For those who have suffered through chemotherapy and radiotherapy, the difference will come as a pleasant surprise. Reportedly, most patients experience improved sleep, a return to normal appetite and a general feeling of well-being by the end of the first week, followed in due time by reduced pain.


## Contraindications and eligibility

Cancer patients are unlikely to benefit from this treatment if:

- Steroids are being administered in high doses. Any blockage of anti-cancer activity is, however, unstable, and therapy with Phenergan could be commenced three days after cessation of steroids.

- There has been brief or intermittent exposure to phenothiazines or to certain chemically related drugs after the onset of disease; this, it might be added, would be unusual.

- Analgesics classified as non-steroid anti-inflammatory drugs (aspirin, Nurofen, etc) are being taken. These particular analgesics should be avoided. Paracetamol in moderation is suitable for pain relief.

- There is dietary supplementation with vitamin E.


The question of vitamin E calls for special mention.

Recent work has shown that, for individuals free from cancer, dietary supplementation (50- 100 international units [iu] daily) is highly beneficial, offering protection not only against the development of malignancy but also against coronary heart disease. Unfortunately, according to Dr. Jones, the same beneficial properties are exploited by cancerous growths, which accumulate vitamin E to protect themselves against successful therapy. Several patients on vitamin E supplements (400mg-1200mg daily) failed to respond. Current advice is therefore to stop supplementation immediately and, if possible, to wait 7-10 days before starting with Phenergan.

Likewise, selenium supplementation above the RDA is not recommended. Patients should be warned that extensive radiotherapy or treatment with certain cytotoxic drugs could lead to a mutation resulting in a partial or complete disablement of the cytotoxic mechanism. Clones of these mutant cells grow rapidly and are generally insensitive to therapy.

Anecdotal evidence suggests that cancer cells regressing under the influence of Phenergan may also be vulnerable to the mutagenic effects of certain anti-cancer drugs. For this reason it is recommended that offers to treat the disease additionally by conventional means with drugs currently used against cancer should be politely but firmly refused. Even if the treatment fails to halt the progress of disease, Phenergan will enhance the quality of life and extend survival. In other words, the therapy places the patient in a no-lose situation.

**Side effects:** Drowsiness in the first few days after commencing Phenergan may be experienced, and normally lasts no more than a week or two. If not, 10mg tablets can be substituted, with two (20mg) taken at night. Sedation is the principal side effect; overall, patients do not find the experience unpleasant, but driving a car and using machinery or sharp tools are not recommended, at least for the first fortnight. Other, less frequent side effects are mentioned in the literature.

**Duration of treatment:** The therapy works slowly; just how long it will be necessary to keep taking Phenergan will depend, among other factors, on the extent of disease when treatment is started and on the state of nutrition. Patience is required. It may be necessary to stay with Phenergan for as long as two years, especially where there are secondary deposits in the bone.

**Precautions:** It is necessary to give up alcohol completely. Exposure to ultraviolet light and sunlight, especially sunbathing, are to be avoided as far as possible. A leaflet is provided with the Phenergan packet; the advice given should be read and, apart from discontinuation, carefully adhered to. The group of drugs known as monoamine oxidase inhibitors must not be taken in conjunction with Phenergan.

See the suggested reading below for further information.

### Further Reading & References

- Notes on the Treatment of Cancer with Low-Dose Phenothiazines, with Special Reference to Promethazine - Based on Dr. Robert Jones DIY Cancer Treatment - Astonishing Facts on How We Totally Controlled Our Cancers, Jill Royce. Obtainable from http://www.realityzone.com/doitcantreat.html

- Promethazine, http://www.ncbi.nlm.nih.gov/pubmedhealth/PMH0000637

- Self-Medication: the Treatment of Cancer with Phenergan Revised," by Robert Jones MA PhD, http://www.whale.to/cancer/jones.html

## Dr. Rosy Daniel/Carctol

Ayurvedic medical expert Dr. Nandlal Tiwari produced the product Carctol®, which is a blend of eight herbs that help detoxify and cleanse acids from the body. The formula has passed strict toxicology tests in India and in Britain, where clinical trials are currently underway. The formula includes:

- Blepharis edulis (200 mg)—also known as thyme-leaved gratiola in English, this small creeping herb is an astringent plant that is also used as an anti-anxiety agent

- Piper cubeba Linn (120 mg)—also called tail pepper; the fruit of this shrub is used to treat a variety of conditions including asthma, diabetes, gonorrhea and rheumatism

- Smilax China Linn (80 mg)—called Chinese sarsaparilla in English, this vine is used extensively in Chinese medicine to reduce inflammation

- Hemidesmus Indicus (20 mg)—known as Indian sarsaparilla, this twining shrub is used to treat syphilis, chronic rheumatism, and urinary diseases

- Tribulus terrestris (20 mg)—this flowering plant is also called cathead or yellow vine; it's known to boost testosterone levels and is also used to soothe nerves

- Ammani vesicatoria (20 mg)—known as blistering ammania because of its acidic leaves, this plant is often used to treat arthritis and rheumatism

- Lepidium sativum Linn (20 mg)—used as a pain reliever and anti-inflammatory remedy

- Rheum emodi Wall (20 mg)—also called Indian rhubarb, the roots of this leafy plant are used as a blood purifier and to cure constipation

According to Dr. Tiwari, Carctol is an excellent daily health tonic. He has been giving it to patients for 25 years.

Renowned oncologist and holistic cancer authority Dr. Rosy Daniel prescribes Carctol for her patients, despite disapproval from the mainstream cancer community. Their objection is based on the lack of clinical data to support the product's effectiveness.

Dr. Daniel bases her decision to prescribe Carctol on anecdotal reports of patients who experienced recoveries and remissions from melanoma, ovarian, and pancreatic cancers. She reportedly met a dozen such people on a visit to India.

According to the claims of success, this Asian herbal blend could be an important preventative measure for people not currently suffering from cancer. This is partly because Carctol helps the body restore a natural pH balance, eliminating excess acid in the body (specifically, hydrogen ions). When the body moves toward a more alkaline state, it is better able to detoxify and energize cells. It's a staple of many different cancer treatment protocols to attempt to render the body less acidic and more alkaline.

The famous nutritionist Dr. Theodore Baroody discussed this imbalance in his revolutionary book *Alkalize or Die*. He says, "The countless names of illnesses do not really matter. What does matter is that they all come from the same root cause: too much acid waste in the body!"

Food is the main reason a person's body chemistry turns acidic. When the body digests food, it leaves an ash as the result. This food ash is acidic, alkaline, or neutral, depending on the minerals in the foods. Acid-producing foods are difficult to digest so the body creates toxic acid wastes as it breaks down these foods. When this acid ash buildup is chronic, it creates the condition called acidosis.

Most healthy individuals have enough alkaline reserves to fight acid ash buildup, but too many processed or sugary foods (a typical Western diet) can quickly deplete alkaline resources. In contrast, eating alkaline-forming foods such as fruits and vegetables helps the body eliminate acids.

Dr. Tiwari recommends using Carctol in tandem with a plant-based, alkaline diet. This creates a hostile environment where cancer cells cannot survive.

The official Carctol website gives you the manufacturer's take on the best alkaline food choices at http://www.carctolhome.com/docs/Carctol_foodlist.pdf. Because Carctol is a proprietary formula available only from doctors, the website also provides a list of recommended doctors willing to prescribe Carctol.

See **Carctol**.

### *Further Reading & References*

- Breast Care (Basel). 2009; 4(1): 31-33. Published online 2009 February 20. doi: 10.1159/000193025

- Carctol website. Retrieved November 23, 2010 from http://www.carctolhome.com/index.php

- Fraser, G. 2010. The Cancer Clinics, Cancer Treatment Centres and Cancer Specialists. Cancer Active website. Retrieved November 24, 2010 from http://www.canceractive.com/cancer-active-page-link.aspx?n=2077

- The official Carctol website food list. Retrieved November 23, 2010 from http://www.carctolhome.com/docs/Carctol_foodlist.pdf

- Klotter, J. "Carctol". Townsend Letter for Doctors and Patients. FindArticles.com. Retrieved November 24, 2010 from http://findarticles.com/p/articles/mi_m0ISW/is_259-260/ai_n10018573/

- Health Creation http://www.healthcreation.co.uk/

- Cancer Active: About Dr. Rosy Daniel, http://www.canceractive.com/cancer-active-page-link.aspx?n=2085

- Dr. Daniel's 'Miracle' Cure, http://www.guardian.co.uk/society/2004/sep/21/lifeandhealth.medicineandhealth

# Dr. Tullio Simoncini Protocol

An Italian doctor, Dr. Tullio Simoncini, was a trained surgeon, oncologist, endocrinologist, and diabetologist, with a University degree in philosophy. He became disturbed by what he viewed as the medical community's blanket acceptance that cancer is 'incurable'. He noted that the 'genetics' paradigm was 80 years old, and had never been proven – and the billions of dollars spent on chemotherapy and irradiation were doing *nothing* to improve survival rates.

Dr. Simoncini contended that psoriasis, an incurable disease, is caused by a fungus, and this inspired him to think that perhaps cancer, another incurable disease, could also be caused by a fungus. There's some evidence for his belief. Many works now document the presence of fungi in cancer patients' tissues, especially in terminal patients.

Of all the fungi that cause diseases in humans, proponents of this theory say that *Candida* is the sole agent responsible for tumors as well as other serious illnesses, such as septicemia. *Candida* is always present in the tissue of cancer patients. Fungi also cause tumors in the plant and insect kingdoms.

Simoncini says most people, including doctors, underestimate the damage that opportunistic fungi can – and will – inflict.

Fungi establish permanent, parasitic colonies. These colonies spread widely all through the body. They're able to communicate with one another and to dominate host organisms.

In most cases, neither patients nor doctors recognize the symptoms of fungal overgrowth. Most doctors will tell a patient the problem is local (for instance, bad digestion or a skin rash), rather than systemic (i.e. affecting the whole body).

The immune system – when it detects a fungal enemy – tries to eradicate it before it can establish high-growth colonies. Unfortunately, a compromised immune system may be unable to do that. Fungi can bypass the epithelia and immune system and penetrate deeply into connective tissue, causing a biological reaction that tries to encapsulate the fungus – to form a container around it – the familiar bulbous tumor. However, the fungus colony not only expands aggressively in the original location, but pursues new habitats (metastasis).

Fungi mutate into different shapes throughout their life cycle – shedding their cell wall to become nearly invisible under a microscope. This is one reason fungal infections can't be detected in blood culture until the patient is nearly dead.

At first, a patient is able to send mature cells to contain the fungi, now a differentiated tumor. But when fungus colonies become more powerful and the tissues become exhausted, they revert to 'simpler' forms that don't require the higher-level functions of healthy differentiated cells such as lung cells or prostate cells.

Advocates of this cancer theory say it's always the same highly-adaptive *Candida* attacking different tissues – each time mutating and adapting itself to its new environment. Scientists think *Aspergillus* is a variation of Candida.

The preferred treatment is to oxygenate the body, because cancer cells thrive in a low- or no-oxygen environment. A number of different cancer protocols attempt to oxygenate the body in different ways.

Cancer cell growth is initiated by fermentation, triggered by the *absence* of oxygen at the cellular level. The body of cancer patients is characterized by an unhealthy acidity. In contrast, a healthy body is slightly alkaline. A high level of acidity prevents oxygen from accessing the tissues in need of it. Acidity also promotes a build-up of carbon dioxide in the tissues, leading to cell death. Many cancer experts besides Simoncini share the belief that a successful treatment plan should render the patient's body more alkaline. But relatively few follow Dr. Simoncini's method for doing so.

Dr. Simoncini's approach is to alkalinize the body with a solution of sodium bicarbonate -- simple baking soda. The Simoncini protocol has earned a devoted following among people who advocate self-treatment, although it's also used by some respected cancer doctors. There are countless testimonials to Dr. Simoncini's protocol available online.

According to the protocol's advocates, sodium bicarbonate shocks cancer cells with massive amounts of oxygen which kills them like a poison, while leaving normal cells unharmed.

It's reported that sodium bicarbonate shrinks a two to four centimeter mass of cancer cells in only 4 to 5 days. Some patients are said to experience complete remission within 5 days.

Sodium bicarbonate can be administered three ways: by mouth, with an aerosol, or intravenously.

The more hard-to-reach cancers are treated by positioning catheters directly into the artery that nourishes the tumor, allowing high doses of sodium bicarbonate to enter the deepest recesses of the cancer mass. Today it's even possible to reach cerebral masses without surgical intervention, in a completely painless way.

Advocates say most tumors can be treated effectively with baking soda therapy – except for bone cancer, due to the lack of blood flow to the bones.

A 2009 study showed sodium bicarbonate increases the pH of tumors, and reduce metastases and lymph node involvement (in breast cancer).

The therapy is said to be extremely effective, painless, free of side effects, and very low risk. With catheterization, there's a small risk of infection.

It's also inexpensive, at least in terms of the equipment and materials required. Catheters cost a bit more, but taking bicarbonate by mouth costs only pennies per day.

Application via catheter, applied directly to the tumor, can be provided only by a mainstream doctor. Most won't be willing to provide such a treatment. Also, full dosages cannot be administered to those with severe heart, kidney, and liver problems.

Based on Simoncini's theory it might seem logical that antifungal drugs would be effective anti-cancer drugs. Advocates say this is not the case. None of the antifungal drugs on the market share the effectiveness of sodium bicarbonate because they cannot penetrate tumor masses. In addition, fungi resist these drugs by quickly mutating into a different form. Finally, it's alleged that the drugs weaken the immune system.

Sodium bicarbonate, on the other hand, reportedly spreads in all directions and fungi cannot easily resist it – largely because it works so fast to disintegrate them that they can't adapt to defend themselves.

Therefore, advocates of this protocol recommend that a strong dosage should be used continuously, without interruption, for at least 7-8 days for the first treatment cycle.

Advocates of this approach advise patients to add 1-2 teaspoons of *aluminum-FREE* baking soda and 1 teaspoon of pure maple syrup to 1 cup of water, and drink. Some sources say to heat it first. The 'sugar' acts as a delivery mechanism to hard-to-reach *Candida* cells. Mark Sircus, Ac OMD suggests doing this every 2 hours for no more than 2 weeks.

This protocol is not recommended if the body is already alkaline. However, most cancer patients are acidic.

Simoncini's theory that fungus is the main cause of cancer is highly controversial, although many support the acid-alkaline theory of cancer causation and treatment.

### Further Reading & References

- *The Germ that Causes Cancer*, by Doug A. Kaufmann

- *Sodium Bicarbonate: Rich Man's Poor Man's Cancer Treatment*, by Dr. Mark Sircus, Ac., O.M.D.

- Dr. Simoncini Web site: http://www.curenaturalicancro.com

- Robey IF, Baggett BK, Kirkpatrick ND, et al. Bicarbonate increases tumor pH and inhibits spontaneous metastases. *Cancer Res.* 2009;69:2260-2268

# Falk Supplementation Schedule

The Falk Supplementation Schedule (from the Falk Oncology Center in Toronto, Canada) comprises:

- Vitamin C (fine crystals, minimum 4 grams (4,000 mg) three times per day. Aim for a dose just below diarrhea level, up to 40 grams per day. 1 level teaspoon = 4 grams. For most Vitamin C, however check the label)

- Niacinamide 500 mg three times per day. (If cholesterol is high, use niacin.)

- Vitamin B Complex (50's) once a day (sublingual B12 is the best form of B12, especially if you are over 35).

- Vitamin E 400 IU once a day

- Beta Carotene 25,000 IU once a day

- Cod Liver Oil 2 capsules once a day

- Zinc Citrate 50 mg twice a day

- Selenium 200 mcg three times per day

- Folic Acid 5 mg twice a day

- Potassium increase to 1 gram once a day

- Magnesium Oxide 420 mg once a day

- Lactobacillus acidophilus.


The now deceased oncology therapist Dr. Rudy Falk also repeatedly stated:
"The greatest use of Poly-MVA is as a cancer prophylactic."


See **Poly-MVA**.


### *Further Reading & References*

- Toronto Advisors: Nutrition — A Cancer Battle Plan, http://www.torontoadvisors.com/Kefir/cancerbattle.htm

- The Medical Journalist Report of Innovative Biologics: Cancer Remission Rates Increase from Use of the Safe and Effective Lipoic Acid Palladium Complex Poly-MVA by Morton Walker, DPM http://www.townsendletter.com/FebMar_2003/polymva0203.htm

# Greek Cancer Cure

The Greek Cancer cure was originated in 1930, by Hariton-Tzannis Alivizatos, MD, a microbiologist. This treatment consists of injections said to contain a combination of organic substances such as sugars, vitamins, amino acids and other ingredients.

Practitioners of the Greek Cancer Cure claim the regular use of the special intravenous injection (which they refer to as a serum) boosts the patient's immune system, enabling it to fight and destroy tumor cells. The inventor of the Greek Cancer Cure claimed to have cured a high percentage of patients who had cancers of the skin, bone, uterus, stomach, and lymph system.

The first stage is a blood test that is said to determine the nature, location, and seriousness of a patient's tumor. The second stage involves daily intravenous injections of the serum. Treatment lasts from 6 to 30 days.

The secret formula is believed to consist of brown sugar, nicotinic acid (also known as niacin or vitamin B3), vitamin C and alanine, an amino acid. An oral supplement is also available.

Patients are also advised to limit their intake of salts and acids, limit physical activities, and avoid drugs such as aspirin and laxatives. They are also asked to stop chemotherapy or radiation therapy before beginning the treatment program.

The cancer cells are excreted with the patient's natural body waste. At the same time, it is alleged that the serum "helps the body rejuvenate those cells or parts of the body that have been destroyed by cancer." Dr. Alivizatos claimed to be successful in treating cancers of the skin, bone, uterus, stomach, and lymphatic system. "His serum - cures the cause of your cancer, dissolves the tumor, restores tissue to its normal healthy state." Despite repeated requests, he did not reveal his precise formula, and today the only treatment available is in Athens, Greece, at an approximate cost of $4000. Independent analysis in the University of Washington claims the primary element in his injections is niacin.

### Further Reading & References

- Hafner AW, editor. Reader's guide to alternative health methods. Milwaukee, Wisconsin: American Medical Association, 1993:128-130.

- National Cancer Institute. Hariton-Tzannis Alivizatos/Greek Cancer Cure. Cancer Facts 1992 Mar 30.

- Silver HKB. Memorandum on Greek cure. Vancouver: BC Cancer Agency, 1986. (BCCA Cancer Information Centre search file 705)

- *Outlines of Greek and Roman Medicine* by James Sands Elliott (2008)

# Homeopathy/Bigelsen Protocol

Homeopathy is the introduction of a small amount of medicine into the body, a medicine chosen to be similar in nature to the problem the patient is having. The concept is that "like cures like" if administered in extremely diluted doses. Proven to be a popular and inexpensive treatment worldwide, homeopathic therapy causes a "vaccination-like" response in the body. Two anti-cancer homeopathic medicines are Nucleic acids 2LC1 and 2LCL1. A number of published studies, conducted around the globe, show a good improvement rate using homeopathy.

Homeopathy is probably the most difficult of the famous alternative methods of healing for conventional doctors to understand. It was derived empirically in the 19th century by Samuel Hahnemann, who discovered that when a substance which causes the symptoms of an illness is given in a small dose, it acts as a trigger to intensify the healing processes that the body's immune system has already begun.

Homeopaths attempt to look at the entire complex presented by a patient by way of the time-honored method of taking a thorough history and performing a complete physical exam (this is rapidly becoming a lost art in the age of specialization.) Then a single homeopathic remedy is chosen, matching the "whole picture" presented by the patient.

These natural remedies are made from plants, minerals, and other natural substances. They are prepared by a process of step-by-step repeated dilution and shaking, which, advocates say, makes them capable of stimulating the body's own immune system. The remedy is usually given one time only, and then allowed to work for a long time. Homeopaths believe that the patient is best served by the least amount of intervention necessary to achieve health. Homeopathy is very common and accepted in England, France, Switzerland, Germany, India and many other countries. The British Royal Family are keen supporters. Homeopathy is less well known in the United States.

It can be used in conjunction with any other approach, including surgery, chemotherapy, and radiation, although the goals are very different. Homeopathic treatment seeks to strengthen and bring into equilibrium the vital force of the cancer patient, in contrast to the conventional approach, which attempts to kill or otherwise remove the cancer but may, unfortunately, weaken the patient.

A homeopath would say that cancer does not arise in a vacuum. There must be susceptibility or fertile ground regardless of whether the cause appears to be genetic, environmental, psychogenic, or other.

If an organism were fully in balance, the cancer could not take hold. The prolific spread of undifferentiated or mutated cells characterized by cancer could not occur. To only cut out or irradiate the cancer with no other treatment or lifestyle change may or may not be effective. If the organism continues to provide a hospitable environment for the cancer cells, a recurrence is possible, depending on many factors.

If, however, the organism is brought into equilibrium, the likelihood of a recurrence is decreased.

Enid Segall, Secretary-General of the British Homeopathic Association states: "Homoeopathy is very supportive to patients with cancer... Certainly, there are people I talk to regularly who have been cured of cancer with the help of homoeopathy."

Most homoeopaths recognize that removal of the end product – the cancerous tumor – may be a useful adjunct to their treatment. However, they do not approve of toxic chemotherapy as a form of treatment.

These days homeopathic practitioners seem reluctant to assert that homoeopathy alone can be effective in curing cancer. Any patient going to a homeopathic hospital with the intention of having homeopathic treatment alone is carefully counseled and reminded that there are limitations to this approach. But this generally defensive attitude to homoeopathy is a modern phenomenon. One hundred years ago, J. Compton Burnett, M.D., wrote a short book entitled *Curability of Tumors by Medicines,* referring to homeopathy. The current cautious attitude may be a reaction to the general hostility that greets alternative cancer treatments.

Dr. A.U. Ramakrishnan, a native of Chennai, has treated over 4,000 patients with cancer, mostly in India, and, more recently, in the United States. He has developed a protocol for administering frequent doses of two homeopathic medicines, often in the 2000 potency, in alternation. The selection of the medicines is based on the type and site of the cancer rather than delving deeply into the mental and emotional state of the patient. Dr. Ramakrishnan's protocol is documented in his book, *A Homeopathic Approach to Cancer.*

*Further Reading & References*

- *Your Cure for Cancer: The Science, the Spirit and the Understanding* by Robert E. Smith, Harvey Bigelsen, Phronda Smith

- *Complete Guide to Homeopathy: The Principles and Practice of Treatment* by Andrew Lockie

- *A Homoeopathic Approach to Cancer* by A. U. Ramakrishnan and Catherine R. Coulter (2001)

- *Comprehensive Cancer Care: Integrating Alternative, Complementary and Conventional Therapies* by James Gordon, Sharon Curtin, and M.D., James Gordon (2000)

# Hydrazine Sulfate

Dr. Joseph Gold's approach to cancer is based on interfering with cachexia, the medical term for the severe malnutrition or emaciation that may affect up to 90% of all advanced cancer patients and account for 50% of all cancer deaths. A layman's term for cachexia would be "wasting away."

Dr. Harold Dvorak, chief of pathology at Beth Israel Hospital in Boston notes: "In a sense, nobody dies of cancer. They die of something else - pneumonia, failure of one or another organs. Cachexia accelerates that process of infection and the building up of metabolic poisons. It causes death a lot faster than the tumor would, were it not for the cachexia."

Dr. Gold drew on the work of two-time Nobel Prize winner, Otto Warburg, who theorized that cancer derives its energy from fermenting glucose. Dr. Gold concluded that cancer imposes a waste recycling system on the liver and kidneys.

The process works like this: cancer uses glucose as its fuel. The waste product that emerges is lactic acid that is excreted into the blood system and is taken up by the liver and kidneys. The lactic acid is then reconverted back into glucose by a process that requires a great deal of energy. The more glucose that is created the more fuel the cancer has to feed on and the more waste products that return to the liver for re-conversion. This process depletes the body and energizes the cancer. When the body cannot keep up, the result is cachexia, or wasting away.

Dr. Gold looked for a drug that would interfere with this process. He settled on **hydrazine sulfate** as the solution. His experiments showed that hydrazine sulfate did indeed have an effect on the cancer energizing process.

His first human volunteer in 1973 was a woman who was expected to die within a matter of days from Hodgkin's disease. She was completely bed-ridden and, not having eaten much for some time, was 'paper-thin'. Administration of the drug resulted in very quick improvement. Within a week, she was shopping, within five weeks she was back in her garden.

Dr. Dean Burke of the National Cancer Institute in Washington declared: "[Hydrazine sulphate is] the most remarkable anti-cancer agent I have come across in my forty-five years of experience of cancer."

Hydrazine sulphate eventually wound up on the American Cancer Society's list of unproven therapies, in effect a list of banned treatments. This was despite the evidence that Gold put forward to support its value.

Dr. Gold analyzed 84 terminally ill cancer patients who had been treated with hydrazine sulfate under a drug company's investigational new drug (IND) license. 70% showed subjective improvements (i.e. decreased pain, improved appetite, weight gain or stoppage of weight loss, and increased strength) and 17% had objective improvements (tumor regression, disappearance of cancer related disorders).

Russian scientists at the NN Petrov Research Institute of Oncology in St Petersburg have replicated these results. In 1974, they used hydrazine sulfate on 48 patients who were considered terminal.

They found that almost 60 per cent felt subjectively much better, indeed euphoric. Their appetites improved and the pain lessened or disappeared. Over half of these had clear signs of tumor control.

The Russian team also found another interesting attribute of hydrazine sulfate. They found that it appeared to make cancers more vulnerable to chemotherapy, even in the case of tumors that had previously been resistant to chemotherapy.

In 1985, Tim Hansen, an eleven-year-old boy with three inoperable brain tumors, was given one week to live. A few weeks later, he was put on hydrazine sulphate. Ten years later, he was alive and still taking the hydrazine sulfate as the tumors were still in evidence.

Studies show that it works against every kind of tumor at every stage. There is an abundance of published, positive, peer-reviewed studies on hydrazine sulfate in the medical literature. Hydrazine sulfate has been demonstrated to produce only few and fleeting side effects. Advocates claim there have been no instances of bone marrow, heart, lung, kidney or immune system toxicity, or death. Hydrazine sulfate has never been shown to be carcinogenic in humans.

Dr. Gold's recommended dosage for adults weighing over 100lbs is 60 milligrams per day for the first three days, then 60 milligrams twice a day for the next three days, and 60 milligrams three times a day thereafter. This treatment must continue for as long as there is evidence of a tumor in the body.

No dose higher than 60 milligrams is to be tried as this can cause nerve damage. Alcohol, tranquilizers, and barbiturates must not be taken during the course of treatment as these inhibit the action of the drug.

For patients weighing less than 100 lbs., the dosage should be halved.

### Further Reading & References

- Syracuse Cancer Research Institute: A New Cancer Treatment, http://scri.ngen.com/hydrazine_sulfate.html

- Recipes for those using the product (tyramine-free, vinegarfree... etc.) are available at http://www.angelfire.com/music/fiddle/recipes/recipesindex.html

- Hydrazine Sulfate Cancer Coverup, http://www.heall.com/medicalfreedom/hydrazinesulphate.html

# Incurables Programs

Dr. Richard Schulze and Dr. John Christopher, master herbalists and healers, developed "Incurables" programs. They believe that disease results from a failure of the immune system, mainly due to bad diet, and their programs are designed to kick the immune system into high gear.

As the name suggests, they helped many who were called "incurable" by medical doctors – people who had been told by their physicians to go home and set their houses in order. Using these two doctors' methods, teachings and herbal remedies, these people brought themselves back to life. Some of the main points are:

- Avoid animal products and adopt a raw vegan diet. Further, when one is very ill, avoid solid food and drink large quantities of freshly squeezed fruit and vegetable juices.

- Cleanse the elimination channels (intestinal cleanse first, then kidney and liver cleanses).

- Massage, exercise and sunshine.

- Hydrotherapy (hot and cold water therapy) and other healing approaches.

Since this is a very intense program, patients should consult a doctor before they begin.

Below is an edited excerpt from 'The First 30 Days' in *Common Sense Health and Healing* by Dr. Richard Schulze. For full details of the program, consult the original:

- **The Food Program**: All food consumed must be 100% total (vegan) vegetarian raw food. This includes all vegetables, fruits, raw nuts and seeds, and soaked and sprouted beans and grains. Try to eat fresh organic produce that is grown locally and in season. Liquids, only distilled water, herbal teas (non-caffeine), and fruit and vegetable juices. No animal flesh, eggs, milk or milk products (cheese, yogurt, butter) can be consumed. No cooked foods (bread, baked potatoes, tofu, etc.) no alcohol, coffee, black tea, or sugar.

- **The Herbal Nutritional Program**: A double dose of SuperFood is suggested every day. This consists of 4 tablespoons per day, 2 tablespoons a.m. and 2 tablespoons p.m. (a double dose). Make the following nutritional drink (mix in a blender): 8 ounces of fresh-squeezed fruit juice, 8 ounces of distilled or pure water, ½ to 1 cup of fresh seasonal fruit and 2 tablespoons of SuperFood.

- **The Cleansing Morning Drinks and Teas**: Every morning must begin with a liver or kidney flush and the herbal tonics and teas from the 5-day cleansing and detoxification program. Alternate these flushes weekly.

- **Hydrotherapy Program**: Use a high enema 2 times a week with an implant afterwards. Use only distilled water for the high enema. The implant can be: 8 ounces of aloe vera gel and 8 ounces of distilled water (soothing) or 2 ounces wheatgrass juice with 16 ounces of water (detoxifying) or 1 - 2 cloves of garlic blended into 8 ounces of raw apple cider vinegar and 8 ounces of distilled water.

- **Hot and Cold Showers**: This is the most effective way to move the blood and create circulation. Once daily, do a complete hot and cold shower. Start with hot water for 1 minute, then cold for 1 minute. Repeat these seven times so the shower should last about 15 minutes. Another time, daily, do a complete hot and cold shower routine again or a partial one just applying the water directly to the affected area.

- **Hot Castor Oil Packs** (breaks up congestion): Use hot castor oil packs in the evening over the affected area and leave on all night long. They can be kept warm with a hot water bottle.

- **The Cold Sheet Treatment:** Do the new cold sheet treatment once weekly.

- **Massage/Bodywork**: Massage the entire body every day with special emphasis on deep foot reflexology and all around the problem areas. Don't be afraid to touch sore or sick parts. Put some life back there. Alternate castor bean oil and olive oil for massage oils. Brush skin with a natural bristle brush and scrub the body thoroughly every day. [*Editor's Note*: most professional cancer massage therapists urge caution in massaging tumor-afflicted areas to avoid rupturing tumors and thereby spreading cancer cells. Having no direct experience of the "Incurables" approach, the editors make no comment on the specifics of its massage protocol.]

- **Exercise:** Exercise every day. Increase the amount every day. Breathe hard and work up a sweat. 1 hour each day is to be the eventual goal.

- **Attitude**: Be responsible for yourself. You created this problem and you can get rid of it. No one ever got better by feeling sorry for himself. The doctors were wrong; you can get well. Forgive everyone in your past, including all the doctors. The main function of the body is to repair and heal, so let's get started. There are NO incurable diseases. Get positive, right now, Believe, start now.

- **Additional Routines**: Walk around naked in the fresh air and sun for 10-15 minutes, lie down on the earth, do deep breathing, use natural soaps, don't use deodorants, etc.

### *Further Reading & References*

- Dr. Richard Schulze official website at http://www.800herbdoc.com

- *There Are No Incurable Diseases: Dr. Schulze's 30-Day Cleansing & Detoxification Program* by

- Richard Schulze (1999)

- *Breaking the Code: A Layperson's Guide to Unlocking The Secret World of Medical Terminology* by Dr. Richard Schulze

- *Cleanse & Heal Your Body with Dr. Schulze's 5-day Bowel Detox* by Richard Schulze (2007)

- *Common Sense Health and Healing* by Dr. Richard Schulze

# Induced Remission Therapy® (IRT)/Dr. Chachoua

According to Dr. Sam Chachoua, a medical doctor credentialed in Australia, "nemesis organisms" both control and provide cures for diseases like cancer and AIDS.

After watching his father die of cancer. Dr. Chachoua pursued fifteen years of research on organ resistance, organism resistance, and spontaneous remission. He developed what he termed to be effective vaccines for the prevention and treatment of multiple killer diseases such as cancer and AIDS and labeled the treatment Induced Remission Therapy, or IRT.

Dr. Chachoua's first beliefs about the cause of cancer stemmed around the popular idea that age, particularly past the point of puberty, was a promoting factor in the decline of the immune system and subsequent higher likelihood of developing cancer. As a person ages, the body experiences a loss of a vital immune-protective agent which normally stems from the thymus gland. The degeneration of the thymus gland, which atrophies in the early teenage years, correlates with an increased likelihood of cancer.

In addition, Dr. Chachoua was intrigued by the seemingly natural resistance of the small intestine in terms of resisting cancer and staying protected from tumors. He points out that the small intestine has lymphoid aggregates known as "Peyer's patches," which are only found in the small intestine. He reasoned the patches could account for the cancer resistance being local. Dr. Chachoua felt that so many researchers were obsessed with theories surrounding the thymus gland that they had overlooked a genuine clue to cancer prevention via the small intestine. Dr. Chachoua further believed that "Peyer's patches would protect the small intestine against direct invasion from the large bowel cancers as well as blood-borne metastases."

In early studies on the reaction of Peyer's patches with cancer, Dr. Chachoua reported that, "Cells from Peyer's patches of mice that had been carrying the cancer surpassed my expectations. As opposed to the 50,000 to 100,000 cells destroying one cancer cell as previously mentioned over a three-day period, it took one lymphocyte from sensitized aggregates to kill 400 cancer cells in a one-hour-or-less time period. The cancer cells would uptake ... red resin dye and soon collapse."

Using non-toxic biological agents that duplicate the activity of Peyer's patches, Dr. Chachoua developed multiple extracts and vaccines using living cultures. These were meant to target the cause of a disease by attaching to cells and then prompting the body to remove the disease and correct any subsequent genetic damage.

In essence, Dr. Chachoua developed a way for immune cells to tag and destroy cancer cells. He essentially changed the appearance of individual cancer cells by developing cultures that attach themselves to cancer organisms so a patient's immune system recognizes them as harmful and destroys them. IRT is, in effect, a system of tagging cancer cells as foreign invaders. He claims to have reversed cancer in more than nine out of ten patients, on average.

According to advocates, Dr Chachoua's serums and vaccines have since been tested and proven to be more effective than anything else in history. His cancer serum has been proven to be 85% effective against cancers while his AIDS serum is 99% effective in putting AIDS into remission for six months to upwards of three years.*

Dr. Chachoua spent five years touring hospitals and institutes all over the world in an effort to share his knowledge, but soon endured personal and professional attack. Dr. Chachoua's therapies have been widely criticized by the conventional medicine establishment which he claims is working to keep his treatments from being known and accessible to the public.

The therapy developed by Dr. Chachoua is available for approximately $10,000, the only requirement being that a physician is found who is willing to administer the therapy.

### Further Reading & References

- *International Wells Directory: The Story of Dr. Sam, http://www.mnwelldir.org/docs/cancer1/sam.htm

- "Induced Remission Therapy: Our Best Hope Against Cancer?" by Dr. Sam Chachoua, http://www.nexusmagazine.com/index.php?page=shop.product_details&category_id=127&flypage=shop.flypage&product_id=1152&option=com_virtuemart&Itemid=44

# Insulin Potentiation Therapy (IPT)/Insulin Therapy/Microdose Chemotherapy

Insulin potentiation therapy or IPT makes use of insulin as a sort of Trojan horse, to "fool" cancer cells into taking in vastly greater amounts of a toxic chemotherapy drug than do healthy cells. The therapy is based on the fact that cancer cells have an extraordinary appetite for glucose (blood sugar) and possess ten times the number of insulin receptors that healthy cells do, thereby enabling them to metabolize sugar at a much faster rate.

For this reason, when insulin is administered to a cancer patient at the same time as a chemotherapy drug, the multiple insulin receptors on cancer cells open wide and take up the chemotherapy drug at a much higher rate compared to healthy cells. This enables the therapist to achieve a lethal effect on the cancer cells many times greater than that felt by healthy cells. The therapist can therefore use a lower dose of the chemotherapy drug, sparing the healthy cells damage, while damaging cancer cells just as much as a high dose of chemotherapy would if delivered without the insulin "boost."

In short, insulin multiplies the killing effect of a chemotherapeutic agent, enabling the use of lower doses and causing less damage to healthy cells.

Insulin was first used as a treatment for diabetes in 1921. By 1928, Dr. Donato Perez Garcia of Mexico City, Mexico, adapted the use of insulin to treat other illnesses, such as syphilis. His treatments centered on the glucose-lowering ability of insulin, which seemed to be beneficial for several diseases.

Dr. Garcia's grandson, Dr. Perez, carries on the practice of insulin-based treatment and uses it for terminal cancer patients. In a staff training workshop at the Hospital Santa Monica, Dr. Perez outlined his method of using micro-doses of chemotherapy at the point of lowest glucose levels, which results in an exceptional uptake of the chemotherapy by cancer cells.

According to Dr. Perez, "I have long taught all my cancer patients that above all, cancer cells need sugar for the energy to divide and grow. In fact, cancer cells have from 10 to 100 times the number of insulin receptors that normal cells do. When the blood glucose reaches its lowest - which can vary from 25 to 45 mg/dl - the cancer cell is desperate for glucose.

"The introduction of minute amounts of chemotherapy, in conjunction with the glucose necessary to bring blood glucose levels back to normal, creates a concentration of the chemotherapy agent in the cancer cell because the extra amounts of insulin receptor sites on the cancer cells means they will receive many times the amount of glucose/chemo as the normal cell. This all makes such good sense to me. It is a way to use the science of chemotherapy that does kill cancer cells but under normal use also kills too many normal cells. This way we concentrate the action in the cancer cells.

"We have used this on many patients to date. Many of them reported, and doctors confirmed, shrinking of cancer mass. The lowering of blood sugar does not cause any side effects other than temporary sleepiness or weakness. All of our physicians feel very comfortable with this therapy."

Chemotherapy drugs are powerful cell-killing agents, which is why they are mainstream American medicine's preferred cancer treatment. In current medical practice, getting these drugs into the inside of cells where they do their work requires that they be administered in doses high enough to force them across the membranes of cancer cells.

A major drawback to this high-dosing strategy is serious dose-related side effects. This happens because chemotherapy agents do not discriminate between cancer cells and other normal cells in the patient's body. They kill both kinds of cells, thus the side effects.

With the development of IPT it is now possible to avoid the dose-related side effects of chemotherapy, while at the same time increasing the effectiveness and specificity of these agents in killing cancer cells.

### Further explanation of the IPT approach

IPT is a non-diabetic use of the hormone insulin to improve the effectiveness and delivery of standard medications dramatically. This slight modification of standard medicine could help many medications act like super drugs, with better results for many millions of patients.

Insulin is the hormone used to treat diabetes. Secreted by the pancreas in healthy people, insulin is a powerful hormone with many actions in the human body, a principal one being to manage the delivery of glucose across cell membranes into cells.

Insulin communicates with cells by joining up with specific insulin receptors scattered on the outer surface of the cell membranes. Every cell in the human body has some of these receptors, with there being from one hundred to one hundred thousand of them per cell. The interesting connection between cancer cells and insulin is that studies report that cancer cells actually manufacture and secrete their own insulin. Related to this is the even more interesting fact that cancer cells have ten times more insulin receptors per cell than any of the normal cells in the body. This fact creates a valuable opportunity because it significantly differentiates normal cells from cancerous ones.

Having ten times more insulin receptors than normal cells means that the effect of administered insulin will be ten times greater on cancer cells than on normal cells. With this difference, an effective dose of chemotherapy drugs, when administered at the same time as intravenous insulin, is able to penetrate the inside of cancer cells — selectively, with a sparing of normal tissues — and this can be accomplished using greatly reduced doses of the toxic chemotherapy drugs, effectively eliminating all their dose-related side effects.

The addition of insulin to a culture medium containing cancer cells has been shown to enhance the cell-killing effect of methotrexate – a commonly used chemotherapy drug – by a factor of up to ten thousand. This striking result was attributed to two effects on the cancer cells.

One was an effect of insulin to increase the trans-membrane transport of the methotrexate into the cell. The other was what the authors called "metabolic modification by insulin" within the cancer cells. It modifies the growth characteristics in tumors, making more of the cancer cells vulnerable to anticancer drug effects.

Just as cancer cells have their own independent secretion of insulin for unlimited access to the fuel they require, they also have their own independent secretion of something called insulin-like growth factor to provide them with an unlimited stimulus for growth. Cancer cells also have ten times more of the receptors for insulin-like growth factor on their cell membranes –just as for the insulin receptors.

The metabolic modification by insulin mentioned above results from the fact that not only can insulin join up with its own specific receptors on cell membranes, but insulin is also able to join up with the receptors for insulin-like growth-factor, and to communicate messages about growth to these cells. While it may seem highly undesirable for a cancer therapy to promote cancer cell growth, this is in fact a valuable effect of insulin in this instance. In IPT, insulin administration has an effect of causing the blood glucose to go down. This is called hypoglycemia. This hypoglycemia is an anticipated side effect of the insulin, one rapidly and effectively controllable with intravenous glucose infusions at an appropriate time, according to the IPT protocol.

Because it is possible to create a clear differentiation between cancer and normal cells using insulin, along with the biologic response modification insulin produces, conventional chemotherapy drugs are targeted more specifically and more effectively inside the cancer cells only, and this can occur with the use of greatly reduced doses of these cell-killing drugs. Cancer cells die, tumors shrink, and no side effects are caused in any other tissues. IPT appears to be an effective new way of treating cancer using nothing other than conventional chemotherapy drugs.

That the NIH lists the therapy as an acceptable mode of treatment speaks for its safety. As they put it, "IPT is 21st century medicine. Cancer treatment with IPT is reported to be gentler, safer, more effective, less expensive, and with usually no side effects."

### Further Reading & References

- *Treating Cancer with Insulin Potentiation Therapy* by Ross A. Hauser, Marion A. Hauser (2002)

- Insulin Potentiation Therapy ( IPT ), http://iptq.com/

- American Cancer Society: Insulin Potentiation Therapy, http://www.cancer.org/ Treatment/TreatmentsandSideEffects/ComplementaryandAlternativeMedicine/ PharmacologicalandBiologicalTreatment/insulin-potentiation-therapy

- Memorial Sloan-Kettering Cancer Center: Insulin Potentiation Therapy, http://www.mskcc.org/ mskcc/html/69265.cfm

- *A Method of Pinpointing Cancer Cells with Microdoses of Chemotherapy without Harming Normal Cells*, As Reported By Kurt W. Donsbach, DC, ND, Ph.D. http://health.dir.groups.yahoo.com/ group/natural_prostate_treatments/message/2367

# Kelley's Program/William D. Kelley/Dr. Nicholas Gonzales Protocol

William D. Kelley, DDS was a dentist who claimed to have healed himself of pancreatic cancer with his own therapy in 1964. The Kelley Anti-Cancer Program combines therapeutic nutrition, supplements, and vigorous detoxification of the body. His healing program was based on metabolic typing with the goal of providing a patient-specific dietary program, detoxification (using coffee enemas – a recognized detoxification therapy – and other therapies), neurological stimulation through chiropractic adjustment, and supplements of vitamins, minerals, and enzymes.

Dr. Kelley believed the root cause of cancer is the body's inability to digest and utilize (essentially, metabolize) protein. He stated: "The person gets cancer because he's not properly metabolizing the protein in his diet. Then, to make matters worse, the tumor has such a high metabolism that it uses up much of the food which is eaten.

"If a person's disordered protein metabolism is not corrected it will give rise to more tumors in the future, even if the first one is successfully removed. This, by the way, is the unfortunate reason why so many seemingly successful cancer operations end up in recurrences a year or two later. The tumor was removed, but the cause — improper protein metabolism — remained."

Dr. Kelley linked faulty metabolism to a deficiency of pancreatic enzymes which he regarded as a fundamental cause of cancer. He believed that certain pancreatic enzymes, especially those that are proteolytic (protein-digesting) enzymes, are the body's first line of defense against malignancy. This theory stands in marked contrast to the view that the immune system, with its natural killer cells, is the body's main line of defense against cancer. (See **Proteolytic Enzymes**.)

The pancreas releases enzymes directly into the small intestine to aid digestion. But Kelley maintained that the pancreas also secretes enzymes into the bloodstream, where they circulate, reaching all body tissues, and killing cancer cells by digesting them. Studies in the clinical literature lend support to this theory, first proposed by Dr. John Beard, a Scottish embryologist working at the turn of the century.

Imbalance of mineral metabolism is another condition that allows malignancy to occur, according to Dr. Kelley. He identified mineral imbalance as a root cause of the breakdown of the immune system. Additionally, he said, cancer cells produce immune-blocking factors and seem to generate an electromagnetic force field that inhibits the proper response of the immune system.

To demonstrate his theories, Kelley divided people into what he called ten metabolic types, with slow-oxidizing vegetarians at one extreme and fast-oxidizing carnivores at the other. Each person is different, he asserted, not only in nutritional needs but also in the way their bodies use food.

Kelley then recommended a different nutritional program for each of the ten different metabolic types. An individualized diet was tailored to match the metabolic character of each patient, taking into account his or her physiology, neurological and physical makeup, basic metabolic rate, and personality. Some common threads ran through the diets, however. The consumption of raw, organic fruits, and vegetables was emphasized, while protein intake was reduced considerably to preserve the enzymes needed to digest fruits and vegetables.

In addition to a diet, Kelley's patients also took as many as 150 supplement pills per day, including pancreatic enzymes, vitamins and minerals, and concentrates of raw beef or organs and glands, believed by Kelley to contain tissue-specific growth factors, hormones, natural stimulants, and protective molecules. A direct anti-tumor effect has been observed repeatedly in patients on various metabolic therapies, who receive enzymes either orally or by injection. According to Kelley, as the enzymes "digest" the tumor, large amounts of cellular debris are released into the bloodstream and surrounding tissues.

These breakdown products from cancer cells are foreign to the normal body and can be very toxic, he maintained. Even though the liver and kidney can filter these substances out of the bloodstream, the wastes from tumor destruction form so quickly during enzyme therapy that the body's normal detoxification processes may become overloaded. To assist their bodies in detoxification, Kelley's patients periodically discontinued their enzymes and other supplements for several days. This rest period, Kelley believed, allows the liver and kidneys to catch up with the body's load of tumor byproducts.

As a second aid in detoxification, Kelley advised all his patients to take at least one coffee enema daily. His reasoning was that coffee enemas clean out the liver and gallbladder and help the body get rid of the toxins produced during tumor breakdown. During a coffee enema, claimed Kelley, the caffeine that is rapidly absorbed in the large intestine flows quickly into the liver. He believed that in high enough concentrations, caffeine causes the liver and gallbladder to contract vigorously, releasing large amounts of stored wastes into the intestinal tract and greatly aiding elimination. Kelley also believed that enemas are important in stimulating the immune system, since most waste products eliminated by detoxification are enzyme inhibitors. Frequent enemas prevent the suppression of protein-digesting enzymes. These enzymes can break down the cancer cells' fibrin (protein) coats, making the cancer cells more vulnerable to the immune system. See **Coffee Enemas**.

The *Merck Medical Manual*, commonly thought to be the "bible of physicians", included coffee enemas as an accepted means of detoxification and constipation relief up through 1977. Despite that, coffee enemas, common also to the Gerson Therapy, became the focal point of opponents who considered Kelley's program unscientific.

The original Kelley program also included purges to cleanse the liver, gallbladder, intestines, kidneys, and lungs. Like many other metabolic therapists, Kelley believed that the functioning of these organs is severely impaired in the cancer patient. Colonic irrigations, liver and gallbladder flushes, and controlled sweating accomplished the cleansing tasks. Kelley also often recommended some form of manipulative therapy, such as chiropractic adjustment or osteopathic manipulation, to stimulate sluggish nerves.

A frequently overlooked part of the Kelley system is its spiritual component. Kelley called his approach metabolic ecology, taking into account the cancer patient's total environment, including physical, mental, emotional, and spiritual aspects. He urged his patients to "accept the fact that you are afflicted with a symptom (malignant cancer) and that recovery is possible. Establish a faith in a power greater than yourself and know that with His help you can regain health and harmony."

Patients were encouraged to conduct a searching self-analysis and to eliminate negative behavioral patterns and emotions.

The Kelley approach boasts extensive documentation with 10,000 medically-verified diagnoses. In one study, all his cases of pancreatic cancer were investigated. With conventional treatment, there were virtually no survivors after 5 years. He had 22 cases on record. Of these, 10 never started the treatment and survived for 67 days. 7 followed it partially and survived an average of 233 days, while the 5 who followed the Kelley treatment all completely recovered.

Interest in Kelley's therapy has increased dramatically in recent years largely due to the work of Nicholas Gonzalez, M.D., a New York City physician who treats cancer patients in advanced or terminal stages using a modified version of the Kelley program. A graduate of Cornell University Medical School, Dr. Gonzalez undertook a five-year case study of cancer patients of Kelley's who did well on the program.

The late Harold Ladas, Ph.D., a biologist and former professor at Hunter College, wrote:

"Gonzalez has given us convincing evidence that diet and nutrition produce long-term remission in cancer patients almost all of whom were beyond conventional help.

"Because the cases [in Gonzalez's study] represent a wide variety of cancers, the implication is that the paradigm has wide applicability to cancer treatment. ...What should happen is that ACS [American Cancer Society] or NCI [National Cancer Institute] should immediately follow up with a half million dollar study to evaluate the rest of Kelley's cancer patients. But don't hold your breath," added Ladas, who concluded, "The evidence is in, and it is stunning. Kelley is vindicated."

In 1987, Dr. Gonzalez set up a private practice in New York City, where he began treating patients with a modified version of Dr. Kelley's program.

A pilot study of Dr. Gonzales treatment in patients with advanced pancreatic cancer was published in 1999. Of the 11 patients included in the study, 9 survived at least 1 year, 5 survived for 2 years, and 4 lived for 3 years. Two of the patients remained alive 4 years later. In contrast, the median survival for patients with inoperable pancreatic cancer who undergo chemotherapy is 5 ½ months. A further clinical study involving patients diagnosed with pancreatic cancer is expected.

Like Kelley, whom the American Cancer Society denounced as a quack, Gonzalez has also been castigated for "departing from accepted practice."

Dr. Gonzales program and its theory are described at http://dr-gonzalez.com/.

### Further Reading & References

- *One Answer to Cancer* by William D. Kelley, http://www.drkelley.com/

- Dr. William D. Kelly's Nutritional-Metabolic Therapy, http://educate-yourself.org/cancer/kellysmetabolictherapy.shtml

- Dr. Gonzalez: Individualized Nutritional Protocols, http://dr-gonzalez.com/

- *The Alternative Cancer Therapy Book* by Richard Walters (1993)

# Koch Treatment/Koch Synthetic Antitoxins

Dr. William F. Koch of Detroit created the Koch method, which is a systematic course of dieting and enemas combined with administration of Koch Synthetic Antitoxins (malonide, glyoxylide, and parabenzoquinone). Koch claimed that "cancer was caused by a germ which resembled a spirochete." He stated that his discovery was also effective against tuberculosis, psoriasis, leprosy, polio, syphilis, appendicitis, and herpes zoster.

The Koch formula, as used for the control of the cancer organism, is a differential poison, which exerts its destructive influence primarily upon the protoplasmic substance within the receptor, and not directly upon the micro-organism. This substance provides an unsuitable soil in which the germ cannot live. Thus the excitant stimulus to cancer is controlled and the mass soon retrogresses. Three weeks after the treatment has been instituted the mass becomes hard, due to calcification prior to absorption. The cancer effort or growth is a histological expression of nature's immunity attempt.

He initially called this substance synthetic anti-toxin; it later became known as "glyoxylide". Apparently, the treatment was also marketed under the auspices of the Christian Medical Research League.

Dr. Koch preferred to deliver glyoxylide only once or twice in the form of intramuscular injections (2 cc), in a highly diluted (possible homeopathic) form. Dr. Koch claimed that the Koch Synthetic Antitoxins stimulate the destruction of the toxins responsible for the growth of cancer tissue.

He reasoned that cells become cancerous because of depletion of the blood's oxygen levels. If sufficient oxygen were continually delivered to the body's tissues, cancer pathology would be virtually impossible.

With the drain on the vital forces of the blood plasma removed, a fairly prompt tonic effect is exhibited. Apparently, a specific action follows, in that the effects show only on the microbic structure and no other action is noted on surrounding structures.

### Further Reading & References

- William F. Koch, Ph. D., M. D. Official Research Page, http://www.williamfkoch.com/

- Diamond WJ, et al. An alternative medicine definitive guide to cancer. Tiburon, California: Future Medicine Publishing, Inc., 1997:34,922

- *Third Opinion* (Fourth Edition) by John Fink (2005)

- *Natural immunity: Its curative chemistry in neoplasia, allergy, infection : a report to the Research Investigation Committee* by William F Koch (1936)

- *Cancer And Its Allied Diseases. Their Common Toxic Cause. Their Cure by Immunization. - Hardcover* by William F. Koch (1929)


# Krebiozen/Carcalon

Krebiozen is a group of remedies specifically designed to stimulate the immune system. It is the commercial name of an alternative cancer formula originally prepared from the blood of horses that have been injected with bacteria. It was claimed Krebiozen cured cancer. Independent studies showed that may be true in 70-80% of the cases. Krebiozen has been manufactured in powder and liquid forms.

Krebiozen was originally developed by Stevan Durovic, a Yugoslavian physician, in Argentina, and brought to the United States in 1949. In the 1950s, it drew the attention of Dr. Andrew C. Ivy, a respected scientist at the University of Illinois, and Krebiozen made headlines in the US, promoted by Dr. Ivy. He began producing his own version of the drug in mid-1959, calling it Carcalon. Ivy published two monographs claiming extensive anticancer benefits. Krebiozen therapy grew in popularity during the 1950s and early 1960s.

One test on the drug claimed the result that it stopped or reduced cancer growth in 88 per cent of a group of 4,227 cancer patients, the vast majority of whom were terminal. Dr. Ivy's "establishment" medical credentials were impeccable. He had authored more than 1,000 articles published in scientific and medical journals, had served as a U.S. representative at the post-World War II Nuremberg trials, and had received bronze, silver, and gold medals from the AMA for his achievements. Even the FDA had sought his medical testimony on occasion in judicial proceedings.

Once Dr. Ivy began advocating an unorthodox cancer therapy, he was promptly derided as a "quack." At the behest of the FDA, he and three associates were indicted in 1964 on 49 criminal counts for violations of the Food, Drug, Cosmetic Act, and many other violations. FDA chemists claimed that krebiozen was simply a common amino acid found in humans and animals. Five hundred doctors used it and 20,000 testimonials of cancer victims stood behind Dr Ivy and his co-workers at their trial. They were acquitted, but the AMA succeeded in blacklisting Krebiozen.

The treatment as sound as it seems to have been, was demolished by mainstream medicine's vicious attack. Unfortunately there is not much evidence the real treatment is currently used anywhere. There are many respected medical journalists and doctors who believe that had Krebiozen been given a place in legal cancer treatments, it would have saved millions of lives.

Assaults on other non-traditional remedies come readily to mind — the case has been laid down in great detail in the book *A World Without Cancer* by G. Edward. Griffin. The jury in its verdicts acquitted Dr. Ivy and the others on all counts. Indeed, the jury added that it believed krebiozen had merit. Yet as journalist and author Michael L. Culbert notes in *Freedom From Cancer*:

"The propaganda campaign paid off, and krebiozen was left in the public mind as another unproven cancer remedy and Dr. Ivy was character-assassinated into the limbo reserved for pioneers who dare operate outside of the medical-governmental axis."

### Further Reading & References

- *Observations on Krebiozen in the Treatment of Cancer* by Ivy, A.C., Ph.D., M.D. et al

- *Krebiozen: The Great Cancer Mystery* by George D. Stoddard (1955)

- *A Matter of Life or Death, The Incredible Story of Krebiozen* by Herbert Bailey

- *Freedom From Cancer* by Michael L. Culbert (1976)

- *A World Without Cancer* by G. Edward. Griffin (2010)

- *Best Alternative Medicine* by Kenneth, Dr. Pelletier, et al (2002)

# Nucleic Acids (Homeopathic 2LC1 and 2LCL1)

"The doctors who pioneered their use in cancer have found that they 're-balance' the weakened immune system, and there are documented cases of recovery which include many advanced cancers – metastatic liver and breast cancer, [leukemias] etc. However, because nucleic acids are usually present in infinitesimal quantities, and high doses are toxic, the principles of homeopathy have been applied to their orthomolecular use."

See **Homeopathy/Bigelsen Protocol**

### *Further Reading & References*

- Survive Cancer: Non-Toxic Complementary Therapies, http://www.canceraction.org.gg/therapies-and-recipes/non-toxic-complementary-therapies

- The Cancer Cure: Alternative Cancer Therapies continued, http://www.cancure.org/choice_of_therapies_continued.htm

# Percy's Powder/Rhomanga

Early on, Percy Weston had experiences involving the health effects of phosphorus, which were striking. At the age of six, he became ill due to inhaling the fumes from phosphorus-impregnated matchstick heads (this is before the days of safety matches). He also had unpleasant experiences with phosphorus in rabbit bait on the family's farm. He saw a school friend collapse in a science laboratory when an experiment involving phosphorus went wrong. These were separate and seemingly unrelated experiences; only later did he realize that phosphorus had been involved on each occasion.

Later, as a farmer, Weston — in common with others in his district — began growing tobacco. This involved very heavy applications of superphosphate fertilizer, at rates as high as a thousand pounds per acre. Subsequently, Weston noticed problems with his sheep: an arthritic condition affecting their knees and cancerous lesions on their ears. Plants grown in the soil so heavily treated with superphosphate exhibited strange mutations.

When he moved the sheep onto poorer pasture, which had not been treated with superphosphate, Weston noticed to his surprise that they recovered. He moved some of them back onto the treated paddock and they developed the same problems again. He moved them off it and they recovered. The pattern was undeniable and impressive. Later again, Weston himself was afflicted with arthritis and a cancerous tumor which developed on his hand. Remembering his early life experiences and realizing that phosphorus had been involved, and recalling his experiences with the sheep, Weston wondered whether reducing his own intake of phosphorus would have any effect. He set about developing a low phosphate diet.

He also further experimented with his sheep by using mineral licks containing supplements of alkaline minerals such as magnesium and potassium, which he believed would counteract the harmful effects of phosphorus and promote its excretion. The results exceeded his expectations; the arthritis eased and gradually disappeared; the cancer tumor dried up, shriveled, separated, and finally broke away from his hand.

Weston continued his experiments with his low phosphate diet for several decades. He became absolutely convinced that exposure to and consumption of phosphorus/phosphate can cause very serious adverse health problems. Later still, he experienced such effects again because of the indiscriminate use of organophosphate sprays in his district. The now infamous Agent Orange, used in the Vietnam War, was an organophosphate herbicide.

His most spectacular success was when he treated his wife with his low phosphate diet and mineral supplements. She had been diagnosed with cancer of the uterus by no less than three doctors, including the top gynecologist in their state (Victoria, Australia). The specialist had advised an immediate hysterectomy. But following strict adherence to the low phosphate diet, the operation, which would have prevented her from ever having children, became unnecessary. Mrs. Weston's tumor reabsorbed. Later she became pregnant and went on to have two healthy children. The specialist, advised of these events, commented that he had never known a woman in the condition Mrs. Weston had been in when he had examined her to survive for twelve months, let alone have children.

Weston's book, *Cancer Cause and Cure* is very informative, covering his experiments and experiences. Percy Weston died at 102 - surviving two personal encounters with cancer and a number of other serious health crises that would seem to bear testimony to the effectiveness of his recipe.

### Further Reading & References

- *Cancer: Cause and Cure* by Percy Weston (2000)

- Percy's Powder, http://www.health-search.com/percyspowder.html (Note: For informational purposes only; not an endorsement.)

# Oncotox®

Oncotox is an essential ingredient in Kurt Donsbach's holistic cancer control program at Hospital Santa Monica. In chemistry, there exists the concept of synergism, where two or more ingredients, when mixed together, equal a result greater than the total results of the individual parts. This is claimed to apply to the Oncotox ingredients.

Oncotox is a liquid concentrate of five separate and effective cancer inhibitors, each with extensive research studies documenting its effectiveness as an adjunct in cancer therapy.

"All of our cancer patients take Oncotox twice a day while at the hospital and it is an important element in their follow-up home protocol," according to Donsbach.

The cancer inhibitors in Oncotox are:

- Resveratrol

- IP-6

- Lactoferrin

- Arginine

- Curcumin

While the ingredients in Oncotox are reputable and well-supported, Mr. Donsbach's own reputation has come under a cloud. He pleaded guilty to a number of felony counts and is barred from practicing medicine in any form. It has been charged that he has never earned a doctor's degree or license of any kind, and Mr. Donsbach did not respond to an invitation from the editors of the book to prove that he is a legitimate doctor.

See **Resveratrol, Arginine, IP-6, Lactoferrin**, and **Curcumin**.

### *Further Reading & References*

- Alpha Medical Institute, http://www.hospitalsantamonica.com

- Cancer Treatment Registry: Oncotox, http://cancer-treatment-registry.org/cancer-treatment/Oncotox.php

# Poly-MVA™

Poly-MVA is a uniquely formulated nutritional supplement designed to provide energy for compromised body systems. It is helpful in increasing energy, reducing fatigue, and enhancing overall health and well-being, and can be particularly helpful in addressing those symptoms in people who are receiving chemotherapy or radiation treatments for cancer. Many people have found Poly-MVA to be helpful in improving quality of life while undergoing a difficult treatment regimen.

The Poly-MVA name comes from the combined terms Poly meaning "many, much, more than one"; M indicating "minerals"; V signifying "vitamins"; and A symbolizing "amino acids." Poly-MVA is a proprietary blend of palladium, alpha-lipoic acid, vitamins, B1, B2 and B12, the amino acids formyl-methionine and acetyl cystiene, and trace amounts of molybdenum, rhodium, and ruthenium.

According to the inventor of Poly-MVA, Merrill Garnett, DDS, PhD, cancer results from the failure of cells to mature. This in turn is caused by a problem of energetics in the cell's metabolic processes. He has developed a chemical compound, palladium lipoic acid, that mimics an energy pathway present in normal cells but missing in cancer cells, and necessary to normal growth and health. As a new principle in the nutritional healing of most cancer types, Poly-MVA assists in correcting malfunctioning nucleic acids in the deoxyribonucleic acid (DNA) of genes.

Dr. Garnett emphasizes that he chose to bind palladium to alpha lipoic acid (ALA) because this amino acid is both water and fat-soluble and able to travel everywhere in the human body, even through the blood-brain barrier, taking the palladium molecule with it.

Dr. Garnett, whose Garnett McKeen Laboratory is located in Islip, New York, has produced a self-published book, *First Pulse: A Personal Journey in Cancer Research*. In it, the author-scientist offers a philosophical, highly technical, but interesting and anecdote-filled discussion of how he came to create his invention.

Dr. Garnett searched for singular substances capable of binding together the various ingredients which make up Poly-MVA. He found the therapeutic component in the platinum-derived palladium mineral, poisonous in the hands of an allopathic dentist, but life saving for someone suffering from cancer. Yet palladium would be poisonous to cancer patients too, if it were not bound tightly to alpha lipoic acid and "sequestered" in the molecule as cobalt is sequestered in vitamin B12. Thus, palladium forms an organic metallo-vitamin-lipoic acid complex that joins with cobalt, a part of the vitamin B12 (cyanocobalamin) complex.

Dr. Garnett created Poly-MVA based on knowledge unknown before he discovered what he calls the Second Genetic Code, regarded by some as a scientific breakthrough. (See the Garnett book for details about the highly complicated Second Genetic Code discovery.)

Dr. Garnett discovered that palladium acts as an excellent catalyst for combining oxygen and hydrogen; the metal absorbs over 900 times its volume of hydrogen. His formula adapts palladium for strengthening the actions of other molecules, too; e.g., iron holds together the active parts of hemoglobin, and its holding action is reinforced in the presence of palladium. Other amino acids besides alpha lipoic acid make up some part of the Garnett formulation.

"Patients I've observed taking Poly-MVA have thrived. Numbers of them are following its protocol now. In my opinion Dr. Garnett and Dr. Sanchez are providing a really well thought out, safe treatment for all types of malignancies. They should be commended," affirms Dr. Stanley R. Olsztyn.

Poly-MVA is manufactured as a liquid mostly for oral ingestion, although some physicians administer it intravenously (see the procedure reported below by David C. Korn, MD(H), DO, DDS, of Apache Junction, Arizona):

"Since PC Spes [a popular prostate cancer treatment] was removed from the market by the FDA almost two years ago, I have substituted the administration of both intravenous and oral Poly-MVA for prostate cancer patients and found it to act effectively. After receiving the new product IV for six or eight weekly injections and simultaneously taking the liquid in water, my male patients find their prostate specific antigen (PSA) markers come down. They go on to take the oral liquid Poly-MVA alone for approximately ten or twelve weeks more. This protocol affords great results. Recently two of my patients dropped down to a PSA of one from much higher markers.

"I believe that saturating the blood with Poly-MVA insures the nutrient's elevated dosage swiftly penetrates into the prostate area, the brain, and other organ sites. The patient with blood saturation of Poly-MVA goes through a physiologic range of reactions illustrated by an elevation of body temperature. I administer the treatment for lymphoma, brain cancer, breast cancer, prostate cancer, and more.

"Insulin potentiation therapy works well in conjunction with Poly-MVA. But for elderly men with bone pain from prostate metastases who are frail, my preference is to administer the Garnett treatment alone. It acts just like a 'smart bomb' for pain relief, requiring four or five hours of the IV Poly-MVA. Based on an educated estimate of tolerated IV liquid, my staff and I gradually increase the dosage to 15 or 20 cc. I additionally include vitamin E, CoEnzyme Q10, lycopene, saw palmetto, and other prostate-specific nutrients.

"My impression is that the Poly-MVA molecule actually behaves like a mild chemotherapeutic agent, but it is safe and not destructive. Moreover, the Lipoic Acid Palladium Complex is highly effective for increasing cancer remission rates," confirms Dr. Korn.

From the established therapeutic effects of its alpha lipoic acid/palladium complex, Poly-MVA provides at least 13 recognized anticancer benefits. The benefits are listed here from observations described by Dr. Merrill Garnett in a series of reports published on his animal studies conducted at the Garnett McKeen Laboratory. He has advised that the lipoic acid/palladium complex:

- Causes an indefinite variety of immune system responses, but with specific manifestations as indicated in the twelve additional attributes listed below.

- Seeks out and destroys cancer cells anywhere in the body by stealing their electromagnetic energy.

- Invigorates normal cells and helps to repair any damage the invasive cancer may have left behind.

- Reduces tumor size or causes the tumor to shrink.

- Produces an idiosyncratic set of effects, which include a pattern of lag-arrest-slow death of cancer cells from an inhibition of their energy metabolism.

- Prevents sterol biosynthesis, thereby preventing new cancer cell plasma membrane synthesis.

- Shows a very large fraction of sensitive cancer cells as a morphological feature.

- Promotes the growth of proliferating normal cells surrounding a core of central tumor necrosis consisting of dead cancer cells.

- Stimulates the infiltration of leukocytes for the removal of cancer cell debris.

- Has absolutely no toxic reaction and no adverse side effects.

- Accomplishes its therapeutic benefits in both animals and humans.

- Works against cancer of many types not only as an orally-administered liquid but also perhaps even more effectively as an intravenous injection.

- Reduces the incidence of cachexia( (the "wasting away" characteristic of cancer patients) with a potential for increased body weight

The late oncologist Dr. Rudy Falk's original anticancer usage protocol strictly for cancer prevention consisted of only 1/2 teaspoonful a day of Poly-MVA. For therapy, a new and updated Poly-MVA protocol is now enthusiastically recommended by the Advanced Medicine and Research Center (AMARC) of Chula Vista, California. The protocol is presented in a publication written by Albert Sanchez, Sr., PhD, EdS, and made available by AMARC.

From the http://www.polymvasurvivors.com website:

"As noted in the letters below, oncologists & physicians are reporting the benefits of Poly MVA when used in conjunction with conventional cancer treatments or as part of other protocol therapies. These physicians are reporting complete remission of aggressive, stage IV cancers that have metastasized as well as continued positive responses in other patients with previously chemo-resistant cancers. Other noted benefits have been significantly improved quality of life and a substantial reduction in the number and severity of side effects from chemo and radiation therapies."

The Cancer Screening & Treatment Center of Nevada, for example, reported a 70% Positive Response Rate in Stage IV Cancer Patients At the same website, the Four Corners Approach is described that apparently has proved very effective for cancer survivors, including those who had been deemed late-stage:

- Destroy anaerobic (cancer) cells

- Improve the immune system

- Detoxify the body

- Reverse acidosis (low body pH)

### Further Reading & References

- Poly-MVA: Palladium Lipoic Complex, http://www.polymva.com/ (Note: For informational purposes only; not an endorsement)

- http://www.polymvasurvivors.com/

- Townsend Letter for Doctors and Patients, Feb-March, 2003: Cancer remission rates increase from use of the safe and effective lipoic acid palladium complex poly-MVA - Medical Journalist Report of Innovative Biologics." http://www.findarticles.com/p/articles/mi_m0ISW/is_2003_Feb-March/ai_97994368

- *Diseases,* 2nd Edition. (Springhouse, Pennsylvania: Springhouse Corporation, 1997), pp. 362-364.

- Sanchez, A. *What You Must Know to Overcome Cancer.* (Chula Vista, California: ARMARC, 2001), pp. 51-54.

- Garnett McKeen Laboratories: *Nucleotide reductase.* U.S. Patent No. 557,637 (October 31, 1995).

- Diamond, W.J.; Cowden, W.L.; Goldberg, B. *An Alternative Medicine Definitive Guide to Cancer.* (Tiburon, California: Future Medicine Publishing, Inc., 1997).

- Garnett, M. *First Pulse: A Personal Journey in Cancer Research,* Second Edition. (New York, New York: First Pulse Projects, Inc., 2001).

- *Poly-MVA Cancer Breakthrough: Palladium Lipoic Complex.* (Chula Vista, California: AMARC, 2001), p. 4.


# Protomorphogens

Dr. Royal Lee's achievement, *The Theory of Protomorphology,* was published in 1947. One enigma in biology that has perplexed scientists for years is how living cells not only repair areas of damage but do it with such precision. In his book, Dr. Lee discusses how he pioneered a unique method of deriving extracts from the "cell determinants" of specific organs and glands for clinical use. Dr. Lee described in detail what these extracts contained and how they functioned with respect to cell regulation, maintenance, and interaction with tissue antibodies.

"Protomorphogens are the tiniest specks of life made specifically by your body for each kind of tissue and are necessary for the control factors involved in disease."

According to Dr. Lee, the protomorphogen (PMG) is the fundamental building block of cell life. It is not DNA or RNA. Nor is it, in its simplest state, a protein, or nucleoprotein. It is a "template" or spatial pattern that determines the production of nucleoproteins or other proteins. This primary unit is cell specific, not species specific. For example, liver protomorphogen is specific as a pattern for liver cell activity. A protomorphogen, properly extracted, is the same throughout all mammalian species. Because it is a mineral substrate, it is indestructible. This theory is not accepted by mainstream medicine.

When an organ develops cancer, the PMG "blueprint" is altered. Cell reproduction becomes uncontrolled. Dr Royal Lee founded Standard Process Labs in Wisconsin (selling only to health care professionals) and patented over 75 PMGs from animal tissue (animals raised organically). In early studies, it was shown that taking PMGs orally (the specific organ PMGs for a specific cancer, *e.g.,* pancreatic PMG for pancreatic cancer) initiated a healing of that organ. Any dietary therapy must contain PMGs and eliminate sugars and all processed foods. The only source of PMGs specifically for an organ that has cancer is from a distributor of Standard Process Labs, or Dr Bruce West.

### Further Reading & References

- *Protomorphology: The principles of cell auto-regulation* by Royal Lee (1947)

# Revici Therapy

Dr. Emanuel Revici developed an original approach to the treatment of cancer. His nontoxic chemotherapy uses lipids (fats), lipid-based substances, and essential elements to correct an underlying imbalance in the patient's chemistry. Lipids, organic compounds such as fatty acids and sterols, are important constituents of all living cells. They are a separate, critical system in the body's defenses against illness, according to research conducted by Dr. Revici early in his career.

The Romanian-born physician applied his wide-ranging discoveries for over sixty years to the treatment of cancer as well as many other disorders, including AIDS, arthritis, Alzheimer's disease, chronic pain, drug addiction, schizophrenia, allergies, shock, and burns.

He based his treatment on correcting an imbalance between fatty acids and sterols in the cancer patient. His approach is called "biological dualism". Revici was considered a very dedicated physician. Among other achievements, he was an early advocate of and developer of selenium as an anti-cancer agent. The effectiveness of selenium is now widely acknowledged.

Dr. Revici viewed health as a dynamic balance between two opposing kinds of activity that occur in all living systems. One process, known as the anabolic or constructive, fosters the growth and build-up of natural patterns. The other process is catabolic, or destructive, involving the breakdown of structure, the liberation of energy, and the utilization of stored resources.

According to Dr. Revici, a long-term predominance of either activity leads to abnormality and disease.

In his "guided lipid" therapy with cancer patients, Revici found two basic patterns of lipid imbalance - one, the result of an excess of sterols, and the other, the result of an excess of fatty acids. Sterols are solid unsaturated alcohols such as cholesterol. In treating cancer, the physician would first check whether the anabolic or catabolic phase of activity is currently progressing unchecked. Then lipid-based compounds to renormalize the balance between the body's opposing forces, were administered.

Revici describes the body's overall defense system as consisting of four successive phases. When an antigen, or foreign substance, such as a virus or microbe, enters an organism, it activates the defense system. In the first phase, the antigen is broken down by enzymes. This is followed by the lipidic phase, followed in turn by the coagulant antibody phase, and succeeded finally by a phase mediated by globulinic antibodies able to neutralize the antigen fully.

The key point about this defense system is that a new phase does not start until the previous phase has been successfully completed. At any point where the agents available are qualitatively insufficient to defend against the noxious influence, the sequence breaks down. Then the body overcompensates by manufacturing excessive amounts of the defense agents from the breakdown point, and it does not progress to the next phase. Revici found that most chronic diseases, including cancer, are characterized by such abnormal conditions. When the body's defense is arrested in the lipidic phase, either fatty acids or sterols are produced in abnormally large quantities, leading to a variety of disorders, including cancer.

Patients diagnosed with an excess of sterols are treated with fatty acids to correct the imbalance. Conversely, patients found to have a predominance of fatty acids are treated with sterols and other agents.

This "biologically guided chemotherapy," as Dr. Revici called it, is highly individualized to suit each person's specific metabolic character and condition.

"There are simply no two cancers which are alike, just as no two individuals are alike," he said. Revici's research demonstrated that lipids have an affinity for tumors and other abnormal tissues. Because of this, the lipids or lipid-like synthetic compounds administered to the patient, either by mouth or injection, travel directly to the tumor or lesion. Cancerous tissue is abnormally rich in free lipids, and the lipidic agents introduced into the bloodstream are readily taken up by the tumor.

Revici's nontoxic cancer therapy has been denied both fair testing and funding in the United States, though it has been studied and put into practice in France, Italy, and Austria.

An unpublished study of the 1,047 cancer patients treated with the Revici regimen between 1946 and 1955 was made by Robert Ravich, M.D., who worked closely with Revici. Most of the patients were far advanced or terminal and most had received prior conventional treatment. Of the 1,047 cases, Ravich found that 100 had favorable response (objective and subjective); 11 had objective response only; 95 had subjective response only; 296 showed no response; and 545 had equivocal or undetermined response (380 of this last group were treated for less than three months).

At the federal level, New York Congressman Guy Molinari held an all-day hearing in March 1988 to address the Revici matter and the whole field of alternative cancer therapies. Dr. Seymour Brenner, a respected radiation oncologist in private practice in New York, testified on Revici's behalf. He had investigated a number of patients in very advanced stages of cancer, incurable by orthodox means, whom Revici had put into long remissions.

Dr. Brenner stated, "Dr. Revici has cured many people of cancer who were otherwise considered incurable. It is my professional opinion that his medicines have worked for many of the patients whose records I have examined."

### Further Reading & References

- *The Doctor Who Cures Cancer* by William Kelley Eidem. (1997)

- *Cancer and Consciousness*, by Barry Bryant, Sigo Press (1990)

- *Research and Theoretical Background for Treatment of the Acquired Immunodeficiency Syndrome (AIDS)*, by Emanuel Revici, M.D.,

- *Townsend Letter for Doctors*, vol. 45, February-March 1987. Contains an indepth discussion of aspects of Revici's treatment for cancer and AIDS.

- Emanuel Revici, MD.: *A Review of His Scientific Work*, by Dwight L McKee, M.D., Institute of Applied Biology, 1985.

- On Emanuel Revici, M.D. by Marcus A. Cohen, Institute of Applied Biology, 1988. Typescript. A valuable source of information on Dr. Revici's life and work.

- Dwight L. McKee, M.D., Emanuel Revici MD.: A Review of His Scientific Work (New York: Institute of Applied Biology, 1985), p. 14.

- Marcus A. Cohen, "On Emanuel Revici, M.D.," unpublished manuscript, 1988.

- Robert Ravich, "Revici Method of Cancer Control. Evaluation of 1047 Patients with Advanced Malignancies Treated From 19461955," unpublished manuscript, undated.

- Revici Therapy, http://www.whale.to/cancer/revici.html

# Sam Biser Treatment

Sam Biser provides a Resurrection Course from his website. He states: "I unmask the dogma of healers, so that those defeated by wrong programs can surge back from the 'dead'."

Here are samples of Sam Biser's discoveries with respect to a cured breast cancer patient: "Breast cancer is a weed that can return to the other breast or to other organs — when its root remains, and that root is defeat: someone or something broke a woman's heart. Doctors cure breast cancers with drugs; alternative healers use herbs; no-one fixes down-deep damage that makes breast cancer return.

"I specialize in defeated people, because for years, I was one, and this website, and my Resurrection Course, are created for such people. Defeated people get the same cancers and diseases as anyone else, but they are more likely to have a reoccurrence, because sitting underneath where their tumors used to be is an active root — a defeated chemistry.

"Defeat begins in a broken spirit — but ends up in the tissues, where all emotions go, and to cure it, I have found that you have to go beyond all the healers's books and programs …

"Emotions are tied to tumors. These emotions have to be extracted as well as the cancer tumor.

"Willpower and alternative healing alone will not reverse a defeated cancer-forming chemistry, but the programs in my Resurrection Course were created specifically for broken people, a group of people who are NOT like others; they are the people I love, the only people I care to write for."

### Further Reading & References

- Cures From The Last Chance Clinic by Sam Biser

- Curing With Cayenne: The Untold, Unknown, and Unpublished Facts About How to Cure with the Greatest Herb of All Time! by Sam Biser (1997)

- Sam Biser's Layman's Course on Curing Last Stage-Diseases, 12 Videos featuring Dr. Richard

- Schulze, includes a 1,370 page manual – Look on E-Bay for these videos. (Previously known as The

- Save Your Life Video Collection)

- Sam Biser: Legendary Health Journalist, http://www.sambiser.com/

# Water Therapy

Water therapy is a simple method to cleanse both the body and mind from toxins. Advocates report that patients who do water therapy get more benefits than one would expect, considering how simple the remedy is. At the physical level, various diseases are healed and at the mind level many negative habits just fade away.

Water therapy is an adjunctive approach that can be used with almost any other approach. According to its advocates, most patients do not drink enough water. Up to 70% of the total body weight is due to water. Normally, our daily diet provides about two-thirds of the body's requirement of water. Some health practitioners suggest that you drink about eight to ten glasses of water every day to meet the remaining one-third of the body's requirement. You may need to drink more water when you are tired, sweating profusely, or when your body has a condition such as cancer.

Some recommend not drinking water while eating food, as the water can dilute the digestive juices in the stomach, thus leading to indigestion. Many recommend the following water cure, including F. Batmanghelidj, M.D., who wrote the book *Your Body's Many Cries for Water*. Dr. Batmanghelidj believed human thirst was a warning signal of disease and labeled the various states of disease as stages of dehydration.

Dr. Batmanghelidj also believed one can't rely on *feeling* thirsty but rather must take pre-emptive action to prevent dehydration before feeling thirsty. By the time a person has a dry mouth, it's already too late.

According to Dr. Batmanghelidj, drinking only after receiving the sign of thirst may be the biggest medical or health mistake people routinely make. He outlined the four false assumptions people make that all tie into this one mistake:

- Treat dry mouth as the only sign of dehydration. In fact, there are many signals of dehydration besides a dry mouth.

- Assume water has no actual chemical properties. In fact, nothing taken orally can even hope to be utilized without water.

- Presuming the body is able to regulate water intake throughout the life span. In reality, older people tend to become dehydrated more quickly without realizing it.

- Assuming any fluid can replace water. Soda, caffeinated coffee, and tea make poor substitutes for water. Coffee and tea are diuretics, *i.e.* they promote urination. Alcohol and caffeine dehydrate the body and flush more water out than they add.

Without enough water to get rid of toxic waste build-up, dehydration quickly manifests in the form of allergies, asthma, and many other diseases.

Dr. Batmanghelidj holds that a 200 pound person needs 100 oz. throughout the day to eliminate toxic waste. That's 12½ cups a day -- far more than the 8 cups often recommended. People who are physically active or live in a hot climate need more than 100 oz. The same is true for people who consume caffeinated coffee or tea, sodas, or alcoholic beverages.

Many water therapy advocates also suggest starting the day with up to five or six glasses of water and then waiting at least an hour before eating or drinking anything. It's best to start slowly and build up to this if the body isn't accustomed to high levels of water consumption.

Some advocates believe it is important to drink water that has not been fluoridated, while other proponents suggest either oxygenating the water or alkalizing it. Ionized water is very alkaline (if your ionizer makes the water alkaline), has a high redox potential (i.e. it is a good antioxidant because its oxidation reduction potential value is very negative), and its water molecules exist in smaller clusters than those typical of normal water. All of these things help inhibit the spread of cancer and aid in killing cancer cells, directly or indirectly, according to advocates of this therapy. However, there is not enough evidence to consider water therapy a stand-alone treatment.

Here is one version of The Water Cure Recipe, according to the Cancer Cure Foundation*:

- Drink 1/2 your body weight of water in ounces, daily. Example: 180 lb body weight implies a need for 90 oz. of water daily. Divide that into 8 or 10 oz. glasses to determine how many glasses you will need to drink, daily.

- Use 1/4 tsp. of salt (non-refined ocean or sea salt) for every quart of water you drink. As long as this isn't prohibited by your physician, you should be able to add the salt.

- Avoid drinks with caffeine or alcohol as they can dehydrate you. Every 6 oz. of caffeine or alcohol requires an additional 10 to 12 oz. of water to rehydrate you.

*Further Reading & References*

- *Cancer Cure Foundation: Water Therapy, http://www.cancure.org/water_therapy.htm

- *Your Body's Many Cries for Water* by F. Batmanghelidj (2008)

- *Water: For Health, For Healing, For Life: You're Not Sick, You're Thirsty!* by F. Batmanghelidj (2003)

# Oxygen Therapies/Hyperoxygenation/ Oxmedicine/Oxidative Therapy/Oxidiology

## Exercise with Oxygen Therapy (EWOT)

Exercise with Oxygen Therapy (EWOT) was developed by Manfred von Ardenne, a German researcher and applied physicist. Von Ardenne believed that any type of stress on the body resulted in a decreased level of oxygen absorbed into the blood. In turn, this decreased oxygen in the body's tissues.

EWOT consists of doing light exercise, such as on a treadmill or stationary bicycle, while breathing pure oxygen. EWOT helps to increase the oxygen level in both the blood and plasma, along with the tissues.

After 15 minutes of EWOT, a patient's skin often begins to gain color, known as "pinking up." The likely explanation for this is that tiny capillaries throughout a patient's body are successfully transporting extra oxygen through the cells of the body. Following an EWOT treatment, some report that vision, mental clarity, and energy levels improve noticeably.

The premise behind EWOT as a cancer treatment is that an oxygen deficiency at the cellular level contributes to chronic illness. From there, cancer develops.

This theory is inspired by two-time Nobel Prize winner Dr. Otto Warburg's findings that cancer loves a low-oxygen environment and cannot exist in an oxygen-rich environment. Some advocates of EWOT claim that chemotherapy and radiation actually encourage the growth of cancer because both interventions rob the tissues of oxygen.

Most EWOT patients participate in multiple sessions over a short period of time; longer if they are suffering from chronic illness. A doctor first assesses the patient's level of physical fitness, and then starts the patient out with mild exercise such as a stationary bicycle or elliptical exerciser. The patient breathes oxygen from an oxygen concentrator while performing the exercise.

It is possible to perform this treatment at home, but the biggest problem lies in getting access to an oxygen bottle. In most states, a doctor's prescription is needed.

Advocates feels EWOT is an excellent preventive tool when it comes to cancer and that it also promotes an improved environment for recovery from the illness.

### Further Reading and References

- *Oxygen and Aging* by Majid Ali, M.S.

- *Stop Aging or Slow the Process: How Exercise with Oxygen Therapy (EWOT) Can Help* by William Campbell Douglass II

- EWOT: Exercise with Oxygen Therapy http://www.advancedinjurycenter.com/2009/08/ewot-exercise-with-oxygen-therapy.html

- EWOT - Exercising with Oxygen Training: http://www.breathing.com/articles/ewot.htm

# Hydrogen Peroxide

Hydrogen peroxide (H2O2) is similar in chemical structure to a water molecule ($H_2O$), except it has an extra oxygen atom. In most households, hydrogen peroxide is used to disinfect small wounds and for other first aid needs.

Hydrogen peroxide is a very common substance and forms naturally in the ozone layer near the outer limit of the earth's atmosphere. Ozone is made up of three oxygen atoms ($O_3$). Ozone is a rather unstable atom and readily gives up one of its oxygen atoms to falling rainwater ($H_2O$), turning that water into hydrogen peroxide (H2O2).

Rainwater has been proven to be more effective in growing plants than tap water, an effect that advocates attribute to hydrogen peroxide. Some farmers even increase crop yields by spraying diluted hydrogen peroxide on their crops.

The white blood cells in the human body are able to make hydrogen peroxide themselves, and do so to oxidize and fend of invading infections.

New research has demonstrated several chemical reactions that take place in the body do so with the help of hydrogen peroxide. Friendly bacteria, such as those found in the colon and vagina, flourish in oxygen-rich environments and so thrive around hydrogen peroxide. Most types of harmful bacteria, on the other hand, cannot survive in the presence of oxygen-rich hydrogen peroxide.

As a cancer treatment, H2O2 is ingested orally or administered intravenously in extremely diluted amounts. Advocates find this a safe, cheap way to treat illness, while opponents state that internal consumption of H2O2 can lead to serious illness or even death. It should be noted that only food grade H202 can be safely ingested, not the antiseptic hydrogen peroxide applied to external wounds to prevent infections.

When H202 is ingested in the body, research shows that the oxygen content of the blood and body tissues increases significantly. In fact, many nutritional supplements intended to help the immune system actually work by increasing cellular oxygen, an effect the supplements sometimes achieve through H2O2 formation. The effectiveness of H202 as well as oxygen-boosting supplements comports well the finding that cancer in the body is directly related to oxygen starvation.

Otto Warburg won the Nobel Prize for his discovery that cancer cells have different metabolic properties than normal cells. Healthy cells are aerobic; they use oxygen in most of their chemical reactions. Cancer cells have reverted to a more primitive metabolic process, called fermentation, which is anaerobic, meaning without oxygen. This means that cancer cells thrive in a low-oxygen environment.

The main energy source for both normal and cancer cells is glucose. However, a cancer cell's anaerobic processing of glucose yields only one fifteenth the energy per glucose molecule, compared with normal cellular metabolism. This is why cancer cells have such a huge appetite for sugar (glucose).

One possible way in which hydrogen peroxide can treat cancer is by releasing pure oxygen in the body. By saturating the cells and tissues with oxygen, hydrogen peroxide promotes healthy, oxygen-based metabolism.

There is a specific $H_2O_2$ program which should be administered and regulated by a physician. It makes use of highly diluted doses of H202, determined by patient symptoms, body weight, and sensitivity to the remedy. The hydrogen peroxide can be administered orally or through IV therapy depending on the severity of the patient's illness.

There are a variety of products on the market, including a hydrogen peroxide Toddy, a tooth gel, a pain gel, a nasal spray and even eardrops. The drugstore variety of H2O2 should never be used internally, because of the chemicals it contains as stabilizers.

A booklet titled *Oxidative Therapy*, published by the International Bio-Oxidative Medicine Foundation (IBOM), a non-profit educational foundation dedicated to supporting research and distributing information, and based in Dallas/Fort Worth, Texas, explains:

"The body uses oxidation as its first line of defense against bacteria, virus, yeast, parasites. It (oxidative therapy) is part of a system, which helps you use the oxygen you breathe. It is a hormonal regulator and is important in the regulation of blood sugar and the production of energy."

Walter Grotz, a proponent of hydrogen peroxide, claims that simple treatment with hydrogen peroxide has been extremely effective in treating even terminal cancer patients. Grotz has stated, ""Hydrogen peroxide is neither toxic nor carcinogenic. But treatment can be tough: it's not easy. I know everybody's looking for a silver bullet these days, but you have to go into it very slowly."

An impressive variety of new ways to introduce oxygen into the body are available, including pressure chambers, liquid oxygen, peroxide, chemical compounds, acid/alkaline balancing, injections, and ozone treatments. Flooding cells with oxygen may retard the growth of cancer cells or even help to return them to normal.

Hydrogen peroxide is now being used intravenously and intra-arterially by a number of doctors in the United States and many foreign countries. IBOM is supporting clinical research in this area.

### *Further Reading and References*

- *The Many Benefits of Hydrogen Peroxide* by Dr. David G. Williams, http://educate-yourself.org/cancer/benefitsofhydrogenperozide17jul03.shtml

- Hydrogen Peroxide Therapy http://drinkh2o2.com/

- *Medical Ozone and Cancer* by Ed McCabe, http://www.oxygenmedicine.com/cancerandozone.html

- *Flood Your Body with Oxygen* by Ed McCabe

- *Oxygen, Oxygen, Oxygen* by Dr. Kurt Donsbach

- *Unmedical Miracle Oxygen* by Elizabeth Baker

- *Hydrogen Peroxide: Medical Miracle* by William Campbell Douglass

- *Oxygen Healing Therapies: For Optimum Health & Vitality* by Nathaniel Altman

- Alternatives Newsletter by Dr. David G. Williams http://www.intelihealth.com/IH/ihtIH/WSIHW000/8513/34968/358849.html?d=dmtContent

- Ed McCabe, Medical Ozone and Cancer, at http://www.oxygenmedicine.com/cancerandozone.html

# Hyperbaric Oxygen Therapy

Hyperbaric oxygen therapy (HBOT) is a means of providing additional oxygen to the tissues of the body. This therapy is inspired by the two time Nobel Prize winner, Dr. Otto Warburg's findings that cancer loves a low-oxygen environment and cannot exist in an oxygen-rich environment.

Hyperbaric oxygen therapy is the primary mode of treatment for gas embolisms (dangerous air bubbles in the bloodstream), the "bends" (a type of gas embolism that occurs when a deep-sea diver surfaces too quickly), carbon monoxide poisoning, and smoke inhalation. It is also generally accepted as supplementary treatment for burns, gangrene, radiation injuries, chronic bone infections, compromised skin grafts, non-healing wounds, destructive soft tissue infections, exceptional blood loss, and crush injuries.

"Hyper" means increased, "baric" means pressure. During hyperbaric oxygen therapy, patients inhale 100% oxygen (versus 21% in the air we breathe) under pressures of up to two atmospheres (pressure at sea level is described as "one atmosphere"). Inhaling pure oxygen at high pressure effectively forces oxygen into tissues it would not normally reach, in large enough quantities to have therapeutic value. The most common environment for this treatment is a specially designed, airtight chamber used for one person only. Large HBOT facilities may feature a multiplace chamber room or series of rooms in which a group of people may receive treatment simultaneously.

Hyperbaric oxygen also has an antibacterial effect. It is poisonous to anaerobic bacteria (bacteria that live without oxygen). In addition, since much of the body's immune system is oxygen-dependent, high oxygen levels can give a boost to the cells that fight off infection, particularly deep in the tissues.

Though this hyperbaric oxygen is effective, ozone or hydrogen peroxide therapy is generally considered to be more powerful. The following statement from Saul Pressman on the question of cancer explains why.

"The answer to why hyperbaric oxygen does not stop cancer whereas ozone and H2O2 does stop it, is related to the nature of the cancer cell.

"Cancer cells are fermenting their sugar anaerobically. This is a wasteful and energy poor process, producing only 150 kjoules of energy. Aerobic oxidation of that same sugar would produce 2870 kjoules of energy for a good cell to use. So cancer cells are perpetually underpowered. This lack of energy means that, among other things, they cannot form the protective enzymes of superoxide dismutase, catalase and glutathione peroxidase. Without this protection, the cancer cell is susceptible to cell lysis (hole in the membrane) which destroys it.

"Oxygen on its own, even pressurised, has too little oxidising power to perform this cell lysis. Hydrogen peroxide has more power and can do the job. Ozone has even more oxidizing power and thus can do it even better. Hydroxyl, OH, is an even more reactive species, with even more oxidative power, which can do an even better job. But it is so powerful, that it causes damage to good cells too, so it is safer to stick with ozone, which is perfectly safe for internal use up to the concentration level of 60 ug/ml."

Hyperbaric oxygen therapy is available in some alternative cancer clinics. It is generally regarded as an adjunct therapy and not a standalone cancer "cure."

### Further Reading and References

- *Dr. Rosenfeld's Guide to Alternative Medicine.* Isadore Rosenfeld, MD. New York: Random House, 1997.

- *Hyperbaric Oxygen Therapy (Walker, Morton. Dr. Morton Walker Health Book.)* by Morton Walker, Richard Neubauer

# Ozone Therapy

Ozone is well known to be present in the upper levels of the earth's atmosphere. It absorbs solar radiation and is made up of three oxygen atoms, unlike the two-atom oxygen molecule that makes up most atmospheric oxygen. Ozone may halt the growth of cancer cells in humans.

To administer ozone, it may be mixed with water and taken by mouth or introduced into a body cavity such as the ear, colon, rectum, or vagina. This is called ozone insufflation. Proponents believe ozone air purification sterilizes and "rejuvenates" room air.

Cupping is a technique that concentrates ozone over a particular area of the body.

Auto-hemotherapy, another type of ozone therapy, is a technique in which blood is withdrawn through a vein, mixed with ozone gas and then injected back into a vein or muscle. Water enriched with ozone has been injected into joints to treat osteoarthritis and rheumatoid arthritis. Ozone or hydrogen peroxide may be injected. Blood may be withdrawn, enriched with ozone, treated with ultraviolet B radiation in a quartz container and then re-injected into the body.

Ozone-enriched water or vegetable oil may also be used to treat wounds, burns, infections and insect bites.

Ozone bagging is a technique in which the body (except for the head) is submerged for up to two hours in a bag containing ozone.

Ozone saunas and ozone-infused drinking water are also commercially available.

There are over 3,000 medical references in the German literature that show the effectiveness and safety of ozone in the course of more than 50 years of application to humans and millions of dosages. The International Ozone Association and the ozone machine manufacturers report over 7,000 doctors in Europe use medical ozone safely and effectively. Some have used it for more than 40 years, yet for the past 20 years, the FDA has prevented human testing and refuses to issue approvals for any ozone-generating device. In the U.S., ozone therapy is taught only by private instruction or in naturopathic schools.

The article by Ed McCabe, *Medical Ozone and Cancer*, at http://www.oxygenmedicine.com/cancerandozone.html is very informative and recommended reading. Here is an excerpt:

"There are no legitimate studies proving ozone doesn't work. It's so simple it befuddles the great minds. Unlike healthy human cells that love oxygen, the disease-causing viruses, bacteria, fungi and parasites-including the HIV and cancer virons, cancer cells, arthritis microbes, colds and flu, and West Nile virus carried by mosquitoes-like most primitive lower life forms, are almost all anaerobic.

"That means these microbes and cancer cells cannot live in high-oxygen concentrations. Therefore, what would happen to these anaerobic viruses and bacteria if they were to be completely surrounded with a very energetic form of pure oxygen for a long time? What if enough of this special form of oxygen/ ozone was to be slowly and harmlessly introduced into the body daily, over the course of a few months, to eventually saturate all the bodily fluids and every cell, including those of the brain, spine, and bone marrow, with it? Wouldn't the disease causing microbes and cells that can't live in oxygen cease to exist?"

### Further Reading and References

- *Flood Your Body with Oxygen* by Ed McCabe

- "Medical Ozone and Cancer," by Ed McCabe http://www.oxygenmedicine.com/cancerandozone. html

- *Oxygen-Ozone Therapy: A Critical Evaluation* by Velio Bocci

- http://www.intelihealth.com/IH/ihtIH/WSIHW000/8513/34968/358849.html?d=dmtContent

- Ed McCabe, Medical Ozone and Cancer, at http://www.oxygenmedicine.com/cancerandozone.html

- Ozone Therapy, http://www.intelihealth.com/IH/ihtPrint/WSIHW000/24479/34968/358849.html?d=dmtContent&hide=t&k=basePrint

- *"Extraordinary Science,"* by Thomas Levy, MD, Jul-Sep 1994

- *Bio-Oxidative Therapies for Treating Immune Disorders : Candida, Cancer, Heart, Skin, Circul* by Nathaniel Altman, Charles H. Farr

- *Oxygen Therapies : A New Way of Approaching Disease* by Ed McCabe

- *The Use of Ozone in Medicine* by Dr. S. Rilling, MD, and R.Viebahn, PhD.

- *The Use of Ozone in Medicine : A Practical Handbook* by Renate Viebahn

- *Oxygen Healing Therapies: For Optimum Health and Vitality* by Nathaniel Altman

# Superoxide Dismutase (SOD)

Each cell of the body has a personalized system for removing toxic matter. The key "cleansing tool" used for this process is the cell's network of enzymes and enzyme systems. These enzymes work to break down toxic materials and flush them out of the cell.

When there are more toxins than a cell's enzymes can handle, or when there aren't enough enzymes in the first place, cells are at risk to become cancer cells. Researchers are looking for ways to fix this problem and maintain a steady count of enzymes.

One enzyme in particular is a major power player in a cell's detoxification system: Superoxide dismutase (SOD). SOD scavenges for and dismantles one of the body's most deadly free radical toxins, superoxide.

Superoxide is a highly reactive particle that damages everything it comes in contact with in a cell. Surprisingly, the superoxide toxin is actually produced by cells themselves, as a byproduct of their metabolic process to produce energy.

Through a series of enzymatic reactions, cells strip away electrons in order to create energy. During the process, electrons attach to oxygen molecules and thereby create the toxic chemical, superoxide. This process of creating energy creates a handful of other toxic radicals too, such as hydrogen peroxide and hydroxyl radicals.

When these toxic radicals are produced, the body's natural supply of cell enzymes including SOD act to shield the cell and quickly eliminate the toxins before they harm the cells. SOD is an antioxidant – a powerful one that the body makes for itself – and the process just described is the familiar antioxidant-free radical reaction.

In addition to breaking down toxins created by cell metabolism, enzymes also neutralize toxins that enter the body by way of air pollution, smoking, or other forms of ingestion.

Each enzyme serves a specific function by attacking an assigned free radical. Superoxide dismutase, for instance, functions solely to attack superoxide and break it up into hydrogen peroxide and oxygen. Hydrogen peroxide itself can be a toxic radical within the cell environment, so another type of enzyme, catalase, is then tasked with decomposing the substance into water and oxygen.

Other cell enzymes are catalase, glutathione, and epoxide hydrolase.

Humans, mammals, and most chordates carry three forms of superoxide dismutase:

- SOD1 (located in the cytoplasm of cells)

- SOD2 (located in the mitochondria)

- SOD3 (extracellular)

In studies on mice genetically engineered to be without these enzymes, SOD was observed to have great importance. Mice without SOD2 died several days after birth from massive oxidative stress. Mice without SOD1 developed hepatocellular carcinoma (age-related muscle mass loss) as well as early-onset cataracts and a shortened lifespan. Mice without SOD3 did not show any noticeable defects.

**SOD's Healing Power**

The more scientists study SOD, the more benefits they find. The enzyme acts as both an antioxidant and an anti-inflammatory. As it breaks down superoxide particles into harmless substances (a process called dismutation), it neutralizes the free radicals and keeps them from damaging cells.

If cells are damaged, they suffer from what's called oxidative stress — which in turn leads to severe health problems including cancer.

The benefits of SOD are much more extensive than just cancer prevention. They include relief from arthritis, prostate problems, inflammatory diseases, burn injuries, inflammatory bowel disease, and fibrosis. Beauty suppliers enthuse about the enzyme and its ability to prevent wrinkles and hair loss. And for those who have cancer, SOD helps prevent damage and side effects from cancer therapy like radiation and chemotherapy.

Research for SOD and its relation to cancer dates back to 1979, when scientists at the University of Iowa noticed the lack of enzyme activity in cancerous cells, plus the proliferation of superoxides and other free radicals. They realized that tumors appeared to produce excessive amounts of superoxide free radicals, so the body's regular production of superoxide dismutase could not effectively compete.

- A 2004 study tested 44 breast cancer patients who developed fibrosis as a result of radiation therapy. An SOD treatment applied to the skin was found to reduce the size of the fibrotic area and significantly decrease pain levels in more than half the patients. The only side effect was one case of a localized allergic reaction.

- A skin cancer study on mice found that topical SOD cream relieved oxidative injury and proliferation of skin carcinomas without affecting the death of healthy cells. A joint study that used oral SOD treatment resulted in decreased tumor sizes by 33% to 57%.

In addition, a 1995 study on colorectal cancer tissue and the significance of superoxide dismutase activity published by the *Journal of Gastroenterology,* aneuploidy (chromosomal abnormality) was found to be high in cancer tissue with high SOD activity. Diploidy (double chromosomes) was high in cancer tissue with low SOD activity. Researchers also found that SOD activity in cancer tissue increased with the progression of each stage of cancer and changed with the depth of invasion. Results of the study suggested that increased use of SOD as an antioxidant defense in cancer tissue could improve cancer treatments.

In another study, manganese-based superoxide dismutase was found to suppress tumors in human prostate cancer. Still another study found that manganese-based SOD expression could suppress the malignant phenotype of human breast cancer cells, meaning as a gene it acts as a tumor suppressor for human breast cancer.

These results are promising, especially considering that SOD is a natural product of the body.

The challenge is that SOD levels decrease as people get older and can't compete with an excess of toxins. How can we best improve the count of SODs in the body if the body isn't making enough? And will synthetic versions be effective?

## Boosting the SOD count

The superoxide dismutase enzyme is one of the body's natural protectors, but there are many cases where additional SODs could help the body's detoxification process.

From a dietary angle, it's important to consume plenty of vitamins and minerals. In particular, vitamin C and copper are needed to help the body produce the natural antioxidant.

Eating more greens may be another way to raise SOD levels. Plants like barley grass, broccoli, wheatgrass, Brussels sprouts, and cabbage are rich in SOD, so eating these might help maintain steady production of superoxide dismutase. But it's not clear whether SOD existing in foods can survive the digestion process. Unfortunately, SOD can't hold up to stomach acid.

When cells need more SODs than they can make on their own, synthetic SOD may be helpful. Synthetic versions of the enzyme can be given by way of injection, topical cream, or oral supplement.

But because of the aforementioned problem with stomach acid, oral supplements should only be taken if they are enteric-coated (a coating that prevents absorption until a pill reaches the small intestine). The enzyme has to get past the stomach intact to reach the small intestine and be properly absorbed into the body.

Another important question is whether synthetic SOD is really as helpful as it could be. The research studies mentioned above about skin cancer and post-radiation breast cancer both used synthetic SOD treatments. Looking at their findings, it seems like synthetic treatments can be useful.

However, there's an opposing view on that matter. According to some authorities, synthetic SOD supplements signal the body to stop its own production of enzymes. This leaves patients reliant on the synthetic versions. More research is needed.

### *Further Reading and References*

- Khan MA, Tania M, Zhang D, Chen H (2010). "Antioxidant enzymes and cancer". Chin J Cancer Res 22 (2): 87–92. doi:10.1007/s11670-010-0087-7.

- Larry W. Oberley and Garry R. Buettner, Role of Superoxide Dismutase in Cancer: A Review1. April 1979. http://www.healthcare.uiowa.edu/corefacilities/esr/publications/buettnerpubs/pdf/cancerres-1979-39-1141-sod.pdf

- Mercola, Antioxidants Extend Lifespan

- http://articles.mercola.com/sites/articles/archive/2000/09/17/antioxidants-aging.aspx

- Mercola, This ONE Antioxidant Keeps All Other Antioxidants Performing at Peak Levels. http://articles.mercola.com/sites/articles/archive/2010/04/10/can-you-use-food-to-increase-glutathione-instead-of-supplements.aspx

- "Phenotypic changes induced in human breast cancer cells by overexpression of manganese containing superoxide dismutase." http://www.ncbi.nlm.nih.gov/entrez/query.fcgi?cmd=Retrieve&db=PubMed&list_uids=7761099&dopt=Abstract

- Robbins, Delira & Yunfeng Zhao. The Role of Manganese Superoxide Dismutase in Skin Cancer, 2010. http://www.sage-hindawi.com/journals/er/2011/409295/

- Satomi A., et al. "Significance of superoxide dismutase (SOD) in human colorectal cancer tissue: correlation with malignant intensity." J Gastroenterol. 1995 Apr;30(2):177-82. http://www.ncbi.nlm.nih.gov/pubmed/7773347

- "Superoxide Dismutase," Memorial Sloan-Kettering Cancer Center, http://www.mskcc.org/mskcc/html/69392.cfm

- Topical superoxide dismutase reduces post-irradiation breast cancer fibrosis, 2004. http://www.rehabco.com/pdfs/studyThermTopicalSuperoxide.pdf

- Venkataraman S, Jiang X, Weydert C, Zhang Y, Zhang HJ, Goswami PC, Ritchie JM, Oberley LW, Buettner GR. "Manganese superoxide dismutase overexpression inhibits the growth of androgenindependent prostate cancer cells." http://www.ncbi.nlm.nih.gov/entrez/query.fcgi?cmd=Retrieve&db=pubmed&dopt=Abstract&list_uids=15543233

- Yumin Hu, et al. Role in Cell Proliferation and Response to Oxidative Stress. http://www.jbc.org/content/280/47/39485.short

# Zell Oxygen

Zell Oxygen is a live yeast cell preparation beneficial in neutralizing free radicals. The preparation contains glutathiones, selenium, vitamins E, and C. Zell Oxygen is reportedly used in Europe and manufactured in Germany. It is said to improve oxygen utilization and keep intestines healthy by supporting the immune and nervous systems.

There is overwhelming scientific evidence that the body's inability to deal with numerous toxins is one of the main causes of cancer. If, as its supporters claim, Zell Oxygen furthers detoxification then it's undoubtedly useful.

Toxins, through several steps, interfere with cell DNA, rendering DNA repair mechanisms defective and inducing mutation. Toxic metals, such as mercury and dioxin, are linked to breast cancer, as are many types of pesticides used in agriculture. Thus if the body is to repair itself, the cancer patient needs to detoxify the cells and tissues by stimulating detoxification mechanisms and relieving toxin accumulation.

Enzyme yeast cells are said to:

- Detoxify, regenerate, and stimulate the small and large bowel

- Stimulate the liver detoxification process

- Reactivate the various biological and chemical processes in the body

Zell Oxygen purportedly contains active enzyme yeast cells that induce strong detoxification and elimination of toxic substances, stimulate the respiratory chain, and increase immune function. According to advocates, it also reduces blood clot formation and platelets, and therefore decreases inflammation, favoring microcirculation and oxygen supply to tissues.

Professor Jurasunas of Lisbon, Portugal, who has reportedly treated thousands of cancer patients, indicates in his study on Zell Oxygen that he has successfully treated numerous cases of anemia, chronic constipation, diabetes, Crohn's disease, and leukemia. He uses Zell Oxygen to reduce chemotherapy and radiotherapy side effects. He recommends the following mixture three times a day:

- 20ml Zell-Oxygen (1 vial)

- 10 ml liquid Chlorophyll (available from health food stores)

- 20 ml fresh red beet juice, Borsch (available in the kosher section of supermarkets)

- 100ml water (rinse vial with filtered water)

Professor Jurasunas says the chlorophyll will increase the oxygenation processes in the body by 20% and that this combination reduces the side effects of chemotherapy. The red beet juice is said to specifically enhance the respiration of damaged cells.

Proponents of Zell Oxygen also say that it increases the blood supply to the brain. It also helps the intestines and the liver, by promoting detoxification and restoration.

### Further Reading and References

- Zell Oxygen, http://www.regenerativenutrition.com/zell-oxygen-therapy-live-cell-yeast.asp (Note: for informational purposes only; not an endorsement.)

# Alkalizing Treatments

## Overview of Alkalizing Treatments

The acid-alkaline theory of cancer treatment enjoys widespread support in the alternative health community.

Herman Aihara, in his book *Acid & Alkaline*, states that:

*"If the condition of our extracellular fluids, especially the blood, becomes acidic, our physical condition will first manifest tiredness, proneness to catching colds, etc. When these fluids become more acidic, our condition then manifests pains and suffering such as headaches, chest pains, stomach aches, etc."*

Advocates of the acid-alkaline theory maintain that disease, and cancer in particular, cannot survive in an alkaline state. Instead, diseased cells thrive in acidic environments with extremely low levels of oxygen and a low pH level. In fact, the two factors always present when cancer cells exist are a lack of oxygen and a low (that is, acidic) pH level.

The abbreviation pH stands for "Potential hydrogen" and measures the hydrogen-ion concentration of any given solution. The pH scale of measurement goes from zero to 14. A number 7.0 is neutral while anything below a 7 is acidic and anything above a 7 is alkaline. A healthy pH level for human blood is 7.365 – slightly alkaline. Some researchers state that healing from chronic illness can only take place if the bloodstream pH levels are restored to normal, slightly alkaline numbers.

Various elements affect the body's pH level, including an acid-forming diet, emotional stress, and toxic overload.

When overcoming illness, it is vital to control the pH levels. With distorted pH levels, microorganisms are able to mutate and may become pathogenic. Enzymes that are normally beneficial can become destructive and delivery of oxygen to cells can decrease. These developments are believed to be the precursors to a host of degenerative conditions.

According to Keiichi Morishita in his *Hidden Truth of Cancer*:

*"If the blood develops a more acidic condition, then our body inevitably deposits these excess acidic substances in some area of the body so that the blood will be able to maintain an alkaline condition. This causes those areas to become acidic and lower in oxygen."*

As this tendency continues, such areas increase in acidity and some cells die; then these dead cells turn into acids. However, some other cells may adapt to the acidic environment. In other words, instead of dying —as normal cells do in an acid environment — some cells survive by becoming abnormal cells. These abnormal cells are called malignant cells.

### The importance of pH Balance

Testing pH is thought by some to be the most significant marker that a person can use daily to monitor his or her healing process. One of the important properties of a dietary approach to treating cancer relates to pH, since the theory is that "cancer cannot grow in an alkaline body."

pH paper is available from many sources including health food stores for about $10 for a 15-foot long roll. It's very easy for patients to measure their own pH. One simply tears a half-inch strip from the roll, wets it with saliva, and compares the color to the chart on the side of the box.

The most significant reading is taken in the morning upon rising and before eating or drinking. This simple test is said to provide a daily reading of the healing process. If one's body is acidic, it is not healing well. Although some people do not get good readings in the morning, they find that their pH is much better in the afternoon when they haven't eaten or drunk anything for two hours. Acid-alkaline measurement is an excellent indicator of progress in treating cancer effectively.

Two primary causes are said to make our bodies acidic: eating meat and stress. In some cases, if a patient deviates from a raw food and juice diet, the pH becomes acidic. After a day or two on a good diet, the body returns to a very healthy pH level.

According to German researcher Dr. Guenther Enderlein, total healing of chronic illness only takes place when and if the blood is restored to a normal, slightly alkaline pH. It is of vital importance to someone who is fighting a disease, overcoming an illness, or just desiring to feel better.

A number of supplements are said to render the body more acidic. The editors of this book have not verified these claims.

According to the book, *The pH Miracle* by Robert O. Young, Ph.D., ""The pH level of our internal fluids affects every cell in our bodies. The entire metabolic process depends upon an alkaline environment. Chronic acidity corrodes body tissue, and if left unchecked will interrupt all cellular activities and functions, from the beating of your heart to the neuron firing of your brain. In other words, over acidity interferes with life itself."

Dr. Young goes on to advocate the following steps:

- **Step 1**: Embark on a transition period in which acid foods are replaced with alkaline foods in the diet. He says that, except in the case of severe disease, which must be immediately and drastically addressed, a slow change in eating habits is more comfortable and is more likely to be maintained.

- **Step 2**: Cleanse ("detox") for one week using some supplements and a mild laxative.

- **Step 3**: Follow a strictly alkaline diet for seven weeks using nutritional supplements.

- **Step 4**: Maintain a diet with 79% to 80% alkaline foods plus a full range of other healthful foods.


His book has a list of acid and alkaline foods and a large selection of recipes and suggestions.

This book is one of many resources that advocate similar programs, which are also practiced in many alternative cancer treatment facilities. The need to alkalize the body can rightly be called a general, widely accepted alternative cancer treatment.

Another interesting book is *Alkalize or Die,* by Dr. Theodore A. Baroody. In Chapter One, he describes the difficulty of getting an accurate pH reading of the body by measuring the pH of urine, saliva, or other body fluids. He also describes how a healthy regimen can actually cause these pH measurements to indicate acid, during the period when the healing process removes the acid-causing materials from the body.

In subsequent chapters, he describes the extreme importance of the body's careful regulation of pH by releasing stored alkaline minerals to balance against the acid produced by an improper diet. He gives recipes, menus and other supporting information.

He describes his 80% alkaline-forming, 20% acid-forming diet, which he considers the ideal diet to restore health. In researching successful alternative healing systems, he discovered that all of them produce alkaline-forming reactions in the diet. He discusses the effects of stress, music, attitude, prayer, and other factors in determining our acid-alkaline balance.

This treatment is a combination of acid-neutralizing minerals like calcium and magnesium to supply proper mineralization and to correct the acid/alkaline balance of the body. Two proponents of this treatment are Carl J. Reich, M.D. and Bob Barefoot. In addition, another approach is the use of potassium, rubidium and especially cesium, which are alkaline elements. When taken, it is believed they alkalinize cancer cells (neutralize their acid nature). Cancer cells do not survive in the higher pH ranges and die off when the body is restored to its normal, healthy alkaline state.

Alkaline environments can absorb oxygen many more times than an acid environment, and as two-time Nobel Prize winner Dr. Otto Warburg proved, cancer cannot exist in an oxygen-rich environment.

### Further Reading & References

- *Acid & Alkaline* by Herman Aihara (1986)

- *The pH Miracle: Balance Your Diet, Reclaim Your Health* by Robert O. Young, Ph.D. (2002)

- *Alkalize or Die: Superior Health Through Proper Alkaline-Acid Balance* by Dr. Theodore A. Baroody (1991)

- Cancer Self-Treatment, http://www.alkalizeforhealth.net/cancerselftreatment.htm

- Complementary Medicine, http://www.alkalizeforhealth.net/complementarymedicine.htm

- "Alternative Cancer Therapies," The Cancer Cure Foundation, http://www.cancure.org/choiceoftherapy.htm

# Alkalize for Health 8-Part Program

The Alkalize for Health website has an 8-step plan to prevent and remove cancer that can be accomplished in the privacy of your own home.

The steps involve body-purification techniques and the creation of a high-oxygen, non-acidic environment that prevents the development of cancer.

Overview of the 8-Step Program:

- Give your body more oxygen

- Raise alkaline levels

- Lower free radicals

- Get more exercise

- Use hyperthermia (heat) to stimulate the immune system

- Supply your body with more enzymes

- Eat a nutrient-dense diet with vitamins B17, F, C, D, and glyconutrients

- Practice transcendental meditation

The emphasis behind this program is that it offers treatments patients can implement on their own to complement the treatments received from practitioners.

A complete description of the program and the logic behind each treatment step can be found on the Alkalize for Health website at http://www.alkalizeforhealth.net/cancerselftreatment.htm.

### Further Reading & References

- Cancer Self-Treatment, http://www.alkalizeforhealth.net/cancerselftreatment.htm

# High-pH Therapy/Dr A. Keith Brewer/Cesium Chloride

Otto Warburg won a Nobel Prize for showing that cancer thrives in anaerobic (without oxygen), or acidic, conditions. Research by A. Keith Brewer, PhD and H.E. Sartori has shown that raising the pH, or oxygen content, range of a cell to an alkaline range of 8.0 creates a deadly environment for cancer. Dr. Brewer found that the use of cesium chloride (CsCl) was an excellent way to boost alkalinity (i.e., oxygen levels).

The pH scale ranges from 0 to 14. Numbers below 7 represent acidic conditions while numbers above 7 represent alkaline conditions, also known as oxygenated conditions.

When cesium is taken up by cancer cells it raises the pH level of the cell, thereby boosting the oxygen content. The cancer cells die and are later eliminated by the body.

In 1984, Dr. A. Keith Brewer explored high-pH therapy through the use of salts of cesium and rubidium together with potassium supplements. He tested the therapy and found it effective on cancers in both mice and humans.

Dr Brewer's findings were described in the article "The High pH Therapy for Cancer — Tests on Mice and Humans." In the article, he reported tumor masses disappeared after several weeks of exposure to cesium chloride. He also stated, "The immediate effect of the cancer therapy is to lessen the pain and side effects of the tumor. This is a result of the cesium neutralizing the effects of toxic enzymes which leak out of the cancer cells … all pains and effects associated with cancer disappeared within 12 to 36 hours.

"There can be no question that [when] Cs and Rb salts [are] present in the adjacent fluids, the pH of cancer cells will rise to the point where the life of the cell is short, and that they will also neutralize the acid toxins formed in the tumor mass and render them nontoxic."

Dr. Brewer's patients ingested 3 to 6 grams of cesium chloride (CsCl) or rubidium chloride (RbCl) daily together with 2 to 4 grams of potassium chloride (KCl) and a variety of other nutritional supplements.

"The toxic dose for CsCl is 135 g. The administration of 6 g per day therefore has no toxic effects. It is sufficient however to give rise to the pH in the cancer cells, bringing them up in a few days to 8 or above where the life of the cell is short. In addition, the presence of Cs and Rb salts in the body fluids neutralizes the acid toxins leaking out of the tumor mass and renders them nontoxic."

The daily dose of mineral salts is divided into three parts, and consumed during or following each meal.

Dr. Brewer writes:

"Many tests on humans have been carried out by H. Nieper in Hannover, Germany and by H. Sartori in Washington, DC as well as by a number of other physicians. On the whole, the results have been very satisfactory. It has been observed that all pains associated with cancer disappear within 12 to 24 hr, except in a very few cases where there was a morphine withdrawal problem that required a few more hours. In these tests 2 g doses of CsCl were administered three times per day after eating. In most cases 5 to 10 g of Vitamin C and 100,000 units of Vitamin A, along with 50 to 100 mg of zinc, were also administered. Both Nieper and Sartori were also administering nitrilosides in the form of laetrile. There are good reasons to believe that the laetrile may be more effective than the vitamins in enhancing the pickup of cesium by the cells.

"In addition to the loss of pain, the physical results are a rapid shrinkage of the tumor masses. The material comprising the tumors is secreted as uric acid in the urine; the uric acid content of the urine increases many fold. About 50% of the patients were pronounced terminal [prior to this treatment], and were not able to work. Of these, a majority have gone back to work.

"Two side effects have been observed in some of the patients. These are first nausea, and the second diarrhea. Both depend upon the general condition of the digestive tract. Nieper feels that nausea can be prevented by administering the cesium in a solution of sorbitol. The diarrhea may, to some extent, be affected by the Vitamin C."

Dr. Brewer described one case history:

"A woman with 2 hard tumor masses 8 to 10 cm in diameter, one on her thyroid and one on her chest, was given 3 to 6 months to live. She had been subjected to chemotherapy, but was discontinued because it weakened her. She was taking laetrile on her own. She was given a 50 g bottle of CsCl and was told to take 4 g per day. She reported her case a year later. Being very frightened she took the entire 50 g in one

week. At the end of that time the tumor masses were very soft, so she obtained another 50 g of CsCl and took it in another week. By the end of that time she could not find the tumors, and two years later there was no sign of their return."

Similarly, he talked about the Hopi Indians of Arizona and natives in Central and South America:

"The incidence of cancer among the Hopi Indians is 1 in 1000 as compared to 1 in 4 for the USA as a whole. Fortunately their food has been analyzed from the standpoint of nutritional values. In this study it was shown that the Hopi food runs higher in all the essential minerals than conventional foods. It is very high in potassium and exceptionally high in rubidium. Since the soil is volcanic it must also be very rich in cesium.

"The Indians who live in Central America and on the highland of Peru and Ecuador have very low incidences of cancer. The soil in these areas is volcanic. Fruit from the areas has been obtained and analyzed for rubidium and cesium and found to run very high in both elements."

It is recommended anyone wishing to take cesium chloride should first consult with a physician, as the mineral must be supplemented by a balance of potassium in order to avoid developing conditions such as ventricular tachyarrhythmia.

### Further Reading & References

- *High pH Cancer Therapy With Cesium* by A. Keith Brewer, available from the A. Keith Brewer International Science Library, 325 N Central Avenue, Richland Center, WI 53581

- *The High pH Therapy for Cancer Tests on Mice and Humans*, first published in Pharmacology Biochemistry & Behavior, v.21, Suppl., 1, pp. 1-5, now available at http://www.mwt.net/~drbrewer/ highpH.htm

- Cesium Therapy, http://www.thewolfeclinic.com/cesium.html

# Enzyme Therapy

## Overview of Enzyme Therapy

Enzymes are of three types: those derived from food, digestive enzymes, and metabolic enzymes.

Food enzymes are abundantly present in all uncooked vegetables, fruits, and grains. They assist in the breakdown of the food in which they are present and perform other useful functions in the body. Food processing commonly employed today destroys nearly all of the enzymes normally present in foods. Whatever enzymes may remain after processing at the factory are destroyed at home in the cooking process.

Cooking by whatever means, except for very light steaming, will completely destroy all enzymes in food — even the foods that were enzyme-rich to start with.

Destroying the enzymes in food places an extra burden on the second group, the digestive enzymes. These are normally made by the pancreas, which produces a specific digestive enzyme for the breakdown and assimilation of each type of food we consume — lipase digest or break down fats, amylase digest carbohydrates or sugars, and proteases or proteolytic enzymes digest different types of protein.

Some familiar examples of proteolytic enzymes are the popular food supplements serrapeptase, bromelain, and papain.

Metabolic enzymes make up the third and most abundant group of enzymes in the body, and these function within the cell to regulate such activity as detoxification, oxygen utilization, and energy production, along with a multitude of life-sustaining and disease fighting functions.

There are over 3000 enzyme systems at work in the body. Performing a vast number of functions, these indispensable substances hold the keys to life. They assist greatly in the rebuilding of all tissues in the body by breaking down ingested protein into its component amino acids, which the body uses as building blocks for repair and rejuvenation. They attack waste materials in the blood and in the tissues, converting them into a form that can be readily eliminated, thereby acting as blood purifiers.

Raw foods are enzymatically rich, which means these foods have active enzymes within them to help digest 40 to 60% of that particular food. Cooked and processed foods are enzymatically dead or denatured, which means there are no active enzymes within that food to help with digestion of that food.

Enzymes also have an activating effect on the immune system and are believed to be an integral part of that system. Studies have shown that cancer is associated with severe deficiencies of many enzymes.

Leukocytosis is defined as an abnormally increased number of leukocytes, or white blood cells (WBCs), in the blood. The WBCs are the blood cells responsible for the immune response. According to Dr. Paul Kouchakoff, the major cause of leukocytosis is eating cooked foods. His research has helped us to understand what develops in the bloodstream when we eat cooked and processed foods.

Dr Kouchakoff's findings:

- Raw foods produce no leukocytosis.

- Commonly cooked food cause leukocytosis

• Man-made, processed, and refined foods, such as carbonated beverages, alcohol, vinegar, white sugar, flour and other foods, cause severe leukocytosis, and eating cooked, smoked, and salted animal flesh brought on violent leukocytosis consistent with ingesting poison

In summary, cooked and processed foods deny essential nutrients to the human body and contribute to illness.

Dr. Edward Howell was one of America's pioneering biochemists and nutritional researchers. His 50+ years of enzyme research shows that most physical problems and disease can be traced back to one source, improperly or not fully digested food. How can the human body function properly if it does not digest food properly?

Advocates of the enzyme theory believe that if the diet consists almost entirely of enzyme-dead, cooked and processed foods, the body's own production of digestive enzymes (by the pancreas) will become exhausted and depleted by the effort to digest food. Essentially the pancreas has to do all the work that should be done in part by enzymes naturally occurring in uncooked food. It's also thought that when digestive enzymes are depleted the body's thousands of metabolic enzymes are diverted to help digest food and are thus not available for their natural function of protecting and repairing the body.

Taking enzyme supplements with food will help digest that food. But enzymes, especially proteolytic enzymes, serve another function. When these digestive enzymes are taken on an *empty* stomach (two hours of no food) the benefits are enormous. Instead of being used to digest food, proteolytic enzymes taken on an empty stomach enter the blood stream and digest foreign bodies in the blood including (according to this theory) invading microbes and cancer cells.

Proteolytic enzymes circulating in the blood will digest any protein they encounter that is not produced by the body itself. The combination of taking digestive enzymes with food for proper digestion AND on an empty stomach thus helps cleanse the bloodstream. It means that the thousands of metabolic enzymes that protect and repair the body are no longer needed to clean up improperly digested nutrients and they can go back into the priority mode of protecting and repairing at full strength. In this priority mode, the protectors and repairers are ready and waiting to utilize the nutrients from the foods we eat and the supplements we take.

Taking enzymes on an empty stomach is reported to:

• Digest proteins

• Assimilate fats

• Increase energy

• Reduce bacteria

• Eliminate yeast

• Break up and dissolve uric acid crystals

• Raise T-Cell activity and production

• Stimulate the Immune System

• Shatter crystalline deposits

• Break up cholesterol deposits

• Increase the white blood cell size and activity

• Increase the surface area of the red blood cells, to carry more oxygen to all the parts of the body

At the Michael Reese Hospital in Chicago experiments were done on two groups of people. The first group was 21 to 31 years old. The second group was 69 to 100 years old. The researchers found the younger people had 30 times more amylase in their saliva than did the older people. This is why young people can handle a diet of sugar, bread, pasta, pastries, and cooked foods without much problem. But because it overworks the body's limited supply of pancreatic or digestive enzymes, this type of diet can cause rapid aging and depletion of our enzyme supplies. The older we get, the more we need enzyme supplementation.

Enzymes digest the cancer cell wall so that other agents can penetrate and kill the rest of the cell. Dr. William Kelley promoted an enzyme therapy that was expensive but, according to his extensive case study records, digested a tumor in four weeks. His work is carried on by Dr. Nicholas Gonzales. See **William D. Kelley**.

These powerfully active natural chemicals are protein-mineral complexes, which occur in all living things and make possible virtually all of the many biochemical reactions in the body. They are indispensable to life and to good health. Whenever there is a significant reduction in the presence or the availability of enzymes, sickness and degeneration begin.

The immune system depends heavily upon enzymes for all of its functions. They are essential to the performance of every function of every organ system in the body.

Many white blood cells produce and utilize enzymes as a necessary part of their function. Another cancer-fighter, the T-lymphocyte, attacks cancer cells in a similar manner, utilizing enzymes in its ability to dissolve and digest tumor cells. These fighters are part of a highly integrated system capable of recognizing cancer cells, then attacking and destroying them. Enzyme therapy is widely used by a great many alternative and integrative doctors who treat cancer patients.

Proteolytic enzymes from the pancreas have the unique ability to break down the muco-protein coating that encases all malignant tumors and protects cancer cells from attack by the body's immune system.

Enzymes also protect the body against cancer, particularly metastatic or spreading cancer, in other ways.

Pre-cancer cells become attached to body tissues by means of fibrin, a protein component necessary for blood clotting. Enzymes digest away the fibrin, preventing the attachment of pre-cancerous and cancerous cells to body tissues, thus releasing these abnormal cells into the circulating blood where they are normally destroyed by circulating enzymes or by the immune system fighters described above.

Some research has suggested that proteolytic enzymes such as bromelain, a protein-digesting enzyme derived from the pineapple, have the power to actually transform cancer cells into normal cells. This and other evidence seems to indicate that, in addition to their many other attributes, enzymes may have a directly normalizing effect on cancer cells.

This knowledge is not new. A century ago, Scottish embryologist John Beard, in spite of having little knowledge of enzymes, discovered that by taking pancreas tissue from young animals he could extract a liquid which was effective in causing tumor reduction.

Practicing in England, Dr. Beard would inject his pancreatic extract either directly into accessible tumors or into the muscle or vein of the patient. Even some advanced cancers considered to be incurable were made to completely disappear. He was reportedly able to help or even cure more than half his patients, most with advanced cancers.

His was a crude preparation, containing impurities and foreign proteins. It caused allergic reactions in some patients. For this, he was roundly criticized and attacked by his peers in the medical profession, not unlike organized medicine's attacks today on alternative physicians.

Dr. Beard's high rate of success in treating cancer patients led to such a demand for his pancreatic enzyme preparation, English physicians were hounded by their patients to be treated with this miraculous substance. Consequently, eight attempts were made to duplicate his preparation, with pharmacists obtaining pancreatic juice from local slaughterhouses.

The trouble was, the pancreases were taken from older animals with far less enzymatic activity than younger animals. Dr. Beard held that it was essential to extract enzymes from the pancreases of healthy young animals because they naturally had higher enzyme levels. The other factor that undermined attempts to duplicate his preparation was the simple passage of time. Enzymes have a relatively short "shelf life," especially if not stored properly.

Dr. Beard had been careful to use only freshly removed pancreases for his material. Thus, physicians who obtained material from slaughterhouses, pharmacists, couriers, etc. found the enzymes useless.

Since Dr. Beard's colleagues had no success with their inactive enzyme material, the concept and method of treatment sadly fell into disrepute and was largely forgotten. Fortunately, in 1907 Beard wrote a book about his experiences in treating cancer patients and his hypothesis of the causation of cancer, now known as the "trophoblast" theory, so his work was not completely lost to future generations.

But for nearly 50 years, there was no significant activity in the area of enzymes and cancer. The medical consensus of the day held that enzymes could not have anything to do with cancer, much less anything to do with curing it.

The next significant advocate of enzyme therapy was Dr. Max Wolf, a faculty member at Columbia University, New York. Dr. Wolf developed an interest in enzymes and cancer and wrote to all of the medical libraries in the US and much of the Western world, seeking information on the subject.

Reading virtually everything that had ever been written about the subject up to that time, Wolf became probably the world's leading authority on enzymes and their relationship to cancer. One of the books he managed to locate and read was John Beard's book, of which only a few copies remained.

Working at his research laboratory at Columbia in the 1950s, Wolf designed a complicated and extensive study of the effect of enzymes on cancer cells. Thousands of cell cultures were prepared with normal cells and cancer cells living and growing together. Each of these cultures was then treated with a particular enzyme or combination of enzymes to determine which was most effective in killing cancer cells while preserving normal ones.

A wide range of enzymes and enzyme combinations was tested in this way to determine which was the most effective against cancer cells, while safely avoiding damage to normal cells. Because of Wolf's connections in Germany (and because of the inhibiting presence of the American FDA), he moved to that country to carry out his clinical work. There he developed the final formula which showed highly favorable results when used to treat human cancer victims.

Dr. Wolf's particular mixture of enzymes survives to this day as Wobe-Mugos, which has been used to treat tens of thousands of cancer patients in Germany over the last 30 years. This enzyme formula, along with a companion product called Wobenzym, has also been used in the US by a few physicians, as well as in several Mexican alternative clinics.

Also available from Germany is an injectable preparation of Wobe-Mugos enzymes, reported to be quite useful in treating accumulations of fluid in the chest, called pleural effusions, when these accumulations are due to cancer. German practitioners have reportedly used this approach for many years with consistent success. Collections of abdominal fluid, called ascites, can be treated in like manner. In addition, any tumor which is accessible by needle may be treated with this material.

These and other similar enzyme products have a wide application in medicine, being effective against many inflammatory conditions, arthritis, autoimmune diseases, injuries, blood clots, and phlebitis, to name a few — as well as being a vital tool in the management and control of cancer.

Of the view of conventional medicine on the value of enzymes, preeminent cancer researcher Ralph W. Moss Ph.D. states:

"For years opponents of alternative medicine have argued that enzymes taken by mouth would be broken down in the stomach and inactivated before being able to do much good at all. This point of view was thoroughly refuted in 2002 when three physiologists at the University of California-San Francisco showed that digestive enzymes can be absorbed into blood, reabsorbed by the pancreas, and reutilized, instead of being reduced to their constituent amino acids in the intestines. This is called an enteropancreatic circulation of digestive enzymes (Rothman 2002). But clearly news of this established fact hasn't reached the implacable opponents of complementary medicine. For instance, an attack on the work of Dr. Gonzalez states, 'Like all dietary proteins, enzymes are dismantled into constituent amino acids by host proteolytic enzymes in the gastrointestinal tract, thus destroying their enzymatic activity'". (Green 1998)

### Further Reading & References

- Enzyme Therapy, http://www.cancer.org/Treatment/TreatmentsandSideEffects/ComplementaryandAlternativeMedicine/PharmacologicalandBiologicalTreatment/enzyme-therapy

- Dr. Gonzalez, Individualized Nutritional Protocols, http://www.dr-gonzalez.com/index.htm

- *One Man Alone: An Investigation of Nutrition, Cancer, and William Donald Kelley* by Nicholas J. Gonzalez, MD (2010)

- *The Enzyme Treatment of Cancer. London,* by J. Beard, Chatto and Windus, 1911.

- *Enzymes and Cancer* by Nicholas J. Gonzalez, MD (2008)

- *The Complete Book of Enzyme Therapy: A Complete and Up-to-Date Reference to Effective Remedies* by Anthony J. Cichoke (1998)

- "Proteolytic Enzymes in Cancer Invasion," *Journal - Enzyme and Protein*, Vol 49, No 1-3 by Liliana Ossowski, R.M. Lopez

- *The Multiple Proteolytic Enzyme Therapy of Cancer* by Dr. Frank. L. Shively (1969)

- *The Immortality Enzyme: Aging, Cancer & Heart Disease* by Phillip Minton (2001)

- *Oral Enzymes - New Approach to Cancer Treatment* by F. Klaschka (1996)

- *Enzyme-Pro-drug Strategies for Cancer Therapy* by Roger G. Melton (Editor), Richard J. Knox (1999)

- *Enzymes for Digestive Health and Nutritional Wealth: The Practical Guide for Digestive Enzymes* by Karen Defelice (2003)

- *Digestive Enzymes: The Key to Good Health and Longevity* by Rita Elkins (1998)

# Pancreatic Enzymes

A 2004 study on the effect of pancreatic enzymes on pancreatic cancer showed that this treatment significantly prolonged survival and slowed tumor growth.

Specifically, porcine pancreatic enzyme extracts, also known as PPE, were used on human pancreatic cancer xenografts in mice. The tumors of the mice treated with PPE became significantly smaller in size than those of the control group. These mice also showed lesser signs of problems like ketonuria and hyperglucosuria. Scientists concluded that PPE significantly prolonged the rate of mice survival, along with slowing tumor growth. It is believed the treatment gave the mice a nutritional advantage over untreated mice.

A number of commercial, over-the-counter enzyme formulas contain selected pancreatic enzymes derived from animals.

### Further Reading & References

- Pancreatic enzyme extract improves survival in murine pancreatic cancer. Saruc M, Standop S, Standop J, Nozawa F, Itami A, Pandey KK, Batra SK, Gonzalez NJ, Guesry P, Pour PM. Pancreas. 2004 May 28 (4):401-12. http://www.ncbi.nlm.nih.gov/entrez/query.fcgi?cm d=Retrieve&db=pu bmed&dopt=Abstract&list_uids=15097858

- Pancreatic Cancer, Proteolytic Enzyme Therapy and Detoxification, http://www.dr-gonzalez.com/clinical_pearls.htm

# Serrapeptase

Serrapeptase is a proteolytic (protein digesting) enzyme produced by certain bacteria that live in the intestinal tracts of silkworms. It is this enzyme that allows silkworms to burn a hole in the cocoon and exit, thereby moving from the larval to the winged stage. Serrapeptase effectively dissolves deadened tissue. It has anti-inflammatory, anti-edema, and fibrinolytic (fibrin dissolving) properties.

Serrapeptase was effectively used by Dr. Hans Nieper in the treatment of clogged coronary arteries. Dr. Nieper reported extensively on the benefits of dissolving layers of blockage within carotid arteries. This treatment meant patients could avoid the drilling or lasering of clogged arteries which often presented the risk of pushing debris into smaller cerebral vessels.

Since that time, Serrapeptase has been found to have powerful anti-inflammatory properties. It can help dissolve or digest blood clots, cysts, and arterial plaque and relieve inflammation of all forms. It is reported to be a faster-acting agent than EDTA chelation when it comes to the removal of arterial plaque.

In addition to its ability to improve blood flow, serrapeptase can help with general pain and healing. In terms of cancer treatment, the enzyme assists in the removal of dead tissue and reduction of inflammation. This makes it easier for the body's natural immune processes to attack cancer cells.

Serrapeptase is available as a nutritional supplement. Patients wishing to take it with other prescription drugs should first consult with a physician.

### Further Reading & References

- Serrapeptase Information, http://www.serrapeptase.info/

- Wellness Watchers MD, https://www.wellnesswatchersmd.com/feature_articles/protect_heart_reduce_inflammation_serrapeptase.php

## Vitalzym™

Vitalzym is a systemic enzyme supplement said to increase overall health and wellness. Systemic enzymes work within organs at the cellular level to fight chronic disease and inflammation. Vitalzym as part of enzyme therapy is intended to increase enzymes throughout the body and contribute to greater health.

Vitalzym is a blend of multiple systemic enzymes, including protease, bromelain, serrapeptase, amylase, lipase, and papain. It is manufactured in Japan by World Nutrition Inc. and is 100% vegetarian. The individual ingredients are found, alone or in combination, in many other commercial enzyme products.

Using Vitalzym as a supplement in conjunction with a healthy diet and exercise is said to help maintain the body's normal enzyme levels. In turn, this balances the body's immune functions.

Vitalzym appears to be relatively safe and has no common side effects. Enzyme supplements in general have few or no side effects. Proteolytic enzymes such as serrapeptase and bromelain act as blood thinners. People taking prescription blood thinning drugs such as Coumadin should consult a physician before taking proteolytic enzymes.

The World Nutrition website says, "Combined with professional healthcare, proper diet and exercise, Vitalzym may help you to maintain proper enzyme levels and balance your body's own repair mechanisms."*

The World Nutrition website also points out that Vitalzym can help reduce inflammation, remove scar tissue and excess fibrin in the blood, and modulate immune function. It has this in common with other enzyme formulas and is not unique.

### Further Reading & References

- Vitalzym Frequently Asked Questions, http://www.energeticnutrition.com/vitalzym/faq_vitalzym.html

- *Vitalzym, http://www.worldnutrition.info/vitalzym

## Wobenzym™/Wobe-Mugos™/Phlogenzym™

Wobenzym, Wobe-Mugos, and Phlogenzym are all closely-related formulations of systemic enzymes with anti-inflammatory and immune-enhancing properties. Wobenzym contains papain, a papaya enzyme, and the animal enzymes pancreatin, trypsin, and chymotrypsin, all secreted by the pancreas. Wobe-Mugos contains papain, trypsin, and chymotrypsin.

Wobe-Mugos, which evolved from an earlier formulation of Wobenzym, is backed by over 50 years of scientific and clinical research. Wobe-Mugos has been used in Europe as an adjuvant treatment to chemotherapy since 1977. Some of its reported benefits include improving the quality of life for patients, reducing symptom severity, and extending lifespan. Other cancer-related benefits, especially where radiation and chemotherapy are involved, include better retention of nutrients.

As an anti-inflammatory and a blood thinner, Wobenzym is commonly used to support joint health and boost circulation, particularly in relation to sports injuries.

Phlogenzym has also been found to be effective as a supplemental treatment to antibiotic therapy. In an experiment following pediatric patients with fevers, Phlogenzym was proven to reduce the time it took the fever to subside by a full day. This evidence supports the ability of the enzyme blend to improve immune function.

All three of these enzyme combinations can be found at health food stores or online supplement retailers.

### *Further Reading & References*

- "New hope for cancer patients," http://findarticles.com/p/articles/mi_m0ISW/is_243/ai_109946496/

- Chemotherapy With or Without Wobe-Mugos E in Treating Patients With Stage II or Stage III Multiple Myeloma, http://clinicaltrials.gov/ct2/show/NCT00014339

- "FDA Grants Orphan Drug Status To Wobe-Mugos For Multiple Myeloma," http://www.cancure.org/Wobe-Mugos.htm

- Phlogenzym Information, http://naturaldatabase.therapeuticresearch.com/nd/Search.aspx?cs=&s=nd&pt=103&id=23839&AspxAutoDetectCookieSupport=1

# Chinese Medicine

## Integrated Chinese and Western Medicine

Many practitioners say that traditional Chinese medicine, with no other therapies, can often treat cancer, pointing to success in cases that proved untreatable by Western medicine. Still, it's rare in the United States for anybody suffering from cancer to be solely treated by Chinese medicine.

"For patients who desire the expertise of a conventional oncologist as well as the benefits of more natural methods," says Roger Jahnke, a doctor of Oriental medicine and director of the Health Action Clinic in Santa Barbara, California, "Chinese medicine can provide an important collaborative resource to link with conventional cancer treatment. Even the National Geographic ran a series on Chinese medicine and cancer, with the remarks of senior oncologists from America. Patients should develop a healing team that could include the oncologist, a practitioner of acupuncture, and herbal pharmacology, and perhaps a nutritionist, psychologist and support group of some kind. The result is a more comprehensive and synergistic therapeutic effect."

When used in tandem with chemotherapy, Chinese herbal medicine can control and minimize the side effects of chemical drugs and may enhance their therapeutic effects. Herbs can also bolster immune-system functions depressed by radiation.

In China, surgery, chemotherapy, and radiation are considered viable treatments for benign and malignant tumors by physicians who are attempting to integrate Eastern and Western methods. Conventional treatments may be required to deal with an urgent situation within the time available to a seriously ill patient, notes Zhang Dai-zhao, a specialist in cancer treatment in Beijing.

Many practitioners in China say that the best results against cancer are obtained by means of a joint attack combining Oriental and Western medicine, with the patient pursuing a suitable diet, Chinese yoga, and therapeutic exercise.

In classic Chinese medicine, there is no specific concept of cancer, though there is of tumors. Many nutritive tonics and herbal medicines were developed to alleviate pain and prolong survival by strengthening the body's life forces and arresting tumor progression. Chinese doctors believe the causes of cancer are multiple, including toxins and other environmental factors, called "external causes," as well as "internal causes" such as emotional stress, bad eating habits, accumulated wastes from food, and damaged organs. Two main factors are stagnant blood and a blockage or accumulation of chi, or qi (pronounced chee). Chi is the vital energy said to circulate along the meridians, or pathways, linking all parts of the body.

Illness is believed to be an energy imbalance, an excess or deficiency of the body's elemental energies. According to the ancient Chinese, chi, the life force, controls the body's workings as it travels along the meridians, completing an energy cycle every twenty-four hours.

A person is healthy when there is a balanced, sufficient flow of chi, which keeps the blood and body fluids circulating and fights disease. But if the circulation of chi is blocked for any reason or becomes excessive or deficient, pain and disease can result. An imbalanced diet or lifestyle, overwork, stress, repressed or excessive emotions, or lack of exercise may disrupt the flow of chi. Imbalances in yin and yang — complementary forces in dynamic flux — also disturb the normal, smooth flow of chi.

In Chinese medicine, cancer, like all other diseases, is regarded as a manifestation of an underlying imbalance. The tumor is the "uppermost branch," not the "root," of the illness. Each patient may have a different imbalance causing what outwardly looks like the same type of cancer.

Each person is unique, so the Oriental doctor attempts to identify the exact individual pattern of excess, deficiency, or blockage that led to the disease. The doctor treats the imbalance rather than a local condition known as "stomach cancer," or "breast cancer," or so on. The prescribed treatment will vary from one patient to the next, depending on the specific imbalances. The Chinese doctor makes a diagnosis in terms of yin and yang, chi, blood, and organ imbalance.

Nearly all of the Chinese herbs used today to treat cancer and other immune-deficient conditions fall into three broad categories. They are often used in combination. Tonic herbs increase the number and activity of immunologically active cells and proteins. Toxin-clearing herbs clear the blood of germs and of waste products from the destruction of tumors and germs. Blood activating herbs reduce the coagulation and inflammatory reactions associated with immune response.

When seeking a doctor in the United States who practices Oriental medicine, cancer patients need to be aware of what doctors can do and what patients can learn to do for themselves.

According to Dr. Roger Jahnke:

"There are four basic things that the doctor of Chinese medicine can do for you: herbal prescriptions, acupuncture, massage, and external chi-gong. At least as important, however, are the things the doctor can teach you to do for yourself. These include guidance in the use of tonic or wellness herbs, in proper nutrition, and in devising a suitable exercise program that may involve activities like swimming or walking. A competent practitioner can also teach the patient self-applied massage, meditation and relaxation techniques, and chi-gong exercises. Finally, the doctor can offer guidance to help patients fulfill their unique spiritual purpose. Prospective patients should look for a doctor who provides all of these things, or one who can help patients network to all of these things, from body care up to the spiritual components of health."


### Further Reading and References

- *Chinese Medicine and Cancer http://www.healthy.net/scr/article.asp?id=2006

- *Between Heaven and Earth: A Guide to Chinese Medicine* by Harriet Beinfield, L.Ac., and Efrem Korngold, L.Ac. (1992)

- *The Web That Has No Weaver: Understanding Chinese Medicine* by Ted J. Kaptchuk (2000)

- *Traditional Medicine in Contemporary China* by Nathan Sivin (1987)

- *Chinese Medicine in Contemporary China: Plurality and Synthesis (Science and Cultural Theory)* by Volker Scheid, Barbara Herrnstein Smith, and E. Roy Weintraub (2002)

- *Traditional Chinese Medicine: An Authoritative and Comprehensive Guide* by Henry C. Lu (2005)

- *Total Health the Chinese Way: An Essential Guide to Easing Pain, Reducing Stress, Treating Illness, and Restoring the Body through Traditional Chinese Medicine* by Dr. Esther Ting and Dr. Marianne Jas (2009)

# Actinidia

"Actinidia is a root that contains the polysaccharide ACPS-R. In one study, when injected into mice, 90 percent of tumors stopped growing. Another study showed a 50 percent success rate with liver cancers."*

### *Further Reading and References*

- *The Herbal Approach: http://www.fightingcancer.com/download/fcpdf/19%20The%20herbal%20approach.pdf

# Chan Su/Toad Venom

Chan Su's active ingredient, bufalin, acts like the glycosides from nerium & digitalis. Bufalin has been shown to effectively induce apoptosis (natural cell death) of human leukemia cells, which is possibly one of the mechanisms for its anti-cancer effect.

### *Further Reading and References*

- "Preliminary study on apoptosis of human leukemic cells induced by bufalin'" Zhongguo Zhong Yao Za Zhi. 2001 Jan Xu RC, Chen XY, Chen L, Qian J. http://www.ncbi.nlm.nih.gov/entrez/query.fcgi?cmd=Retrieve&db=pubmed&dopt=Abstract&list_uids=12525125

- "Induction of apoptosis by bufalin in human tumor cells in associated with changes of intracellular

- concentration of Na+ ions," J. Biochem. 1999,126 pp. 278-86. www.ncbi.nlm.nih.gov/entrez/eutils/elink.fcgi?dbfrom=pubmed&cmd=prlinks&retmode=ref&id=10423518

# Fu Zhen Therapy

The leading cause of death in China is cancer, followed by stroke. Conventional Western cancer therapies—chemotherapy, radiation, and surgery—have been increasingly used since the 1960s in Chinese hospitals. However, the side effects of these treatments have been, there as here, often highly debilitating.

This has led the Chinese government to fund research into the traditional herbal medicines. One result is the routine use of Fu Zhen therapy, an immune-enhancing herbal regimen, as an adjunct to chemotherapy and radiation. Fu Zhen therapy is reported to protect the immune system from damage and to increase survival rates, sometimes dramatically, when used in conjunction with the modern cancer therapies. The principal Fu Zhen herbs strengthen the body's nonspecific immunity and increase the functions of T-cells. The most commonly used Fu-zhen herbs are astragalus, ligustrum, ginseng, codonopsis, atractylodes, ganoderma, actinidia and rabdosia.

Studies of Fu Zhen therapy in the United States and China have demonstrated its value in treating a wide range of immune-compromised conditions, including cancer, leukemia, AIDS and ARC, and chronic Epstein-Barr virus. In a study of seventy-six patients with Stage II primary liver cancer, twenty-nine of the forty-six people receiving Fu Zhen therapy in combination with radiation or chemotherapy survived for a year, and ten survived for three years.

Only six of the thirty patients who received radiation or chemotherapy alone survived one year, and all died by the third year. In laboratory studies, Fu Zhen herbs have prevented the growth of transplanted tumors.

### Further Reading and References

- Chinese Medicine and Cancer http://www.healthy.net/scr/article.asp?id=2006

- *Between Heaven and Earth: A Guide to Chinese Medicine* by Harriet Beinfield, L.Ac., and Efrem Korngold, L.Ac. (1992)

- *The Web That Has No Weaver: Understanding Chinese Medicine* by Ted J. Kaptchuk (2000)

- *Traditional Medicine in Contemporary China* by Nathan Sivin (1987)

## Golden Book Tea or Six Flavor Tea

"Doctors at the Beijing Institute for Cancer Research have found that an herbal tonic usually prescribed for kidney ailments, known variously as Golden Book Tea or Six Flavor Tea had a highly significant effect when combined with chemotherapy against small cell lung cancer."

### Further Reading and References

- The Herbal Approach, http://www.fightingcancer.com/download/fcpdf/19%20The%20 herbal%20approach.pdf

## Tang Kuei/Angelica sinensis

"The most highly praised blood tonic in the East, Tang kuei (Angelica sinensis), has been used clinically in China to treat cancer of the esophagus and liver with good results.

"The Chinese have claimed dramatic success using this herb both alone and in combination with other medicinal agents in treating cervical cancer and, to a lesser extent, breast cancer in women. It can be administered in either infusion or douche form. Many other Chinese herbs could be cited for their documented antitumor effects."

### Further Reading and References

- Chinese Medicine and Cancer, http://www.healthy.net/scr/Article.asp?Id=2006

# Acupuncture

Acupuncture is a Chinese therapeutic method for changing the flow or quality of the life force and rebalancing body energies. The Chinese say that chi circulates within fourteen major meridians, or energy channels, traversing the body from the top of the head to the tips of the fingers and toes. Each meridian is connected to an internal organ.

Specific points on each invisible channel, when stimulated, affect the flow of chi in that and other channels or in the associated organs. By stimulating these points with extremely fine needles or massage, acupuncture unblocks energy or adjusts its flow. Inserting and manipulating the needles—hairlike slivers of stainless steel—is believed to correct the imbalances that underlie disease.

Acupuncture has been used to treat persistent pain, arthritis, asthma, infertility, and acute and chronic diseases. In cancer, it can alleviate the pain and functional disorders associated with the illness, for example, improving the ability to swallow in victims of esophageal cancer. Acupuncture is also used to mitigate the side effects of chemotherapy and radiation, and has been employed as a primary treatment for very early signs of breast and cervical cancer, though the Chinese are more likely to utilize herbal remedies to support immunity and control malignant growth. Acupuncture can also be helpful in stress reduction and the alleviation of pain following surgery.

Some practitioners advise against acupuncture in the treatment of cancer, arguing that the increased energy flow and circulation pose a risk of spreading the disease. Most others disagree, however, pointing to the benefits already cited. Leukemia has been successfully treated with acupuncture therapy. In addition, acupuncture has exhibited a wide range of actions in boosting immunity, including increasing the number of white blood cells, boosting natural killer cell activity, and increasing the amount of B-cells, which manufacture antibodies, chemicals that help destroy foreign invaders in the body. Acupuncture also elevates the levels of circulating immunoglobulins and stimulates the production of red blood cells.

Nobel Prize-nominee Robert Becker, M.D., a pioneer in tissue repair and regeneration through electrotherapy, has theorized that the meridians are electrical conductors and the acupuncture points, amplifiers. With the help of a biophysicist, Dr. Becker proved to his satisfaction that "at least the major parts of the acupuncture charts had an objective basis in reality.'"

Two French physicians have done a series of intriguing experiments that they claim make visible the acupuncture meridian system. Jean-Claude Darras, M.D., and Professor Pierre de Vernejoul, M.D, injected radioactive isotopes into the acupuncture points of patients and traced the isotopes' uptake by gamma-camera imaging.

They found that the isotopes migrated along the classical Chinese meridian pathways. In contrast, injecting the isotopes into random points on the skin produced no such results. Further tests demonstrated that the migration was not through the vascular (blood vessel) or lymphatic systems. The research, conducted at the Nuclear Medical Section of Neckar Hospital in Paris, was reported at the World Research Foundation Congress in 1986.

At least two different schools of acupuncture practice their trade in the United States. In traditional or five-element acupuncture, the needles are inserted and withdrawn within seconds, and a relatively small number of points are treated in any given session. In the other school, sometimes called simply Chinese acupuncture, a large number of needles are inserted at once and may be left there anywhere from ten to 30 minutes. Chinese acupuncture seems to be most common among ethnic Chinese and may more accurately represent acupuncture as practiced in China.

Contrary to what a new patient might expect (or fear), the needles are not painful and the treatment is soothing and relaxing.

*Further Reading and References*

- *The Web That Has No Weaver: Understanding Chinese Medicine* by Ted J. Kaptchuk (2000)

- *Acupuncture for Everyone: What It Is, Why It Works, and How It Can Help You* by Ruth Kidson, et al (2000)

- *A Manual of Acupuncture* by Peter Deadman, et al (2007)

- *Chinese Acupuncture and Moxibustion* (Revised Edition) by Cheng Xinnong (2010)

- *The Body Electric: Electromagnetism and the Foundation of Life* by Robert Becker and Gary Selden (Jul 22, 1998)


# Black Tree Fungus/Mo-her/Auricularia polytricha

"The Chinese black tree fungus is an anticoagulant available in most Asian markets. It provides a protective effect against the spread of cancer – it interferes with platelet function similar to aspirin."


See **Anticoagulants**.


*Further Reading and References*

- New England Journal of Medicine article by Dale Hammerschmidt (vol. 302, pp1191-1193, 1980).


# Chinese Tian Xian Herbal Treatment

Tian Xian is the name of a Chinese herbal formula containing a number of different ingredients selected to control, inhibit and/or destroy cancer cells. It's marketed by a number of different vendors (and with varied spellings of the name) that generally describe it as a dietary supplement. Most of the websites selling Tian Xian (cancer-central.com, tian-xian.com, tianxian.com, etc.) contain stern warnings about counterfeit versions of Tian Xian, making it difficult if not impossible to discern the customer is getting the "real" Tian Xian or not.

To make things even more confusing, another website sells what appears to be the same product in the U.S. under the name Tien Hsien liquid (tienhsien.com). This is in addition to distributors in 15 or so other countries.

To keep things simple, in this article the remedy will be called Tian Xian, and references will be to the info found on the tian-xian.com website.

Tian Xian has been heavily promoted with testimonials. While testimonials can provide valuable information, they should be the starting point for more investigation, not the last word – especially when dealing with a serious disease like cancer.

The editors of this book were unable to find any scientific publications in PubMed or in scientific journals regarding Tian Xian.

**The website clearly states that its function is as a *complement* to Western therapies. That's one**

**reason it's difficult to assess how well it works, in the absence of published studies.**

The company lists its Tian Xian liquid ingredients as:

- Radix Ginseng (12.5%)

- Radix Astragali (15%)

- Cordyceps (24%)

- Ganoderma (17%)

- Rhizoma Dioscoreae (11%)

- Herba Scutellariae Barbatae (2%)

- Margarita (4%)

- Fructus Lycii (9%)

- Fructus Ligustri Lucidi (0.5%)

- Radix Glycyrrhizae (5%)


Some of the ingredient lists on the other websites differ from this. For the most part, these are respected Chinese herbs, highly regarded for their healing capabilities throughout the ages.

Three show particular promise for cancer treatments. They belong to a long-lived ancient Chinese tradition – and are in fact supported by scientific research.

- **Cordyceps sinensis** (also called caterpillar mushroom) – one of the better known Chinese herbs, grows above 10,000 feet in the highlands of China, Tibet, and Nepal. a broad range of biological effects on the liver, kidneys, heart, and immune system. A search under the topic "Cordyceps sinensis cancer" *PubMed* 85 listings.

- **Ganoderma (also reishi)** – has been used for 2,000 years in Chinese medicine, and is respectfully called the "Mushroom of Immortality."

  *PubMed* has 189 entries on ganoderma's impact on cancer. One promising study (Gao 2003) showed a positive impact of ganoderma on cancer immune function, increasing the beneficial cytokines IL-2, IL-6 and interferon-gamma, and significantly decreasing pro-inflammatory ones. Natural killer (NK) cell activity also increased 8%. The authors concluded that ganoderma enhanced immune function in late-stage cancer patients.

- **Astragalus** – used in traditional Chinese medicine for thousands of years, highly regarded as an immune booster. It's an adaptogen, meaning it helps the body adjust to physical and emotional stressors. What's more, it's an anti-bacterial and an anti-inflammatory. *PubMed* 416 articles on astragalus and cancer.


The Tian Xian seller's website lists a number of side effects that you might experience when taking its remedy, such as:

- Constipation

- Diarrhea (may contain blood)

- Stomach pain

- Dizziness

- Racing pulse, high blood pressure

- Loss of appetite

- Aches and pains

- Rash

- Darkened skin (if you have liver cancer)


Since no toxicity studies have been done on Tian Xian, it's impossible to know whether drug interactions are likely.

As of this writing, a 28-day supply of Super Tian Xian Liquid sells for $1,280. A brief search of the Internet found one of the ingredients, sinensis, available as a supplement for as little as $7 for a 60-day supply. Another ingredient, reishi (organic), was available for under $10 for a 45 day supply. Astragalus could be purchased for $9 to $10 for a 60 day supply.


# Ginseng/Zhu-xiang

Ginseng has been the most valued herb in China since the dawn of that country's written history. It is probably also the most studied medicinal plant in the world. Since the turn of the century, over 3,000 papers on ginseng and its constituents have appeared, mostly in Russia and China. Most of this research has not been published in the West.

The peculiarity of such medicine is that although an entire civilization has been using it for very long time periods, people mainly use it as a home remedy, and therefore documentation in the form of clinical studies, the core of medical practice in the west, does not exist.

Ginseng is considered in the Chinese tradition to be a "tonic" herb, or one that "builds chi." In Chinese medicine, chi is defined as the vital life force or life energy.

According to Paul Bergman in his book *The Healing Power of Ginseng and the Tonic Herbs*:

"When [chi] becomes blocked, disease may result. Imagine a garden hose with water flowing through it. If the hose becomes crimped, the water pressure above the crimp increases and the hose swells there.

"Below the crimp, the flow is decreased. Similarly, stuck chi can result in too much chi in one place and not enough in another.

"Chinese physicians consider stuck chi to be one of the major causes of pain and tension in the areas of the body where chi has become stagnant, the part of the hose above the crimp. Organs or tissues below the site of obstruction may also not function properly due to a local deficiency of chi, like the end of the hose with its diminished water flow."

According to Chinese medicine, chi obstruction is very important to consider when taking ginseng or other chi-building herbs. To build up the chi when it cannot flow freely would be the equivalent of turning up the water pressure in a hose that is crimped. For this reason, the chi-building herbs are not taken when pain, tension, inflammation, emotional frustration, anger, high blood pressure or other signs of chi obstruction are present.

Medicinally, Asian ginseng has been used to increase strength in those who are weak, to help build the blood in cases of anemia, to improve respiration in those short of breath from weakness, to calm the spirit and nerves, as a remedy for impotence and to increase wisdom in spiritual pursuits.

Bergman describes the first real breakthrough in Western ginseng research as being the work of Russian scientist Itskovitz I. Brekhman and his colleagues in the late 1940s and early 1950s. Their research was significant in that they devised a way to describe the action of ginseng and the other tonic herbs in Western terms. Previously, there had been no vocabulary in the West to describe the Chinese understanding of ginseng's activity.

Brekhman and his colleagues coined the term "adaptogen" to describe a substance that enables the body to respond to a non-specific stress, not through adaptogen's own chemical activity, but by strengthening the body's own innate response mechanisms. Other properties of adaptogens in the Russian model were that they were non-toxic and could be taken as foods. They also tended to normalize bodily functions, enhancing those that are deficient and reducing those that are in excess.

Bergman cites research in humans with cancer using ginseng, which demonstrated increased survival. A group of 100 cancer patients suffering from gastric, colon, and pancreatic cancers were treated for three months with a ginseng constituent called prostisol. In about 75% of cases, the injections prevented the recurrence of cancer and growth of tumors and also boosted red cell counts and blood measures of immune factors. In another trial with 150 patients with rectal, breast, and ovarian cancer, oral doses of ginseng taken for 30 to 60 days prevented progression of disease. White cell counts and other measures of immunity also improved.

In addition to the intriguing evidence for its role in supporting immune function during conventional therapies and possible direct anticancer effects, ginseng has also been prescribed for relief of menopausal symptoms in breast cancer patients because it contains phytoestrogens.

Ginseng has very low toxicity compared to most over-the-counter pharmaceuticals available in the United States. Despite the fact that perhaps ten million people in the United States regularly consume ginseng, it is claimed that no life threatening side effects have appeared in the medical literature.

Bergman cautions that having the guidance of a practitioner of Chinese medicine is important, not only because of the contraindications described above, but also in terms of obtaining a high quality ginseng product.

Boik speculates in his textbook *Cancer & Natural Medicine* that ginseng use may be counterproductive during radiotherapy because it is a free radical scavenger, and the use of antioxidants during radiation therapy is widely discouraged by oncologists who believe that it they may protect neoplastic tissues as well as normal tissues from the effects of ionizing radiation.

There are many commercial sources of quality ginseng. It's reported that American sources produce a higher quality product, in general, because they use a better grade of ginseng. Bergman describes the various forms in which ginseng may be taken, including the technique for making tea or the traditional Chinese alcohol extract with jujube dates.

The jury is certainly still out in terms of ginseng as a treatment for cancer. As things stand, this therapy may fall into a large category that includes many other complementary approaches for cancer — that is, while not intrinsically a cancer cure, when used skillfully it is relatively safe and inexpensive, and it may well enhance the general level of health. More importantly, it may be quite useful for the control of symptoms and side effects of other therapies. Generally, ginseng is available in powder form, tablets, capsules, liquid extracts and teas, though the quality is uneven.

The major active ingredients of ginseng root are considered to be a family of about 30 triterpene saponins called ginsenosides. Ginseng products vary in the amount of ginsenosides they contain. Commercial ginseng products typically are standardized to contain about 4 to 7% ginsenosides.

*Consumer Reports* analyzed 10 different brands of ginseng and found a wide variation in the content of ginsenosides, from 0.4 milligrams/capsule in one brand to 23.2 milligrams/capsule in another.

Ginseng capsules or tablets usually provide about 100 to 400 milligrams of dried extract, equivalent to 0.5 to 2 grams of ginseng root per day. Generally there are no side effects observed with the use of ginseng, although some people report feeling overstimulated. It is suggested that for effectiveness, ginseng be used no longer than three months and then discontinued for one month. Ginseng is contraindicated with stimulants, including the excessive use of caffeine-containing foods and beverages. The safety of use during pregnancy has not been established.

In a 2004 study, a herbal formula called Zhu-xiang that contains ginseng was shown to inhibit breast cancer:

"The inhibitory effect of an herbal formula comprising ginseng and carthamus tinctorius on breast cancer.

A compound (Zhu-xiang) from herbal extracts containing ginseng and carthamus tinctorius was used to treat the MDA-MB-231 breast cancer cell and normal human mammary gland cell lines. The inhibition of cell proliferation by Zhu-xiang, epirubicin, 5- fluorouracil and cyclophosphamide was determined by WST-1 assays. The apoptotic effect was studied …The proliferation index as well as cell cycle progression were also evaluated …The Zhu-xiang showed significantly inhibition in cell proliferation and the inhibition was dose dependent. The inhibitory effect of Zhu-xiang was significantly greater than commonly used cytotoxic drugs. The inhibitory effect is a result of the induction of apoptosis, which is concentration-and-time-dependent. …. The three different concentrations of Zhu-xiang all exhibited the ability to inhibit proliferation in solid tumour. Zhu-xiang could be a useful anti-cancer compound against breast cancer."

### Further Reading and References

- *The Healing Power of Ginseng* by Paul Bergman (1996)

- *Cancer & Natural Medicine: A Textbook of Basic Science and Clinical Research* by John Boik (1995)

- *Miracle Cures : Dramatic New Scientific Discoveries Revealing the Healing Powers of Herbs,*

- *Vitamins, and Other Natural Remedies* by Jean Carper (1997)

- Life Sci. 2004 Nov 26;76(2):191-200.The inhibitory effect of a herbal formula comprising ginseng and carthamus tinctorius on breast cancer. Loo WT, Cheung MN, Chow LW.

# Korean Red Ginseng

Korean red ginseng has been reported to support the immune system. This herb contains polyacetylene compounds that promote inhibiting effects on the growth of cancer cells by suppressing mutation and metastasis, while promoting the activity of natural anti-cancer cells. Korean red ginseng promotes good health by acting on restoring the immune system debilitated by cancer.

### *Further Reading and References*

- Red Ginseng: What is it and where does it come from? http://www.redginseng.com/

- *The Ancient Wisdom of the Chinese Tonic Herbs* - Paperback by Ron Teeguarden (2000)

# PC SPES

PC-SPES is a combination of eight Chinese herbs. It was extremely popular with American prostate cancer patients but was banned by the authorities when it was found to contain a prescription drug not disclosed on the label. (A conflicting lab test suggested that the alleged prescription drug was, in fact, a similar natural chemical that has the same effect as the drug.)

Notwithstanding the charge that PC-SPES was adulterated with a drug, it mainly contained herbs that do apparently possess anti-cancer, anti-inflammatory, antiviral, and immune enhancement properties.

PC-SPES was developed in the early 1990s by a chemist named Sophie Chen, PhD, who claimed to have developed the formula by integrating modern science and ancient Chinese herbal wisdom. By the mid 1990s, the formula became widely promoted in the United States. Its withdrawal from the market was controversial. Many prostate cancer patients were dismayed by the government decision to deny them access to this remedy.

The disclosed components of PC SPES are:

- Isatis indigotica

- Glycyrrhiza glabra and Glycyrrhiza uralensis (licorice)

- Panax pseudo-Ginseng (ginseng)

- Ganoderma lucidum

- Scutellaria baicalensis (skull cap)

- Dendranthema morifolium Tzvel (chrysanthemum)

- Rabdosia rubescens

- Serenoa repens (saw palmetto)


PC-SPES was said to arrest the growth of prostate cancer cells by ten different biological mechanisms:

- Suppresses cancer cell growth

- Reduces intracellular PSA

- Reduces level of PSA secreted into blood

- Decreases the number of androgen receptors

- Decreases the intensity of binding to the androgen receptor

- Decreases clonogenicity (ability of cancerous cells to grow a colony of new cells)

- Slows the cell cycle and prevents tumor cells from going into the S phase (where

- DNA replication occurs)

- Causes programmed cell death (apoptosis)

- Down regulates BCL-2, which is a gene that resists cell death (apoptosis)

- Sensitizes radiation effects (Makes radiation therapy ineffective)

PC-SPES showed some promise as a treatment for prostate cancer, hence its popularity and word-of-mouth reputation. PC-SPES reportedly lowers the level of prostate specific antigen (PSA), a protein secreted by cancerous prostate cells. A small study involving use of PC-SPES for at least 3 months in 9 patients with prostate cancer found that 5 of them responded to treatment as measured by an average decline in PSA levels of 62%.

A decrease in PSA production often means that a prostate tumor is shrinking, but the study did not show that PC-SPES reduced tumor size or slowed the rate at which tumors spread. The study concluded that PC-SPES may prove to be useful in treating hormonally sensitive prostate cancer; but when used with conventional treatments, it may have mixed results.

PC-SPES exhibits strong estrogenic activity. Therefore, side effects of PC-SPES include breast tenderness and/or enlargement, leg and muscle cramps, diarrhea, fatigue, and impotence. More serious side effects are blood clots (in the legs or lungs), heart attack, and stroke.

However, these side effects are typical for high-dose estrogen treatment. Some patients have had allergic reactions to PC-SPES. These patients experienced difficulty breathing and swelling of the face and tongue.

Reports from three laboratories showed that DES, a carcinogen, was present in their samples of PC-SPES. On the opposing side, the California State Health Authorities did not find any DES in samples of PC-SPES.

At this time, PC-SPES has been recalled by its manufacturer due to an FDA ban.

### Further Reading and References

- *Beating Cancer With Nutrition* by Patrick Quillin, et al. (2005)

- Cedars-Sinai: PC-SPES for Prostate Cancer, http://www.cedars-sinai.edu/Patients/Programs-and-Services/Urology-Center/Prostate-Cancer/Nutritional-Information/PC-SPES-for-Prostate-Cancer.aspx

# Sophora

Sophora is a genus of about 45 species of small trees found on several continents. Some species from this genus are said to have medicinal properties.

Injection of sophora extract, containing mainly the alkaloids, was used as an adjuvant to standard medical therapy in 200 cases of lung cancer, with reportedly good effects.

The injection at 200–400 mg each time, once daily, was reported to counter leukopenia induced by radiation therapy. Leucopenia is a deficiency in the number of white cells in the blood. It places a patient at increased risk of infection. The sophora extract was said to improve the white blood count or WBC for 21 out of 25 patients. The total dosage of alkaloids used (sum of daily treatments) ranged from 2.8 to 18 grams. The same basic result was found in patients who suffered from leukopenia due to either radiation therapy or chemotherapy, at a dose of 200–400 mg each time, once or twice daily for 4–37 days (total alkaloid dose ranging from 1.6– 29.6 grams). It was reported that the effects were rapid: the improved WBC could be detected within one week of therapy in nearly all responding patients. In yet another study, a dose of 400 mg once daily for less than three weeks total time was sufficient to improve WBC in women with gynecological tumors (26 of 30 cases).

According to *Anticancer Medicinal Herbs*, in the treatment of cancer, Sophora subprostrata has the function of stimulating the immune mechanism rather than inhibiting cancer cells directly.

### Further Reading and References

- Sophora, http://www.itmonline.org/arts/sophora.htm

# Qian-Hu/Peucedanum Root

Qian-hu is a traditional Chinese medicine that "completely suppressed tumor formation" for up to 20 weeks, without toxic side-effects, according to an article in *Carcinogenesis* 1990:11:1557-61. It contains a form of coumarin called Pd-II. Coumarin is a fragrant chemical found in a number of plants and said to have blood-thinning, fungicidal, and anti-tumor activities. Coumarin can be toxic when used in high doses or for a long period.

See **Anticoagulants**.

### Further Reading and References

- Carcinogenesis 1990:11:1557-61.

- *Integrating Conventional and Chinese Medicine in Cancer Care: A Clinical Guide* by Tai Lahans (2007)

# Ayurvedic Medicine

## MAK-4 (Amrit) and MAK-5

MAK-4 and MAK-5 are Ayurvedic health-promoting, therapeutic herbal preparations developed by the Maharishi Mahesh Yogi. MAK-4 is also known as Maharishi Amrit Kalash Nectar and MAK-5 is also known as Maharishi Amrit Kalash Ambrosia. The two are reported to be effective in the control of side effects during chemotherapy and to inhibit both tumor formation and the spread of tumors.

A 1992 study conducted in Florida found that MAK-4, when given to mice with Lewis Lung Carcinoma, prompted a reduction in the number of metastatic cancer cells along with a reduction in nodule size.

In another study the same year, an ethanol extract of MAK-5 showed signs of reversing the malignant process in 75% of murine neuroblastoma cells while in culture. The same ethanol extracts also appeared to induce neurite formation in neuroblastoma cells. Neuroblastoma is a form of brain cancer.

"[MAK-4] contains potent phytochemicals and has many beneficial properties, without any toxic side effects. Research has shown that it decreases the toxic effects of chemotherapy in cancer patients. This herbal mixture has also been shown to decrease tumor formation and its spread under experimental conditions, in the areas of breast cancer, lung cancer, liver cancer, neuroblastoma (a tumor of the nervous system), and melanoma."*

"The book *The Answer to Cancer* goes into detail about the research conducted on Amrit and we give instructions on how to take it."

MAK-4 and MAK-5 are widely available through nutritional supplement companies specializing in Ayurvedic Medicine.

### Further Reading & References

- "Reduction of Metastases of Lewis Lung Carcinoma by an Ayurvedic Food Supplement [MAK-4] in Mice," Nutrition Research, Vol. 12, pp. 31-61, 1992. Nutrition Research, Vol. 12, pp. 31-61, 1992, http://www.ayurveda-florida.com/Research_non_ayurvedic_topics_health_disease_related/cancer_research_3.htm

- "Ayurvedic (Science of Life) Agents [MAK-4 and MAK-3] Induce Differentiation in Murine Neuroblastoma Cells in Culture," Neuropharmacology, Vol. 31, No. 6, pp. 599-607, 1992, http://www.ayurveda-florida.com/Research_non_ayurvedic_topics_health_disease_related/cancer_research_3.htm

- *Interview with Dr. Sharma and Total Health News on "Cancer," http://www.ayurveda.ie/html/ayurveda_news%20letter_cancer2.htm

- *The Answer to Cancer: Is Never Giving It a Chance to Start*, by Hari Sharma, James G. Meade, and Rama K. Mishra (2002)

# Carctol®

Carctol is an Indian Ayurvedic formula developed by Dr. Nandlal Tiwari, Ayurvedic specialist. Dr. Tiwari has been treating terminally ill cancer patients with his special herbal cancer therapy for the past 20 years. He claims a fair measure of success based on hits treatments.

The eight herbs that make up Carctol are recognized in India for their medicinal properties. Dr. Tiwari developed the formula following research on herbs gathered in the Assam forests of India. Both Dr. Tiwari and additional scientists in the United Kingdom ran tests on the herbs within Carctol and found them to be effective as a healing agent for people with cancer, excluding cancer where ascites is present.

Ingredients within each capsule of Carctol are:

- Blepharis Edulis 200 mg

- Piper Cubeba Linn 120 mg

- Smilax China Linn 80 mg

- Ammani Vesicatoria 20 mg

- Hemidesmus Indicus 20 mg

- Lepidium Sativum Linn 20 mg

- Rheum emodi Wall 20 mg

- Tribulus Terrestris 20 mg

Carctol is most often used as an adjunct treatment for cancer sufferers already taking conventional medicine. It can also be taken as a preventative treatment for those without cancer.

Dr. Tiwari claims Carctol works by changing the pH of the body so that it is less acidic and more alkaline, making it hard for acidic cancer cells to survive. In many ways, Carctol is a form of detoxification that helps the kidneys, liver, and bowels excrete toxins. Proponents also claim that it strengthens the immune system. These benefits supposedly help neutralize the toxicity often experienced with chemotherapy and radiation treatment.

A study in India of 1,900 cancer patients who followed the Carctol program reported a 75% or higher improvement in 2% of the patients. A 25%-75% benefit was seen in 50% of the patients and little improvement was seen in the remaining 25%.*

See **Dr. Rosy Daniel**.

### *Further Reading & References*

- The Official Carctol Website: http://www.carctolhome.com/

- *The Cancer Prevention Book: Holistic Guidelines From the World-Famous Bristol Cancer Help Centre*, by Rosy Daniel and Rachel Ellis (2002)

- "What is Carctol?" http://www.cam-cancer.org/CAM-Summaries/Biologically-Based-Practices/Carctol/What-is-it

- *"Carctol," Townsend Letter for Doctors and Patients, Feb-March, 2005 by Jule Klotter, http://findarticles.com/p/articles/mi_m0ISW/is_259-260/ai_n10018573/

# Urine Therapy

## Dr. Danopoulos/Carbatine

Dr. Evangelos Danopoulos, professor at the Medical School of Athens University in Greece, reported in 1954 on the healing potential of urine for cancer. He went on to create the drug Carbatine to battle skin cancer.

Carbatine combines creatine hydrate and urea, a chemical derived from urine. Urea is the main substance excreted in urine and stems from protein metabolism, with approximately 30g per day excreted by individuals through urine. The specific combination in Carbatine is 25 grams of creatine hydrate mixed with 15 grams of urea in a quart of water.

Professor Danopoulos reportedly enjoyed a 99% success rate in treating skin cancers by injecting Carbatine directly into skin cancer tumors along with applying urea powder directly to ulcerated skin tumor areas.

Carbatine also appears to be effective against liver cancer because of its ability to penetrate the water-like substance that surrounds and protects cancerous cells. Once this is done, the body's immune system is able to take over.

In oral doses, urea appears to reach such high concentrations that it can inhibit cancer growth in the liver. It also prevents the formation of new blood vessels in tumors, thus cutting off the food source for the tumor.

Throughout an 11-year period during which Dr. Danopoulos treated liver cancer patients with Carbatine, 15 of 22 patients reported significant healing.

It is unknown whether Carbatine could be effective against cancers other than skin and liver cancer. The liver is the only organ that shows high concentrations of urea after oral administration.

Carbatine can be consumed orally, although it is important to monitor Blood Urea Nitrogen (BUN) levels on a daily basis. BUN levels must be kept around 35-40.

A 1977 report from *Clinical Oncology* stated that of those patients who took oral doses of carbatine following bowel surgery, only 25% developed lung or liver metastases in the first two years after surgery.

### Further Reading & References

- What modern science knows about a miracle medicine (and isn't telling), http://health.centreforce. com/health/urea.html

- *Alternatives In Cancer Therapy*, by R.Ross, P. Pelton, and Lee Overholser, http://curezone.com/ diseases/cancer/urea.asp

# H-11

English Professor James H. Thompson first devised this form of urine therapy in the 1930s after studying the parathyroid gland which normally controls the body's calcium and phosphorus metabolic ability. He was searching for something he called a "growth inhibitor" within the gland which, he contended, keeps a fully-grown body functioning and able to maintain normal processes without further growth or development.

Thompson believed this same growth inhibitor could be injected into the body where it would travel throughout all systems. In a healthy body, the inhibitor would have no effect. In an unhealthy body such as one with cancer, the growth inhibitor would be drawn to the place of cancerous growth and assume its inhibiting ability.

Thompson and his colleagues first experimented on animals with tumors. After injecting them with the parathyroid extracts, he noted that the tumors halted growth within days. With further injections, the size of the tumors decreased. Microscopic biopsies showed the tumors appeared to be encapsulated and so could not multiply or spread to other organs.

Thompson's next course of action was to isolate the same growth inhibitor in humans. He found what he was looking for in human urine where extracts proved to effectively retard tumor growth. Thompson was able to isolate a polypeptide from the urine of healthy adults, called H-11, and put it to clinical use testing it as a treatment for cancer patients.

Urine extracts in fact turned out to be retardants of tumoral as well as normal tissue as numerous investigations have shown, including those by Nobel Prize winner Szent-Györgyi. All investigations point in the direction of the growth and tumor-inhibiting property of urine extracts.

By 1950, treatment of 2,277 humans showed a halt in the growth of primary tumors which effectively extended the survival rate of many patients. Some patients showed tumor regression and a few even experienced a return to normal tissue where the tumor once had been. Thompson reported satisfactory results in 70% of his cases.

Administration of H-11 was given orally via liquid or tablets or intravenously, just above the muscle layer. Suppositories and salves were also provided for local application.

No evidence has been found to support the use of H-11 for leukemia, but it is considered effective therapy for bronchial carcinomas, breast carcinomas, tumors found in the cervix, ovaries, or uterus, and carcinomas of the alimentary tract.

Brain tumors, bladder tumors that have not metastasized, and kidney cancers also reacted favorably to treatment, as did lymphosarcomas and malignant skin melanomas. Osteosarcomas respond less favorably.

### Further Reading & References

- *Golden Fountain: The Complete Guide to Urine Therapy* by Coen Van Der Kroon, Volker Moritz (1996)

- Cancer chemo(toxico)therapy revisited and alternative ways of healing. "The H-11 Therapy," http://www.karlloren.com/biopsy/book/p9.htm

- Urine and Urea Therapy, http://cancerresourcecenter.com/articles/alt114.html

# Urea

Urea, which comes from urine, is used to destroy the "water" matrix surrounding and protecting cancer cells. Once the cancer is unprotected, the natural defenses of the immune system are better able to attack the cancer.

The use of urine for medicinal purposes is not new. In fact, it has been used for centuries by many older cultures where it was taken internally to heal disease or applied topically to heal skin problems. Some cultures even recommend the regular consumption of urine as a preventative measure for illness.

Over the years, several scientists have investigated the merits of urea as an anticancer treatment. J.H. Lawrence, a British scientist during World War II, found that a substance in urine seemed to have anti-tumor activity in animals.

J. W. Armstrong, author of *The Water of Life: A Treatise on Urine Therapy*, promoted the concept of a three-week long urine fast (plus some water). Using this treatment, Armstrong regarded cancer as easy to cure. Armstrong's book relays several cases of diagnosed cancer that appeared cured following this urine fast.

Greek Internal Medicine professor E.V. Danopoulos was one of the first to proclaim urea to be the potent anti-cancer factor in urine. His work focused on the treatment of liver cancer and skin cancer patients (Dr. Danopoulos created Carbatine, mentioned above in an earlier entry).

Dr. Stanislaw Burzynski, creator of antineoplaston therapy, procures peptides from urine and claims it is not really waste material. Instead, Dr. Burzynski sees it as a complex chemical mixture that delivers crucial information about the body. In fact, he calls urea "a treasure of information."

In 1996, a conference on the benefits of auto-urine therapy (that is, drinking one's own urine) was held. At the conference, Chinese research Dr. Ming Chen Liao claimed that 47% of his cancer patients treated in this way were cured of their cancer.

Dr. Shigeyuri Arai, a Japanese researcher attending the same conference, boasted a success rate of 73% with cancer patients.

The ingestion of urine is most common in Asia but is increasingly found in Europe. Several hundred thousand Japanese are said to gargle with or drink urine on a daily basis.

Several animal studies have been conducted in which urea was directly injected into tumors. Those tumors reportedly stopped growing or disappeared altogether (this is consistent with the research of Dr. Danopoulos).

The average adult human excretes about an ounce of urea a day. Urea appears to have no side effects and is virtually non-toxic, though some researchers suggest using a concentration no stronger than 40%.

Urea appears to work especially well with liver cancers. Because it can be taken orally, it is believed to have a strong beneficial effect on the liver as well as the lungs. Mixing the urea with creatine hydrate is one way thought to render it more effective by facilitating its distribution to other tissues and organs. Creatine hydrate is a chemical that has its own history as a cancer remedy, being the supposedly active ingredient of a much maligned anti-cancer drug known as Krebiozen. See **Krebiozen.**

### *Further Reading & References*

- *The Water of Life: A Treatise on Urine Therapy*, by J. W. Armstrong (2005)

- *Golden Fountain: The Complete Guide to Urine Therapy* by Coen Van Der Kroon, Volker Moritz (1996)

- *Miracles of Urine Therapy* by Beatrice Bartnett and Margie Adelman (1988)

- *Second World Conference on Urine Therapy* by Coen Van Der Kroon (2000)

- *Urine Therapy* by John F. Oquinn (1980)

- *Urine-Therapy: It May Save Your Life* by Beatrice Bartnett (1993)

- *Urine Therapy: Self-Healing Through Intrinsic Medicine*, by C.P. Mithal (1978)

- The Diversity Of Natural Cancer Cures, http://www.alternativehealth.co.nz/cancer/diversity.htm

- *Alternatives In Cancer Therapy*, by R. Ross, P. Pelton, and Lee Overholser, http://curezone.com/diseases/cancer/urea.asp

# CDA-II

CDA-II (short for cell differentiation agent II) is a substance that can be isolated from healthy human urine. CDA-II is believed to have anticancer properties and has undergone testing against human acute myeloid leukemia cell lines.

Using urine and urine extracts for their medicinal properties is a practice that has been around for many centuries. Only recently did urine therapy gain popularity in Asia, where individuals use it to treat a wide variety of illnesses.

The inventor of CDA-II, Dr. Ming C. Liau hypothesized on the effect of methionine in cancer cell differentiation, "Methionine obstructs the differentiation of cancer cells, thus allowing cancer cells to live much longer than the normal cells. Ordinary meats from the animals are much higher in methionine content compared to vegetables, grains and fruits. This is one of the reasons why a vegetarian diet helps in cancer treatment."

Dr. Liau believes methionine content may be a cancer marker in the treatment that uses a cell differentiation agent such as CDA-II. With the success of CDA-II in early clinical trials, hopefully Dr. Liau's hypothesis will be pursued and verified in further research.

In 1996, after reading the seventh volume of the *Miraculous Urine Therapy* edited by Dr. Kamataro Sano, Dr. Liau contacted Dr. Sano in Japan to discuss the feasibility of adding CDA-II to Dr. Sano's urine therapy. Dr. Sano was very receptive and immediately used CDA-II in his protocol for cancer patients. The results were very positive. Following are the clinical results of using urine therapy, laetrile therapy, Gerson therapy, and CDA-II at Dr. Sano's Hospital from 1996-1997. Dr. Sano's protocol reportedly included laetrile, vitamin C and a Gerson-type diet, in addition to urine therapy and CDA-II, so the results cannot be considered definitive as regards CDA-II alone.

Of 50 patients treated, 46 patients were regarded as capable of evaluation, having been treated with CDA-II for more than 4 weeks. These are data provided by Dr. Sano of Sano Surgical Hospital, 22-4. Aosawa 2 Chome, Kofu, Japan:

- Complete remission: Total eradication of tumors. Dramatic increase of appetite, also dramatic improvement on respiration, pain, and cough. (4 patients, 8.7%)

- Partial remission: Decrease of tumor size over 50%. Good appetite, also good improvement on respiration, pain, and cough. (16 patients, 34.8%)

- Improvement: Decrease of tumor size less than 50%. Recovery of appetite, also noticeable improvement on respiration, pain, and cough. (13 patients, 28.2%)

- No change: No significant change of symptoms. (8 patients, 17.4%)

- Disease progressive: Tumors increasing. Worsening to result in death. (5 patients, 10.9%)

- Total: 46 patients

In a study reported by the *American Journal of Chinese Medicine,* CDA-II appeared to halt growth in leukemic cells without causing cytotoxicity in peripheral blood cells.

Along with slowing the growth rate of tumors, CDA-II appears to prolong the survival rate of cancer sufferers.*

In another study, CDA-II was found to be effective against cancer thanks to its ability to induce differentiation of neoplastic cells.

Phase III trials in China completed in 2004 showed CDA-II was definitely helpful as a supplement to chemotherapy by modulating abnormal methylation enzymes. It increased the therapeutic efficacy rate by a significant amount and reduced the toxic manifestation of cytotoxic chemotherapy on breast cancer and NSCLC.

### Further Reading & References

- *Miraculous Urine Therapy* edited by Dr. Sano

- *"Effect of CDA-II, Urinary Preparation, on Lipofuscin, Lipid Peroxidation and Antioxidant Systems in Young and Middle-Aged Rat Brain," http://findarticles.com/p/articles/mi_m0HKP/is_1_29/ai_73711325/

- **"CDA-II, a urinary preparation, induces growth arrest and apoptosis of human leukemia cells through inactivation of nuclear factor-kappaB in a caspase-dependent manner," http://www.sciencedirect.com/science?_ob=ArticleURL&_udi=B6T6P-4T5TPRJ-1&_user=10&_coverDate=01%2F31%2F2009&_rdoc=1&_fmt=high&_orig=search&_origin=search&_sort=d&_docanchor=&view=c&_searchStrId=1560766252&_rerunOrigin=google&_acct=C000050221&_version=1&_urlVersion=0&_userid=10&md5=ff89f9479ebaf663c9824009e6990efe&searchtype=a

- Urine Therapy and CDA-II In Cancer Treatment, http://www.brave-souls.com/learn-from-others/

- Fengyi Feng, et al. "Phase III clinical trials of the cell differentiation agent-2 (CDA-2): Therapeutic efficacy on breast cancer, non-small cell lung cancer and primary hepatoma1," *Chinese Journal of Clinical Oncology* Volume 2, Number 4, 706-716, DOI: 10.1007/BF02819536.

# Topical Treatments

## Bloodroot/Sanguinaria canadensis

Bloodroot is a perennial flowering plant found throughout eastern North America. It is the only species in the genus *Sanguinaria*. Bloodroot is a vital ingredient in many types of topical salves used to treat skin cancer. It has been shown in several studies to have antimicrobial, anti-inflammatory, and antioxidant properties.

Bloodroot has been used successfully for over a hundred years in the treatment of skin cancer. Researchers believe the anticancer ingredient in the plant is sanguinarine, an alkaloid salt extract.

Early studies of sanguinarine showed cancerous cells decreased depending on dosage level.* Other studies showed prostate cancer cells responded to sanguinarine treatment, resulting in inhibition of cell growth, arrest of cells, and induction of apoptosis (natural cell death).** The success of the treatment was dose-dependent.

Other research shows sanguinarines has antiseptic properties that help prevent bacteria from forming plaque. If further developed, this could be an effective treatment against oral bacteria and a way to reduce dental plaque.

Researchers believe sanguinarine has potential as an anticancer drug.

Some believe bloodroot should not be taken internally, even in small doses.

Sanguinarine is also found in the Greater Celandine (Chelidonium majus), an herb common along roadsides in Europe and elsewhere.

See **Cansema** and **Ukrain/Greater Celandine**.

### Further Reading & References

- Cancer Tutor: "Over 200 Alternative Cancer Treatments…", http://www.cancertutor.com/Other/Big_List.htm

- *"Differential antiproliferative and apoptotic response of sanguinarine for cancer cells versus normal cells," http://www.ncbi.nlm.nih.gov/pubmed/10778985?dopt=Abstract

- **"Sanguinarine causes cell cycle blockade and apoptosis of human prostate carcinoma cells via modulation of cyclin kinase inhibitor-cyclin-cyclin-dependent kinase machinery." http://www.ncbi.nlm.nih.gov/pubmed/15299076?dopt=Abstract

# Cansema/Can-X/Cansema/Bloodroot Paste/Silver Aloe Healing Salve

*Cansema* is the brand name of a popular alternative treatment for cancer that is also known as "black salve." It was first developed by Alpha Omega Labs but was banned after the FDA stopped the company's operations in September 2003, at the same time incarcerating Greg Caton, the company's chief herbalist. (Note: Caton tells his version of the story at http://www.goodhealthinfo.net/cancer/fda_panacea.htm.)

Cansema is classified as an escharotic, which means it burns and destroys tissue when applied to the skin. Typically, it leaves a black scar called an eschar. Supporters of the remedy believe it is an effective treatment for skin cancer.

Escharotics were commonly used to treat skin problems in the 1900s but have been largely replaced by what the medical establishment deems to be safer and more effective treatments. Escharotics are still commonly prescribed by mainstream dermatologists to remove warts.

Spokesmen for Alpha Omega Labs claimed that every single empirical case study they followed showed successful removal of malignant carcinoma, adenocarcinoma, and melanoma, following treatment with Cansema. The company backed its product with a refund guarantee.

Alpha Omega Labs also stated that Cansema, when applied to healthy skin, would warm the skin slightly and possibly cause a pink color, but that it attacks malignant lesions.

Opponents of Cansema warn against the use of any kind of black salve or escharotics, citing serious consequences, such as disfigurement, for using these treatments in place of standard cancer treatments.

Some independent cancer experts do not recommend bloodroot and similar salves for the treatment of melanoma -- the serious, life-threatening type of skin cancer. The over-the-counter salves are reportedly safe and effective for less-serious basal cell carcinomas and squamous cell carcinomas. Other experts maintain the salves are indeed effective for melanoma. As melanoma is an aggressive, life-threatening form of cancer, the reader will need to weigh the risks accordingly.

One testimonial from the Alpha Omega website reads, "[Case #091403: Cansema Salve / Quikheal Green & BCC's] … This was my 4th basal cell carcinoma in about 20 years. Previously had surgery, but this last one on the tip of my nose, did not have much underlying tissue. I assumed a dermatologist's care would involve skin grafting and a fairly large scar. So for 2 years I, at various times, attempted to treat the lesion with a poultice of vitamin C and DMSO or a salve which contained a glycoalkaloid. These applications produced a scab but no erosion of the basic lesion. And gradually the lesion was getting larger. Then I learned of Cansema on the Internet.

"One 24-hour application of Cansema. After 16 hours I experienced slight discomfort. It felt as if someone were pinching my nose just slightly with pliers. Enough to make me aware. This minor discomfort persisted for 3 days. There was also slight edema and a large area of redness.

"Because I'm a practicing chiropractor, meeting people, I kept a light bandage over the not too attractive eschar. Exactly 7 days after the first and only application of Cansema, the eschar, about 3mm in diameter, fell off. I was using Quikheal Green around the eschar and it caused a very slight itching. I was just lightly stroking around the eschar and it fell off. I was very pleasantly surprised!

"Within 2 days a not too objectionable scab formed which I continued to treat with Quikheal Green. Exactly 7 days after the eschar fell out or off, the scab fell off. I now have a slightly discolored, 3mm in diameter, excavation or depression on my nose which doesn't look bad at all and which I continue to treat with Quikheal Green. I'm confident this depression will gradually even out with the adjoining tissue.

"I could not be more pleased with this very simple solution to what could have been an involved problem. Imagine, 14 days in all and I fooled around for 2 years."

Alpha Omega also provides the following guarantee: "If instructions are followed, Alpha Omega guarantees 100% success in the removal of dermal or epidermal malignant lesions, including basal cell, squamous cell epitheliomas and even melanomas -- regardless of type or size... or the treatment is free and payment is refunded."

Original formula Cansema and additional alternatives are obtainable from Centreforce Australia, PO Box 227, Gin Gin Qld 4671 Australia Phone +61 (7) 41574262 Fax +61 (7) 41574446, Website http:// health.centreforce.com. Here are the ingredients for most of the formulations:

- *Centreforce Cansema Black Salve*
  "Ingredients: Bloodroot, Galangal, Red Clover, Sheep Sorrel, Graviola. This Black Salve is similar to the well known Can-X, an alternative product to Cansema, formulated without the aggression and proven effects of Chaparral and Zinc Chloride."

- *Centreforce Cansema Deep Tissue*
  "Ingredients: Bloodroot, Galangal, Chaparral, Ginger root, Zinc Chloride, Graviola, Emu Oil and pharmaceutical-grade DMSO. True to the original "Cansema Deep Tissue" from Alpha Omega Labs, with its proven effectiveness when you need to penetrate further than skin deep."

- *Centreforce Cansema Salve for Cats, Dogs & Horses*
  Ingredients: Bloodroot, Galangal, Chaparral, Ginger root, Zinc Chloride, Graviola, Emu Oil and pharmaceutical-grade DMSO. True to the original "Cansema Salve for Cats, Dogs & Horses" from Alpha Omega Labs, with the same proven effectiveness of penetration as "Cansema Deep Tissue", formulated specifically for Animals."

- *Centreforce Bloodroot Paste*
  "Ingredients: Purified water, bloodroot powder, red clay, glycerine, zinc chloride. Bloodroot (Sanguinaria canadensis) has long been known for its strong medicinal properties, especially with respect to its curative action in treating a wide variety of skin disorders."

- *Centreforce SilverAloe Healing Salve*
  "Ingredients: Aloe Vera, Colloidal Silver, Manuka Honey. Purified Water Centreforce SilverAloe Healing Creme profoundly stimulates healing in skin and other soft tissues in a way unlike any known natural process, kills the most stubborn infections of all kinds, including surrounding bacteria and fungus."

### Further Reading & References

- Alternative Cancer Therapies, http://www.mnwelldir.org/docs/cancer1/altthrpy.htm#cansema

- Cansema, http://en.wikipedia.org/wiki/Cansema

- *Alternative Medicine: Medical Uses of Silver, Radiesthesia, Chiropractic Controversy and Criticism, Colorpuncture, Cansema* by Greg Caton (2010), http://www.amazon.com/Alternative-Medicine-Radiesthesia-Chiropractic-Colorpuncture/dp/1156763487/ref=sr_1_1?s=books&ie=UTF8&qi d=1291592944&sr=1-1

# Castor Oil Packs

A castor oil pack is made from a cloth (usually flannel, folded into four layers) soaked in cold-pressed castor oil and then placed on the skin. The oil-soaked flannel is often covered with a piece of plastic to prevent dripping and staining on either the patient or the bedding. Heat, in the form of a hot water bottle or heating pad, is then applied over the pack and the plastic. A blanket or towel can be placed over the heat source to keep everything in place. The patient then relaxes while the castor oil pack is left for a minimum of 60 minutes up to a maximum of 3 hours.

Proponents of the therapy believe it increases circulation and promotes healing for the tissues and sometimes the organs underneath.

According to a study of 36 healthy subjects that was described (or presented) at the Annie Appleseed Project 4th Annual Evidence-based Complementary and Alternative Cancer Therapies Conference in May 2010, castor oil was identified as an anti-toxin that impacts the lymphatic system and helps enhance immunological function. A castor oil pack applied for a minimum of two hours helped increase the number of T-11 cells within the 24-hour period following treatment. This increase meant a boost in the body's immune function, helping to increase the number of lymphocytes that formed antibodies against toxins such as bacteria and cancer cells.

Castor oil, also known as Palma Christi, has been used as a medicinal treatment for centuries, dating back to ancient Egypt. It is derived from the castor bean and used to be commonly administered internally. Now it is only used topically due to potential toxicity problems when ingested.

### Further Reading & References

- *Castor Oil! It's Healing Properties*, by Beth M. Ley (2003)

- *A Physician's Diary: Case Histories of Hope and Healing with Edgar Cayce's and Other Natural Remedies* by Dr Dana Myatt (1994)

- Castor Oil Cures, http://www.earthclinic.com/Remedies/castor_oil.html

- "Castor Oil: Uses," Annie Appleseed Project, http://www.annieappleseedproject.org/castoroiluses.html

# Escharotic Salves

Escharotic salves, also known as botanical surgery, represent an aggressive approach to the treatment of certain cancers compared to other natural and alternative treatments.

An escharotic salve is a thick salve, or paste, made of Native American herbs placed on a small spot on the skin, close to a diagnosed or suspected malignancy. According to practitioners, the salve causes a reaction in the skin only if there is some type of malignancy. When a malignant tumor is present within the tissue under the selected spot, the salve reportedly helps bring the tumor to the surface until it fully emerges and detaches itself from the skin.

The therapy has shown efficacy with several cancers such as melanoma and other skin cancers. It is also said to be highly effective against breast cancer. Escharotic salves have also reportedly been used successfully on inoperable tumors including pancreatic cancer, lung cancer, and colon cancer. It is recommended by some alternative cancer practitioners, usually as a last resort.

Escharotic salves often include herbal extracts of chaparral (Larrea tridentata), zinc chloride, cayenne (Capsicum frutescens), bloodroot (Sanguinaria canadensis), red clover (Trifolium pratense), birch bark (Betula alba), burdock root (Arctium lappa), Irish moss (Chondrus crispus), and sometimes DMSO (dimethyl sulfoxide). The salves are often used in conjunction with internal preparations.

Although they have a long history in North American and English medicine, escharotic salves have been totally eradicated from standard medical practice.

The most common form of orthodox therapy for melanoma is to surgically remove or burn the lesions. All too often this is a temporary solution at best, and the recurrence rate is very high. Melanoma often metastasizes to internal organs and is often fatal.

Escharotic salves may represent an alternative for this highly aggressive and life-threatening type of skin cancer, but they remain somewhat controversial even within the alternative health community. They should be used, if at all, only in conjunction with systemic (whole body) cancer treatments designed to change the body environment that made the patient vulnerable to cancer in the first place.

Escharotics belong to a group of compounds capable of producing a scab when applied to the skin. More specifically, when an escharotic is applied to visible cancer areas, the following sequence of events may occur:

- Attack on cancerous cells but not normal cells

- Puss formation with a scab forming over the area

- Sloughing off of the scab, leaving a non-cancerous "pit" or cavity

- Once healed, a slightly de-pigmented area with a slight scar will remain

The entire procedure takes between 5 to 15 days.

It is reported that the following phenomenon takes place with the use of an escharotic salve: If a patient has a suspicious skin growth, he or she can apply the escharotic ointment once and then observe it for a period of several days. If an eschar (puss which scabs over) forms, it is cancerous. If it doesn't, the growth is benign. Some doctors reportedly use this method to diagnose suspicious growths.

Although the escharotic ointment is said to be capable of removing larger tumors from beneath the skin, it is not recommended for home use without the guidance of a qualified professional. Anecdotally, the editors of this report know of at least one case in which a serious internal tumor of some size was literally drawn out of a patient's body by the use of a topical salve. The Stage IV patient then experienced complete remission. But the treatment is by no means common among alternative health practitioners.

It is important to heed warnings when using this salve, as it may produce scarring or holes in the skin when not administered properly.

See **Cansema**.

### Further Reading & References

- *Cancer Salves: A Botanical Approach to Treatment* by Ingrid Naiman (1999)

- *Beating Cancer With Nutrition* by Patrick Quillin (2005)

- Escharotic salves, http://www.cancure.org/salves.htm

- Cancer Salves: "Types of Escharotics," http://www.cancersalves.com/introduction/escharotics. html

# Glycoalkaloids/Skin Answer/Curaderm/Devil's Apple-Solanum sodomaeum

Glycoalkaloids come from the family of flowering plants *Solanum dulcamara*, also known as nightshade. Glycoalkaloids themselves are a family of poisons and potentially toxic to humans. Glycoalkaloid-based treatments were once sold in the U.S. as a way to prevent skin cancer but was banned in 2004 by the FDA as an unapproved drug.

However, as a cream formulation with up to a 10% concentration of solasodine glycosides, this treatment was shown in a 1991 Australian study to be effective toward malignant and benign human skin tumors. Specifically, the study authors report,

"A cream formulation containing high concentrations (10%) of a standard mixture of solasodine glycosides (BEC) has been shown to be effective in the treatment of malignant and benign human skin tumours. We now report that a preparation (Curaderm) which contains very low concentrations of BEC (0.005%) is effective in the treatment of keratoses, basal cell carcinomas (BCCs) and squamous cell carcinomas (SCCs) of the skin of humans. In an open study, clinical and histological observations indicated that all lesions (56 keratoses, 39 BCCs and 29 SCCs) treated with Curaderm had regressed. A placebo formulation had no effect on a smaller number of treated lesions. Curaderm had no adverse effect on the liver, kidneys or haematopoietic system."*

This study has an interesting background. In the early 1980's, a veterinarian alerted an Australian medical researcher to the effectiveness of the juice from the Devil's Apple weed in stopping the growth of cancer around the eyes in cattle. This plant is also known as Kangaroo Apple. It is part of the *Solanum* genus.

When the juice from this weed is applied to skin cancer, the glycoalkaloids, and in particular the Solasodine glycoalkaloid, have the ability to attach to cancer cell receptor cites, permitting the Solasodine to attack lysosomes and mitochondria within the cancer cell causing cell rupture and death.

Many fruits and vegetables produce glycoalkaloids as a defense against insects and other animals. Medical literature on the use of glycoalkaloid-rich plants in the treatment of cancer go back to Galen in the Second Century A.D. Recently, in vitro and in vivo studies have shown anticancer effects in glycoalkaloids extracted from a variety of plants in the Solanum family.

The glycoalkaloid cream only produces the redness, inflammation, and ulceration that are the signs of cell death when abnormal cell types are present. Healthy cells at the margins of lesions are unaffected.

In a 1987 human study of 42 females and 44 males, the compound was applied twice a day for a period of three months. Three kinds of cancer-type lesions, including keratoses, basal cell carcinomas, and squamous cell carcinomas were apparently 100% cured with no scarring:

"A cream formulation containing glycoalkaloids purified from the plant species Solanum sodomaeum L. is effective in the treatment of the malignant human skin tumours; basal cell carcinomas (BCCs), squamous cell carcinomas (SCCs) and the benign tumours; keratoses and keratoacanthomas.

Histological analyses of biopsies taken before, during and after treatment give compelling evidence of the efficacy of the formulation. The treated lesions did not recur for at least 3 years after cessation of therapy. ... There were no adverse effects on the liver, kidneys or haematopoietic system during treatment. Normal skin treated with the formulation likewise was free from adverse histological or clinical effects. The data indicate that glycoalkaloids of this type are therefore potentially useful in the treatment of several types of human skin cancers."**

In one case, a woman had several basal cell carcinomas on her nose; physicians told her that she would likely lose her nose and have it replaced with a plastic prosthesis. After treatment with the compound formulated into a cream called Curaderm, the cancers began to ulcerate and slough off, leaving the cartilage in her nose visible. By the end of 13 weeks, her nose had entirely regrown to its original shape with no evidence of any tumors remaining.

One clinical trial tested a group of patients with 13 keratoses, 12 basal cell carcinomas and 3 squamous cell carcinomas. After 4 to 8 weeks of treatment, 27 out of 28 patients showed complete recovery. All post-treatment biopsies could detect no cancer.

The Curaderm cream is a well-known brand of glycoalkaloid salve. It comes in a kit form that includes one bottle of antiseptic and a small bottle of the Curaderm cream.

- Apply the antiseptic to the lesion.

- Apply and rub a small amount of cream directly on the lesion.

- Cover with a small band-aid.

- Repeat the process twice daily.

Some burning or stinging and ulceration are experienced as the cancer cells are being sloughed from the skin. Some people experience complete removal in two or three weeks. Others reportedly take longer.

In clinical use, patients are told their therapy is completed when applying the glycoalkaloid cream daily no longer produces a reaction, indicating that normal healthy cells have replaced all the skin cancer cells.

In spite of tremendous opposition from the medical community, glycoalkaloids have been used for years now and with no serious or long-term side effects reported.

### *Further Reading & References*

- *"Topical treatment of malignant and premalignant skin lesions by very low concentrations of a standard mixture (BEC) of solasodine glycosides." http://www.ncbi.nlm.nih.gov/entrez/query.fcgi?cmd=Retrieve&db=pubmed&dopt=Abstract&list_uids=1913614

- **"Glycoalkaloids from Solanum sodomaeum are effective in the treatment of skin cancers in man." http://www.ncbi.nlm.nih.gov/pubmed/3621146

- IndiaDivine.org, http://www.indiadivine.org/audarya/ayurveda-health-wellbeing/978774-glycoalkaloids-squamous-cell-carcinoma.html

- "The Skin Cancer Self Treatment from Weeds in the Australian Bush," http://rastaseed.com/2007/11/13/the-skin-cancer-self-treatment-from-weeds-in-the-australian-bush/

- "Breakthrough Treatment for Skin Cancer, BEC5," by Jeffrey Dach MD, http://jeffreydach. com/2007/07/16/breakthrough-treatment-for-skin-cancer-bec5-by-jeffrey-dach-md-2.aspx

## Pyridoxal (Vitamin B6) Cream

Vitamin B6 has been reported to be particularly effective in inhibiting melanoma cancer cells. Based on this experimental evidence, one research team developed a topical pyridoxal cream that produced a significant reduction in the size of subcutaneous nodules and complete regression of cutaneous papules when applied to patients with recurrent malignant melanoma. The results were considered preliminary, but they may lead to a more successful topical treatment of this highly lethal cancer.

### Further Reading & References

- Robert D. Reynolds, "Vitamin B6 Deficiency and Carcinogenesis." In Poirier, et al., eds., Essential Nutrients in Carcinogenesis, 339-45.

## Radium Weed/Milkweed/Petty Spurge

Radium weed, also known as petty spurge, milk weed or Euphorbia peplus has been used as a folk treatment for skin conditions, including corns and warts, for hundreds of years.

Extracts from Euphorbia peplus have been shown by scientists at the Queensland Institute of Medical Research, Australia to have promise as a treatment for squamous and basal cell carcinomas and other non-melanoma skin cancers.

The study, conducted on behalf of Peplin Biotech, a company which has patented the active compounds in the weed, showed complete removal of the lesions in 90% of the cases. Patients involved in the trial were mainly the very elderly for whom surgery was considered inappropriate, or others for whom conventional therapy had failed.

Limited local inflammation appears to be the only side effect of the radium weed treatment. The researchers maintain that more extensive trials over several years are necessary to confirm the long-term effect and ensure patient safety. However, the sap of the plant is well known as a folk remedy for skin lesions.

Experts point out that attempts at self-treatment with the plant could be dangerous. The milky sap causes irritation to normal skin and can cause blindness if it comes in contact with the eyes. Anyone with skin lesions should always seek advice from a medical practitioner

In a more recent *British Journal of Dermatology* study, 36 patients were treated for different types of non-melanoma skin cancer: basal cell carcinomas, squamous cell carcinomas, and intraepidermal cell carcinomas. After applying sap from the Euphorbia peplus plant for one month, the study found that cure rates for the three types of cancer were 57%, 75%, and 50%, respectively, 15 months after treatment.

The BJD study suggests mild pain is fairly common. 43% of the patients in the study reported no pain and 14% reported enough pain to call it "moderate." One patient complained of "severe pain." It may depend on how frequently the Euphorbia sap is applied. In the British study, the sap was applied once a day for only three days. That was enough to completely get rid of 41 of the 48 cancers within a month.

The novel class of natural compounds purified from Euphorbia peplus shows great potential in the laboratory as a potent treatment for a wide range of human cancers including breast and prostate cancer, leukemia, melanoma and other skin cancers, as well as lung, colorectal and cervical cancer.

### *Further Reading & References*

- Radium Weed Kills Skin Cancers, by Brian McDermott, http://www.rense.com/general69/skin.htm

- Brisbane Times: Old wives' tale to fight skin cancer, http://www.brisbanetimes.com.au/queensland/old-wives-tale-to-fight-skin-cancer-20090518-bca6.html

- "Home treatment of basal cell carcinoma." http://www.ncbi.nlm.nih.gov/entrez/query.fcgi?cmd=Retrieve&db=pubmed&dopt=Abstract&list_uids=979751

- "The sap from Euphorbia peplus is effective against human nonmelanoma skin cancers." J.R. Ramsay, A. Suhrbier, J.H. Aylward, S. Ogbourne, S.J. Cozzi, M.G. Poulsen, K.C. Baumann, P. Welburn, G.L. Redlich, P.G. Parsons. Published online 27 Jan 2011, DOI: 10/1111/j.1365.2133.2010.10184.x

# Raspberry Skin Cream

Raspberry Skin Cream was developed by Dr. Peter Pugliese. It is marketed as a topical cream for skin cancers and keratoses that utilizes the proven ability of ellagic acid (transformed in the body from the ellagitannins in raspberry seeds) to fight cancer. Taken internally, ellagic acid extracted from raspberries, strawberries or other plants, is a well-accepted cancer remedy. It acts by inhibiting the proliferation of cancer cells. Its efficacy as a topical remedy, however, is not well-established.

Raspberry Skin Cream ingredients include the following, excerpted from advertising material:

- Ellagitannins from raspberry seeds.

- Ascorbyl palmitate and allantoin:

- Shitake mushroom extract

- Three moisturizers

- Linoleic esters

- Three component sunblock

- Oat protein


The cream does not include any of the following substances for the given reasons:

- Mineral oil - mineral oil clogs pores

- Diazolidinyl urea - formaldehyde producing preservative

- Sodium lauryl sulfate (sls) - questionable toxicity

- Propylene glycol - processing aid which adds nothing for the skin

*Further Reading & References*

- Ellagitannins from raspberry seeds. http://www.smdi.org/new_page_22.htm (Note: for informational purposes only; not an endorsement.)

- "Raspberry Skin Cream gets rid of skin cancers with no pain or scarring..." http://www.cancer-prevention.net/skincancer.html

# Alternative Technologies

## Robert Beck/Beck Electrifier

The Beck Electrifier is an electronic device originally invented by Robert Beck (but since improved) that is claimed to reverse many "incurable" viral and bacterial conditions, including AIDS, cancer, chronic fatigue syndrome, gastritis, herpes, hepatitis, lupus, and Gulf War Syndrome.

It delivers a low frequency, low current, alternating polarity signal, which neutralizes (stops reproduction of) viruses and bacteria in the bloodstream and organs so the microbes can be eliminated from the body.

Research from MIT & Albert Einstein College of Medicine has revealed the effectiveness of electric currents on all viruses, even on the AIDS virus. The treatment succeeds by deactivating a virus's ability to penetrate cells, and its ability to reproduce in cells it has already penetrated. If viruses are kept out of the cells and in the blood serum, the immune system can easily remove them from the body.

The Beck Electrifier attaches to 2 cloth-covered metal electrodes which are strapped over arteries on the wrists or ankles. Typical usage is 1 to 2 hours daily for 6 weeks. The theory is that putting small, unfelt, safe amounts of electric charge into the blood (via the wetted cloth electrodes placed over the arteries) will disable viruses and bacteria from being able to reproduce. In patent #5139684, laboratory results were listed which showed that 100ua of electric current was sufficient to reduce the infectivity of the HIV-1 virus by 99%.

Self-treatment starts at 10 minutes daily. Over a 1 month period it increases to 1 hour daily, which is sustained for the second month. The advocates of the device claim that daily treatment will render a patient free of any virus and/or bacteria infecting the body within 2 months.

If the infection is extensive, then the microbes will probably also be present in the lymphatic fluids. According to advocates, this requires the use of a Magnetic Pulser, which forces the stagnant lymph fluid to circulate into the bloodstream where the microbes can be disabled by the electricity from the blood electrification unit.

### Further Reading & References

- *The Body Electric: Electromagnetism and the Foundation of Life* by Robert Becker and Gary Selden

- Further information about Bob Beck at http://toolsforhealing.com/CD/Articles/B/BobBeck/BobBeckInfo.html

- Cancer Tutor: Bob Beck Protocol, http://www.cancertutor.com/Cancer02/BobBeck.html

## Bioresonance Therapy/BICOM Device

Bioresonance therapy is an aid to diagnosis and treatment that makes use of a diagnostic tool, the Bioresonance device. Bioresonance therapy deals with the patient's own electromagnetic frequency patterns. The patient's electromagnetic oscillations are received by electrodes working as an antenna and fed into the device.

With the help of special electronic systems, the BICOM device changes the body's own information into therapy signals, which are returned to the patient by the output cable. According to advocates, by this method the electromagnetic pathologic information in the body is eliminated or reduced. The patient and the therapy device respond to one another in a feedback cycle.

The premise is that cells communicate with each other by means of certain wavelengths (frequencies). Where this form of communication remains unimpaired by disturbance frequencies, the person in question is considered healthy. For example, when a toxin enters the body, it disturbs an individual's frequency patterns, and thereby interferes with the body's own regulatory powers and in turn impairs the body's functions. The BICOM device transforms these frequency patterns, which cause illness, into therapeutically effective frequency patterns.

As a diagnostic tool, the device can be used to test a patient for bacteria, candida, fungi, heavy metals, pesticides, environmental pollutants and for vitamin and mineral deficiencies. The device can also be used to measure energy on acupuncture points on the hands and feet, which correlate to twenty organs in the body: liver, kidneys, lungs, large intestine etc.

The screening is carried out quickly, and is completely safe and painless. A small, flat probe is used to take readings on the surface of the skin. The readings give a comprehensive picture of the body's energy balance and organ function in order to identify persistent health problems.

Bioresonance Therapy may be likened to electrical acupuncture without the use of needles.

After completion of the full body screening, the results can be used to correct imbalances in the body's energy field. The machine takes electromagnetic energy information from the body, modifies it, and feeds it back in a way that counteracts energy imbalances. Advocates claim this process enhances regulation and detoxification of the body, which raises the immune system and ultimately improves health.

Bioresonance is said to be very helpful for chronic illnesses like arthritis, fibromyalgia, allergies, addictions, herpes, candida, chronic pain, chronic fatigue, irritable bowel syndrome, indigestion, excess weight and bloating, sinus and migraines.

The German physicist Dr. F.A. Popp and his team of bio-photon researchers produced a great quantity of evidence in support of the hypothesis that all life is controlled by electromagnetic oscillations. Some of the results of Popp's research are presented in his book entitled *How Cancer Can Occur - How Cells Communicate with Each Other*. Dr. Popp said the following about his hypothesis:

"We need to reconsider the concept of illness. I am referring to illness as an interruption of the electromagnetic field of the body before physical symptoms appear.

"We can imagine the illness as a storing of improper oscillations. It is already known that the biological systems have the characteristic of being capable of storing improper oscillations that remain stubbornly stored within the organism and produce regulatory disorders.

"The many thousands of successful therapies in the area of ultrafine bioenergy (BioResonance) also testify to the correctness of the statement that the electromagnetic oscillations of the biological processes are of great importance. The electromagnetic oscillations cause and control the biochemical processes. Whether an organism or organ is healthy or ill is determined, in the final analysis, by the electromagnetic oscillations."

*Further Reading & References*

- BICOM2000, http://www.biotecnoquimica.com/BIOingles.HTM

- BICOM: Bioresonanzmethode, http://www.bicom2000.com/ (Note: site in German)

# Chondriana/Life Crystals

George Merkl claimed that he had discovered a new form of life that destroyed cancer and repaired damaged organs. He called this form of life Chondrianas. Life Crystals Inc. was the distributor.

*Further Reading & References*

- George Merkl, Chondriana & Life Crystals http://www.rexresearch.com/merkl/merkl.htm

- An Ancient, Sacred Knowledge, by Dr. George Merkl, Ph.D. http://www.sun-nation.org/merkl-life-crystals.html

# Cold Laser Therapy

Cold laser therapy uses a beam of low-intensity laser light to initiate a series of enzymatic reactions and bioelectric events that stimulate the natural healing process at the cellular level.

According to Marvin Prescott, D.M.D., of Los Angeles, cold laser therapy, sometimes referred to as soft or low-level laser therapy, utilizes a beam of low-intensity laser light to initiate a series of enzymatic reactions and bioelectric events that stimulate the natural healing process at the cellular level.

Dr. Prescott states: "Cold laser therapy has been successfully applied to pain control, orthopedic myofascial syndrome (inflammation of the muscles and their surrounding membranes), neurology, trauma, dermatology, and dentistry. The effects on microcirculation, increased synthesis of collagen in the skin, production of neurotransmitters, and pain relief have all been documented."

Dennis Tucker, Ph.D., L.Ac., of Nevada City, California, uses cold laser therapy to stimulate acupuncture points as an aid to healing wounds, and to reduce inflammation and balance the energy flow in the acupuncture meridians. Dr. Tucker also finds cold laser therapy very effective in treating infections under teeth. According to advocates, cold laser therapy is applicable with little prior knowledge, either by a health provider or by self-application, with no demonstrable side effects when used properly. With the development of microelectronics, pen-sized, low-level laser instruments are now available.

*Further Reading & References*

- American Cancer Society: Cold Laser Therapy, http://www.cancer.org/Treatment/TreatmentsandSideEffects/ComplementaryandAlternativeMedicine/ManualHealingandPhysicalTouch/cold-laser-therapy

- Laser Therapy relief for chronic pain, http://www.thorlaser.com/

# Colored Light Therapy

There is significant evidence that different colors of light have different effects on the body. In 1942, the Russian scientist S. V. Krakov demonstrated that red light stimulates the sympathetic nervous system, while white and blue light stimulate the parasympathetic nervous system. Earlier experiments revealed that certain colors stimulate hormone production, while other colors inhibit it. Specific colors have effect on specific diseases.

In the late 19th and early 20th centuries, it was noted that symptoms of acute eruptive diseases such as smallpox and measles were relieved when patients were put in a room with red windows. Melancholiacs also recovered after a few hours in such rooms. Norman Shealy, M.D., Ph.D., of Springfield, Missouri, uses flashing bright lights and colored lights to treat pain and depression. According to Dr. Shealy, these treatments have been shown to alter neurochemical production in the brain and this may account for their positive effects. Dr. Shealy believes the brain has specific responses to different frequencies of flashing light and the different wavelengths of various colors.

"Sleep problems can often be cured in one day by this method," he says, "but mood alteration usually takes one to two weeks of treatments." Dr. Shealy believes that it is the relaxation induced by these methods that is responsible for the effects seen in patients suffering from pain. "I believe tension is a primary factor in 100% of pain," he says, "and once you relax the tension, the pain eases."

Dr. Shealy has found that photo-stimulation with flashing opaque white or violet lights induces relaxation, reducing stress and chronic pain. "Photo-stimulation, or brain wave synchronization, has been used as a tool to assist relaxation and the induction of hypnosis since 1948," he says. "It has been used with the EEG (electroencephalogram) as an adjunct to the diagnosis of epilepsy."

Another method of colored light therapy known as monochromatic red light therapy is used to treat a range of problems, including shoulder pain, endocrine problems, dysmenorrhea, diabetes, gastrointestinal problems, depression, impotence, and frigidity. Gerald Hall, D.C., of El Paso, Texas, uses monochromatic red light therapy to treat the acupoints of the ear and elsewhere on the body.

Ray Fisch, Ph.D., C.H., of Los Angeles, uses monochromatic red light therapy for headaches (applying the light across the brow), arthritis, allergies, sore throats, sinus problems, stress reduction, and wound healing. The red light is also applied to acupressure points or to sites of localized pain. For localized pain such as tendinitis, two five-minute applications directly to the painful area are followed by ten to fifteen seconds to the surrounding area. This is followed by a gentle massage of the area. Treatment is repeated two to three times a day for a week, then twice a day for a week followed by once a day for another week.

According to Dr. Fisch, there are "virtually" no side effects and the patient can administer this treatment at home.

### Further Reading & References

- Krakov, S. V. "Color, Vision and the Autonomic Nervous System." Journal of the Optical Society of America 31 (Apr, 1944): 335-337.

# Cytoluminescent Therapy/Photoluminescence/PDT - Photodynamic Therapy/Phototherapy

Cytoluminescent Therapy is an advanced form of Photodynamic Therapy (PDT). In essence, it utilizes a photosensitizer -- a chemical substance that becomes active only in the presence of a certain type of light. Once light of the appropriate wavelength hits the photosensitizing agent (which accumulates in cancer cells) it damages or kills those cells.

The procedure consists of injecting a photosensitizer into the patient's body that finds its way into the cancerous cells wherever they are. Then, light of a particular frequency is shone onto the location of the cancer, activating the photosensitizing agent, which kills the cancer cells.

The procedure does little or no harm to health cells. Once in the body, the photosensitizing agent is rapidly eliminated from normal tissue but selectively accumulates in neoplastic and dysplastic (i.e., cancerous) tissue. This is followed by irradiation with light of the specific wave length that activates the photosensitizer. The result is selective damage or elimination of tumor cells while normal tissues are unharmed.

This treatment is also variously called "Therapeutic Light Therapy" or "Photoluminescence". It has far-reaching clinical implications in the treatment and/or prevention of infectious diseases. "Photo" refers to light, and "luminescence" refers to the emission of light.

Advocates of this therapy note that two photosensitive amino acids are present in all cells to varying degrees. Bacterial and viral cells contain at least five times as much of these amino acids as do healthy blood cells. Thus, bacterial and viral cells absorb five times as much photonic energy as their healthy counterparts. The healthy cells remain intact while the diseased cells are killed and marked. If accurate this would help explain the reported effectiveness of PDT in the treatment of infectious diseases.

This method, used intermittently, has produced no known serious and adverse side effects. PDT is a minimally invasive treatment with great promise in malignant disease. It can be applied before or after chemotherapy, ionizing radiation, or surgery, without compromising these treatments or being compromised itself. Unlike radiotherapy and surgery, it can be repeated many times at the same site. Response rates and the durability of response with PDT are as good as, or better than, those with standard loco-regional treatments. Furthermore, there is less morbidity and better functional and cosmetic outcome.

PDT is reportedly valuable for premalignant conditions such as mucosal dysplasia and carcinoma-in-situ. The excellent cosmetic outcome makes it valuable for skin lesions and for lesions of the head, neck, and oral cavity, where another advantage is that PDT has negligible effects on underlying functional structures. With endoscopic delivery of light to hollow structures such as the stomach, PDT has been successful in the treatment of early gastrointestinal cancers, such as esophageal cancer and lung cancer.

Preclinical studies have shown that photodynamic therapy (PDT) of tumors augments the host antitumor immune response.

The momentum behind Photo-Dynamic Therapy as a cancer treatment has been growing rapidly. It is currently being used and studied in Russia and the USA.

Cancer Research UK, working with the Gray Cancer Institute in Middlesex, has reported highly promising results. They found that a colorful combination of red light, blue dye, and a plant hormone can be used to kill cancer cells. Their study reported in the prestigious journal *Cancer Research* shows the treatment could be much more effective when combined with a plant hormone that in nature helps plants grow towards the sun.

Scientists at the Institute treated cancer cells with a special blue dye that becomes chemically energized in response to light. When they shone red light on to the cells treated with dye and the plant hormone, the hormone shattered to produce toxic chemicals called free radicals. These form poisonous byproducts with the potential to kill cancer cells. Sir Paul Nurse, Chief Executive of Cancer Research UK, says, "This is fascinating work in that it combines using clever technology with something provided by nature — the plant chemicals. It is a further step in the direction of producing a therapy that directly targets the tumor."

Another study has shown, "Photodynamic therapy, according to a research paper, increased the expected lifespan of many of the 16 pancreatic cancer patients who underwent it. There are two stages to the treatment. Firstly, a drug is given which 'sensitizes cells to the effects of light. If these cells are exposed to strong light, they die.

"Then, a fiber-optic cable is placed near the target tumor, and light is precisely aimed through it. When the beam hits the tumor cells, it kills them, hopefully without damaging too many surrounding cells. The research, carried out at University College London and detailed in the journal *Gut*, involved patients with inoperable advanced cancer, who were not expected to live long."

### Further Reading & References

- The Moss Reports, by Ralph W. Moss http://www.cancerdecisions.com/121904_page.html

- The Moss Reports Part II, by Ralph W. Moss http://www.cancerdecisions.com/122604_page.html

- "Photodynamic therapy: a clinical reality in the treatment of cancer." Hopper C. Lancet Oncol. 2000 Dec;1:212-9. Related Articles, Links http://www.ncbi.nlm.nih.gov/entrez/query.fcgi?cmd=Retrieve&db=PubMed&list_uids=11905638&opt=Abstract

- Cancer Res., March 15, 2002; 62(6): 1604-8.

- BBC News: "Light Therapy Tackles Cancer," http://ews.bbc.co.uk/1/hi/health/1871474.stm

## Dr. John Holt/Tronado machine

Dr. John Holt stated to millions on Australian television in August 2004 that he cures 25% of his cancer patients. Dr. John Holt's controversial treatment works, in layperson's terms, by giving the patient an injection of a glucose-blocking agent. He then shines "radio waves" into the body at a specific frequency. He does not guarantee success with every patient. At the time this information was gathered the cost of the treatment was about AUS$6500, much of which was covered by medical insurance.

Born in Bristol 80 years ago and a member of the Royal Colleges, Dr. Holt has 26 medical letters after his name. For more than a decade, he was in charge of Western Australia's main cancer institute, until the late 1970s, when he was blacklisted by his medical colleagues and politicians. While working as a radiotherapist at the Sir Charles Gairdner Hospital in Perth, with the help of the then Premier of Western Australia, John Tonkin, he bought Tronado machines for both the hospital and his private clinic. Dr. Holt treated more than seven thousand cancer patients with the Tronado—with remarkable results, according to his supporters... At the same time, he continued to treat cancer patients at the hospital with normal radiotherapy.

In a published trial with head and neck cancers (for easy verification of results), a 34% initial success rate was achieved with radiotherapy and 17% were still in remission three years later. With the Tronado the initial success was 92% with 68% still in remission after three years.

"The doctors took up such an action initially, they said the treatment was fake and useless," said former WA Premier John Tonkin, but added, "There is no doubt whatsoever in my mind that this is the most advanced form of cancer treatment in the world today."

### Further Reading & References

- RightHealth, http://www.righthealth.com/topic/Tronado_Machine

- Australian Dr. John Holt's Cancer Treatment, http://www.cam.net.uk/home/aaa315/healing/john-holt-cancer-treatment.htm

# Elanra

Elanra is the brand name of a unique device reported to reduce pain, raise energy levels, and increase survival. Apparently, many health practitioners recommend it to their patients.

The device increases the levels of negative ions of oxygen in the ambient air of a room or enclosed dwelling. Inhaling such air is said to benefit the body's fluids and tissues. As two-time Nobel Prize winner Dr. Otto Warburg said, "Cancer cannot survive in an oxygen-rich environment". Additionally, the device utilizes specific frequencies that may enhance the immune system and eradicate bacteria and viruses linked to cancer.

The Elanra therapeutic ionizer is reported to be the only ionizer available today capable of generating the small negative ions of oxygen that can be inhaled to enter the bloodstream and produce biologically beneficial effects.

Furthermore, it has the ability to modulate frequencies down to as low as IOHz for relaxation and the magical 7.83Hz, which is the Schumann Resonance - or the Earth's own "brainwave", according to enthusiasts for this approach. Dr. Robert Beck, the father of electro-medicine, wrote in the *Archaeus*, Volume 4 1986:

"it has been speculated that frequencies in the 7.83Hz. range may be the universally permeating 'clock frequencies' or carriers on the which 'mind' or 'consciousness' states can be impressed and in which they may interact with other life forms in the nebulous realms of ESP, psychotronics, distant healing, radiesthesia and related paranormal phenomena".

### Further Reading & References

- Hidden Cures: under "Air," http://www.hiddencures.com/hiddencures.htm

# Electrotherapy/Electro Cancer Treatment (ECT)/Dr. Björn Nordenström/Galvano Treatment

Electrotherapy, also known as electro-cancer treatment (ECT), electrochemical tumor therapy, and Galvano treatment was developed in Europe by the Swedish professor Björn Nordenström and the Austrian doctor Rudolf Pekar. The therapy employs galvanic electrical stimulation to treat tumors and skin cancers.

ECT is used most often as an adjunct with other therapies. Using local anesthesia, the physician inserts a positively-charged platinum, gold or silver needle into the tumor and places negatively-charged needles around the tumor. Voltages of 6 to 15 volts are used, dependent upon tumor size. To enhance the cancer-cell-killing power of ECT, sometimes small amounts of chemotherapy agents are applied to the skin and driven into the tumor by a kind of sweating effect of the electric current ("iontophoresis").

ECT works by influencing the acid/alkaline (pH) levels within the tumor and causing electrolysis of its tissue, which is more susceptible to direct current than normal tissue is. The pH change depolarizes cancer cell membranes and causes tumors to be gently destroyed. The ECT process also appears to generate heat shock proteins around the cancer cells, inducing cell-specific immunity. This process triggers Natural Killer (NK) cells, thought to be key anticancer immune system cells.

Electro medicine has been widely used for many years, especially in orthopedics where it has been used for regeneration, i.e., to accelerate the healing process in broken bones, and also for treating pain. In oncology, however, the use of electromedicine (ECT) is relatively new and certainly not accepted by conventional oncologists.

Direct current can be directed into tumorous tissue (skin metastases, lymph node metastases or isolated organ metastases) through the application of electrodes. If the total amount of direct current is high enough, this procedure results in the destruction of cancerous cells.

As soon as direct current is connected to the electrodes, different electrochemical reactions influence the pH-value and can cause electrolysis of tumor tissue. Depolarization of the cell membranes changes the cellular environment, forcing the tumor cells to gently disintegrate. The interruption of certain functions within the cancerous cells can lead to the destruction of these cells.

The body's own catabolic processes remove the destroyed malignant tissue from the body.

It is also hypothesized that through this process the immune system is activated and starts attacking all other cancer cells within the body. Once ECT is successfully completed and the cancerous area is treated, the area heals and is replaced with scar tissue.

One practitioner states that ECT is suitable for all types of superficial or deep seated tumors, which can be reached by needle electrodes. Specifically, however, it is used for small mammary carcinomas or isolated axillary, supraclavicular and thoracic nodes, all tumors of the ENT area, especially after radiation or chemotherapy, skin carcinomas e. g. Basaliome, Spinocellular carcinoma, Melanoma etc. gynecological carcinomas, soft tissue tumors.

The destructive effect of the direct current on tumorous tissue can be enhanced by the simultaneous administration of cytotoxic substances (chemotherapy drugs), for example, Mitomycin, Adriamycin, Epirubicin, and Cis-Platinum.

Cytotoxic substances are best applied to hollow organs, for example, esophagus, bladder, stomach, and rectum. The membrane potentials are changed to such an extent by the current that the cells open and absorb cytotoxic substances more rapidly.

Normally, the treatment is carried out under local anaesthetic and on an outpatient basis. The size of the tumor determines how many needle electrodes are required. However, a minimum of 2 are always used. These are introduced into the tumor through the skin. The electrodes should not be further than 1.5cm apart.

These methods are used at the Klinik St. Georg in Bad Aibling, Germany, where the therapy is often combined with hyperthermia (either local or whole body) and low dose chemotherapy. Full treatment programs are available in either China or Germany. Electrical therapy is painless unless a large tumor is being dealt with.

### Further Reading & References

- The electro-cancer therapy (ECT) according to Dr. med. Rudolf Pekar, http://www.dr-baltin.de/en/cancers/approaches-therapies/electro-cancer-therapyp-pekar.html

- Exclusive Report: Electro-Cancer Therapy (ECT/BET), a gentle alternative to cancer therapy, http://www.german-news.de/news/news+article.storyid+2833.htm

# Far Infrared Therapy/Near Infrared Therapy/Nanoshells

Over the last 25 years, Japanese and Chinese researchers and clinicians have completed extensive research on infrared treatments and report many provocative findings. In Japan, there is an "infrared society" composed of medical doctors and physical therapists dedicated to further infrared research. Their findings support the health benefits of infrared therapy as a method of healing.

Infrared energy penetrates tissues to a depth of over one inch. Its energy output is tuned to correspond closely to the body's own radiant energy so that body tissues absorb close to 93% of the infrared waves that reach the skin.

There have been over 700,000 infrared thermal systems sold in the Orient for whole-body treatments. An additional 30 million people have received localized infrared treatment in the Orient, Europe, and Australia with lamps, which emit the same 2-25 micron wave bands as employed in a whole-body system. In Germany, physicians have used whole-body infrared therapy for over 80 years.

More recently, infrared heat has been used in cancer therapy. This is a new experimental procedure that shows great promise in some cases when used properly. American researchers favor careful monitoring of the tumor temperature; whereas, the successes reported in Japan make no mention of such precaution.

One of the newest treatments for fighting cancer with infrared technology is the use of an infrared sauna. These saunas penetrate up to 1-1/2 inches below the surface of the skin, effectively detoxifying and revitalizing cells. This results in a deep, detoxifying sweat that eliminates toxins at the cellular level.

Infrared energy is powerful, yet safe. It remains the energy of choice used in hospitals to warm newborn infants. The mechanism behind infrared heat ability to fight cancer has to do with its high temperature. High temperatures are known to kill cancer cells, usually without damage to normal tissues.

In an article in the *Townsend Letter for Doctors and Patients*, Lawrence Wilson, MD writes, "If I were to single out one method to combat cancer, it is the sauna. It assists removal of chemical toxins and heavy metals, increases oxygenation, enhances the immune system, and reduces the radiation burden in the body."

Dr. Wilson notes that infrared sauna therapy for cancer offers a combination of healing mechanisms. They act simultaneously to support the fight against cancer. These include:

- **Hyperthermia:** Heating the body is a well-known and underused method of killing cancer cells, says Dr. Wilson. Cancer cells are weaker than normal cells and more susceptible to damage from heat. Infrared saunas are superior for this purpose, he says.

- **Eliminate Toxins:** Saunas also help purge the body of toxins, such as heavy metals and chemicals.

- **Improving circulation**. Cancer often grows in tissues with poor circulation and thus poor nutrition and oxygenation. Infrared saunas boost overall circulation. This brings nutrients, hormones, oxygen and other substances to all body tissues.

- **Decongesting the internal organs.** The liver, kidneys and other internal organs can become burdened with estrogen, chemicals, and toxic metals. Infrared saunas cause blood to move toward the body surface. This helps cleanse the internal organs.

- **Care for your body's largest organ:** The skin is a major organ for eliminating body wastes. But in most people, it's inactive because they don't sweat enough. Infrared saunas help cleanse the body from the inside. They encourage sweating and free up toxins stored beneath the skin.

In a clinical study published in the *Journal of Cancer Science and Therapy*, scientists studied far infrared's effects on human cancer cells *in vitro* (lab cultures) and on cancer cells in mice. Far infrared therapy reduced tumor volumes 86% in 30 days. The tumor-suppressing effects were also seen without high temperatures, even as low as 77 degrees Fahrenheit.

In another study, researchers in Japan discovered that whole-body hyperthermia induced far infrared radiation (essentially, deep heat) strongly inhibited the growth of breast cancer tumors in mice without deleterious side effects. Researchers believe this therapy is promising for long-term studies of a noninvasive treatment of breast cancer.

The deep penetration of infrared heat releases toxins from the fat layers just beneath the skin. It also helps the body eliminate toxins from the internal organs. These toxins pass from the organs to the fat tissue under the skin and are then eliminated in perspiration.

In an effort to explain this phenomenon, researchers analyzed the sweat from both traditional and infrared saunas. Sweat from traditional saunas was roughly 97% water and 3% toxins. In contrast, infrared saunas produced a sweat that was only 80-85% water. The remaining 15-20% was made up of heavy metals, sulfuric acid, sodium, ammonia, uric acid, and fat-soluble toxins.

Infrared saunas are typically accessible at local health clubs and spas. They can also be purchased for home use.

### Further Reading & References

- *Pain Free With Far Infrared Mineral Therapy: The Miracle Lamp* by Kara Lee Schoonover (2003)

- Far Infrared Medical, http://www.farinfraredmedical.org/

- van der Zee J. Heating the patient: A promising approach? *Annals of Oncology* 2002; 13:1173-1184.

- Wilson, L. Saunas and Cancer, *Townsend Letter for Doctors and Patients*, June 2004

- Tatsuo I, Ishibashi, J. et al Non-Thermal Effects of Far-Infrared Ray (FIR) on Human Hepatocellular Carcinoma Cells HepG2 and their Tumors, *J Cancer Sci Ther Volume* 1(2) : 078-082 (2009) - 078 http://www.omicsonline.org/ArchiveJCST/2009/December/01/JCST1.78.pdf

- Udagawa Y, Nagasawa H, Kiyokawa S, Inhibition by Whole-Body Hyperthermia (WBH) with Far-infrared rays of the Growth of Spontaneous Mammary Tumours in mice. *Anticancer Res.* 1999 Sep-Oct;19(5B):4125-30

- Dr. A. J. Adams, International Institute of Holistic Healing: What is Far Infrared Therapy and How Does it Work Toward Healing the Body? www.drajadams.com/SaunaDomeInfrared

# Hyperthermia/Heat Treatment

Hyperthermia is a type of therapy where the body's temperature is raised by an artificial device. Hyperthermia can be administered either locally or over the whole body.

The theory behind hyperthermia (heat therapy) is that raising the temperature of the body increases circulation and also increases the supply of oxygen to the cancer site. Cancer cells do not thrive in the presence of oxygen. Tumors and cells located near the surface of the body are more vulnerable to heat treatments than those protected deep inside.

In local hyperthermia, a device is placed over the specific area of the body to be heated. For example, the doctor applies the hyperthermia device to the breast of a breast cancer patient to heat up the area. This kind of hyperthermia can take place every other day.

Whole-body hyperthermia is somewhat more extreme. The patient, wrapped in towels, lies naked on a hyperthermia bed. The patient's body temperature is gradually raised to about 105 degrees Fahrenheit and kept at that temperature for about two hours. In some instances, the temperature may be raised as high as 107 degrees, known as "extreme hyperthermia." Unlike local hyperthermia, whole-body hyperthermia is generally done no more than once a week.

There are three kinds of whole-body hyperthermia:

- Moderate hyperthermia, in which the patient's core temperature is raised to 101-103 degrees Fahrenheit for two hours, which simulates a natural fever.

- Systemic hyperthermia, which raises the core temperature to 105 degrees F.

- Extreme hyperthermia, which goes up to 107 degrees F.

Throughout the procedure, the patient is carefully monitored. A good machine for whole body hyperthermia costs well over a quarter of a million dollars and is generally complicated to operate. Few medical practitioners are trained to use these machines.

Hyperthermia is a commonly used therapy in German and Mexican alternative cancer clinics. In Germany, local hyperthermia is done with radio frequencies (short waves), which penetrate deep into the body (often as much as 18 centimeters, or about seven inches). This novel kind of hyperthermia is available only in Germany, which is one reason cancer patients from all over the world go there for treatment.

Another German innovation is transurethral hyperthermia for prostate cancer. This approach to local hyperthermia, which applies heat only to the prostate gland by way of a catheter inserted through the urethra (the urinary passage), shows promise of becoming the most effective treatment known for early stage prostate cancer (*i.e.* prostate cancer that has not spread to other parts of the body).

Clinics in other countries offer local hyperthermia using microwaves, which only penetrate the body about five centimeters, or approximately two inches. This is far less effective than the deeper penetrating radio frequencies that German doctors use. Hyperthermia with radio frequency waves is not yet available in the United States. Whole-body hyperthermia is not available in the United States, due to hostile medical regulations, and local hyperthermia is available in only a few clinics and doctor's offices.

Some patients opt to have a low dose of chemotherapy administered in conjunction with hyperthermia treatment. Patients suffer none of the typical chemotherapy side effects when they receive this mild form of dual treatments.

In a 1999 study published in *Anticancer Research,* 80 patients were treated for colorectal cancer with liver metastases. The treatment was a combination of hyperthermia and low-dose chemo. The study found that the average survival time was "twice as high as expected" — compared to patients treated with chemotherapy alone.

Many physicians who offer hyperthermia treatment believe that a strong immune system is key to the success of the treatment. Because of that, patients are given a number of immune-supportive therapies prior to undergoing their first hyperthermia treatment. The immune-strengthening therapies used include mistletoe, thymus peptides, vitamin C by IV, magnetic-field therapy, ozone therapy, and oxygen therapy.

### Further Reading & References

- North American Hyperthermia Society, http://www.thermaltherapy.org

- *Application of Hyperthermia in the Treatment of Cancer* by R.D. Issels (1988)

- Hyperthermia In The Treatment Of Cancer, http://www.thelancet.com/journals/lancet/article/ PIIS0140-6736%2879%2990594-4/abstract

- Hager, Dieter. "Deep Hyperthermia with Radiofrequencies in Liver Metastases," *Anticancer Research* 19: 3403-3408 (1999).

- Hager, Dieter. "Intraperitoneal hyperthermic perfusion chemotherapy (IPHC) for patients with chemotherapy-resistant peritoneal disseminated ovarian cancer." *International Journal of Gynecologic Cancer* 2001;11 (Suppl. 1): 57-63.

# Magnets/Magnetic Field Therapy

Dr. William Philpott of Choctaw, Oklahoma treated a 20-year-old patient with an inoperable glioblastoma – a form of brain cancer. He placed the north pole of a ceramic magnet on the back of the patient's head at the point where the tumor had initially started to grow. The magnet was left in this position for 24 hours a day.

At the beginning of the treatment at the American Biologics hospital in Tijuana, Mexico, this patient was incapable of making any response to his environment. After three days of continuous treatment, he was able to wiggle his fingers in response to questions. Three weeks later, he reportedly walked out of the hospital with the assistance of only a walker. The patient continued magnetic-field exposure of the brain five hours a day and was reported to be well six months later, except for a residual imbalance problem.

Obviously an ordinary magnet is of no use for this kind of treatment as both north and south poles appear on the same side. What is needed is a flat bar magnet, magnetized so that opposite poles are on opposing flat sides. Note that biomagnetic south fields must be avoided. To check the north and south poles of a magnet a magnetometer is needed. North pole reads negative, south positive.

It is also possible to buy magnetic beds to sleep on. Japanese beds are based on normal magnets that have an alternating current force field. These can give temporary benefits, but advocates claim that for long term benefits a direct current negative field bed is required. One developed by Dr. Bonlie, marketed by Magnetico, reportedly has a force field nearly ten times stronger than the earth's.

Bonlie's research produced evidence that the magnetic force of the earth is depleting at a rate of 5 per cent every century – and his bed therefore gives off a magnetic force equal to that prevalent on earth some 4,000 years ago. The flow of this magnetic energy through the body for eight hours a day has had, he claims, a remarkable effect on healing, particularly with arthritis, but more interestingly with regard to cancer. It has a demonstrable and powerful effect on the oxygen levels in the blood and the efficiency of the body's biochemical reactions.

Clinical experiments indicate that magnetic therapy is safe, non-addictive, and there are no known harmful exposure levels. Clinical tests have suggested that magnets are effective to reduce pain. Magnetic fields deeply penetrate the flesh with a field that energizes, alkalizes, and oxygenates the blood, improving the immune system performance and the body's healing abilities, according to advocates.

Dr. Albert Roy Davis, Ph.D., noted that positive and negative magnetic polarities have different effects upon biological systems of animals. He found that magnets could be used to arrest and kill cancer cells in animals, and could also be used in the treatment of arthritis, glaucoma, infertility, and diseases related to aging. He concluded that negative magnetic fields have a beneficial effect on living organisms, whereas positive magnetic fields have a harmful effect.

A number of practitioners offer different types of magnetic therapy based on different theories and their own clinical experience. There appears to be no uniform, generally accepted protocol among the many advocates of this approach. Nonetheless, there are many impressive anecdotes of successful treatment.

### Further Reading & References

- The Magnetic Answer For Cancer, http://www.alternativehealth.co.nz/cancer/magnetic.htm

- Magnetico Sleep Pads, http://www.magneticosleep.com (Note: For informational purposes only; not an endorsement)

- Alternative Options, http://www.fightingcancer.com/download/fcpdf/21%20A-Z%20of%20 alternative%20options.pdf

# Multi-Wave Oscillator (MWO)/Dr. Lakhovsky

There has been a recent surge of interest in a Russian made electromagnetic machine called the "Multi-Wave Oscillator." George Lakhovsky, a Russian doctor, reputedly had a 98% success rate in treating fatal cancers over an 11-year period with his machine. Lakhovsky's device was used in the U.S. until 1942 and in Europe for about another 15 years. It was ordered removed from the US hospitals that were using it shortly after Lakhovsky was hit by a car and died in 1942.

There are Multi-Wave Oscillators for sale on the Internet that claim to be based on Lakhovsky's work.

### Further Reading & References

- Georges Lakhovsky, Bioelectric Pioneer, http://educate-yourself.org/be/lakhovskyindex.shtml

- Georges Lakhovsky, Bioelectric Pioneer, http://alternativehealingtools.com/Lakhovsky/

- *Lakhovsky Multiple Wave Oscillator Handbook: Comprising the Borderland Sciences Research Foundation Lakhovsky Multiple Wave Oscillator & Radio-Cellular Oscillator Research Files* by Thomas J. Brown, Tom Brown (1990)

- *Secret of Life: Electricity Radiation & Your Body* by Georges Lakhovsky (1988)

# Orgone/Orgone Accumulators/Orgone Beam/Wilhelm Reich

Austrian-born Wilhelm Reich began his career as a conventionally trained scientist who studied medicine at Vienna University. His main theme was that sexual energy was of vital importance not only to the creation of life but to its complete fulfillment, and that sexuality was "the center around which revolves the whole of social life as well as the inner life of the individual."

Reich eventually concluded that almost all sickness —including psychological ailments such as schizophrenia and depression — was the result of failing to achieve "true orgasm", complete sexual satisfaction.

He was an important member of Freud's Psychoanalytic Society in Vienna, but later broke with Freud. In 1939, forced to leave Austria following the Nazi takeover, he settled in New York.

In 1935, he announced that he had succeeded in producing what he called 'bions' from certain substances (such as coal), and that these were capable of developing into protozoa (single-cell organisms). In short, he claimed to have produced life from inanimate materials – merely one of many unusual claims he made during his controversial career.

Biologists rejected this finding, but Reich worked on, and in 1939 announced that the radiation given out by 'bions' produced from sterilized sea sand was a hitherto unknown form of energy. He called this energy orgone, and described it as "the basic life-stuff of the universe." In 1942, he founded the Orgone Institute, a center for development of his theory that the lack of repeated discharge of this energy through "true orgasm" led to both individual and social neuroses.

Reich claimed orgone was a radiating energy, blue in color and universally present, that was emitted from organic materials and life forms and could be accumulated, observed, and measured. Reich also believed that in specified doses, orgone energy had positive healthful properties, and could help in the treatment of cancer, although not cure it.

Reich conducted a study between 1937 and 1939 on 178 healthy mice. He injected some with T-bacilli, some with PA-bions, some with T-bacilli and then PA-bions, and some with PA-bions and then T-bacilli. The T-bacilli injected group had many more deaths than the PA-injected group.

Also, his data suggested that the PA-bions had an innoculatory effect against the T-bacilli, although damage did not seem to be reversed when the T-bacilli were injected first. Of the 30 mice that died from T-bacilli injections alone, Reich claimed to find cancerous cells in 20. Reich theorized that the T-bacilli he injected acted as a cancer agent.

In the early 1940's Reich soon found that T-bacilli were present in people who were perfectly healthy as well. Reich observed T-bacilli in both the blood of healthy people and cancer patients, and he observed that in the blood of the cancer patients, the T-bacilli developed easily and rapidly. He also found that the red blood cells disintegrated much more rapidly in the cancer patients, and when they did they formed shrunken granules as opposed to the large uniform granules of healthy people.

Reich observed similar findings in the sputum, excrement and vaginal secretions of patients. He claimed he could identify patients at a high risk for cancer by the high levels of T-bacilli in their blood. Interestingly, at the time, no cancer researchers had observed or noted finding evidence of cancer in the blood or other bodily fluids of their patients. It wasn't until 1955 that classical cancer pathology discovered that cancer cells could be found in the sputum of cancer patients.

Reich had earlier observed the deteriorating effects of the PA-bions, which he believed to be charged with orgone energy, had on T-bacilli, which he now believed was an agent of cancer. He decided to see how orgone energy collected in his accumulator affected mice with cancer. He found that the average life span of the untreated cancer mice was four weeks, whereas the average life span of the mice that had been treated with the accumulator was eleven weeks.

"The very first tests revealed an astonishingly rapid effect; the mice recuperated rapidly, the fur became smooth and shiny, the eyes lost their dullness, the whole organism became vigorous instead of contracted and bent, and the tumors ceased to grow or even receded."

Reich began experimenting with the use of orgone accumulators on cancer patients. In the fifteen cases he worked with between 1941 and 1943, all were in advanced stages of cancer. Three of them died in the time expected by their doctors, six of them lived five to twelve months longer than expected, and the rest were still alive when Reich published his paper on them in 1943. In all cases, he claimed that their pain was greatly alleviated and their use of morphine was lessened or eliminated altogether.

Reich claimed that orgone could be measured, collected in an "orgone box", and used for the treatment of serious diseases, including cancer. However, the United States Food and Drug Administration declared it a fraud and, in 1956, he was sentenced to two years imprisonment for contempt of court and violation of the Food and Drug Act. He died in prison a year later.

Orgone accumulators are easy to build with alternating layers of metal and organic material. The Orgone beam works on the orgone principle of cell vibration. According to Reich's theory, every living cell vibrates at a specific rate and when the body is low on orgone energy the cell is unable to vibrate at its natural rate. This disturbance in cell vibration enables disease to arise.

### Further Reading & References

- Galactic Orgonomy Exchange, http://www.orgone.org/

- *The Orgone Accumulator Handbook: Construction Plans Experimental Use and Protection Against Toxic Energy* by James DeMeo

- Radionics & Radiesthesia: *A Guide to Working With Energy Patterns* by Jane E. Hartman (2004)

- *The Book of Secrets* by Osho (1998)

- *The Function of the Orgasm: Discovery of the Orgone (Discovery of the Orgone, Vol 1)* by Wilhelm Reich, Vincent R. Carfagno (1986)

- *The Cancer Biopathy (The discovery of the orgone, v.2)* by Wilhelm Reich

- Emotional Armoring: *An Introduction to Psychiatric Orgone Therapy* by Morton Herskowitz D.O.


# PAP Ion Magnetic Induction (PAP-IMI) Device

The PAP ion magnetic induction (PAP-IMI) device developed by Professor P.T. Pappas is an ultra fast, short duration, magnetic and induced electric pulse generator. The PAP-IMI device uses pulsed electromagnetic fields to generate or induce electric pulses inside biological matter.

The PAP-IMI device is most commonly used to treat pain. It has also reportedly been used to treat cancer.

"Nanopulses tweak the innards of cells: a method that would allow doctors to tweak the innards of cells without even touching a patient's body is being developed in the US. The technique is still in its infancy, and it is still not clear exactly what it does to cells. But initial experiments suggest it might one day be possible to use the technique to treat cancer, speed up healing or even tackle obesity," says an article on the PAP-IMI website.

The following is an interesting transcript of an interview with Dr. Michael Cargile, Emeritus Chair of Research for the American Association for Acupuncture and Oriental Medicine:

"Our research group has been using the PAP-IMI with respective areas of dimensions of integrated healing because it seems to cross all lines of physiological, bio-chemical, and electro-chemical phenomena that pertain to the proper operation of a living cell. The National Library of Medicine, in a report that I generated for the healthcare task force in 1993, pursuant to declassifying acupuncture and electro-medicine out of investigational, experimental, and unscientific status into mainstream understanding with the respect of modern science. In that report the National Library of Medicine clearly states that several converging view points from these various disciplines of science have clearly shown and indicated that the body is far more than simply a collection of molecules and cells. That in fact the body is comprised of a set of standing stabilized electromagnetic oscillations or oscillatory patterns and that these electromagnetic patterns, the changes in these patterns, occur before any morphogenesis or pathogenesis, that is, they precede the morphogenesis and pathogenesis."


### Further Reading & References

- Papimi NanPulse Therapy, http://www.papimi.dk (Note: for informational purposes only; not an endorsement)

- Pap-Ion Magnetic Inductor, http://en.wikipedia.org/wiki/Pap-Ion_Magnetic_Inductor

# Radiofrequency Ablation (RFA)

Radio frequency ablation (RFA) is a medical procedure where part of the electrical conduction system of the heart, tumor or other dysfunctional tissue is removed using high frequency alternating current to treat a medical disorder.

High-frequency electric current is used to heat tumors from within, a process referred to as "cooking the tumor to death" (McCullough 2001). In cardiology, high frequency radio waves have been used for decades to ablate cardiac nerves in patients with dangerous heart rhythms that resisted drug therapy. The concept merged into oncology with radiofrequency ablation (RFA) initially used to provide palliative relief to inoperable, terminal patients, particularly those with liver cancer.

Momentum is growing for the technique, and the therapeutic focus is changing as well. So strong are the prospects for RFA that this pioneering treatment appears (according to researchers) to have the potential to replace both surgery and radiation therapy. Because of its therapeutic value and cost effectiveness, along with its noninvasive, low-risk profile, RFA has the attention of both physicians and patients.

The National Institutes of Health consider RFA the most predictable, safest, and simplest method for thermal ablation in bone, liver, kidney, prostate, breast, and brain cancers.

Using open MRI, doctors gain access to the tumor through a needle puncture, a process requiring no surgery. Using specially designed titanium or stainless steel instruments, doctors are directed by the MRI image to the site of malignancy. A titanium electrode is guided to the tumor and enough heat is generated (just below the boiling point) to kill the cancerous cells. After 10-12 minutes of continuous contact with the tumor tissue, the radiofrequency energy "cooks" a sphere of 1-2 inches. By "cooking" adjacent spheres, larger tumors can be treated.

Dr. Jonathan Lewin, director of magnetic resonance imaging at University Hospitals of Cleveland, says that tumorous areas that earlier appeared white are now black, a black hole of dead tumor tissue. It is immediately possible to determine the amount of tumor destruction and to plan treatments (should additional treatment be necessary).

The dead cells are not removed, but become scar tissue and eventually shrink. The procedure is done under local anesthesia, with minimal discomfort to patients. There are no cumulative dose effects as with radiation therapy, so patients can be treated repeatedly if the cancer returns to other sites. Hospitalization is usually limited to several hours rather than days.

Dr. Patrick Sewell (University of Mississippi Medical Center) performed this procedure on nine lung cancer patients in China, ranging in age from 38-78 years. Five had primary tumors, two had primary lung tumors with metastasis, and two had metastasized cancer that had spread to the lungs from other locations. When the PET scans came back (3 days following treatment), all tumors had been killed (Sewell 2000).

At the 85th Annual Meeting of the Radiological Society of North America (Chicago), Dr. Tito Livraghi of Vimercate Hospital, Italy, presented the results of a study designed to evaluate the efficacy of RFA in breast cancer-to-liver metastasis. The study consisted of 15 lesions in 10 patients (average age 51 years). Eight of the patients had progressive metastatic disease following chemotherapy; two patients with hepatic metastasis had not undergone chemotherapy.

Following RFA, the value of the treatment was assessed by biphasic helical computed tomography (CT) performed at 4-month intervals. Complete necrosis was obtained in 14 out of 15 lesions (93%). Follow-up imaging studies (at 4-30 months) were unable to detect a recurrence in any of the 14 lesions. Four patients have remained disease free; five (later) have developed new hepatic and/or extrahepatic metastasis; and one has died with diffuse metastasis. RFA resulted in no treatment-induced complications (Pullen 1999).

Early results (from an NIH Clinical Center Study) look promising for the use of RF energy in patients with certain kidney and adrenal tumors. Of 18 kidney tumors treated, 13 (72%) showed no x-ray evidence of residual tumors immediately following treatment. One patient remained cancer-free 2 years following treatment. In a related NIH study involving adrenal gland tumors, 7 of 11 tumors (64%) showed no active disease following RFA. Though the remaining 36% of patients had evidence of residual tumors on follow-up imaging, all patients treated had x-ray confirmation that most of the targeted tumor was killed by treatment (Healthlink 2000).

### Further Reading & References

- "Radiofrequency ablation of hepatocellular cancer in 110 patients with cirrhosis." http://www.ncbi.nlm.nih.gov/entrez/query.fcgi?cmd=Retrieve&db=PubMed&list_uids=10973388&dopt=Abstract

- "Radiofrequency ablation of 40 lung neoplasms: preliminary results." (18 patients with inoperable lung cancer experienced a 94.4% success rate), http://www.ncbi.nlm.nih.gov/entrez/query.fcgi?cmd=Retrieve&db=pubmed&dopt=Abstract&list_uids=15269026

# Radionics

Radionics is a form of energy medicine. It was created by Dr. Albert Abrams (1863-1924), who claimed he could detect distinct energies or vibrations (radiation) emitted from healthy and diseased tissue in all living things.

### Further Reading & References

- *Radionics and the Subtle Anatomy of Man* by David V. Tansley (2004)

- *Radionics & Radiesthesia: A Guide to Working With Energy Patterns* by Jane E. Hartman (1999)

- *Chakras-Rays and Radionics* by David V. Tansley (2004)

- *Radionics Interface With the Ether Fields* by David V. Tansley (2004)

- *The Secret Art: A Brief History of Radionic Technology for the Creative Individual* by Duncan Laurie (2009)

# Royal R. Rife/Rife Frequency Generator

Dr. Royal R. Rife developed the Rife device in the 1930s. Dr. Rife's machine uses a variable frequency, pulsed radio transmitter to produce mechanical resonance within the cells of the physical body. The Rife machine was, in its time, a pioneering front-runner for what is today the basis of energetic medicine. He is one of the most famous and colorful figures in the history of alternative cancer treatment.

The Rife device utilizes the law of resonance. Its main mode of action is to destroy pathogenic microorganisms i.e. viruses, bacteria, fungi (e.g. Candida) and other pathogens without harming healthy tissue. This is done through the use of electro-magnetics. Rife discovered he could use a specific electro-magnetic frequency to kill a particular strain of bacteria or virus, thus destroying the target diseased organism, causing no damage to the surrounding tissue.

It was Rife's belief that cancer is caused by a microscopic organism with the ability to change from a virus to a bacterium to a fungus. Mainstream medicine has not accepted the existence of these organisms but the theory remains popular among advocates of alternative cancer treatments.

Though the first machines were used on diseases such as tuberculosis, arthritis, and ulcers, it is more commonly known for its use on cancer, as many authors have reported, including Barry Lynes in his book *The Cancer Cure that Worked*. Rife machines work on the principle of sympathetic resonance. This principle states that if there are two similar objects, and one of them is vibrating, the other will begin to vibrate as well, even if they are not touching. In the same way that a sound wave can induce resonance in a crystal glass and shatter it, and ultra-sound can be used to destroy gallstones, Dr. Rife's instrument aims to use sympathetic resonance to physically vibrate the cells of the cancer-related parasite, resulting in possible elimination.

Vibration between two objects can be seen in everyday life, from a tuning fork to a guitar string, or as in an opera singer's voice causing a glass to shatter. In this instance, the musical tone sets the glass into motion, and that motion builds until the glass shatters. Mechanical resonance is created when a small periodic stimulus (in Dr. Rife's case, a pulsed wave) of the same natural vibration period of a cell, tissue, or even a molecule, is used to produce a large amplitude vibration of the cell, tissue, or molecule. If the induced resonant vibration is intense enough, the cell, tissue, or molecule will be destroyed. It is claimed that Rife was the first person in history to actually physically prove pleomorphism in micro-organisms. Pleomorphism is the phenomenon of mutating into distinctly different life forms; similar to caterpillars turning into butterflies, and challenges modern biology theory. Pleomorphism has also been observed by other cancer researchers including Dr. Virginia Livingston and Gaston Naessens. All used powerful microscopes that examined living material (unlike current microscopes that examine nonlive material).

From Rife's 1953 article:

"We have classified the entire category of pathogenic bacteria into 10 individual groups. Any organism within its group can be readily changed to any other organism within the ten groups depending upon the media with which it is fed and grown. For example, with a pure culture of bacillus coli, by altering the media as little as two parts per million by volume, we can change that microorganism in 36 hours to a bacillus typhosis showing every known laboratory test even to the Widal retraction. Further controlled alterations on the media will end up with the virus of poliomyelitis or tuberculosis or cancer as desired, and then if you please, alter the media again and change the micro organisms back to a bacillus coli."

Rife was fiercely persecuted for his unorthodox views and the original design for his machine was reportedly lost. A number of Rife-like machines are now on the market that claim to be based on reconstructed versions of his design — or to be improvements in his design. These claims cannot be verified.

Various patients and practitioners use these machines and there are extensive anecdotal reports of successful treatment.

### Further Reading & References

- *The Cancer Cure that Worked* by Barry Lynes (1987)

• The Rife Way, by Mark Simpson, http://www.keelynet.com/biology/rifeway.htm

# SCENAR/ENAR

SCENAR stands for Self-Controlled Energy Neuro-Adaptive Regulator. It is one of a new generation of electrotherapeutic, biofeedback devices. SCENAR technology was first invented in Russia in the mid-1980s by A. Karasev. Originally, it was developed under the umbrella of the Russian space and military program. SCENAR Therapy was first introduced to the UK in 1995 and then spread across the world to the US, Europe, Canada, Australia, South Africa and Asia.

Electrical impulses from the device generate informational input in the body. The SCENAR, through the skin, communicates with the nervous system on three levels:

• Locally, where you touch

• To the zone or spinal segment related to where you touch

• To the central nervous system, including the brain.

In response to a SCENAR impulse, regulative neuro-peptides and the body's own endorphins are released. Cancer patients are reportedly said to receive long lasting pain relief. SCENAR therapy would seem to be a useful supportive therapy throughout the course of chemo- and radiotherapy. It helps to diminish side effects from therapy and releases energy in the body. The patients feel emotionally uplifted as well.

SCENAR therapy was given to 17 cancer patients suffering with chronic pain. All of them were registered as stage four cancer patients. The group consisted of 9 women and 8 men between the ages of 41 and 73. All patients had been suffering pain for at least 3-6 weeks; in 3 cases there had been pain for over 2 months. Before starting SCENAR therapy, all 17 patients had been receiving continuous medical treatment for pain (14 of them with nonnarcotic medication, 3 with promedol injections). As a rule, SCENAR treatment consisted of 9-10 sessions.

Fourteen of the 17 patients (82%) felt pain relief with SCENAR therapy. Patients reduced the use of pain medication; some of them completely stopped taking medication. Patients also enjoyed better sleep with longer dream cycles, better appetite and improved motor activity.

Z. K. Milkevich concludes after observing SCENAR-applications in various cancer clinics: "SCENAR-therapy can become an independent treatment method and can be effectively used at the different stages of the oncological patient's treatment, in combination with the universally accepted techniques. It is absolutely necessary for fourth-stage patients for the improvement of their life quality."

The SCENAR is typically used in a professional setting, but the ENAR (Energy-Neuro- Adaptive-Regulator) is a personal device version of the SCENAR. Macquarie University in Sydney, Australia has completed a randomized control trial on chronic neck pain and dysfunction that shows the ENAR not only gives swift relief from chronic pain and improved functionality but also, coincidentally, improves mental and emotional health. Importantly, these improvements were shown to be sustained at the six months review, well after the end of the six-week treatment period.

This research suggests the ENAR hand-held therapy device has been confirmed as a significant new tool for hands-on body-workers of all types and for use as a personal / family therapeutic device.

*Further Reading & References*

- Bogdanova E.R., Zaidiner B.M., *Scenar Therapy In Oncology*

- Enlightened Therapies, http://www.enlightenedtherapies.com (Note: for informational purposes only; not an endorsement)

- Scenar Therapy, http://invet.net/scenar-therapy.php

# UHF Pulsing to Increase Cell Energy of Cancer Cells

UHF Pulsing is a new concept based on the energy resource deficiency that proponents think is central to the carcinogenic mechanism. They contend the hypothesis offers a new explanation of cancer cell metabolism and suggests methods for the prevention and cure of cancer based on the direct application of high amplitude, plasma-generated pulses of UHF oscillations to cancer cells. It is said to be supported by clinical observations of satisfactory results.

References to the relationship of cell energy level and cancer are found throughout the literature; however, advocates contend that this may be the first definition and characterization of cancer cells as cells with low internal energy.

When a cell becomes cancerous, the following facts relating to the internal energy of the cell are:

- The number of mitochondria is diminished, thus reducing the activity and energy level of the cell.

- The ATP-producing function of oxidation-phosphorylation is diminished causing further reduction in available energy.

- Anaerobic metabolism (glycolysis) increases, acquiring a smaller number of ATP molecules, resulting in limited energy production and reduced thermal energy.

- The internal level of $Na+$ ions is increased relative to the $K+$ ions

Tumor growths of nearly all types have been seen to reduce and even to calcify with UHF pulsing. While the theory has appeared in scientific papers the world over, it awaits a thorough cycle of human clinical trials as of this writing.

See **PAP-IMI Device**.

*Further Reading & References*

- "Effects Of Pulsed Magnetic Field Oscillations In Cancer Therapy," http://www.rife.org/otherresearch/oscillationsincancer.html

# Ultraviolet Light Therapy

Ultraviolet light is known to have antibacterial properties and has been used to sterilize medical equipment.

The healing properties of ultraviolet light were first demonstrated in the 1880s by Niels Ryberg Finsen. He reportedly provided ultraviolet radiation therapy to patients with skin disease or mucous membrane disease. Finsen and his followers are said to have treated more than 2,000 patients with a success rate of 98%. For that he earned the Nobel Prize in 1903.

In the 1930s, ultraviolet therapy was used as a blood treatment. Physicians would essentially "clean" a patient's blood by withdrawing a sample, irradiating it with ultraviolet light to kill unwanted particles in the blood, and then re-injecting it back into the patient. The cleansing process was believed to lower infection levels. It also had a side effect of strengthening the patient's immune system.

From there, ultraviolet light therapy was used successfully in California to cure multiple cases of polio. Despite the positive outcome of the treatment, it was largely abandoned by the medical community once antibiotics were developed.

In the therapy, a small amount of blood, from 60 to 250 CC's, is drawn from the patient and passed through a chamber where it is exposed to ultraviolet light. The blood is then returned to the patient. To those unfamiliar with the therapy, it's surprising and counter-intuitive that exposure of such a small amount of blood to UV light can affect the whole patient, even granted that UV light is a known microbe-killer. The amount of blood exposed, and presumably the microbes killed, are a tiny percentage of the whole.

It's reported that, once stimulated by a UV irradiation of the blood, the immune system continues its activity for hours and sometimes days after the treatment. The number of treatments needed is determined by factors such as the state of the patient's immune system and the length and seriousness of the illness. The usual treatment is about 30 minutes, and is almost painless.

According to Dr. William Campbell Douglass, II, ultraviolet light therapy has been proven in extensive studies and has a "fabulous" record of safety. He reports it has eased the suffering and prolonged the lives of thousands of patients with cancer and other ailments and that he has personally used it in his practice with excellent results.

In 2007, researchers at Newcastle University in the U.K. devised a way to use ultraviolet light to activate antibodies that then target specific tumors. They begin by coating the surface of an antibody with an organic oil that is photocleavable. This prevents the antibody from being activated within the patient until it is specifically illuminated by ultraviolet light. When that happens, the activated antibody binds to T-cells, triggering them to target the surrounding tissue.

When the antibodies are activated near a tumor, the tumor is killed. This means ultraviolet light therapy can be used to steer antibodies directly toward killing cancer tumors, thus sparing attack on healthy tissue and resulting in fewer side effects.

Professor Colin Self, one of the lead researchers in the study, describes the treatment as " … the equivalent of ultra-specific magic bullets. This could mean that a patient coming in for treatment of bladder cancer would receive an injection of the cloaked antibodies. She would sit in the waiting room for an hour and then come back in for treatment by light. Just a few minutes of the light therapy directed at the region of the tumor would activate the T-cells causing her body's own immune system to attack the tumor."

Today, ultraviolet light therapy is said to be a common treatment for multiple ailments in Russia, where drugs are expensive and hospital budgets are severely limited.

The American College for Advancement in Medicine (ACAM) retains a list of doctors who offer this treatment.

### *Further Reading & References*

- *Light directed activation of Human T-Cells*. Colin H. Self, Alexander C. Self, Jacqueline A. Smith, David J. Self and Stephen Thompson. *Journal of ChemMedChem*. 2007.

- *Light activation of anti-CD3 in vivo reduces the growth of an aggressive ovarian carcinoma*, Stephen Thompson, Robert Stewart, Jacqueline A. Smith and Colin Self. *Journal of ChemMedChem*. 2007.

- *Hidden and Forbidden but for REAL: Medical Miracles Nobody Told You About*, by Dr. William Campbell Douglass, II

- *UV Light Improving Chances of Fighting Cancer*, Science Daily, 3 Nov. 2007, http://www.sciencedaily.com/releases/2007/10/071030080626.htm

- The Nobel Prize in Physiology or Medicine, 1903: Niels Ryberg Finsen, http://nobelprize.org/nobel_prizes/medicine/laureates/1903/finsen-bio.html

# Zappers

Many cancer patients now use electronic zappers and magnetic pulsers with apparently good success. The most commonly used varieties are the Hulda Clark zapper and the Beck zapper. They are used in combination with a number of other cancer therapies, not as a standalone cancer treatment.

The Zapper is an electronic device that generates a positive offset frequency that kills bacteria, viruses and parasites simultaneously. The protocol calls for three treatments of 7 minutes each to kill everything, with 20-30 minutes intermission. The Zapper is the size of a regular transistor radio. It operates on a 9-volt battery. Hulda Clark believed that bacteria, viruses, and parasites are a major cause of cancer, and eliminating them is essential to restoring health. (See **Hulda Clark**.)

Killing harmful bacteria and other invaders through electricity is a welcome solution when the time-investment is only three 7-minute sessions. This eliminates the need to go through a range of frequencies, one KHz at a time, as with some similar therapies. It also saves the patient from having to single out specific frequencies as with Rife. Regardless of where the frequency is set (within reason), it will be able to eliminate both small and large aggressors such as flukes, roundworms, mites, bacteria, viruses, and fungi.

Every living thing emits a characteristic range of frequencies (bandwidth), according to the theory. In general, the more primitive the organism, the lower its bandwidth. Advanced animals have higher frequencies and the range is wider. The human range is from 1520 KHz to 9460 KHz. Pathogens (molds, viruses, bacteria, worms, mites) range from 77 KHz to 900 KHz. Thus, humans can work on zapping pathogens in the lower ranges without affecting themselves in the upper range.

Applying an alternating electrical voltage within an organism's bandwidth injures it. Small organisms with narrow bandwidths are extinguished readily (three minutes at five volts). Positively offset frequencies can kill the entire range of small organisms. According to the treatment's proponents, it takes three treatments to kill everything because the first zapping kills viruses, bacteria, and parasites. But a few minutes later, bacteria and viruses (different ones) often recur. They had been infecting the parasites, and killing the parasites released them. The second zapping kills the released viruses and bacteria, but soon a few viruses appear again. The hypothesis is that they infected some of the last bacteria. After a third zapping no viruses, bacteria or parasites are found, even hours later.

For this reason, practitioners say a single treatment with a frequency generator or "Zapper" frequently gives the patient a cold (partial detoxification with re-infection) and can leave him or her fatigued. The Dr. Clark Research Association asked Prof. Henry Lai from the University of Washington in Seattle to find out whether the zapper had any effect on cancer cells in the laboratory. The research work took six months but confirmed that the Zapper selectively kills cancer cells. That is to say, healthy cells are not affected while cancer cells are killed. The research showed that in the lab culture, after 24 hours there were 42% fewer cancer cells than in a control culture that was not subjected to the Zapper.

"To be quite frank when I started the research project I expected that the zapper would do nothing" said Prof. Lai. But when he saw how effective the minimal zapper current was on the cancer cell cultures, he stated:

"Now we must find the mechanism how the cancer cells are killed. If we can do that then I think we can improve the treatment and make it more effective. If we can reduce cancer cells by 42%, we should be able to reduce them by 100%."

### Further Reading & References

- Dr. Clark Information Center, http://www.drclark.net/

- Dr. Hulda Clark Zappers, http://www.huldaclarkzappers.com/php2/index.php (Note: for informational purposes only; not an endorsement)

# Mental, Emotional and Spiritual Approaches

## Behavior Therapy/Psychotherapy

Behavior therapy and related therapies are methods proven in several randomized trials to prevent cancer (and coronary heart disease) and produce a significant reduction in mortality in people suffering from these degenerative diseases. The following article is an extract from a presentation "Evaluating Cancer Therapies and Developing a Cancer Program" by Don Benjamin, Convenor/Research Officer, Cancer Information & Support Society Inc. (CISS), St Leonards (Sydney, Australia), 2003.

"Because of their learned behavior/temperament, people either are susceptible to getting cancer (cancer prone) – sometimes called a Type C personality, or are susceptible to getting coronary heart disease (CHD prone) – sometimes called a Type A personality, or have emotional problems but don't get cancer or CHD, or are emotionally healthy and don't get cancer or CHD (the healthy 'autonomous' type).

The evidence includes a study of 3,235 people diagnosed with stress. Each was given a questionnaire to determine his or her personality profile. The results showed that

- 901 were categorized as cancer-prone

- 818 as coronary CHD-prone

- 570 displayed a mixture of psychological tendencies but were not deemed likely to develop either cancer or CHD

- 946 were the healthy autonomous type


When researchers followed up thirteen years later, the results included the following:

- Of the 901 cancer prone, 39% had died of cancer, 7% of CHD, and 61% were still alive.

- Of the 818 CHD-prone, 25% had died of CHD, 4% of cancer, and 75% were still alive.

- Of the 570 not likely to develop cancer or CHD, 19% had died, and 81% were still alive.

- Of the 946 healthy autonomous type, only 5% had died, and 95% were still alive.


These results give credence to the idea that cancer, CHD, and other degenerative diseases are tied to emotions. Researchers went on to discover how best to apply these results and their implications to prevention and treatment programs.

## Prevention

When the cancer prone type of person was treated with a particular type of individual behavior therapy, results were dramatic. For example:

- Cancer incidence treated dropped from 42% to 26%

- Cancer mortality dropped from 32% to 0%

- Using group therapy, results were still good but not as dramatic (incidence down from 56% to 32%, mortality down from 47% to 7.5%).


It is, therefore, clear that behavior therapy can be used to affect a person's learned behavior and significantly reduce his or her risk of getting cancer and other degenerative diseases.

Results of behavior therapy on people who have already been diagnosed with cancer:

- **Effect of behavior therapy on terminal cancer patients:** This study involved 24 pairs of cancer patients with six different types of inoperable cancer, including scrotal, stomach, bronchiolar, corpus uteri, cervical, and colorectal. Survival times of the treated group averaged 5.07 years (ranging from 1.7 yrs for bronchiolar to 9.5 yrs for colorectal). For the control group, survival averaged 3.09 years (ranging from 1.0 yrs for bronchiolar to 4.9 yrs for colorectal). This is an increase in survival of 64%.

- **Effect of adding behavior therapy to chemotherapy for metastasized breast cancer:** Fifty women with metastasized breast cancer, for whom chemotherapy had been proposed, were divided into pairs matched for age, social background, extent of cancer and medical treatment. One of each pair was then randomly assigned to receive psychotherapy in addition to chemotherapy. Thirty hours of psychotherapy were given to one group of 25 women. The other group of 25 received only chemotherapy. Mean survival times for the 25 patients who received chemotherapy plus psychotherapy was 22.4 months compared with 14.08 months for the 25 who received chemotherapy alone, an increase of 59%.

- **Effect of adding psychotherapy to no treatment for women with metastasized breast cancer:** Fifty of those who refused chemotherapy in the trial above were matched, then one of each pair was randomized to receive psychotherapy. Mean survival for the 25 patients who received psychotherapy was 14.9 months compared with 11.28 months for the 25 who received no treatment, an increase in 32%. It was also observed that the lymphocyte count of those receiving psychotherapy continued to rise over time, whereas in those not receiving psychotherapy it fell, suggesting that the psychotherapeutic intervention may have had its effect through the involvement of the immune system.

- **Effect of structured psychotherapy on women with metastasized breast cancer:** Randomized trials measured survival after structured psychotherapy for late stage breast cancer patients. Eighty Six patients with metastatic breast cancer were randomized into two groups, a study group of 50 and a control group of 36. Both groups received routine oncological care, but the study group was offered a 1½ hr weekly supportive group therapy and self-hypnosis for pain for a one-year period. Average survival for the study group was 36.6 months compared with 18.9 months for the control group, a 94% increase in survival.

- **Effect of structured psychotherapy on people with malignant melanoma:** Twenty eight men and 33 women with melanoma were randomized into two groups, a study group of 35 and a control group of 26. The study group was given a structured psychotherapy group intervention which lasted about 1½ hours per week for 6 weeks. After 6 years there were only 3 deaths out of 34 (9%) in the treated group compared with 10 out of 34 (29%) in the control group (corrected for smaller size) - a 69% reduction in mortality.

It seems apparent that specific forms of structured psychotherapy such as behavior therapy have a dramatic effect on survival or mortality, far greater than that observed with any orthodox therapy.

The mechanism of this connection between the mind/emotions and the body is now becoming more widely understood. For example, unexpressed or inappropriately expressed emotions give rise to circulating protein peptides. Cell receptors on the brain or other organs respond to these peptides, and they enter the cells of the organ. Cell metabolism is disrupted, the immune system becomes weakened, and health deteriorates.

According to Eysenck, author of *The Causes and Cures of Neurosis,* the personality profile that is predisposed to cancer is characterized by an absence of autonomy, i.e. emotional dependence, which prevents such people from making independent decisions in the light of their own best interests.

### *Further Reading & References*

- "Evaluating Cancer Therapies and Developing a Cancer Program" a presentation by Don Benjamin, Convenor/Research Officer, Cancer Information & Support Society Inc. (CISS), St Leonards Sydney, Australia, (2003)

- *The Causes And Cures Of Neurosis: An Introduction To Modern Behaviour Therapy Based On Learning Theory And The Principles Of Conditioning* by H. J Eysenck (1967)

- *The Best of Behaviour Research and Therapy* by S. Rachman, et al (1997)

- *Molecules of Emotion* by Candace Pert (1999)

- Fawzy FI et al. Malignant melanoma. Effects of an early structured psychiatric intervention, coping, and affective state on recurrence and survival 6 years later. Arch gen Psychiatry Sep 1993; 50 (9): 681-9.

- Spiegel, D. et al. Effects of psychosocial treatment on survival of patients with metastatic breast cancer, *Lancet*, October 14, 1989

# Emotional Freedom Techniques (EFT)

EFT was designed and developed by Gary Craig, a Stanford engineer, based on Dr. Roger Callahan's Thought Field Therapy (TFT). Craig describes it as this: "In simple terms, EFT is an emotional form of acupuncture except that we don't use needles. Instead, we tap with the fingertips to stimulate certain meridian points while the client is *tuned in* to the problem. We are still learning why EFT (and its many cousins) work so well. The existing theory is that the cause of all negative emotions is a disruption in the body's energy system."

"Western scientists have largely ignored the subtle energies that circulate throughout the body (until recently). As a result, our use of them for emotional and spiritual healing has been sparse at best. With EFT, however, we consider these subtle energies to be the front running cause of emotional upsets and issues. As a result, EFT professionals claim results that go far beyond those of conventional methods."

The simple, drug-free technique may help patients to deal with the emotional aspects connected to cancer. It may also even bring about physical improvements.

Based on impressive new discoveries involving the body's subtle energies, emotional freedom techniques (EFT) has been clinically effective in thousands of cases for trauma & abuse, stress & anxiety, fears & phobias, depression, addictive cravings, children's issues and hundreds of physical symptoms including headaches, body pains and breathing difficulties. Proponents claim that, properly applied, over 80% achieve either noticeable improvement or complete cessation of the problem.

As can be seen from the home page of the main EFTsite, many doctors are supportive of the use and benefits of these techniques.

### Further Reading & References

- "EFT: Healing the Emotional Roots of Disease," http://www.emofree.com/

# Emotional Trauma and Stress Reduction/Psycho-Oncology/ Psychoneuroimmunology (PNI)

According to some researchers, the power of the mind is apparent from the fact that tumors frequently become evident about a year after an emotional trauma, such as the loss of a close relative. Before, the tumor may have been dormant or slow growing, but the temporary suppression of the immune system through excessive grief or mental depression allows the tumor a growth spurt.

E.M. Reiche et al, state that, "The links between the psychological and physiological features of cancer risk and progression have been studied through psychoneuroimmunology. The persistent activation of the hypothalamic-pituitary-adrenal (HPA) axis in the chronic stress response and in depression probably impairs the immune response and contributes to the development and progression of some types of cancer. ... In general, both stressors and depression are associated with the decreased cytotoxic T-cell and natural-killer-cell activities that affect processes such as immune surveillance of tumors, and with the events that modulate development and accumulation of somatic mutations and genomic instability."

Rene Mastrovito, in a chapter on behavioral techniques in the *Handbook of Psycho-Oncology*, reports that:

"The last two decades have seen a dramatic rise in the use of behavioral therapies for control of symptoms. Especially in cancer, they are now extensively applied to control psychological distress and pain. The behavioral techniques, encompassing hypnosis, meditation, autogenic training, progressive relaxation, and biofeedback, are also called by some cognitive-behavioral, holistic, and alternative modes of therapy.

"Such therapeutic interventions generally are characterized by two basic stages in which the patient is first guided through a primarily cognitive activity that creates the second stage, an altered state of consciousness. By far, the most widely used technique in cancer is relaxation therapy, which promotes an altered state of awareness through reducing distressing emotions and producing a physiologically quiescent state in which there is selective awareness of specific sensory stimuli to the exclusion of others."

Rigorous studies support the use of such behavioral therapies to help patients reduce the nausea and vomiting they often experience at the mere thought that they are about to undergo chemotherapy. 25%

to 65% of patients both anticipate and experience nausea once signed up for protracted chemotherapy, as reported by William Redd, Ph.D. and leading authority in the field of behavioral interventions. He has studied interventions to diminish anticipatory nausea and vomiting that included hypnosis with imagery, biofeedback with imagery, systematic desensitization, progressive relaxation with imagery, and attentional or cognitive distraction.

Dr. Redd says, "For some patients, any event or stimulus that is repeatedly associated with post-treatment side-effects becomes an elicitor of anticipatory reactions ... clearly the most potent stimulus for the chemotherapy patient is the smell of the rubbing alcohol used to clean the skin in preparation for an infusion. After four or five infusions, the nurse's perfume, the hand soap the doctor uses, and the odor of coffee may elicit it."

Consistent, positive results have been reported by multiple studies that showed significant reductions in both nausea and vomiting despite the type and stage of cancer, despite the chemotherapy procedure, and across multiple researchers and research methods.

Similarly, Cannici and colleagues found progressive muscle relaxation training reduced the insomnia side effects often faced by people with cancer. Fifteen patients suffering from cancer-related insomnia saw a reduction in the time it took them to get to sleep, from 124 minutes prior to treatment down to 15 minutes following treatment, compared to almost no improvement in a control group that did not receive treatment. The improvement lasted for three months.

Mastrovito and colleagues conducted a series of hypnosis studies on pediatric patients undergoing bone marrow aspiration. Using hypnotherapy or imagery, the children experienced less pain during medical procedures. Mastrovito says that painful diagnostic and treatment procedures which typically provoke fear and apprehension are ideal situations for progressive relaxation, both for children and adults.

Mastrovito opined, "It is shocking that these simple procedures are not universally used for children undergoing these painful procedures."

T.G. Burish and colleagues report that behavioral relaxation techniques "alleviate some conditioned side effects of chemotherapy including nausea, vomiting, and negative emotions such as anxiety and depression. These behavioral techniques are generally inexpensive, easily learned, and have few if any negative side effects." Techniques include systematic desensitization, electromyogram (EMG) biofeedback, progressive muscle relaxation training, and hypnosis.

According to the book *Hypnosis and Behavioral Medicine* by Daniel P. Brown and Erika Fromm, "Numerous studies have shown that animals in which tumors have been induced (by means of chemicals, transplantations, or radiation) and were then exposed to acute stressors (electrical shock, bright lights, extreme temperatures, rapid rotation, immobilization, isolation, overcrowding, confrontation with other--feared--animals) suffered from immunosuppression. Rapid tumor growth was facilitated in the stressed animals. The accumulated data for humans, although not so extensively documented, are similar and suggest that acute stressors result in immunosuppression or tumor facilitation in humans."

Janice R. Kiecolt-Glaser and Ronald Glaser are two leading researchers in the field of behavioral therapy as it relates to multiple emotional challenges such as bereavement, divorce, depression, chronic stress, and academic stress. After conducting human studies that show how immune function becomes depressed in these situations, they summarized their research in the *Journal of Psychoneuroimmunology*.

In their article, they pointed out the large body of literature that ties stressful life events and negative life changes to increased risk of disease. Kiecolt-Glaser and Glaser say the research is "remarkably consistent across populations and different kinds of events. In particular, events associated with the loss of important personal relationships appear to put individuals at greater risk."

Bereavement and divorce are two of the largest life stressors with the biggest negative health impact. Mortality rates increase for bereaved individuals, as does the incidence of cancer. Divorce appears to have even greater health risks than bereavement. However, though there is good evidence of an increase in morbidity and mortality associated with major negative life events, there is not a large body of robust evidence that these events result in a disproportionate increase in the incidence of cancer specifically.

Regardless, it appears that behavioral techniques have a place as a complementary treatment for cancer patients.

See **New Medicine/Dr. Hamer**. Dr. Hamer is perhaps the best known (and most controversial) advocate of the theory that cancer is almost always triggered by a major emotional trauma. Most of the controversy arises from Dr. Hamer's a most exclusive focus on emotional trauma. Other advocates tend to see it as one cause of cancer among many.

### *Further Reading & References*

- "Stress, depression, the immune system and cancer." http://www.ncbi.nlm.nih.gov/entrez/query.fcgi?cmd=Retrieve&db=pubmed&dopt=Abstract&list_uids=15465465

- "Treatment of insomnia in cancer patients using muscle relaxation training," http://www.ncbi.nlm.nih.gov/entrez/query.fcgi?cmd=Retrieve&db=pubmed&dopt=Abstract&list_uids=6358270

- "Behavioral intervention for cancer treatment side effects." Redd WH, Montgomery GH, DuHamel KN. Program for Cancer Prevention and Control, Derald H. Ruttenberg Cancer Center, Mount Sinai School of Medicine, New York, NY http://www.ncbi.nlm.nih.gov/entrez/query.fcgi?cmd=Retrieve&db=pubmed&dopt=Abstract&list_uids=11390531

- Redd WH, Montgomery GH, DuHamel KN. "Effects of fentanyl on natural killer cell activity and on resistance to tumor metastasis in rats. Dose and timing study." Shavit Y, Ben-Eliyahu S, Zeidel A, Beilin B. http://www.ncbi.nlm.nih.gov/entrez/query.fcgi?cmd=Retrieve&db=pubmed&dopt=Abstract&list_uids=15249732

- *Handbook of Psychooncology: Psychological Care of the Patient With Cancer* by Jimmie C. Holland, Julia H. Rowland Psycho-Oncology by Jimmie C. Holland, William Breitbart.

- *Massachusetts General Hospital Guide to Primary Care Psychiatry*, Second Edition by Theodore A. Stern, et al.

- Handbook of psychooncology. New York: Oxford University Press. Weisman, A.D. (1979).

- *Cancer and the Family Caregiver: Distress and Coping* by Ora Gilbar, Hasida Ben-Zur.

- *Hypnosis and Behavioral Medicine* by Daniel P. Brown, Erika Fromm

- *Group Therapy for Cancer Patients: A Research-based Handbook of Psychosocial Care* by David Spiegel, et al.

- The Human Side of Cancer: Living with Hope, Coping with Uncertainty by Jimmie Holland, Sheldon Lewis. http://www.fightingcancer.com/download/fcpdf/21%20A-Z%20of%20alternative%20options.pdf

- *Choices In Healing: Integrating The Best of Conventional and Complementary Approaches to*

*Cancer* by Michael Lerner (1996) http://www.commonweal.org/pubs/choices/10.html

- Redd, William H. and Christin Morrell, "Management of Anticipatory Nausea and Vomiting." *New England Journal of Medicine*, 1982; 307:1476-1480.

- T.G. Burish, et al., "Behavioral Relaxation Techniques in Reducing Distress of Cancer Chemotherapy Patients," Oncology Nursing Forum 10:32-5 (1983). Abstract cited in Steven E. Locke, Psychological and Behavioral Treatments Associated with the Immune System: An Annotated Bibliography (New York: Institute for the Advancement of Health, 1986), 234.

- D.F. Campbell et al., "Relaxation: Its Effect on the Nutritional Status and Performance of Clients with Cancer," Journal of the American Dieticians Association 4:201-4 (1984). Abstracted in Locke, Psychological and Behavioral Treatments, 235.

- Daniel P. Brown and Erika Fromm, Hypnosis and Behavioral Medicine (New Jersey: Lawrence Erlbaum Associates Publishers, 1987), 135.

- Kiecolt-Glaser and Glaser. "Emotions, Morbidity, and Mortality: New Perspectives from Psychoneuroimmunology" Annual Review of Psychology, 2002.

# Group Support/Group Therapy

There is strong evidence that those who live within a network of strong social relationships live longer and healthier lives.

Authorities and clinicians in cancer treatment increasingly view it as vitally important for the cancer patient to seek and receive support from other people in his or her life who can share the experience of cancer. This is particularly true of cancer patients interested in psychological work that may extend their survival.

Holland and Rowland, editors of the *Handbook of Psycho-Oncology: Psychological Care of the Patient with Cancer*, endorse this view and reflect that it "not only softens the psychological impact of cancer but may 'modulate' survival as well." The theory is that personality and social support likely interact to curb the psychological and biological stressors that may be related to both the incidence and progression of some cancers.

In effect, it serves as a buffer against the harmful effects of the stress that accompanies a cancer diagnosis. When there is someone within the cancer sufferer's environment who can empathize with and share the experience, then, as Rowland writes, "the presence of positive social support not only diminishes ... but may be important in modulating survival as well."

Evidence for this proposition now also comes from research in psychoneuroimmunology. Sandra Levy and her colleagues (1985, 1987) examined psychological and biological variables in women with breast cancer. Levy looked at the psychosocial condition of the women and immunological status both at the time of their mastectomies and again three months later. She and her team found that NK cell status was a significant predictor of the number of positive axillary nodes the women had. This was noteworthy as the number of positive nodes is a significant predictor both of survival and the likelihood that the disease will recur.

At least 51% of the variance in the activity of NK cells (the immune system's natural killer cells) could be explained by what they termed "distress factors." These included lack of adjustment, lack of social support, and fatigue, all of which are depressive symptoms. This meant anybody having difficulty coping with cancer who, on top of that, lacked social support and frequently felt melancholy and tired, would likely have a depressed physiological response from the NK cell component of their immune system which would result in more positive nodes. This example shows the convergence of personality and social support with the body's biological and psychological response to the stress of cancer.

Jimmie Holland, author of *Psycho-Oncology,* commented that "The Levy studies are of particular interest because of the findings from studies of Kiecolt-Glaser and colleagues that NK activity is negatively perturbed in physically healthy individuals under the stresses of examinations (1984), and loneliness (1986) in medical students. Their reports are also important in that NK-cell activity is important in response to tumors of viral origin, such as herpes virus and cervical cancer. The affective state described as 'helplessness-hopelessness' as an outcome predictor in human cancer has received considerable attention, in part because of animal studies (Sklar and Anisman, 1981). Animals that lacked control over environmental stress (such as electric shocks from which they could not escape) survived tumors for a shorter time than did animals that were provided the means to control the shocks.

Holland continues, "Cox and Mackay (1982) have used these studies to hypothesize that helplessness is associated with depletion of catecholamine [the 'fight or flight' hormones released by the adrenal glands in response to stress]; in turn adrenocorticotrophic hormone (ACTH) release [a pituitary gland hormone released in response to stress] stimulates the release of corticosteroids, which suppress immune function. The intense need to regain control of events in patients with cancer has led to extrapolation of these concepts to the clinical area. Regaining a sense of control has been seen as not only promoting coping but also enhancing host resistance to tumor growth."

In one study on the effect of group support for cancer patients, a randomized trial measured survival after structured psychotherapy for late stage breast cancer patients: Eighty Six patients with metastatic breast cancer were randomized into two groups, a study group of 50 and a control group of 36. Both groups had routine oncological care, but the study group was offered a 1½ hr weekly supportive group therapy and self-hypnosis for pain for 1 year.

Average survival for the study group was 36.6 months compared with 18.9 months for the control group, a 94% increase in survival. The patients receiving group therapy and pain-control support survived nearly twice as long.

### Further Reading & References

- *Effect of psychosocial treatment on survival of patients with metastatic breast cancer,* Spiegel, D. et al., The Lancet, October 14, 1989.

- *Group Therapy for Cancer Patients: A Research-based Handbook of Psychosocial Care* by David Spiegel, et al. Excerpt from page 49 "... to investigate the incidence within the last five years of divorce /separation, bankruptcy/unemployment of major wage ... a relationship between stress and cancer. Social Relationship Effects On Health ... Leproult et al., 1996), immune (Glaser, Kiecolt-Glaser et al., 1985, 1998; Glaser and Kiecolt-Glaser, 1986; Cohen, ..."

- *The Human Side of Cancer: Living with Hope, Coping with Uncertainty* by Jimmie Holland, Sheldon Lewis (2001)

- *Psychiatric Aspects of Symptom Management in Cancer Patients* by William Breitbart, Jimmie Holland (1993)

- *Meeting Psychosocial Needs of Women With Breast Cancer* by Maria Hewitt, et al (2004)

- *Psychosocial Aspects of Oncology* by Jimmie C. Holland, et al (1998)

- *Handbook of Psychooncology: Psychological Care of the Patient With Cancer* by Jimmie C.

Holland, Julia H. Rowland (1990)

- *Psycho-Oncology* by Jimmie C. Holland, William Breitbart (1998)

- *Choices In Healing: Integrating The Best of Conventional and Complementary Approaches to Cancer* by Michael Lerner (1996)

- Levy, Sandra M.; et al., "Prognostic risk assessment in primary breast cancer by behavioral and immunological parameters." *Health Psychology*, Vol 4(2), 1985, 99-113.

- Levy, S., et al., "Breast conservation versus mastectomy: Distress sequelae as a function of choice*." Breast Cancer Research and Treatment*. 10, 1987, p. 123.

- *Handbook of Psychooncology: Psychological Care of the Patient with Cancer*, edited by Jimmie C. Holland (Editor), Julia H. Rowland, (1990)


# Meditation

There is scientific evidence that the mind, in meditation, can effect physiological changes in the human body. One study entitled "Suppressing tumor progression of in vitro prostate cancer cells by emitted psychosomatic power through Zen meditation" reported remarkable evidence that when "Human prostate cancer PC3 cells were treated in vitro with psychosomatic power emitted by a Buddhist-Zen Master. A significant decrease of growth rate was observed as determined by MTT assay after 48 hours. These cells also had two- to three-fold higher levels of prostatic acid phosphatase (PAcP) activity, a prostate tissue specific differentiation antigen. In addition, the treated cells formed fewer and smaller colonies in soft agar as compared with control cells, which displayed anchorage-independent growth.

"These observations provide insight into the suppressive effects of healing power through the practice of Buddhist-Zen meditation on tumor progression. The emitted bioenergy may be suggested as an alternative and feasible approach for cancer research and patient treatment."

Meditation is a well-established technique for controlling and reducing stress, which in itself inhibits the immune system and thereby diminishes the body's ability to resist cancer. Experienced meditators are able to control their blood pressure, heartbeat, and other common physical signs and symptoms. Such evidence as there is suggests that meditation in other religious traditions besides Buddhism has similar physiological effects.

## Further Reading & References

- 'Suppressing tumor progression of in vitro prostate cancer cells by emitted psychosomatic power through Zen meditation' by Yu T, Tsai HL, Hwang ML. Department of Applied Chemistry, National Chiao Tung University, Hsinchu 300, Taiwan.

- *The Complete Book of Zen* by Wong Kiew Kit. (1998)

- *Meetings with Remarkable Women: Buddhist Teachers in America* by Lenore Friedman. (2000)

- *Meditation for Dummies* by Stephan Bodian. (1999)

- *In This Very Moment: A Simple Guide to Zen Buddhism* by James Ishmael Ford. (2006)

- *Healing Words: The Power of Prayer and the Practice of Medicine* by Larry Dossey (1995)

# New Medicine/Dr. Hamer

Dr. Ryke Geerd Hamer, a German medical doctor, reportedly achieved an exceptionally high success rate with his cancer therapy, among the highest seen in any therapy. During one of several trials of the persecuted Dr. Hamer, the public prosecutor (Wiener-Neustadt in Austria) had to admit that after four to five years, 6,000 out of 6,500 of his patients – most of them suffering from advanced cancer - were still alive.

That is over 90%, almost a reversal of the results to be expected following conventional treatment of advanced cancer.

Dr. Hamer started his cancer research when he himself developed testicular cancer after his son was shot dead. He wondered if his son's death was the cause of his cancer.

"Since I had never been seriously ill, I wondered if my (cancer) condition had anything to do with the death of my son. Three years later, as chief of internal medicine in a so-called gynecology-oncology clinic at Munich University, I had the opportunity to study female patients with cancer and to compare my findings to see if the mechanism was the same as mine; if they too had experienced such a terrible shock. I found that all of them, without exception, had experienced the same type of biological conflict as I had. They were able to recollect the shock, the resulting sleeplessness, weight loss, cold hands and the beginning of tumor growth. At the time, my point of view was very different from all the current medical concepts, and when I presented these discoveries to my colleagues, they gave me an ultimatum: either to deny my findings or leave the clinic immediately."

Subsequently he investigated and documented over 15,000 cases of cancer and always found the following characteristics to be present, which he termed the five biological laws of the German New Medicine:

- The Iron Rule of Cancer is the law that every disease has two phases of development to the extent that there is a resolution of the conflict. It involves the ontogenetic system of tumors and cancer-equivalent diseases as well as that of microbes in disease. The criterion is that every cancer originates from a very difficult, dramatic, highly acute, and isolating shock, also known as Dirk Hamer Syndrome (DHS). The experience of the shock affects the psyche, the brain, and the organs.

  The type of conflict caused by experiencing DHS determines the location of the Hamerschenherd (HH) in the brain along with the location of the cancer or other disease. (Note: "Herd" roughly translates to "center of disturbance.")

- Both "cold" and "warm" diseases exist, as identified by medical textbooks. Cold diseases have been described as cancer, MS, angina pectoris, neuro-dermatitis, diabetes and mental and mood disorders, and are brought on by situations of protracted stress, weight loss, and sleep disorders. Warm diseases are purportedly rheumatic, infectious, allergic, and especially exanthematous (characterized by skin eruptions or rashes).

  In new medicine, both cold and warm diseases are recognized, but not as separate entities. Instead, they each represent one of two phases of an illness with the cold phase coming first and the warm coming second.

- The ontogenetic system of tumors and cancer-equivalent diseases relates to interconnections and relationships. Criteria include conflict at the embryonic level, old-brain directed conflicts, and cerebral-directed conflicts. In addition, every illness is a meaningful biological occurrence to be understood through embryology and behavioral research. This means that the illness presents with the challenge of solving an unusual and unforeseen biological problem.

• Embryonic-layer related organ groups correspond without exception to embryonically related microbe groups. Microbes are not the harbingers of the symptoms but rather the optimizers of the healing phase. Microbes are steered from the brain and follow instructions from the brain, actually playing a more important role than the typically-imagined immune-system response of microbes battling cancerous cells. Following instructions from the brain, the pathogenic microbes become benign apathogenic microbes that retreat into a part of the organism where they are no bother and can be recalled and reactivated in the PCL phase on specific organs.

• Disease no longer exists as it has been defined up till this point. Rather, so-called diseases should be recognized as having biological meaning. This law is the soul of the German New Medicine and achieves the connection between what can be investigated scientifically and what can be called transcendental, supernatural, parapsychological, or understandable only from a religious point of view. Things that are felt and experienced from a scientific point of view and that cannot be explained become puzzling or nonsensical.

With the fifth biological law, the human connection to the cosmos is understood.

At the moment, of the conflict-shock a short circuit occurs in a pre-determined place of the brain. This can be photographed with computed-tomography (CT) and looks like concentric rings on a shooting target or like the surface of water after a stone has been dropped into it. Later on, if the conflict becomes resolved, the CT image changes, an edema develops, and finally scar tissue.

How specific and precisely located these brain lesions are may be seen from the following. After a professional lecture, a doctor handed Dr. Hamer the brain CT of a patient and asked him to explain it. From this, Dr. Hamer reportedly diagnosed the patient to have a fresh bleeding bladder carcinoma in the healing phase, an old prostate carcinoma, diabetes, an old lung carcinoma and sensory paralysis in a specific area, in addition to the corresponding emotional conflicts.

Dr. Hamer was able to show that at the same time a concentric brain lesion appears, the corresponding target organ may show such a concentric lesion. According to Dr. Hamer, this happens instantly when the psychic shock hits the subconscious level - and this same second is the start of cancer. Other diseases can be caused by the same mechanism. Also, the severity of a disease may depend on other psychological, energetic, and nutritional factors - but its nature and location are determined by the content of the conflict shock.

Hamer believes that the correlation between key emotional shock events, the target brain areas, and the related organs has developed as an adaptation of our human evolution from similar programs in the animal world. When we unexpectedly experience emotional distress, an emergency repair program is set in motion, a biological conflict program with the aim of returning the individual to normal. Such programs can even apply to families or other groups.

Hamer gives the following example: A mother sees her child in a bad accident. In evolutionary terms, small children recover faster when they receive extra milk. Therefore, the biological conflict program tries to stimulate milk production by increasing the number of breast cells. If the mother is right-handed, that will instantly cause the appearance of a Hamer Herd in a specific part of her right brain, which in turn relates to the left breast. When the child is well again, conflict resolution begins and extra milk is no longer needed. The mother gets a benign form of tuberculosis in that breast which breaks up the excess breast cells. However, if the mycobacteria required for this are lacking, then the area may just calcify and remain as a dormant tumor.

If instead a person is diagnosed with cancer, even if the diagnosis is wrong, the same biological program is set in motion by the fear of death. The stress level jumps and the brain-lung connection is activated but there is nowhere to run. Until the conflict is resolved, which may take years, there will be constant stress as well as brain-induced stimulation of lung activity, which now takes the form of increasing lung capacity by the incessant division of cells.

Only switching off the trigger in the brain by defusing the original conflict shock can stop this process. This happens when the patient subsequently has surgery or natural therapy, which he or she fully believes will lead to a cure. However, the same procedure in a patient who has doubts about its effectiveness will leave the conflict unresolved and allow the disease to progress. According to Dr. Hamer and his supporters, this is no longer just an unsubstantiated assumption, but rather scientific fact that can be verified anytime with a CT brain scan.

The selection of the conflict focus occurs by subconscious association. For instance, biological conflicts involving water but also other fluids, such as milk or oil, lead to kidney cancer, fear of death leads to lung cancer and psychologically swallowing a bigger chunk then we can digest leads to stomach or intestinal cancer.

Other typical situations that may lead to biological conflicts are loss situations, such as loss of a loved one, of a job, a valued possession or a territory.

Dr. Hamer believes that the cancer-fear or death-fear resulting from giving the patient a cancer diagnosis or a negative prognosis causes most metastases or secondary tumors. However, the resulting conflict shock may not be fear of death but rather anger, resentment or a conflict resulting from separation from partner or children —in which case tumors would appear in different places. Also, a diagnosis of colon cancer commonly leads to liver cancer because of a subconscious fear of starvation.

Generally, hopelessness, despair, and meaninglessness create chronic stress, which prevents healing from cancer and other diseases, but it is not the primary cause of cancer. According to Hamer, the real cause of cancer and other diseases is an unexpected traumatic shock for which we are emotionally unprepared.

The following list purportedly shows some of the relationships between conflict emotions and impact on different organs resulting in cancer.

- Adrenal cortex - Wrong direction, gone astray

- Bladder - Ugly conflict, dirty tricks

- Bone - Lack of self-worth, inferiority feeling

- Breast milk gland - Involving care or disharmony

- Breast milk duct - Separation conflict

- Breast, left (right-handed) - Conflict concerning child, home, mother

- Breast, right (right-handed) - Conflict with partner or others

- Bronchials - Territorial conflict

- Cervix - Severe frustration

- Colon - Ugly indigestible conflict

- Esophagus - Cannot have it or swallow it

- Gall Bladder - Rivalry conflict

- Heart - Perpetual conflict

- Intestines - Indigestible chunk of anger

- Kidneys - Not wanting to live, water or fluid conflict

- Larynx - Conflict of fear and fright

- Liver - Fear of starvation

- Lung - Fear of dying or suffocation, including fear for someone else

- Lymph glands - Loss of self-worth associated with the location

- Melanoma - feeling dirty, soiled, defiled

- Middle ear - Not being able to get some vital information

- Mouth - Cannot chew or hold it

- Pancreas - Anxiety-anger conflict with family members, inheritance

- Prostate - Ugly conflict with sexual connections or connotations

- Rectum - Fear of being useless

- Skin - Loss of integrity

- Spleen - Shock of being physically or emotionally wounded

- Stomach - Indigestible anger, swallowed too much

- Testes and Ovaries - Loss conflict

- Thyroid - Feeling powerless

- Uterus - Sexual conflict

The start of a DHS or conflict-shock experience is different from other conflicts that we experience in our daily lives. It causes a continuous stress resulting in a tendency to develop cold hands and feet, lack of appetite and weight loss, sleeplessness and dwelling all the time on the unfortunate life-changing event. If the conflict is not resolved soon, the long-lasting stress will lead to specific symptoms and the development of cancer or another disease.

When the conflict resolves, the patient is no longer occupied with the unhappy event, the appetite returns, hands are warm again and also normal sleep returns, but the patient may also experience weakness, fatigue and a need to rest. These effects show that the parasympathetic nervous system is now in control. This is the beginning of the healing phase, which can be long and difficult.

During the first part of the healing phase, water retention and inflammations are seen but the tumor stops growing. This eventually leads to a healing crisis, which Hamer calls an epileptic or epileptoid crisis because it is caused by an edema in the Hamer Herd brain lesion. It shows unique symptoms for each illness.

After this, the body starts to expel the accumulated water, the patient gradually regains strength, and body functions become normal. The connective tissue in the brain starts repairing the Hamer Herd. This may be interpreted by conventional radiologists as a fast-growing brain tumor and treated accordingly. Hamer writes that real brain tumors do not exist, as nerve cells in the brain cannot divide.

According to Hamer, these conditions are generally self-limiting and only get out of control when additional conflict shocks occur or the body is too old or weak, or through the methods of conventional medicine. In contrast, natural healing methods aim to support body and mind during this trying time. Most healings proceed without major problems, but about 10% need the full support of an experienced therapist, especially at the time of the healing crisis.

The main task in every case of cancer is to find the original emotional shock experience and make sure that it has been healed or is being healed. In many cases it will have corrected itself and the patient suffers from an effect of the healing phase.

According to Hamer, animals in the wild get cancer from the same responses to shock as humans. However, 80 to 90% survive and do not notice much because the healing phase can take its natural course. Those that die are mainly old animals that cannot resolve a conflict, such as regaining their territory from a rival or replacing a lost cub.

It is different in human society, as the natural healing process is routinely interfered with. Intervention often starts with prescriptions for tranquilizers or antidepressants during the active conflict phase, which prevent the patient from fighting back and regaining his or her "lost territory." This may then lead to a cancer diagnosis that causes an additional active conflict (or emotional shock) and ends with morphine, which totally disables healing responses.

While Hamer does not believe that health foods, medicinal remedies, cleansing or healthy living in general can cure cancer, these certainly can be important in order to survive the ordeals of the healing phase. Actually, Hamer regards all diseases as consisting of two phases, the first being an active conflict, followed (if possible) by a healing phase that reverses the conflict program.

He no longer calls these phenomena diseases but rather special biological programs. It is claimed that he has worked with over 31,000 patients and found his theories confirmed in every single case without exception. Hamer claims that overall the New Medicine has a 95% success rate with cancer.

But doctors and natural therapists in Europe who practice according to the principles of the New Medicine face persecution. In Austria, Belgium, France, Germany, and Spain authorities have initiated proceedings against such doctors to take away their right to practice.

However, in 2001, a prominent neurologist, Dr. Therese von Schwarzenberg, openly defended Dr. Hamer by publishing a book about the New Medicine and demanding that his theories be officially tested.

### Further Reading & References

- The German/Germanic New Medicine®, http://www.newmedicine.ca

- "Excerpts from Summary Of The New Medicine," by Dr. R. G. Hamer

- http://www.newmedicine.ca/excerpt.php

# Prayer

Studies show that religious people tend to live healthier lives. It's said, "They're less likely to smoke, to drink, to drink and drive." In fact, people who pray tend to get sick less often, as indicated by separate studies conducted at Duke, Dartmouth, and Yale universities.

Prayer activates hope. Research by Greer on coping styles shows that those who react to a cancer diagnosis with hopelessness and helplessness have a much lower chance of survival than similar patients with a fighting spirit.

There have now been numerous studies on the benefits of being prayed for by others, perhaps one of the most well known being conducted by cardiologist Randolph Byrd and published in 1988. Byrd's work took place with coronary care unit patients and was scientifically rigorous, using a randomized, double-blind protocol. Over ten months, 393 patients in the unit were, with consent, admitted to a prayer group (192 patients) or a control group (201 patients). They were prayed for by Christians outside the hospital.

Neither the doctors nor the patients knew who was receiving prayer. Although when the study began the patients were all of a similar state of health, over time the patients receiving prayer showed much better recovery rates than the others. The prayed-for patients were five times less likely than control patients to require antibiotics and three times less likely to develop pulmonary edema. While twelve of the control patients needed intubation to help with breathing, none of the prayed-for patients did.

Another impressive study was conducted more recently in 1998 by Dr. Elisabeth Targ at the California Pacific Medical Centre in San Francisco. Her study (again a double-blind experiment) was conducted with patients suffering from advanced AIDS. Those patients receiving prayer had six times fewer hospitalizations, which were also of a significantly shorter duration, than those people who received no prayer. Even Dr. Targ was surprised, "I was sort of shocked," she said in an interview with ABC News:

"In a way it's like witnessing a miracle. There is no way to understand this from my experience and from my basic understanding of science."

Yet another study was done by Dr. Mitchell Krucoff at Duke University Medical Center in North Carolina. He studied the effects of prayer on patients undergoing cardiac procedures such as catheterization and angioplasty. His findings show that patients receiving prayer have up to 100% fewer side effects from these procedures than people not prayed for.

A leading researcher in this field is Dr. Larry Dossey, who has written extensively about the power of prayer. On his website, he cites examples from the plant and animal world. When bacteria are prayed for they grow faster; when seeds are prayed for, they germinate quicker; when wounded mice are prayed for they heal faster. He says: "I like these studies because they can be done with great precision, and they eliminate all effects of suggestion and positive thinking, since we can be sure that the effects are not due to the placebo effect."

### Further Reading & References

- *Prayer Is Good Medicine: How to Reap the Healing Benefits of Prayer* by Larry Dossey (1997)

- *Healing Words: The Power of Prayer and the Practice of Medicine* by Larry Dossey (1995)

- *You Are Never Alone: Prayers and Meditations to Sustain You Through Breast Cancer* by Maureen Murray (2003)

- *When Hope Is Tried: Meditations for Those Who Are Ill and the People Who Love Them* by Carol Winters (2001)

- Larry Dossey, MD: Official Website, http://www.dosseydossey.com/larry/default.html

- Religious Tolerance: "Effectiveness of personal prayers used in addition to medical treatment," http://www.religioustolerance.org/medical4.htm


# Psychic Surgery

Various cancer patients claim to have been cured by psychic surgery, especially in the Philippines. Few, if any, serious students of alternative cancer treatment believe it is valid. Psychic surgery is a modern expression of traditional Filipino shamanism. Practiced also in North America by visiting Filipino shamans, psychic surgery involves the extraction of "tumors" from the body through a bloody but painless and invisible 'incision' in the patient's abdomen.

The main treatment appears to be the application of external Qi Gong energy through the fingers of the right-hand, in combination with Shiatsu Massage and a procedure using the hands and resembling chiropractic manipulation. It is estimated that there are more than 400 psychic surgeons in the Philippines. Reportedly, there is one in every big hotel in Manila.

Reverend Tony Agpaoa was the most famous. Now deceased, "he put faith healing on a multi-national footing with his own travel agency, Diplomat Tours, which organizes groups from Europe, North America, Japan, Australia, and New Zealand." He was unable to organize tours from the U.S. where he was indicted for fraud in connection with psychic surgery in 1967. He forfeited a $25,000 bond when he jumped bail and returned to the Philippines.

Psychic surgeons claim to be able to cure many diseases including diabetes and cancer. Agpaoa talked of imbalances in the body, biofeedback, and mental consciousness. "Our healing is secondary, we bring back the natural way of life to make people healthy again."

According to Agpaoa, "We guarantee that, physically and spiritually, people will leave here better, but we can't guarantee we will cure them. Becoming a psychic surgeon is not something that one can choose to do. It is something that comes upon one often during a period of illness."

A report on psychic surgery made by the Yukon Medical Association notes that many individuals who had undergone psychic surgery showed marked subjective improvement. All of these cases had chronic, poorly defined, nonspecific disorders, such as headaches, abdominal pain, or back pain. Dr. Hirota, a psychic surgeon from Brazil, claims to treat 1,000 to 2,000 patients daily between 9 am and 12 noon.

The strongest opponent of faith healing is the Philippine Medical Association (PMA). The PMA claims that, "they (the surgeons) take advantage of the gullibility of people. We know that they are fooling the people, but it is hard to do anything about it. Patients won't complain. Either they are ashamed that they have been made fools of, or they have died - so we usually have no proof against faith healers.

"The Canadian Embassy in Manila had signed three death certificates for people who would never return alive from their miracle tours (although not from Agpaoa's tours). Of more than 20 known cancer cases who went to Baguio from Vancouver three and four years ago, not one is still alive according to the BC Cancer Agency."

In 1974, Donald F. Wright and Carol Wright testified before a U.S. Federal Trade Commission hearing in Seattle investigating travel agents promoting tours to visit the Philippine healers. The Wrights, from Iowa, students and believers of ESP and magnetic healing, traveled to the Philippines in 1973 to study psychic surgery. Eventually they were convinced that what they saw was not surgery but trickery, and they learned the methods from their surgeon teacher. They were taught how to shop for animal parts used to make up a 'bullet'.

A bullet is actual animal tissue or a clot of animal blood and cotton, which is made to appear like tissue coming from inside the body. They were taught how to make the bullet, wrap it, prepare the tissue, how to hide the bullet and then how to transfer it onto the patient.

Donald Douglas, who had a healthy heart, claimed to have a "bad heart" on the list of ailments he prepared for psychic surgeons. The healer then purported to yank a "tumor" the size of a peach pit out of Douglas' heart. "I didn't get a good look at it because he threw it in the bucket". The "surgery" involved blood, but Douglas reports that he was sure that it was chicken blood and tissue, not human.

### Further Reading & References

- Azuma N, Stevenson I. "Psychic surgery" in the Philippines as a form of group hypnosis. American Journal of Clinical Hypnosis 1988 July;31(1):61-67.

- American Cancer Society: Psychic Surgery, http://www.cancer.org/Treatment/ TreatmentsandSideEffects/ComplementaryandAlternativeMedicine/ ManualHealingandPhysicalTouch/psychic-surgery

# Simonton Method/Guided Imagery

Imagery is one of the most powerful tools in use with cancer. It is practiced extensively by cancer patients and therapists who work with them.

O. Carl Simonton, M.D., and Stephanie Matthews Simonton were the pioneers who first used imagery with the goal of physically reversing the development of cancer. Their approach is well-regarded in the alternative cancer treatment community. Their best-selling book, written with James Creighton, *Getting Well Again*, was a major, though controversial, contribution to this area when it was first published in 1978. It remains one of the most useful and comprehensive psychological self-help books for people with cancer.

The Simontons recommended that a person first put himself into a deeply relaxed state. Then, the patient should mentally picture the cancer in either realistic or symbolic terms.

The treatment begins by asking the patient to "think of the cancer as consisting of very weak, confused cells. Remember that our bodies destroy cancerous cells thousands of times during a normal lifetime. As you picture your cancer, realize that your recovery requires that your body's own defenses return to a natural, healthy state.

"If you are now receiving treatment, picture your treatment coming into your body in a way that you understand. If you are receiving radiation treatment, picture it as a beam of millions of bullets of energy hitting any cell in its path. The normal cells are able to repair the damage that is done, but the cancer cells cannot because they are weak." (This is one of the basic foundations of radiation therapy.)

"If you are receiving chemotherapy, picture that drug coming into your body and entering the bloodstream. Picture the drug acting like a poison. The normal cells are intelligent and strong and don't take up the poison so readily. But the cancer cell is a weak cell so it takes very little to kill it. It absorbs the poison, dies, and is flushed out of your body. Picture your body's own white cells coming into the area where the cancer is, recognizing the abnormal cells, and destroying them. There is a vast army of white blood cells. They are very strong and aggressive. They are also very smart. There is no contest between them and the cancer cells; they will win the battle.

"Picture the cancer shrinking. See the dead cells being carried away by the white blood cells and being flushed from your body through the liver and kidneys and eliminated in the urine and stool. Continue to see the cancer shrinking, until it is all gone. See yourself having more energy and a better appetite and being able to feel comfortable and loved in your family as the cancer shrinks and finally disappears.

"If you are experiencing pain anywhere in your body, picture the army of white blood cells flowing into that area and soothing the pain. Whatever the problem, give your body the command to heal itself. Visualize your body becoming well.

"Imagine yourself well, free of disease, full of energy. Picture yourself reaching your goals in life. See your purpose in life being fulfilled, the members of your family doing well, your relationships with people around you becoming more meaningful. Remember that having strong reasons for getting well will help you get well, so use this time to focus clearly on your priorities in life.

"Give yourself a mental pat on the back for participating in your recovery. See yourself doing this mental imagery exercise three times a day, staying awake and alert as you do it."

The Simontons stressed that it was not necessary to see the imagery if you could sense, think, or feel it.

Among other benefits, it is claimed that relaxation and imagery can:

- Decrease fear

- Bring about attitudinal changes and enhance will to live

- Effect physical changes to enhance the immune system and alter the course of a malignancy

- Serve as a method to evaluate current beliefs and alter those beliefs, if desired

- Be used as a tool for communicating with the unconscious

- Serve as a way of decreasing tension and stress

- Help to confront and alter the stance of hopelessness and helplessness. Again and again, this underlying depression is a significant factor in the development of cancer.


In the Simontons' and some other imagery techniques, the immune system is considered to be the mechanism by which the body actively combats cancer. Some researchers believe that other host resilience factors may contribute to life extension. The immune system may or may not turn out to be the most important system by which psychological practices modulate cancer survival.

According to the Simontons' research, the content of the imagery appeared as critical to positive outcomes as the regular practice of imagery. People with negative imagery in which the cancer appeared more powerful than the treatment or the response of their bodies often did not do well. Together with the assistance of Dr. Jeanne Achterberg, a research psychologist, they developed a list of criteria that can be used to evaluate the content of one's mental imagery:

Representing cancer cells as ants, for instance, is generally a negative symbol. Have you ever been able to get rid of ants at a picnic? Crabs, the traditional symbol for cancer, and other crustaceans are also negative symbols. These beasts are tenacious, they hang on.

Interpreting mental imagery is similar to interpreting dreams: It involves a highly personal, symbolic language. The emotional meaning of a particular symbol may be different for different individuals, so that a symbol that means strength and power to one person may mean anger and hostility to someone else.

### Further Reading & References

- *Getting Well Again: The Bestselling Classic About the Simontons' Revolutionary Lifesaving Self-Awareness Techniques* by O. Carl Md Simonton, et al. (1992)

- *Cancer: 50 Essential Things to Do* by Greg Anderson, O. Carl Simonton (1999)

- *Dr. Carl Simonton's Getting Well: A Step-By-Step, Self-Help Guide to Overcoming Cancer for Patients and Their Families* by Carl Simonton (Audio Cassette) (1987)

- *A Feather in My Wig: Ovarian Cancer Cured, Seventeen Years and Going Strong!* by Barbara Van Billiard. (1998)

- *The Healing Journey* by O. Carl Md Simonton (2002)

- *The Human Side of Cancer: Living with Hope, Coping with Uncertainty* by Jimmie Holland, Sheldon Lewis. (2001)

- *Getting Well Again: A Step-By-Step Self-Help Guide to Overcoming Cancer* by Carl, Et Al Simonton

- *New Choices In Natural Healing: Over 1,800 Of The Best Self-Help Remedies From The World Of Alternative Medicine* by Bill Gottlieb. (1997)

- *Healing Images for Children: Teaching Relaxation and Guided Imagery to Children Facing Cancer and Other Serious Illnesses* by Nancy C. Klein, Matthew Holden

- *Imagery in Healing: Shamanism and Modern Medicine* by Jeanne Achterberg Fighting Cancer

- *From Within: How to Use the Power of Your Mind For Healing* by Martin L., Md. Rossman.

- *Rituals of Healing: Using Imagery for Health and Wellness* by Jeanne Achterberg, Barbara Dossey. (2002)

- *Wellness Book: The Comprehensive Guide To Maintaining Health And Treating Stress-Related Illness* by Herbert Benson, Eileen M. Stuart (1993)

- *Women's Bodies, Women's Wisdom* by Christiane Northrup. (2002)

- *Consciousness, Bioenergy and Healing: Self-Healing and Energy Medicine for the 21st Century*

- *(Healing Research, Vol. 2)* by Daniel J. Benor.

- *Healing Words* by Larry Dossey. (1995)

- *Guided Imagery for Self-Healing: An Essential Resource for Anyone Seeking Wellness* by Martin L., MD Rossman. (2000)

# Stress Alleviation

There is a recognized association between the strength of the immune system and the cancer process.

"In general, both stressors and depression are associated with the decreased cytotoxic T-cell and natural-killer-cell activities that affect processes such as immune surveillance of tumors, and with the events that modulate development and accumulation of somatic mutations and genomic instability."

Chronic stress seems to trigger the premature aging of immune system cells, a study reported in 2004 suggests. Although people who are under stress for long periods often look haggard, scientists didn't understand how chronic stress causes damage at the cellular level.

Telomeres are the focus of a new study on stress and aging. Cells divide a certain defined number of times and then die, a natural healthy process called apoptosis. The new research focused on one sign of biological aging – caps of DNA and protein at the end of chromosomes called telomeres, which shorten as cells reproduce over time. With each cell division, the telomeres become shorter until the cell dies by apoptosis. Young people have an enzyme that regenerates the ends, but this process stops late in life.

Researchers studied 39 healthy, premenopausal women who cared for a child with a chronic illness, compared to 19 mothers of the same age who had healthy children. Among women caring for a sick child, the telomeres shortened by the equivalent of 10 years of premature aging compared to the control group, according to the study published in the Proceedings of the National Academy of Sciences.

Lead researcher Elissa Epel, a professor of psychiatry at the University of California at San Francisco, and her team evaluated stress using a standardized questionnaire, and measured the length of telomeres from blood samples.

Epel stated: "Chronic stress appears to have the potential to shorten the life of cells, at least immune cells."

Previous studies have shown a link between chronic stress and heart disease and weaker immune function. The new findings point to a cellular mechanism behind the link.

"The goal now is to determine how to reduce the effects of stress at the physical level," wrote Robert Sapolsky of Stanford University in a commentary accompanying the study. Epel's team is now conducting a long-term study on telomere length. They also want to do clinical trials to see if stress reduction techniques like meditation slow the rate of telomere shortening.

Al Sears, M.D., of Primal Force, Inc. in Royal Palm Beach, FL, claims to have identified a nutrient, TA-G5, that preserves the length of the telomere by activating the enzyme telomerase.

An additional study in 2004 showed that written emotional disclosure buffers the effects of social constraints on stress among cancer patients.

"The aims of the present study were to examine whether written emotional disclosure would reduce distress among cancer patients and whether it would buffer the effects of high levels of social constraint (negative social responses to patients' expressions of emotion regarding their cancer) on distress. …. Results showed that written disclosure buffered the effects of social constraints on stress at the 6-month follow-up and that avoidance partly mediated these effects."

Meditation and prayer have been shown to relieve stress. See **Meditation and Prayer**.


*Further Reading and References*

- *Mind-Body Cancer Wellness: A Self-Help Stress Management Manual* by Morry D., Ph.D. Edwards

- *Fighting Cancer From Within: How to Use the Power of Your Mind For Healing* by Martin L., Md. Rossman (2003)

- *Stress Management Intervention for Women With Breast Cancer* by Michael H. Antoni, Roselyn Smith (2003)

- *Success From Stress: Is It a Cause of Cancer?* by Ralph Wilkerson

- Reiche EM, Nunes SO, Morimoto HK. Lancet Oncol. 2004 Oct;5(10):617-25. "Stress, depression, the immune system, and cancer." http://www.ncbi.nlm.nih.gov/entrez/query.fcgi?cmd=Retrieve&db=pubmed&dopt=Abstract&list_uids=15465465

- Epel, E. Proceedings of the National Academy of Sciences, Nov. 30, 2004. News release, University of California, San Francisco.

- Zakowski SG, Ramati A, Morton C, Johnson P, Flanigan R.Rosalind Franklin University of Medicine and Science, Department of Psychology, North Chicago, IL, US.

- "Written emotional disclosure buffers the effects of social constraints on distress among cancer patients." "http://www.ncbi.nlm.nih.gov/entrez/query.fcgi?cmd=Retrieve&db=pubmed&dopt=Abstract&list_uids=15546223

# Suggestion/Hypnosis/Autogenic Training

The object of visualization is to tell the mind what to think and thereby to tell the mind what to do in the body. The idea is to let thoughts and messages filter from the conscious to the subconscious regions of the mind.

Many athletes improve their performances through mental gymnastics, or mental tennis, and so on. There is scientific study to back that the mind becomes what it thinks — and so too does the body. By actively guiding the imagination, the body can be led to a state of health. It's claimed that if a person wants something enough, then he has simply to imagine it over and over again while in a deeply relaxed frame of mind.

Some people may find this a difficult idea to accept. The story of psychiatrist Milton Erikson shows what can be achieved through thought alone. Erikson was paralyzed by polio as a young boy and forced to spend a lot of time on his front porch in a rocking chair watching the world go by. One day, left at home strapped to a rocking chair he found he was too far from the window to look out.

Suddenly he became aware that his obsession with getting to the window was causing his chair to rock. He started to concentrate his thoughts on getting to the window. The more he did so the more the rocking increased. He soon found that he could direct the movement of the chair by working on his thoughts. It took him all afternoon but he managed to reach the window.

This experience led him to the idea that he could influence other movements by concentrating his thoughts. He was reportedly able to overcome the paralysis completely and began to walk again!

How can a person use this visualization to help stay healthy? By letting himself dwell inwardly on a healthy positive image. What follows is an example of the kind of creative visualization that can, it is claimed, restore or maintain the body's health.

With eyes closed, imagine your very favorite place. Maybe this is near where you live or a place that you remember from your youth or a place that you have visited on your holidays. It may even be a totally imaginary place —wherever it is, it is a place where you are happy. Reflect on the happiness you feel being there. Feel the warmth of the sunlight.

Feel the glow of the sun on your body. How comfortable you feel with the warm living rays of the sun permeating your whole body. It is filling your body with health and happiness, energy and love. It suffuses through all the limbs and through the whole of your being. With each breath, the warmth and the light grow stronger and lighter. You release yourself into the heart of this feeling and you sit and feel this and let your mind sense these sensations. Then, when you're ready, you can return to normal consciousness.

Some people visualize the cancer and watch in their minds as their body's immune defense system attacks it and slowly destroys it. Some people focus their visualization on the chemotherapy drug or the radiation they are receiving.

They imagine the drug eating up the tumor. They imagine the radiation rays like the healing rays of the sun dissolving the tumor. Or, as one patient did, they imagine the radiation as golden bullets. This man had a nearly-always fatal form of throat cancer at a late stage of development, his weight having dropped from 130 to 98lbs. He was barely able to swallow. He was given radiation treatment, but was not expected to benefit greatly from it - perhaps just some short-lived relief from a temporarily radiation-shrunk tumor. In addition to the radiation treatment, he was asked to visualize the radiation as millions of little bullets bombarding the cancer tumor. He also imagined the cancer cells as being weak and unable to repair themselves —while he imagined the normal cells as being strong and repairing themselves quickly.

He visualized the white blood cells swarming over the dead and dying cancer cells and carrying them out of the body through the liver and kidney. He did this three or four times a day. The result? He not only recovered but suffered very little associated radiation damage. His doctor, O. Carl Simonton, had similar success with a large number of patients who were considered incurable. Of a group of 156 people with 'incurable cancers', 63 were still alive four years later and in 43 of these the cancer had either disappeared, was regressing, or had stabilized.

Dr. David Sobel, co-author of *The Healing Brain*, describes being plagued by warts on his hand when he was young. Standard medical treatments did nothing. In a newspaper article with a headline that read, "Warts Cured by Suggestion," he read that hypnosis and suggestive thinking could eliminate warts. A specific treatment protocol was not described so he came up with his own method, which involved concentrating intensely on the warts every day for four weeks while repeating the phrase, "Warts go away," ten times. At the end of the four weeks, all the warts had vanished.

Dr. Bruno Bloch, known as the 'famous wart doctor of Zurich,' also tells an interesting success story. He built a machine with flashing lights and a noisy motor and then instructed patients to put their hands in the machine. They had to leave their hands there until being told the warts were dead. At that time, Dr. Bloch would add a pink vegetable dye to the warts and tell the patients not to wash or touch the wart until it was gone. At least 30% of Dr. Bloch's patients were cured after one session. Such is the power of suggestion.

Warts are similar to tumors and relate to cancer in the sense that they are growths caused, as are some cancers, by a viral infection. Anything that can work for warts may have a good of working for cancer tumors.

Dr. Christina Liossi of the University of Wales in Swansea, says, "Hypnosis improves the quality of life for children and adults with cancer. It may also improve the length of life, though we are not yet sure on that. We need to put it into clinical practice."

Dr. Liossi made this statement after reviewing the outcome of a study with 80 children in Greece who clearly showed less reaction to pain when hypnosis techniques were used. In contrast, children who did not undergo hypnosis but instead took part in comforting conversation, both reported and displayed more pain than hypnotized ones.

Hypnosis has also been shown to reduce hot flashes in breast cancer survivors. "Hot flashes are a significant problem for many breast cancer survivors and can cause discomfort, insomnia, anxiety, and decreased quality of life. In the past, the standard treatment for hot flashes has been hormone replacement therapy. However, recent research has found an increased risk of breast cancer in women receiving hormone replacement therapy, at least when using hormones not derived from a human source (non-bioidentical hormones). As a result, many menopausal women and breast cancer survivors reject hormone replacement therapy and many women want nonpharmacological treatment. In this critical review we assess the potential use of hypnosis in reducing the frequency and intensity of hot flashes. We conclude that hypnosis is a mind-body intervention that may be of significant benefit in treatment of hot flashes and other benefits may include reduced anxiety and improved sleep. Further, hypnosis may be a preferred treatment because of the few side-effects and the preference of many women for a non-hormonal therapy."*

See **Simonton Method**.

### *Further Reading & References*

- *"Can hypnosis reduce hot flashes in breast cancer survivors? A literature review." http://www.ncbi.nlm.nih.gov/entrez/query.fcgi?cmd=Retrieve&db=pubmed&dopt=Abstract&list_uids=15376607

- *The Healing Brain: Breakthrough Discoveries About How the Brain Keeps Us Healthy* by Robert Ornstein, David Sobel

- Self-Hypnosis for Cancer Patients by Lee Overholser (Audio CD)

- *Hypnosis for Change* by Josie Hadley, Carol Staudacher

- *Self-Hypnosis: The Complete Manual for Health and Self-Change* by Brian M. Alman, Peter T. Lambrou

- *The Cancer Survival Cookbook: 200 Quick & Easy Recipes with Helpful Eating Hints* by Donna L. Weihofen

- *Cognitive Behaviour Therapy for People With Cancer* by Stirling Moorey, et al.

- Ericksonian Approaches by Rubin Battino, et al.

- *Soul Healing* by Bruce Goldberg

- *Autogenic Training: A Mind-Body Approach to the Treatment of Fibromyalgia and Chronic Pain Syndrome* by Micah R. Sadigh Ph.D.

- *Holistic Nursing: A Handbook for Practice* by Barbara Montgomery Dossey, et al

- *The Creation of Health: The Emotional, Psychological, and Spiritual Responses That Promote Health and Healing* by Caroline Myss, C. Norman Md Shealy

- *Capturing the Aura: Integrating Science, Technology and Metaphysics* by C. E. Lindgren

- *Healing Mind, Healthy Woman: Using the Mind-Body Connection to Manage Stress and Take Control of Your Life* by Alice Domar

- *The Subconscious Mind: A Source of Unlimited Power* by Erhard F. Freitag, Hans Sechelman

- *Blackwell Complementary and Alternative Medicine: Fast Facts for Medical Practice* by Mary A.

- Herring, Molly M. Roberts

- *Good News About High Blood Pressure: Everything You Need to Know to Take Control of Hypertension...and Your Life* by Thomas Pickering

- Alternative Options to Fighting Cancer, http://www.fightingcancer.com/download/fcpdf/21%20 A-Z%20of%20alternative%20options.pdf

- "A pilot randomized trial assessing the effects of autogenic training in early stage cancer patients in relation to psychological status and immune system responses." Hidderley M, Holt M. Southern Derbyshire Acute Hospitals NHS Trust, UK. http://www.ncbi.nlm.nih.gov/entrez/query.fcgi?cmd= Retrieve&db=pubmed&dopt=Abstract&list_uids=15003745

- *Cancer: The Complete Recovery Guide,* by Jonathan Chamberlain (2008)

# Exercise and Bodywork

## Exercise

Frequent physical exercise has been found to decrease cancer risk. Exercise stimulates circulation, improves muscle tone, improves cardiac function, and boosts immunity. It is also a way to eliminate toxins from the body. Exercise is a critical component in the elimination of "poisons" - such as the myriad toxins that build up due to regular bodily processes and exposure to man-made chemicals. Exercise eliminates toxins by a several different mechanisms. The first is that when we exercise we breathe more deeply, more forcefully and more often. In doing so, we release toxic byproducts through the lungs.

When we exercise we also perspire. Perspiration is another means of eliminating metabolic waste material from the body. And muscular activity is the only way to move waste material through the lymphatic vessels. If we don't sweat, don't breathe heavily and don't move our muscles, these toxins must find another way out. Unfortunately, they usually remain in the body, only to befoul the biochemical machinery that makes our immune system operate efficiently. The result: susceptibility to illness.

Experts on exercise as a cancer treatment put special emphasis on the need to pump toxins out of the lymph glands. While the circulatory system has its own pump – the heart – to constantly keep blood on the move, nothing moves lymph fluids except our own voluntary exertions. If lymph fluids are kept on the move and filtered through the kidneys, the foreign matter they carry is eliminated. A sedentary lifestyle undermines this process of elimination and results in the accumulation of toxins in the lymph glands.

A man with a rare documented recovery from metastatic colon cancer from Memorial Sloan-Kettering Hospital in New York said that he attributed his recovery to his iron determination to keep playing tennis even when chemotherapy made him feel he could not take another step. Indeed, many cancer patients have intuitively made some regular form of exercise part of their recovery effort.

Josef Issels, one of the great pioneering German alternative cancer therapists, regularly instructed the patients who came to his clinic in the Bavarian Alps to "go climb a mountain." And yet, as with every other major component of intensive health promotion, a few cancer experts dissent from incorporating exercise or certain types of exercise in their cancer protocols.

Max Gerson, the pioneering German nutritional cancer therapist strongly opposed exercise for his cancer patients. He believed they needed deep rest and that exercise was counterproductive. Practitioners of yoga and meditation do not oppose exercise in health and healing but believe that aerobic activity brings the "heat" to the surface of the body, while yoga and meditation bring heat to the internal organs, which, they believe, is more important for healing than is aerobic activity.

In human studies, some of the most important work has been done by Rose E. Frisch of Harvard. Frisch and colleagues surveyed 5,398 women ages 21 to 82.3. According to a summary in *Oncology Times*, they found that:

"in every age group, the non-athletes had a higher life-time occurrence of cancers of the reproductive system, which covered cancers of the uterus, ovary, cervix, and vagina. The non-athletes had 2.5 times the risk of the athletes."

Frisch also found that exercise by these females during their college years was far more protective against cancer than exercise initiated by non-athletes in later life, although exercise initiated later did have some effect. Of non-athletes who exercised later in life, 50% had a reduced risk of cancer.

Dr. Frisch postulates reasons for the lower risk in former athletes. First, the athletes may have made less estrogen because they were leaner and had less adipose tissue, which converts androgen to estrogen. A decrease in estrogen, which causes breast and reproductive tissue to divide, would result in less tumor cell division. Secondly, the estrogen athletes made may have been less potent. It has been previously shown that the leaner one is, the more one's estrogen metabolism produces a less potent estrogen, which inhibits the division of uterine and breast cells.

That vigorous exercise reduces body levels of the highly active form of estrogen was confirmed in a study by Rachel Snow, a graduate student working with Frisch, who measured body fluids of athletes and nonathletes. She found that girls and women with anorexia and an irregular menstrual cycle develop an excess of the inactive form of estrogen.

Frisch also found that hard exercise is often associated with the delay of the onset of menstruation. She believes this may be protective against breast and reproductive system cancers. In fact, she postulates that the higher the total number of ovulatory periods in a woman's lifetime, the greater her susceptibility to cancer may be.

In another study, Frisch found that cancers of the digestive system, thyroid, lung, and other sites, as well as the hematopoietic cancers (lymphoma, leukemia, myeloma, and Hodgkin's disease), were also lower for the college athletes. The rates of malignant melanomas and skin cancers did not differ significantly between the two groups.

Another protective pathway by which exercise may modulate the development of cancer is through its effect on depression. In a number of studies, exercise has been shown to have an antidepressive effect, and depression is a common precursor and concomitant factor in cancer. Moderate exercise can have a powerful protective effect against depression, which in turn may work through complex mind-body pathways to help prevent or modulate the development of a cancer.

Some researchers have hypothesized that at high exercise levels the body may experience an increase in free radicals and peroxide production in the body, which might account for the increase in cancer in some animal studies and the increase in humans, particularly in smokers.

Still another interesting perspective on cancer and physical activity comes from Ron E. LaPorte, Associate Professor of Epidemiology at the School of Public Health at the University of Pittsburgh. LaPorte believes physical activity rather than exercise may be the important protective factor against cancer.

As *Oncology Times* reported, LaPorte believes: "there is...some evidence...that increased physical activity alters bowel transit time. Decreased transit time might be related to reduced colon cancer risk, said Dr. LaPorte, because there is less time for carcinogens to be produced. He also cited evidence for decreased cancer risk related to physical activity via increased thermal effects, and increased concentrations of vitamin A."

Indirect evidence shows the benefits of physical activity for people with cancer. The line of reasoning is that enhanced functional status or performance status is a predictor of better outcomes in some cancers, and "functional status" is a synonym for capacity to be physically active. Similarly, most oncologists regard a person who is in good physical shape as potentially more resilient to treatment.

Also, a study has found that for breast cancer patients, a home-based moderate-intensity walking exercise program may effectively mitigate the high levels of fatigue prevalent during cancer treatment.

*Further Reading & References*

- Huang XE, Hirose K, Wakai K, Matsuo K, Ito H, Xiang J, Takezaki T, Tajima K. "Comparison of lifestyle risk factors by family history for gastric, breast, lung and colorectal cancer." Asian Pac J Cancer Prev. 2004 Oct-Dec;5(4):419-27. http://www.ncbi.nlm.nih.gov/entrez/query.fcgi?cmd=Retrieve&db=pubmed&dopt=Abstract&list_uids=15546249

- R.A. Yedinak, D.K. Layman, and J.A. Milner, "Influences of Dietary Fat and Exercise on DMBA-Induced Mammary Tumors." Meeting abstract, Federation Proceedings, 46(3):436 (1987).

- Rose E. Frisch et al., "Lower Prevalence of Breast Cancer and Cancers of the Reproductive System

- Among Former College Athletes Compared to Non-Athletes," British Journal of Cancer 52(6):885-91 (1985). Mock V, Frangakis C, Davidson NE, Ropka ME, Pickett M, Poniatowski B, Stewart KJ,

- Cameron L, Zawacki K, Podewils LJ, Cohen G, McCorkle "Exercise manages fatigue during breast cancer treatment: a randomized controlled trial." http://www.ncbi.nlm.nih.gov/entrez/query.fcgi?cmd=Retrieve&db=pubmed&dopt=Abstract&list_uids=15484202

# Massage

Massage therapy offers profound benefit to both hormonal and immunologic systems. It also stimulates the lymphatics to get rid of toxins found in the body. Cancer patients who undergo massage tend to report relief from the five most common symptoms of cancer and cancer treatment: pain, nausea, fatigue, depression, and anxiety.

Several research studies support a decline in anxiety due to massage. A 2005 study in the *International Journal of Neuroscience* proved that when women diagnosed with breast cancer received three 30-minute massages a week for five weeks, they ended up less depressed, less angry, and with more energy than the control group. More importantly, dopamine levels, natural killer cells, and lymphocytes reportedly increased for the massage therapy group.

In the literature on massage for cancer patients, a number of nursing studies show that slow-stroke back massage enhances relaxation or the feeling of general well-being. For example, an article by K. Warren in *Nursing Times* recommends slow-stroke back massage, along with distraction, guided imagery, progressive muscle relaxation, systemic desensitization, hypnosis, and dietary adjustments, to help patients with chemotherapy-induced nausea and vomiting.

In the same journal, S. Sims reports a pilot study with six breast cancer patients undergoing radiotherapy for whom back massage resulted in fewer symptoms, more tranquility and vitality, and less tension and tiredness. L.A. Barbour, in a descriptive study in *Oncology Nursing Forum*, found that patients can use an array of non-analgesic methods to control pain that include heat, deep breathing, massage, and exercise.

B.Z. Dobbs in *Nursing Mirror* reports that reflexology was helpful to advanced cancer patients both in comforting them and controlling pain. Reflexology involves massage of the hands and feet based on the theory that pressure points there correspond to different parts of the body, including the internal organs.

In physical therapy, massage is frequently a necessary part of the management of lymphedema, in which the protein-rich fluids of the lymph system accumulate in tissue after breast surgery or radiotherapy. One key to the treatment of lymphedema is to identify and treat it early, since prolonged presence of lymphedema in the tissue can break down the structure of the tissue so that it loses the elasticity necessary to squeeze out lymphatic accumulations.

At Sir Michael Sobell House in London, which specializes in the treatment of lymphedema, diuretics are no longer used (they reduced edema at the expense of dehydration). Instead, massage combined with a variety of sleeves and stockings is used to control the movement of lymphatic swelling.

Another benefit to massage is that it energizes the lymphatic system. This means it prompts the flow of fluid in the body's arteries and veins that pass through a patient's lymphatic system. The lymph tissues then trap waste products from this fluid and carry them out of the body. By prompting blood flow up to a healthy level and increasing the rate of function, the body can eliminate toxins more quickly and effectively.

A study published many years ago in the *Journal of Clinical Investigation* showed lymphatic drainage increased in dogs after having only their foot pads massaged. The same is true for massage in humans, only the benefit increases dramatically with full-body massage.

For many years there was a widespread myth that all massage was contraindicated (i.e. bad) for anybody with cancer. This was based on the underlying fear that massage could speed along the process of cancer metastasis.

This is largely because massage promotes circulation and because it is a known fact that cancerous cells travel throughout the body via the bloodstream. To many, it made sense that better circulation would simply move cancerous cells more quickly through the body. The reality is that although cancerous cells are loosely attached to tissues within the body and are more likely to break off than normal tissue cells, the act of increasing blood flow through massage simply promotes healthy circulation. Such circulation is similar to what one would get from cardiac activity which is commonly recommended for cancer patients.

Though massage is proven to help cancer patients have a more bearable experience with cancer treatment, there are certain times when a patient should either wait to have a massage or at least make sure to have a therapist skilled in oncology massage designed specifically for cancer patients.

The first contraindication is the actual tumor site of the cancer. The tumor site should never be massaged as pressure on the site might disturb tissues in the vicinity of the tumor.

Surgeon Bernie Siegel stated in the *Massage Therapy Journal*, "Massage therapy is not contraindicated in cancer patients; massaging a tumor is, but there is a great deal more to a person than their tumor."

When a patient has cancer in an internal organ, there is little worry in getting a comforting massage to the head, neck, shoulders, limbs, and upper chest.

In some cases, it may be necessary to see how cancer progresses in order to assess how one's body is affected by the cancer and whether bones or vital organs are involved. Until then, it is difficult to provide enough instruction for a massage therapist to create a treatment plan.

The final contraindication is if massage hurts. Some cancer treatments leave patients aching, in which case a massage is unlikely to bring pleasure. Eventually, massage might help a patient overcome this, but in the first few days following chemo, radiation, or especially surgery, it may hurt too much to be touched.

Massage therapists can provide seriously ill cancer victims with powerful relief and healing. A growing educational movement supports this approach, and the list of training programs for oncology massage has more than doubled in the past few years. In addition, the length of training is getting longer now that more research is being conducted on the benefits for cancer patients.

Because it can be individualized for a wide variety of symptoms and complications, massage therapy is beneficial in terms of treating different types and stages of cancer. In effect, that means this treatment is one of the most promising for helping the greatest number of people.

### Further Reading and References

- *Medicine Hands: Massage Therapy for People With Cancer* by Gayle MacDonald (2007)

- Hernandez-Reif, M. (2005). Natural Killer Cells and Lymphocytes Increase in Women with Breast Cancer Following Massage Therapy. *International Journal of Neuroscience*, 495-510.

- Murray, M. (2002). *How to Prevent and Treat Cancer with Natural Medicine.* New York: Penguin Group.

- Oz, M. (1998). *Healing from the Heart: A Leading Surgeon Combines Eastern and Western Traditions to Create the Medicine of the Future.* New York: Penguin Group.

- Walton, T. (2006). Cancer & Massage Therapy: Essential Contraindications. *Massage Therapy Journal*, 119-134.

- B.Z. Dobbs, "Oncology Nursing 6: Alternative Health Approaches," Nursing Mirror 160(9):41-2 (1985).

- K. Warren, "Will I Be Sick, Nurse?" Nursing Times 84(12):53-4 (1988).

# Qigong and Tai Chi

The term Qigong (pronounced "chee gung" - sometimes spelled "chi kung") literally means "energy practice." It refers to a family of practices for health, fitness, energy development, and stress relief.

Qigong includes more than just movement exercises. It also includes standing and sitting meditations, massage, therapeutic healing techniques, and other practices designed to build health and energy. Qigong is also sometimes referred to as "Chinese yoga."

Tai Chi is actually just one form of Qigong. Tai Chi is an exercise that focuses on natural physical movement, breathing, and mental concentration. The exercises and practices of Tai Chi come directly from "kung fu" (Chinese martial arts). Tai Chi is graceful, slow, and relaxing, and these days, most people practice Tai Chi not for self-defense, but for the great health and stress relief benefits it provides.

Tai Chi has a number of exercises, but the basic practice of Tai Chi is "sets" or "forms." Sets are a series of movements done in a precise order to help facilitate energy flow, fitness, relaxation, and mental concentration. Some sets are short, taking just a few minutes to practice, while others are longer and require more time to practice. More important than the length of the set, though, is how well the set teaches you the principles of natural movement, body structure, and internal energy.

Tai Chi and Qigong are used in clinics in China and around the world to treat diseases ranging from cancer to hypertension. Doctors, hospitals, research studies, and participants in Tai Chi and Qigong say that it:

- Lowers blood pressure

- Builds greater aerobic capacity

- Improves strength, mobility, and endurance

- Relieves stress and improves nervous system function

- Promotes deeper relaxation and better sleep

- Produces a marked increase of immune response (blood t-cell) during and after practice

- Benefits chronic illness

- Improves posture and back and spine problems

- Clears negative emotions and reduces anxiety

- Lowers stress hormone (salivary cortisol) levels

- Increases respiratory capacity

- Increases joint flexibility

Dr. Feng Li-da, professor of immunology at Beijing College of Traditional Chinese Medicine, has done many experiments on external chi transmission and claims that a chi-gong expert can destroy uterine cancer cells, gastric cancer cells, flu virus, and colon and dysentery bacilli with varying degrees of success.

In *The Scientific Basis of Chi-gong*, Professor Xie Huan-zhang of Beijing Industrial College states that chi effects detected with scientific instruments include magnetic fields, infrared radiation, infrasound, and ion streams of visible light and superfaint luminescence.

### *Further Reading & References*

- *The Scientific Basis of Chi-gong* by Professor Xie Huan-Zhang

- *The Way of Qigong : The Art and Science of Chinese Energy Healing* by Ken Cohen (1999)

- *Qigong Empowerment: A Guide to Medical, Taoist, Buddhist, Wushu Energy Cultivation* by Shou-Yu Liang, Wen-Ching Wu (1996)

- *The Healing Promise of Qi: Creating Extraordinary Wellness Through Qigong and Tai Chi* by Roger Jahnke (2002)


# Therapeutic Touch

Therapeutic Touch can be seen as a modern version of the ancient practice of laying on of hands. Many of our ancestors - in antiquity and throughout the Middle Ages - believed that touch had a magical quality for healing, particularly if it were administered by a holy man or healer. Today, the laying on of hands is being revived in many churches.

Therapeutic Touch, however, is a systematic protocol for healing with the hands, originated by Dora Kunz, a famous healer, and Dolores Krieger, Professor of Nursing at New York University.

According to Krieger, although it had its historical origins in the laying on of hands, Therapeutic Touch takes its theoretical basis from modern physics.

"Physics posits that energy fields are the basic units of all matter, that the human being extends beyond what we perceive as a physical boundary and is, through energy, interconnected with everything in the environment. This is further substantiated by the Eastern theories of qi and prana, the Chinese and Indian concepts of the life energy" says Krieger.

Eastern literature states that a healthy person has an overabundance of "Prana" or "Qi", and that an ill person has a deficit. Indeed, having a deficit of Prana is the Eastern definition of illness. Prana or Qi can be channeled from a healthy person to an ill one if– and this is very important– the healer has the conscious intent to do so. This transfer of energy will help the ill person to buttress his own energy system in the service of self-healing. Krieger believes that anyone can learn therapeutic touch:

"It's a natural potential in all human beings and this potential can be developed."

There are three major phases in the procedure:

- Centering - a short period in which the therapist enters a meditative state of awareness and washes away all the "busy-ness" of her own thoughts, becoming acutely open to any input from the client.

- The therapist then "listens passively" with the hands as they scan the client's body a few inches above the skin, and "tunes in" to any disturbances in the energy field around the body. In this phase, they search for temperature changes or other energy differences as clues to underlying energy imbalances. This is called assessing.

- In the third phase, with hands still above the client's skin, the therapist "unruffles" or smoothes out the energy field surrounding the body and begins to concentrate on areas where the therapist has sensed accumulated tension. She helps redirect the energy flow so that it is no longer congested and begins to move smoothly through the body. This is known as re-balancing.

Normally, the whole process takes no longer than 15 to 20 minutes. "The basis of Therapeutic Touch," says Krieger, "lies in intelligently directing healing energy through the healer to the healee."

Therapeutic Touch is now used by nurses in many major medical centers, hospices, and in home care throughout this country and abroad, albeit not without resistance from conservative physicians.

In an innovative study by Daniel Wirth, M.S., J.D., president of Healing Sciences International in Orinda, California, small experimental wounds were administered to the arms of college students, who then placed their arms through a special armhole in a wall and were randomized into a group that received Therapeutic Touch and a group that did not.

The group receiving Therapeutic Touch experienced significantly faster wound healing. Wirth and his colleagues obtained similar results in a subsequent replication of the original study.

Whatever the merits of its theory, Therapeutic Touch has been demonstrated in careful research to have efficacy in physical and psychological healing. What is different about Therapeutic Touch is that it is employed systematically by nurses and researchers in a nonsectarian manner and that a strong effort has been made to develop systematic research on its effectiveness. Recent studies have shown that Therapeutic Touch is effective in reducing pain, mood disturbance, and fatigue in patients receiving cancer chemotherapy and radiation therapy.

### Further Reading & References

- *Hands of Light: A Guide to Healing Through the Human Energy Field* by Barbara Brennan (1988)

- *The Spiritual Dimension of Therapeutic Touch* by Dora Kunz, Dolores Krieger (2004)

- *The Therapeutic Touch: How to Use Your Hands to Help or to Heal* by Dolores Krieger (1979)

- *Quantum Touch: The Power to Heal* by Richard Gordon, et al (2006)

- *Healing Touch: A Guide Book for Practitioners* by Dorothea Hover-Kramer (2001)

- Post-White J, Kinney ME, Savik K, Gau JB, Wilcox C, Lerner I. University of Minneapolis, Minnesota, USA."Therapeutic massage and healing touch improve symptoms in cancer." Integr Cancer Ther. 2003 Dec;2(4):332-44

# Yoga

The term yoga means 'union'. Many people mistakenly believe this term refers to a union between the body and mind or the body, mind and spirit. However, the traditional acceptance is that it represents a union between the Jivatman and Paramatman. These terms mean, respectively, one's individual consciousness and the Universal Consciousness.

Yoga refers to a certain state of consciousness. It also represents methods that help one reach the goal of achieving a state of union with the divine. Additional benefits to yoga include increased strength and flexibility, improved circulation, the promotion of well-being, and relief for common postural and chronic pain problems.

Yoga is increasingly being used as a form of breast cancer therapy, and there are a growing number of instructors and yoga classes specifically dedicated to breast cancer survivors. Breast Cancer patients utilize yoga to improve mind, body and spirit. Yoga helps to reduce stress as well as increase strength, flexibility, energy, balance and concentration. It helps to alleviate chronic pain and aides in the relief of back and neck pain.

Yoga offers cancer patients relief from the stress of treatment, while also assisting with the rehabilitation of their weakened bodies. In fact, at the country's most prestigious cancer centers, yoga mats and other yoga products are a common sight. Yoga has become an increasingly popular part of cancer wellness programs both in professional rehabilitation programs as well as in patients' homes.

U.S. researchers said the use of Tibetan yoga helps cancer patients to sleep. The researchers, at the University of Texas M. D. Anderson Cancer Center, said lymphoma patients who practiced Tibetan yoga for seven weeks went to sleep faster, slept longer, had better overall sleep quality, and used less sleep medication, compared with a "control" group of patients with lymphoma who did not use yoga.

There were, however, no differences between the groups in other "quality of life" measures, they said, including anxiety, depression and fatigue. The most likely reason for this is the study's brief time frame.

Two Tibetan practices in particular, "Tsa lung" and "Trul khor," incorporate controlled breathing and visualization, mindfulness techniques and postures. Little is known about this form of yoga and no research has examined its benefits, the researchers added.

### Further Reading & References

- *Healing Yoga for People Living with Cancer* by Lisa Holtby (2004)

- Cohen L, Warneke C, Fouladi RT, Rodriguez MA, Chaoul-Reich A. Psychological adjustment and sleep quality in a randomized trial of the effects of a Tibetan yoga intervention in patients with lymphoma. Cancer. 2004 May 15;100(10):2253-60.

# Drugs

## Anticoagulants/Coumarin/Heparin/Warfarin

Anticoagulants are drugs that reduce the clotting ability of blood. Coumarin, heparin and warfarin are examples of such drugs.

It has been observed that stopping clotting also stops metastases. When cancer cells break away from the original tumor and enter the bloodstream they attract platelets, which bind to sugarcoated molecules called mucins on the cancer cell surface, forming a cloak. This platelet cloak appears to protect the tumor cells from the body's natural defense systems, enabling them to establish new tumors in other parts of the body. Heparin interferes with formation of the platelet cloak, apparently leaving tumor cells exposed to attack by white blood cells.

In research at the University of California, San Diego Cancer Center, experimental mice received a single dose of heparin, which lasted for only a few hours, yet this early exposure resulted in markedly reduced cancer cell survival and metastasis when the mice were examined several weeks later.

Warfarin has been shown to prolong survival for patients undergoing conventional therapy – especially for lung cancer patients and for post-menopausal women with breast cancer. However, a side-effect is that immunity is suppressed; therefore anticoagulants work best together with drugs that enhance NK cell activity.

### Further Reading & References

- Alifano, M., Benedetti, G., Trisolini, R. (2004). Can Low-Molecular-Weight Heparin Improve the Outcome of Patients With Operable Non-Small Cell Lung Cancer?: An Urgent Call for Research. Chest 126: 601-607

- Zielinski, C. C., Hejna, M. (2000). Warfarin for Cancer Prevention. N Engl J Med 342: 1991-1993 [Full Text]

- Borsig, L., Wong, R., Feramisco, J., Nadeau, D. R., Varki, N. M., Varki, A. (2001). Heparin and cancer revisited: Mechanistic connections involving platelets, P-selectin, carcinoma mucins, and tumor metastasis. Proc. Natl. Acad. Sci. U. S. A. 98: 3352-3357 [Abstract] [Full Text]

- Collen, A., Smorenburg, S. M., Peters, E., Lupu, F., Koolwijk, P., Van Noorden, C., van Hinsbergh, V. W. M. (2000). Unfractionated and Low Molecular Weight Heparin Affect Fibrin Structure and Angiogenesis in Vitro. Cancer Res 60: 6196-6200 [Abstract] [Full Text]

- Ma, Y.-Q., Geng, J.-G. (2000). Heparan Sulfate-Like Proteoglycans Mediate Adhesion of Human Malignant Melanoma A375 Cells to P-Selectin Under Flow. J Immunol 165: 558-565

- Letai, A., Kuter, D. J. (1999). Cancer, Coagulation, and Anticoagulation. Oncologist 4: 443-449

# Benzaldehyde/BG/Zilascorb

Benzaldehyde, the essential oil of bitter almond, is naturally found in peach and apricot kernels as a byproduct of amygdalin. Its presence is rendered obvious by the bitter almond taste. Amygdalin, or laetrile – one of the most famous alternative cancer remedies -- is a naturally occurring phytochemical found in hundreds of plants. A molecule of amygdalin consists of a unit of benzaldehyde, a unit of hydrogen cyanide, and two units of glucose. The amygdalin is broken into its constituent parts, including benzaldehyde, in the presence of a certain enzyme.

Benzaldehyde has a history of being investigated as an anti-cancer agent. In the 1960's and 70's, it was often combined with chemotherapy. Using a modified form of benzaldehyde, Dr. M. Kochi treated 65 patients who had inoperable cancers. "The overall objective response rate was 55%" Japanese doctors said. "7 patients achieved complete response, 29 achieved partial response, 24 remain stable, and 5 showed progressive disease."

A derivative of benzaldehyde called BG has also been shown effective in stopping cancer. Like benzaldehyde, it was also non-toxic. Toyama scientists show that in 24 patients with advanced cancer there was an overall response rate of 58%. An ascorbic acid form of benzaldehyde called zilascorb has been shown to be more effective than pure benzaldehyde or other derivatives. Its effects were shown to be reversible – even after protracted therapy, including destruction of more than 99% of the cancer cells. The few surviving cells appear to be undamaged after removal of the drug, showing how basically safe this drug is.

Additionally, benzaldehyde seems to be able to transform malignant cells back to normal, according to a Norwegian report. It had been postulated in the early 1980's that benzaldehyde, as well as betacarotene, interferon and antineoplastons, could be considered a new type of therapy which stops cell growth and transforms cancer cells back to normal without harming the patient.

Dr. Hans Nieper, an unconventional German physician, utilized benzaldehyde for its "paralytic effect" on tumor growth. Dr. Nieper found that benzaldehyde "is one of the most valuable anti-cancer substances which is currently and practically available" but he also went on to claim that "acetaldehyde, a related substance, is clearly "superior for melanoma".


See **Laetrile/Amygdalin**.


### Further Reading & References

- *Cancer Therapy: The Independent Consumer's Guide to Non-Toxic Treatment and Prevention* by Ralph W. Moss (1992)


# Clodronate

This treatment reportedly stops breast cancer from spreading to the bones.

"The Food and Drug Administration's suppression of clodronate may have caused the premature or needless death of about 30,000 American women each year, based on the Aug. 6, 1998, New England Journal of Medicine study. Since clodronate could have been made available 15 years ago, about 517,000 American breast cancer victims were forced to suffer agonizing bone metastasis, and a total of 450,000 women probably died prematurely because the FDA aggressively denied this drug to cancer patients."*

"In 1998, the *New England Journal of Medicine* published impressive data indicating that clodronate reduced the incidence and number of metastases in bone and viscera (organs enclosed in the abdominal, thoracic, or pelvic cavity) in high-risk breast cancer patients by 50%."**

### Further Reading & References

- *"Battling Back Against Cancer-Induced Bone Metastasis and Pain," by William Faloon, *LE Magazine*, January 1999, http://www.lef.org/magazine/mag99/jan99-cover.html

- **Diel et al. "Reduction in New Metastases in Breast Cancer with Adjuvant Clodronate Treatment." *The New England Journal of Medicine*. 6 Aug 1998.

- Alternative Cancer Therapies: http://www.mnwelldir.org/docs/cancer1/altthrpy.htm

# Clomipramine

Existing anti-cancer drugs are unable to cross the blood-brain barrier, and some types of brain tumor are usually difficult to treat. Experience indicates that for these patients clomipramine (Anafranil) is more effective than Phenergan.

Clomipramine is a prescription drug; treatment therefore requires a participating doctor. At the time of writing details of the treatment have not been published, but its use is expected to be described shortly.

From the Samantha Dickson Research Trust: "Clomipramine is a major breakthrough in cancer treatment and 350 patients have already been treated, providing 'anecdotal evidence' that the drug crosses the blood brain barrier and attacks the tumor. The majority of patients have shown an improvement in their condition, and a promising amount has seen a reduction in tumor mass on their latest MRI scans. Sadly, some patients have died for a variety of reasons, some of whom either had not been given the right dosage, or others whose illness had progressed too far for any real effect."

### Further Reading & References

- Excerpt from Samantha Dickson Research Trust May 21, 2004 'Finding a Cure for Brain Tumors for Children and Adults' http://www.sdrt.co.uk/

- Cancer Active: Using Clomipramine to treat brain tumors, http://www.canceractive.com/cancer-active-page-link.aspx?n=1096

# Diethylstilbestrol (DES)

This drug is a synthetic hormone that was found to be present in an alternative treatment for prostate cancer manufactured in China called PC-SPES. As the drug is available in the United States by prescription only, it could not be sold in an over-the-counter formula, and PC-SPES was removed from the market. Two other drugs were allegedly present in PC-SPES.

DES can cause blood clots. Some doctors think the DES was the element of PC-SPES that made it so effective on advanced prostate cancer patients. One of the other manufactured drugs found in PC-SPES was a blood thinner. While PC-SPES was removed from the market, doctors are now looking at DES as a treatment for advanced prostate cancer.

While comparing PC-SPES to DES, Glenn Bubley, MD, director of genitourinary oncology at Harvard Medical School and Beth Israel Deaconess Medical Center, stated:

"DES was the first drug prescribed for prostate cancer in 1950. We got rid of it because it caused blood clots. We need to know that PC-SPES is not just garden-variety DES."

See **PC-SPES**.

### Further Reading & References

- National Cancer Institute, http://www.cancer.gov/cancertopics/causes/des

# Dimethyl Sulfoxide (DMSO)

Related to MSM, DMSO is different enough to be placed in its own category. It is a solvent with the ability to penetrate living tissue and thereby transport different medicines in their original state to other areas within the body. It is most commonly used as a vehicle for topical drugs.

Research has shown that DMSO may slow the progression of cancer cell proliferation, though conclusive proof is lacking. DMSO has also been used to prevent the accidental administration of intravenous-infused chemotherapeutic agents from leaking into surrounding tissues.

Many researchers view DMSO's capabilities as a new principle in medicine that is, as yet, largely untapped.

See **DMSO and MSM**.

### Further Reading & References

- DMSO Dimethyl Sulfoxide, http://www.dmso.org/

- Dimethyl Sulfoxide - DMSO Cancer Benefits, http://www.xyz-wellbeing.com/the-xyz-services-we-offer/xyz-alternative-cancer-retreat-facility-services/dimethylsulfoxidedmsocancer.html

- Memorial Sloan Kettering Cancer Center: Dimethylsulfoxide, http://www.mskcc.org/mskcc/html/69205.cfm

- Bertelli G. Prevention and management of extravasation of cytotoxic drugs. Drug Saf 1995; 12:245-55.

- Dorr RT. Antidotes to vesicant chemotherapy extravasations. Blood Rev. 1990; 4:41-60.

- Jacob SW,.Herschler R. Pharmacology of DMSO. Cryobiology 1986; 23:14-27.

- Brayton CF. Dimethyl sulfoxide (DMSO): a review. Cornell Vet. 1986; 76:61-90.

# Doxycycline

Research conducted by scientists at the Stanford University School of Medicine, suggests that turning off just one cancer-causing gene is enough to eliminate aggressive, incurable liver tumors in mice in just four weeks.

The researchers led by Dean Felsher studied mice whose liver cells had been altered to carry a modified Myc gene. Myc protein acts as a cellular conductor, orchestrating messages that tell a cell to divide. The Myc gene churns out the Myc protein until it is turned off by feeding mice the antibiotic doxycycline, a form of tetracycline.

The mice remained cancer-free as long as they maintained their diet of the antibiotic. But as soon as doxycycline was withheld, the gene was back on; Myc protein accumulated in the liver cells, and the animals developed aggressive liver cancer within an average of 12 weeks.

The doxycycline diet again turned off the production of Myc protein and eliminated the cancer in mice as was confirmed by the appearance of normal liver cells. The researchers found that turning the Myc gene on and off acted like a tap, releasing the cancerous cells to divide uncontrollably, then shutting off their cancerous progression.

Felsher said:"The exciting thing is that you can turn cancer cells into something that appears to be normal."

In previous mice studies, doxycycline was shown to reduce— by 70% in mice—the spread of some types of human tumors to the bone. "Doxycycline not only shrank breast and prostate tumors that had metastasized (or travelled) to the bone, but it also showed an ability to prevent the spread of cancer in the first place", says Dr. Gurmit Singh, Director of Research at Hamilton Regional Cancer Centre and a Professor at McMaster University.

The research team had an additional surprise: doxycycline not only reduced bone tumors and stopped bone loss, but it actually promoted the growth of new bone tissue. "This might be very useful for breast cancer patients because they get a lot of fractures when the disease goes to the bone," said Dr. Singh. For unknown reasons, between 70% and 80% of breast cancer metastases and 70% of prostate cancer metastases go to the bone. It is these secondary tumors that often cause pain and death. "People give up hope and the will to live when they are in so much pain," said Dr. Singh. "I think there is something to be said for the will to live, and this drug may actually provide pain relief, which in turn might even increase the survival of individuals."

### *Further Reading & References*

- New Scientist http://www.newscientist.com/news/news.jsp?id=ns99996511 Journal reference: Nature (DOI: 10.1038/nature03043)

- Doxycycline decreases tumor burden in a bone metastasis model of human breast cancer. Duivenvoorden WC, Popovic SV, Lhotak S, Seidlitz E, Hirte HW, Tozer RG, Singh G. Hamilton

- Regional Cancer Centre and McMaster University, Hamilton, Ontario, L8V 5C2 Canada.

- "Doxycycline decreases tumor burden in a bone metastasis model of human breast cancer."http://www.ncbi.nlm.nih.gov/entrez/query.fcgi?cmd=Retrieve&db=PubMed&dopt=Abstract&list_uids=11912125

- Effects of doxycycline on human prostate cancer cells in vitro. RS Fife, GW Sledge Jr, BJ Roth, and C Proctor Cancer Lett 1998;127(1-2): 37-41 UI:98281155

- Cancer Care Spring/Summer 2002 http://www.cancercare.on.ca/pdf/
  cco02springsummer(ENG).pdf

# Gossypol

Gossypol is a pigment isolated from cotton seed in 1937. It has been found to stop rapidly dividing cells. It has been shown to cause a 60% decline in blood flow to pancreatic cancers in mice. It has also been observed to actually punch holes in the surface of mouse leukemia cells, after only two days of treatment.

Gossypol has also been studied as a tumor fighting agent for breast cancer, and was shown to have a strong inhibitory effect on the growth of breast cancer cells.

NIH scientists gave the drug to a patient with adrenal cortex cancer who had multiple metastases to the liver and lungs. After three weeks, scans showed a complete resolution of lung metastases and more than 50% decrease in the size of liver metastases.

Its toxicity in animal studies was found to be formidable, and a narrow effectiveness range needs to be established in humans. Observed side effects in the above patient consisted mainly of fatigue, dryness of the mouth and tremors.

### Further Reading & References

- "Cottonseed Drug Boosts Cancer Treatment in Mice," http://psa-rising.com/med/chemo/
  gossypol1004.htm

# Insulin-induced Hypoglycemic Therapy (IHT)

The BioPulse clinic in Mexico began using IHT in June, 1999.

"The exact mechanism is unsure but cancer cells die and the tumors shrink, that much we know. When glucose (sugar) levels are lowered by insulin, the body's metabolic state slows; oxygen accumulates in the blood and carbon dioxide decreases. The reason for this is thought to be a decrease in oxidation of carbohydrates and thus an increase of available oxygen. This in turn increases the pH of the blood and tissue.

These things we know about cancer cells: "They don't live well in highly oxygenated environments. They carry out anaerobic glycolysis of glucose and thus if increase of oxygen they don't survive. They die if the pH gets high enough. If the sugar gets low enough, cancer cells die." The FTC subsequently obtained a $4.3 million judgment against BioPulse International Inc, and the results of this treatment are unconfirmed.

### Further Reading & References

- Insulin-Induced Hypoglycemic Therapy, http://www.annieappleseedproject.org/inhypther.html

# Low-Dose Naltrexone/LDN

Clinical trials and anecdotal evidence confirm that low dose naltrexone (LDN) can arrest cancer progression, reduce symptoms, and help the body heal itself.

Burton Berkson, M.D., Ph.D., reports LDN's impressive effect on cancer, as well as arthritis, lupus, MS, and other autoimmune diseases.

LDN is inexpensive and FDA approved, but not, so far, for conditions other than dependence on alcohol and opium-derived drugs. For off-label purposes including cancer treatment, LDN is effectively being kept under wraps and few people know it exists.

Naltrexone is a pharmacologically active opiate antagonist used to treat drug and alcohol addiction, typically at doses of 50mg to 300mg. It was FDA approved in 1984 for those purposes.

More recently, researchers discovered that low dosages of LDN (3 to 4.5mg) could modulate the immune system, and ***were valuable for treating various kinds of cancer*** as well as a wide range of autoimmune diseases, including[1]:

- Rheumatoid arthritis

- Multiple sclerosis (MS)

- Parkinson's

- Fibromyalgia

- Crohn's disease

- Ulcerative colitis

- Lupus

- Diabetic neuropathy

- Dermatomyositis (an inflammatory muscle disease)

- Hepatitis C

One physician, Dr. Jacquelyn McCandless, even found that LDN helped children with autism.

Dr. Bernard Bihari – the discoverer of the clinical effects of LDN in humans – began to treat cancer patients with LDN in 1999.[2] Most of these patients had failed to respond to standard treatments and in many cases they were already gravely ill when first seen by Dr. Bihari.

Although not considered a controlled clinical trial, medical records suggest that Bihari's clinical 'off-label' use of LDN on 450 cancer patients significantly benefited more than 60% of them.

Of 354 patients with whom Dr. Bihari had regular follow-up, 86 showed at least a 75% reduction in tumor size. Another 125 patients were stabilized or moving toward remission. Those who showed the best progress toward remission had never received chemo.

LDN therapy thus looks like a very promising alternative. It offers the possibility of long-term stabilization and/or gradual reduction of the size of the tumor.

Unfortunately, Dr. Bihari lacked up-to-date follow-up data on 96 patients. Of the other 354 patients – those for whom we know the results -- 84 died (all but 4 due to cancer-related causes). Most of these deaths occurred within the first 8-12 weeks on LDN, among patients who were extremely ill and had exhausted all other treatment options by the time they saw Dr. Bihari.

The apparent remissions among Dr. Bihari's patients included[3]:

- 2 children – neuroblastoma

- 6 – non-Hodgkin's lymphoma

- 3 – Hodgkin's disease

- 5 – pancreatic cancer metastatic to the liver

- 5 – multiple myeloma

- 1 – carcinoid

- 4 – breast cancer metastatic to bone

- 4 – ovarian cancer

- 18 – non-small cell lung cancer

- 1 – small cell lung cancer

- 5 – prostate cancer (with no prior hormone-blocking therapy


Recently-diagnosed prostate cancer patients *without* previous therapies appear to do well on LDN. But those with prior hormone-related therapies, including testosterone-blocking drugs and PC-Spes, were unresponsive to LDN. LDN appears promising for prostate cancer prevention and early treatment, given that *all* anecdotal cases not previously receiving hormonal treatments went into remission.[4]

Overall, it appears plausible that about 60% of cancer patients could benefit from LDN. This is underscored by Dr. Bihari's observation that earlier treatment with LDN seemed to improve results.

The National Cancer Institute is aware of LDN. In June 2002 an oncologist reviewed some 30 charts of Dr. Bihari's cancer patients. About half were said to have responded to LDN beyond doubt. With patient permission, medical records went to the NCI for further analysis and for consideration for NCI's Best Case Series.

Dr. Bihari had 88 patients with cancer in partial or total remission whose outcome appeared to be clearly attributable to LDN alone. Some LDN-only patients had been on the medication up to 4 years at the time of this report. However, most of Dr. Bilhari's cancer patients were on other treatments besides LDN.


**How LDN works**

LDN boosts immune system function.

Scientifically, endorphins are neurotransmitters in the brain that regulate immune function, cell growth and pain sensation. They bind to neuroreceptors. According to the *Journal of Immunology,* the release of endorphins can boost the immune system.

Scientists have discovered that the beta-endorphin activates NK cells (natural killer cells) which are believed to kill cancer cells. Beta-endorphins also relieve pain, reduce stress, and postpone the aging process.

LDN works by inhibiting these endorphins for a short time – resulting in a rebound effect in endorphin production.

Those higher levels then up-regulate vital elements of the immune system and promote corresponding increases in T-lymphocytes. Apparently the increase restores the body's normal balance of T-cells to reduce the impact of some diseases including cancer.

The potential benefit of LDN for cancer arose largely from the work of Penn State's Dr. Ian Zagon and his colleagues.

Dr. Ian Zagon and his team at Penn State University researched naltrexone and other opiate antagonists. They found that one particular endorphin, met-enkephalin, inhibited cell proliferation, reducing inflammation in autoimmune and neurological disorders, and **stopping cell growth in tumors**.

Zagon published evidence that LDN:

- Reduced neuroblastoma tumor incidence by 66%

- Retarded tumor development by 98%

- Extended survival by 36% over controls.


LDN arrested B-cell lymphoma in one published case[5]. Along with alpha-lipoic acid, it stopped metastasized pancreatic cancer for 3 years in another case.[6]

LDN is available by prescription only. Any physician can ethically and legally prescribe LDN as an off-label prescription. But at present, few doctors know about it. It may be useful to show them the references with this article and also refer them to www.lowdosenaltrexone.org, a doctor-managed website.

LDN is reportedly compatible with other medications except narcotics or immunosuppressive drugs. It is said to be free of toxicity and to have few or no side effects. To date, the adverse effects from clinical studies have only amounted to temporary insomnia and vivid dreams. "Long-acting" or "slow release" varieties of naltrexone should be avoided. The drug is contraindicated for some types of thyroid disease and for people who have had organ transplants or are taking immunosuppressive drugs.

Solid evidence for the safety of long-term use of LDN was demonstrated in recent trials for Crohn's[7] and MS[8], and in more than three decades of FDA approved daily 50mg doses for alcoholism.


### *Further Reading and References*

- [1] www.lowdosenaltrexone.org, a doctor-managed website.

- [2] www.lowdosenaltrexone.org/ldn_and_cancer.htm

- [3] www.lowdosenaltrexone.org/ldn_and_cancer.htm

- [4] www.lowdosenaltrexone.org, a doctor-managed website.

- [5] Berkson BM, Rubin DM, Berson AJ. Reversal of signs and symptoms of a B-cell lymphoma in a patient using only low-dose naltrexone. Integ Cancer Therapy, 2007; 6:293-6.

- [6] Berkson BM, Rubin DM, Berkson AJ. The longer-term survival of a patient with pancreatic cancer with metastases to the liver after treatment with the intravenous alpha-lipoic acid/low-dose naltrexone protocol. Integ Cancer Therapy 2006; 5:83-9.

- [7] Smith JP, Stock H, Bingaman S, Mauger D, Rogosnitzky M, Zagon IS. Low-dose naltrexone therapy improves active Crohn's disease. Am J Gastroenterol 2007: 102:1-9

- [8] Gironi M, Martinelli-Boneschi F, Sacerdote P, Solaro C, Zaffaroni M, Cavarreta R, Moiola I, Bucello S, Radelli M, Pilato V, Rodegher M, Cursi M, Franchi S, Martinelli V, Nemni R, Comi G, Martino G. A Pilot Trial of Low Dose Naltrexone in Primary Progressive Multiple Sclerosis. Mult Scler 2008; 14(8):1076-83

- www.HonestMedicine.com

- www.ldners.org

- www.ldn.com

- www.ldnresearchtrust.org

- www.KeepHopeAlive.com

- www.lowdosenaltrexone.org

- http://articles.mercola.com/sites/articles/archive/2009/05/26/Powerful-Breakthrough-Beats-Cancer-and-AutoImmune-Diseases.aspx

- http://articles.mercola.com/sites/articles/archive/2009/01/13/can-ldn-really-help-multiple-sclerosis-rheumatoid-arthritis-and-other-autoimmune-diseases.aspx

- http://www.youtube.com/watch?v=XbYC0R5uKzE&feature=related

- http://www.youtube.com/watch?v=DAZ1fQKdOC8&feature=related

- (Numerous YouTube videos discuss ongoing clinical trials, speakers from professional LDN conferences, and more. Each of the above two videos will lead you to similar ones.)

# Megace

Megace is a synthetic form of the hormone progesterone. It was used as a palliative drug to treat metastatic breast cancer. It was noticed that the drug seemed to produce weight gain in some of the patients. Various studies have shown how the drug combats cachexia -- the severe malnutrition and wasting seen in many cancer patients.

In a University of Maryland Cancer Center study, a quarter of women with advanced breast cancer gained weight with conventional doses of the drug and almost all gained weight with high doses (480mg to 1600mg per day). Almost all also had subjective improvement in appetite and all those on high doses reported an increased sense of well being. NIH scientists conducted a study in 1990 and found that Megace "can stimulate appetite and food intake in patients with anorexia and cachexia associated with cancer, leading to significant weight gain in a proportion of such patients".

In 1990, German doctors giving fairly high doses of Megace to 26 cancer patients for eight weeks, found that half gained weight and those receiving higher doses responded more frequently with greater weight gain. Only in the high dose group was there an increase in both fat and lean body mass.

*Further Reading & References*

- *Cancer Therapy: The Independent Consumer's Guide to Non-Toxic Treatment and Prevention* by Ralph W. Moss (1992)

- National Cancer Institute: Megace, http://www.cancer.gov/dictionary/?CdrID=413949

# Methylene Blue

Methylene blue is a synthetic dye that inhibits rather than kills bacteria. Scientists at the Beijing Tuberculosis and Thoracic Tumor Research Institute, China, found that methylene blue inhibited the growth of three kinds of animal cancer. The average lifespan of the treated animals was longer than that of the controls.

When the conventional chemotherapy drug adriamycin was given to mice at the same time as methylene blue, its acute toxicity was decreased and survival time was prolonged. Methylene blue has been shown to make phototherapy effective faster. Six kinds of cancer cells were studied in a test tube. Phototherapy worked within sixty minutes, but the time was halved if the cells were first stained with methylene blue.

Furthermore, methylene blue has been found to effectively inhibit free radical activity.

*Further Reading & References*

- *Cancer Therapy: The Independent Consumer's Guide to Non-Toxic Treatment and Prevention* by Ralph W. Moss (1992)

- Skin and fat necrosis of the breast following methylene blue dye injection for sentinel node biopsy in a patient with breast cancer," http://www.ncbi.nlm.nih.gov/pmc/articles/PMC1308848/

- "Sentinel Lymph Node Biopsy for Breast Cancer Using Methylene Blue Dye Manifests A Short Learning Curve Among Experienced Surgeons," http://www.medscape.com/viewarticle/704817

# Nafazatron

Nafazatron is a drug produced by Miles Laboratories of West Haven, CT. It prevents blood clots and has also been shown to be a potent inhibitor of metastasis. Mice with tumors treated with nafazatron showed a remarkable six fold reduction in secondary metastases in their lungs compared to controls. The drug halted a process of cellular breakdown that leads to metastases.

*Further Reading & References*

- *Cancer Therapy: The Independent Consumer's Guide to Non-Toxic Treatment and Prevention* by Ralph W. Moss (1992)

# Sulindac

Sulindac, a nonsteroidal anti-inflammatory drug (NSAID), has been shown to cause the regression of benign colon polyps, thereby helping to prevent development of colon cancer. The drug inhibits the growth of laboratory-grown cancer cells that do not express cyclooxygenase, which synthesizes inflammatory mediators known as prostaglandins.

Dr. Richard Gaynor, director of the Harold C. Simmons Comprehensive Cancer Center and colleagues believe sulindac and its breakdown products inhibit cell growth by promoting programmed cell death – a mechanism by which potentially cancerous cells commit suicide. They found that sulindac prevented the activation of the cellular regulatory protein NF-kB. It is known that NF-kB is critical in regulating cellular growth and stimulating the inflammatory response. High levels of NF-kB have been found in the nucleus of some types of tumor cells, implying a role for NF-kB in the stimulation of cancer-cell growth.

"We found that sulindac inhibits a kinase (an enzyme that adds phosphate onto its target), which in turn prevents the activation of NF-kB," Gaynor said. "This kinase should be an excellent target not only for the development of novel anti-inflammatory agents but also for the development of agents to inhibit the growth of cancer cells."

Sulindac derivatives also can cause growth inhibition and induce apoptosis in human prostate cancer cells by a COX-1 and -2 independent mechanism, and this occurs irrespective of androgen sensitivity or increased expression of bcl-2. These compounds may be useful in the prevention and treatment of human prostate cancer.

### Further Reading & References

- Journal of Biological Chemistry, Sept. 17 1999

- Lim JT, Piazza GA, Han EK et al. Sulindac derivatives inhibit growth and induce apoptosis in human prostate cancer cell lines. Biochem Pharmacol 1999;58:1097–107.

- CBS News: Pain Killer Kills Cancer? Anti-Inflammatory Drug Sulindac Makes Tumor Cells Commit Suicide, Study Says, http://www.cbsnews.com/8301-504763_162-20008306-10391704.html

- The Medical News: Sulindac shuts down cancer cell growth, initiates cell death: Study, http://www.news-medical.net/news/20100615/Sulindac-shuts-down-cancer-cell-growth-initiates-cell-death-Study.aspx

# Onconase®/Ranpirnase

Onconase is a purified anti-tumor protein derived from early stage embryos of the common North American leopard frog. It shows anti-tumor activity in mouse tumor models and is effective on several tumor lines. It is currently in clinical trials.

In animal tests and clinical trials, Onconase shows lesser toxicity and fewer side effects compared to most chemotherapeutic drugs. "Onconase may act as a 'Trojan Horse' inside tumor cells," states research scientist, Dr. Darzynkiewicz.

Onconase slows down cancer cell growth by decaying RNA. Without certain RNA strands, cancer cells cannot make certain critical proteins and therefore cannot replicate. This slows down the growth of the tumor. Normally, high doses of chemotherapy are needed to affect cancer cells. However, Onconase is able to make cancer cells more susceptible to lower doses of chemotherapy, and therefore reduce side effects.

### Further Reading & References

- Mesothelioma: "Onconase® May Target Small RNAs That Regulate Cell Proliferation and Death'"
http://www.mesotheliomaweb.org/trojanhorse.htm

- Mesothelioma Options, http://www.mesotheliomaoptions.com/onconase.htm

# Tetracycline/COL-3 /CMT-3

A cancer treatment is being developed that is relatively safe, cheap, and almost completely effective, according to its advocates. It has been around for decades but no one ever thought about using it to fight the cancer.

The treatment is tetracycline, a family of inexpensive acne antibiotics. The drug is being researched for its ability to prevent metastases, the migration of cancerous tumor cells that migrate throughout the body, creating secondary tumors.

Dr. Gurmit Singh of the Hamilton Regional Cancer Centre is leading research on the drug. Singh learned that tetracycline is not only effective at preventing metastases from forming in bones, it also has the ability to kill tumor cells in the bone. A man whose Doberman suffered bone cancer, osteosarcoma, worked with his vet using this protocol — in this dog's case, 250mg. tablets, 3 capsules 4 times a day. Time passed and an x-ray eventually showed that the mass in the bone was almost gone.

In tests on mice, his team found the drug cut the spread of certain cancers to the bone by 70%. "This was very exciting to us so we continued on with our experiments and what we found was that it actually improved the bone itself. In some ways, it healed the bone," says Dr. Singh.

Tetracycline has been used to treat acne and periodontal disease. The drug is absorbed by teeth and bones, and blocks a group of enzymes called matrix metalloproteinases, a cause of gum degradation. But its efficacy at inhibiting the growth of cancerous osteoclasts in bone has not been fully researched.

The problem may be the drug's price - its low price. Because the medication is generic and cheap, there is not much incentive for drug companies to fund research. "Pharmaceutical companies, understandably, may not be willing to invest resources in developing research that won't result in a profit for their companies," says Dr. Robert Bell of the Princess Margaret Hospital.

Claudia Huettner can switch off deadly leukemia in mice simply by putting tetracycline in their drinking water. Her system even causes regression of advanced stages of the cancer. When the antibiotic-spiked water is withdrawn, the cancer returns. "I have reversed leukemia as much as three times in some animals" she says.

A study at the University of Iowa suggests tetracycline may help prevent cancer recurrence. Interestingly, a form of tetracycline has recently been used in prevention of cancer recurrence. Chemically modified tetracyclines such as COL-3 are derived from antibiotic tetracyclines, but because of their modifications, do not act as antibiotics. Instead, they inhibit certain enzymes and processes that normally encourage cancer growth. By making cancer cells less aggressive, these drugs may show potential for long-term management of some cancers.

Investigators at the University of Miami School of Medicine have shown that tetracycline compounds traditionally used as antibiotics, have been shown to inhibit many tumor cell functions such as growth and invasion. Additionally, tetracycline compounds are known to accumulate in the bone, a tissue also adversely affected by metastatic prostate cancer. Miami researchers have found CMT-3, a synthetic tetracycline, to be toxic to prostate cancer cells, to inhibit their growth, and to block enzymes that are needed to clear a path for cell invasion.

Robert Rowen, M.D., a well known alternative doctor who edits *Second Opinion*, a popular newsletter, has spoken favorably of Dr. Singh's work with tetracycline.

### Further Reading & References

- "Tetracycline offers promise for halting cancer," http://www.ctv.ca/servlet/ArticleNews/story/CTVNews/20030119/tetracycline030119/

- Harvard University Gazette: "Researchers Switch Cancer Off and On — in Mice," http://www.news.harvard.edu/gazette/2000/02.10/leukemia.html

# Theophylline

It has been reported that asthma patients with a history of theophylline use enjoy a lower mortality rate from lung cancer than expected. Theophylline is often used to treat asthma. Theophylline belongs to the family of drugs responsible for relaxing respiratory smooth muscles. It is an inducer of cyclic AMP.

Joseph Wybran and Andre Govaerts of the Hospital St. Pierre in Brussels, Belgium, were among the first to suggest, in 1975, that the same doses of theophylline used to treat asthma should be used to treat cancer. They referenced a report out of England (*The Lancet* in 1974 ii p. 1475 by Michael Alderson) on cancer among asthma patients that read, "Alderson had demonstrated that cancer deaths from all cancer except from lung cancer was only about 65% that of the general population among patients with asthma. Records on asthma patients were kept on 765 male patients and 1,127 women. In all cancers other than lung cancer, there were 43 cancer deaths when 65.8 such deaths had been expected. This was an indicated reduction of 35% in cancer deaths. There was a smaller reduction in lung cancer deaths, 16 when 20 had been expected. It was said that this reduction in lung cancer deaths was not significant.

"...Reference was made to the work of T.T. Puck of the Eleanor Roosevelt Institute for Cancer Research published in the Proceedings of the National Academy of Science USA, October, 1977 pp. 4491-95. Puck said that cyclic AMP converts cancer cells back to normal cells or at the very least, restores contact inhibition to cancer cells thus making them non-invasive and hence harmless."

### Further Reading & References

- Townsend Letter for Doctors and Patients: "On theophylline and evening primrose oil in the treatment of cancer - Letters to the Editor," http://www.findarticles.com/p/articles/mi_m0ISW/is_2002_June/ai_86387594

# Thioproline

Thioproline has proven successful in treating human cancer. It provides a completely non-toxic approach and may feasibly be used as a first treatment in cancers where it is acceptable to delay orthodox treatment (because the delay will not affect the prognosis). Cancer cells in vitro (lab culture) can be induced to undergo reverse transformation to normal cells by exposure to cyclic AMP, prostaglandin (PG) and certain drugs such as thioproline.

## *Further Reading & References*

- The reversibility of cancer: the relevance of cyclic AMP, calcium, essential fatty acids and prostaglandin E1 Med Hypotheses 1980; 6(5): 469-86.Horrobin, D.F. http://www.ncbi.nlm.nih.gov/pubmed/6251348

- The Lancet: "Thioproline And Reversal Of Cancer," http://www.thelancet.com/journals/lancet/article/PIIS0140-6736%2883%2991947-5/fulltext?version=printerFriendly

# Detoxification, Antimicrobial and Antiparasite Therapies

## Anti-Fungals

There is a body of thought that some fungal infections are misdiagnosed as leukemia. In 1997, Mark Bielski linked leukemia with the yeast candida albicans and in 1999 Dr. Meinolf Karthaus detailed how three of his young patients with leukemia went into remission after being treated with a cocktail of three anti-fungal drugs.

Doug Kaufmann in his book *The Germ that Causes Cancer* asserts that not only fungi, but grain, sugar and peanuts also contain cancer-causing fungal poisons. He explains how even antibiotics may play a role in the disease process. Antibiotics destroy the normal, protective gut bacteria, allowing intestinal yeast and fungi to grow unchecked. These internal, intestinal yeast make toxins, too. This can lead to immune suppression, symptoms of autoimmune disease, or even cancer.

"If the onset of any symptom or disease -- cancer included -- was preceded by a course of antibiotics," he maintains, "then look for a fungus to be at the root of your problem."

Autopsies show that fungal infections are found in about 10% of cancer patients and 25% of acute leukemia and bone marrow therapy patients.


See **Candida Eradication**.


### Further Reading and References

- Karthaus, M. Treatment of fungal infections led to leukemia remissions. Sept. 28, 1999

- Cancer is a Fungus - Know The Cause - Alternative Cancer Treatments, http://www.healthsalon. org/373/cancer-is-a-fungus-alternative-cancer-treatments/

- Preventative use of antifungal drugs in patients treated for cancer, http://jac.oxfordjournals.org/ content/53/2/130.full

- "Antifungal prophylaxis in cancer patients after chemotherapy or hematopoietic stem-cell transplantation: systematic review and meta-analysis." http://www.ncbi.nlm.nih.gov/ pubmed/17909198

# Candida Eradication/ThreeLac/Oxygen Elements Plus/Coconut Oil

There are several associations between cancer and Candida organisms. Candida infection compromises immune and systemic body systems. This, it is thought, allows cancer to gain a foothold. Chemotherapy also suppresses the immune system, allowing Candida to gain a foothold. As low levels of Candida are present in everybody, Candidemia "infection" in this context means overgrowth of this microorganism leading to toxicity or inappropriate immune-system reactions.

Candidemia can severely complicate the care of cancer patients:

"Candidemia is a serious infection that can severely complicate the care of children with cancer. ... Death attributed to the fungal infection occurred in 21% of episodes, with nearly all the deaths occurring in patients with C. albicans and C. tropicalis."

Candida appears notoriously difficult to control. Numerous treatment protocols are said to eradicate this infection or overgrowth. A large number of enthusiastic consumers attest to the ability of ThreeLac and Oxygen Elements Plus to eradicate these infections.

Unlike other dietary supplements, which are unregulated in the U.S., ThreeLac was formulated by scientists in Japan and is manufactured at a pharmaceutical company under strict government regulations. This particular combination of bacterial strains will not be found in any other product.

The company bringing it into the US, Global Health Trax, is an FDA-approved, GMP manufacturing facility in Vista, California.

ThreeLac is a proprietary formula containing three strains of live lactic acid bacteria that eat yeast. ThreeLac is designed to get the yeast-fighting live bacteria safely past the acidic environment of the stomach so that, once in the intestinal tract, these friendly bacteria can devour candida yeast. ThreeLac also reputedly makes body pH more alkaline which makes it hard for candida yeast to thrive.

Ingredients are spore-forming lactic acid bacteria (Lactobacillus sporogenes), spore-forming bacteria (Bacillus subtilis), lactic acid bacteria (Streptococcus faecalis), lemon juice powder, refined yeast powder, and castor oil. Yeast is included in ThreeLac packages in order to feed and sustain the live lactic acid bacteria.

Lactobacillus Sporogens is the main lactic acid bacterium in Threelac. It is naturally occurring in the intestinal tract and constitutes a major part of the intestinal flora. Lactobacillus Sporogens is responsible for the synthesis of B-complex factors, Vitamin K, and digestive enzymes. It also produces lactic acid, prevents the uncontrolled growth of putrefactive bacteria and creates an environment that promotes normal functioning of the gastrointestinal tract.

Lactobacillus Spores: These spores provide protection from pathogenic invasions into the intestinal tract and help to restore the normal balance of intestinal flora after antimicrobial drugs treatment, and can limit the activity of harmful pathogenic bacteria such as E. coli, and Salmonella.

Advocates recommend taking Oxygen Elements Plus at the same time as Threelac.

"The USP challenge test conducted by Bioscreen Testing Services showed that Oxygen Elements Plus (formerly Hydroxygen Plus) completely destroyed Candida albicans yeast and four other pathogens: A. niger, E. coli, P. aeruginosa, S. aureus. And that they did not return during the entire 28 day testing period."

Virgin coconut oil and other coconut products are also effective in fighting Candida. Caprylic acid is one of the fatty acids found in coconut oil that has been effective in fighting candida yeast infections. Besides caprylic acid, two other medium chain fatty acids in coconut oil have also been found to kill

Candida albicans. People generally work up to taking a tablespoon of oil three times a day.

A study done at the University of Iceland showed that "Capric acid, a 10-carbon saturated fatty acid, causes the fastest and most effective killing of all three strains of Candida albicans tested, leaving the cytoplasm disorganized and shrunken because of a disrupted or disintegrated plasma membrane. Lauric acid, a 12-carbon saturated fatty acid, was the most active at lower concentrations and after a longer incubation time."

The "die-off effect" or Herxheimer Reaction would be expected from undertaking the above treatments. It refers to the symptoms generated by the body dealing with the dead yeast microbes. Eventually these symptoms recede as Candida is eliminated.

### Further Reading and References

- Mullen CA, Abd El-Baki H, Samir H, Tarrand JJ, Rolston KV. Support Care Cancer. 2003

- May;11(5):321-5. Epub 2003 Mar 11."Non-albicans Candida is the most common cause of candidemia

- in pediatric cancer patients." http://www.ncbi.nlm.nih.gov/entrez/query.fcgi?cmd=Retrieve&db=pubmed&dopt=Abstract&list_uids=12720076

- Gudmundur Bergsson, et. al., In Vitro Killing of Candida albicans by Fatty Acids and Monoglycerides,

- Antimicrobial Agents and Chemotherapy, November 2001, p. 3209-3212, Vol. 45, No. 11

# Chelation

Chelation therapy is a medical treatment performed intravenously in a doctor's office or by oral medication. It is intended to remove toxic substances and thereby improve metabolic function and blood flow through blocked arteries throughout the body.

The human body needs regular cleaning of toxic material such as heavy metals, excess calcification, and arterial plaque build up. Chelation (pronounced key-lation) therapy is a common form of detoxification. According to its advocates, it also stimulates the immune system, sharpens the appetite (digestion), and generally helps to eliminate the by-products of metabolism. Because of all this, many consider it an excellent treatment for cancer.

Used by some alternative doctors for heart patients, chelation is a method by which unwanted metals are purged from a system by putting another substance through the system, which binds to the metals and flushes them out. Conventional medicine accepts chelation as a treatment for heavy metal poisoning (lead, mercury, et al.) but not for artery disease, much less cancer.

Manufacturers identified the need for a chelating substance before the Second World War. Paint, rubber, petroleum, and electro-plating industries all needed substances that would bind and eliminate corrupting substances. Research in pre-war Germany came up with an extremely good substance: Ethylene-diamine-tetra-acetate, an amino acid, known since then as EDTA for short.

In 1947 it was first used for medical purposes to clear the bloodstream of a cancer patient suffering toxic side effects of chemotherapy. It reportedly worked. In the early 1950s, EDTA was used in a number of circumstances where large numbers of workers were suffering from heavy metal poisoning. According to Harold and Arline Brecher who have written a number of books on chelation therapy, it worked very well in every case.

Most chelation protocols today administer EDTA by an intravenous infusion using a small 25-gauge needle. This protocol for administering EDTA was developed and refined by Elmer M. Cranton, MD, author of *Bypassing Bypass Surgery* and editor of *A Textbook on EDTA Chelation Therapy*.

Since the first use in humans, hundreds of studies have consistently shown the benefits of chelation therapy, particularly for atherosclerosis - a problem for which the heart bypass operation was designed.

Additionally, it appears that chelation therapy has a possible cancer preventative action. A Swiss study, led by Dr. W. Blumer and Dr. T. Reich, investigated the link between lead-based gas fumes and cancer incidence based on the health records of 231 Swiss citizens living next to a heavily used highway. It showed that cancer mortality among this group was indeed significantly higher than among persons living in a traffic-free section of the same town. In both groups, the subjects studied were lifelong inhabitants of their respective areas.

However, there was a curious exception. One group of the fume-exposed population had developed such severe symptoms of lead poisoning that they had been detoxified with the usual treatment for lead poisoning: EDTA. As a result, Blumer and Reich were in a position to compare long-term death rates in a matched population of chelated and non-chelated patients. They found a significant mortality difference between the two groups. Of the 231 people in the study, 59 adults had chelation; 172 matched controls did not. Only one (1.7%) of the chelated persons died of cancer, as compared with thirty (17%) of the non-treated. After exploring all possible explanations for this statistical disparity in cancer mortality, the authors concluded that chelation was the sole reason for the 90% decrease in cancer deaths.

This supports the experience of doctors who use chelation in their practices. Dr E.W. McDonagh, founder member of the International Academy of Preventive Medicine, found that of 25,000 patients that he had treated with chelation, only one of those who had not previously had cancer was later diagnosed as having cancer. Taking this as an interesting indication of chelation's merits, he looked for cases of Vietnam veterans who had been severely poisoned by Agent Orange.

This group is known to suffer very high incidences of cancer. He found 63 veterans who had later had EDTA. Not one of them subsequently developed cancer. Not all doctors are convinced of this anti-cancer effect. Chelation may not be so effective if cancer has already started to develop before the chelation treatment starts. "I have personally seen cancer develop in three people who were undergoing chelation therapy. In these cases the cancer was present at the start of the chelation but unrecognized at that time," according to Dr Harold Steenblock.

Chelation works against cancer by removing toxic metals, a source of free radicals. It is therefore a preventive measure. For patients who already have cancer, it improves blood circulation by clearing arterial obstructions and so allows greater supplies of oxygen to reach the cancer site. Cancer tumors do not thrive in high oxygen environments, as Nobel Prize winner Otto Warburg discovered.

Also, some advocates believe that EDTA strips away the protein coat that surrounds tumor cells. This protein shield is what protects the cancer cells from T-lymphocytes, the white blood cells whose job is to kill invaders. Because of the protein layer, T-lymphocytes do not identify the tumor as an enemy to be overcome.

Once the cancer cells' protein layer has been stripped away, the T-lymphocytes can start kill them. During chelation, the patient is hooked up for 2-3 hours per session to an intravenous drip, which contains not only EDTA but also mega-doses of vitamins.

Increasing numbers of people are undergoing chelation treatments as a general preventive health measure. One caution is that chelation needs to be carefully administered. There can be kidney complications from the extraction of too much toxic metal in a short time. A careful graduation of chelation treatments is therefore required. A typical treatment includes 20 sessions. Also, high supplementation of minerals such as magnesium, zinc and selenium is needed, as good metals are taken out with the bad.

Some infrequent effects of chelation may include: low blood calcium, cardiac arrhythmia, fever, headaches and inflammation of the veins. However, these side effects are not common. Chelation is contraindicated in the cases of damaged kidneys, liver disease, TB, brain tumors and pregnancy.

Oral chelation has become widely popular and available in recent years. While over-the-counter chelating agents can be purchased, it is not recommended that patients undertake a course of chelation without a doctor's supervision. Medical tests (typically a special urine analysis) should be administered before chelation to determine whether it's warranted, and the test should be repeated during or after chelation to determine if the desired result has been achieved. The patient needs to supplement with a wide range of minerals to replace those (such as magnesium) that chelation removes. The patient should be examined beforehand to ensure that he or she doesn't have a medical condition that precludes chelation.

### Further Reading and References

- Everything You Should Know About Chelation Therapy by Morton Walker, Hitendra Shah (1998)

- Bypassing Bypass Surgery: Chelation Therapy: A Non-Surgical Treatment for Reversing Arteriosclerosis, Improving Blocked Circulation, and Slowing the Aging Process by Elmer M. Cranton, Elmer, M.D. (2001)

- Questions from the Heart: Answers to 100 Questions About Chelation Therapy, a Safe Alternative to Bypass Surgery by Terry Chappell, Julian Whitaker (1995)

- A Textbook on Edta Chelation Therapy by Elmer M. Cranton, Elmer M., M.D. (2001)

- If EDTA Chelation Therapy is so Good, Why Is It Not More Widely Accepted? by Dr. James P. Carter,

- MD, DrPH

- Chelation Critics Deceive the Public by Elmer M. Cranton, MD

- The Chelation Answer: How to Prevent Hardening of the Arteries & Rejuvenate Your Cardiovascular System. - Paperback by Morton Walker, Robert Atkins, Steven E. Kroening, and William Campbell Douglass (1993)


# Clay Treatment

Clays have been used both internally and externally for detoxification purposes. Advocates report that specially formulated clay baths are able to literally pull pollutants out like a magnet, getting rid of years of toxic accumulation in just one bath.

Detoxification symptoms are reportedly less severe than from internal chelation methods, and results can happen much more quickly. Clay baths have been scientifically proven to release toxic metals and chemicals from the body, and they are inexpensive, advocates say.

According to Lauana Lei, an active advocate and user of the clay bath, "A few years ago, I was diagnosed with heavy metal and chemical poisoning. Among the many toxic substances in my body, mercury from the fillings in my teeth was a major culprit. Having neither health insurance nor the money to pay for these expensive treatments, I began searching for alternative ways to eliminate these poisons — a major cause of immune system breakdown — and thus, the source of various diseases. Eventually, my search led me to a book, *Using Energy to Heal*, by Wendell Hoffman. Through his own research, Hoffman found that a special bentonite (a very fine volcanic clay) used in a bath can actually draw out toxic chemicals through the pores of the skin. After many experiments, he concluded that optimum results are obtained by immersing oneself in a tub of very warm water mixed with a special bentonite clay for exactly 20 minutes!"

Clay is sometimes applied as a poultice, as in the research experiment described at http://www.silvermedicine.org/clay-cansema-silver1.html that treated a skin cancer with healing clay, Cansema and colloidal silver. Graphic photographs track the healing process.

### Further Reading and References

- *Using Energy to Heal* by Wendell Hoffman (1979)

- *The Healing Clay: The Centuries Old Health and Beauty Elixir/Amazing Cures from the Earth Itself* by Michel Abehsera (1986)

- Our Earth, Our Cure — Clay Therapy, http://www.shirleys-wellness-cafe.com/clay.htm

- "Medicinal Clay Bath Treatment for Health and Detoxification," by Lauana Lei, http://www.shirleys-wellness-cafe.com/clay.htm

- Article: Skin Cancer Treated with Clay, http://www.aboutclay.com/info/Articles/skin_cancer.htm


# Coffee Enemas

Coffee enemas are one of the most widely used and generally accepted treatments to detoxify the body in alternative cancer protocols. They are employed in many of the world's top alternative cancer clinics. They are also used safely at home by many people.

Coffee enemas were an accepted mainstream medical therapy, included in the Merck Manual — the profession's guide to treatments — until the 1970s when it was dropped without explanation.

Dr. William D. Kelley, DDS, MS stated, "A coffee enema should be given every morning for one month; then twice a week for eight months. The coffee enema is very stimulating to the liver, and is the greatest aid in eliminating its toxic poisons."

From the book *Alternatives in Cancer Therapy: The Complete Guide to Non- Traditional Treatments:*

"Recent research shows that certain chemicals in coffee called palmitates stimulate an important liver enzyme called glutathione-S-transferase, which is capable of removing a variety of free radicals from the bloodstream. A coffee enema increases the glutathione- S-transferase enzyme activity in the liver from 600 percent to 700 percent above normal. During the time that the coffee enema is being held in, all the blood in the body passes through the liver at least five times, since all the blood in the body goes through the liver every three minutes.

"Other chemicals in coffee, including caffeine, theobromine, and theophylline, cause blood vessels and bile ducts to dilate, increasing the elimination of toxic bile. Additionally, some of the water absorbed through the intestinal wall goes directly to the liver, diluting the bile and increasing bile flow.

"A choleretic is any substance that increases bile flow. The coffee enema is the only pharmaceutically effective choleretic noted in the medical literature that can be safely used many times daily without toxic effects."

### Further Reading and References

- Alternatives in Cancer Therapy: The Complete Guide to Non-Traditional Treatments by Ross Pelton with Lee Overholzer (1994)

- *What Your Doctor Won't Tell You: Today's Alternative Medical Treatments Explained* by Jane

- Heimlich (1980)

- Coffee Enemas Reverses Cancer by Waste Removal and Detoxifying http://www.treating-cancer-alternatively.com/Coffee-enemas.html

- A Discussion By People Who Are Using This Detoxification Method, http://www. annieappleseedproject.org/coffeeenemas.html

# Dr. Clark Clean-Ups

See also **Dr. Hulda Clark/Dr. Clark's Treatment** for how to eliminate the cancer.

After cancer is under control, one can get well if the toxins that invited parasites, bacterial, and viral invaders are removed. Removing toxins from the affected organs lets them heal. For example, lung lesions will not heal unless cigarette smoking, Freon, asbestos, and fiberglass exposure are stopped.

Carcinogens draw the cancer to the organ: nickel draws cancer to the prostate, barium draws cancer to the breast. Dr. Clark considers the most serious threats to be: freon (CFCs or refrigerant), copper from water pipes, fiberglass or asbestos, mercury from amalgam tooth fillings, lead from joints in copper plumbing, formaldehyde in foam bedding and new clothing, and nickel, usually from dental metal.

Dental, diet, body, and home clean-ups aim to remove parasites and pollutants at their source. The body constantly fights to remove pollutants, but if the patient is being 're-supplied' with them, the body cannot heal.

Silver or amalgam fillings contain 48-55% mercury, 33-35% silver, and various amounts of copper, tin, zinc, and other metals that corrode and seep into the body. Mercury is continually released from mercury fillings in the form of mercury vapor and abraded particles, which can be increased 15-fold by chewing, brushing, and hot liquids. Research has shown that mercury, even in small amounts, damages the brain, heart, lungs, liver, kidneys, thyroid, pituitary and adrenal glands, blood cells, enzymes, and hormones, and suppresses the body's immune system.

The materials which have entered our food chain and body by way of personal care products —particularly petroleum products, alcohol, asbestos, colorings, dyes, formaldehyde, and perfume — should not be there and were not there fifty years ago. The tested ingredients in 99% of perfumes are labeled as toxic hazards and not allowed in the agriculture industry, according to Dr. Clark. So, apart from avoidance of processed foods, Dr. Clark warns against commercial salves, ointments, lotions, colognes, perfumes, deodorants, toothpaste, soaps, washing powders etc. and gives recipes for homemade substitutes, e.g. borax powder for cleaning.

She suggests if you have been quite ill to move to a warm climate where you can avoid heating and cooling, and sit outside in the shade all day.

Dr. Clark also says that syncrometer testing makes it possible to know exactly which toxins and parasites cause the patient's cancer. The syncrometer can be used for diagnosing and monitoring progress until cured. It consists of an audio oscillator circuit, which includes the body as part of the circuit. Dr. Clark maintained that every living and non-living entity produced certain specific frequencies which can be heard with the audio oscillator. Every living creature broadcasts its presence like a radio station. The syncrometer tests for parasites or pollutants in any product or body tissue, by using samples of those parasites or pollutants. Cancerous tumors grow in the body for at least three years before they are big enough to be detected by medical imaging techniques, but the syncrometer can detect them long before that.

For detoxifying the body, Dr. Clark recommends vitamins, minerals, and herbs from safe sources. Apart from the parasites and dental cleanses, she gives detailed instructions for liver, kidney, and bowel cleanses. She recommends that the liver cleanse should not be done if the liver contains living parasites, and is best carried out after a parasite cleanse and then a kidney cleanse. The liver cleanse is reported as the single most important thing you can do for your health. Medical herbalists, naturopaths and other natural healers speak highly of her cleanses.

### Further Reading and References

- *The Cure and Prevention of All Cancers* by Hulda Regehr Clark and Ph.D. N.D. (2008)

- Curing Cancer, http://www.lightsv.org/cancer.htm

# Liver-Gallbladder Flush

Dr. William D. Kelley, DDS, MS stated, "The importance of cleansing the debris from the liver and gall bladder, thus keeping the bile free flowing, cannot be overemphasized. This can be effectively accomplished by doing the Liver-Gall Bladder Flush (a form of which at one time was widely used at the world famous Lahey Clinic in Boston, MA), which is necessary even if one has had their gall bladder removed."

Liver-Gallbladder flushes, of which Kelley's is but one variant, are widely popular among alternative health therapists and consumers. Despite this, they are not universally accepted and are reputed to be quite harsh to endure. In patients who already have gallstones, a flush can induce a gallbladder attack, which is extremely painful and can lead to immediate surgery to remove the gallbladder.

The four basic active principles in Kelley's procedure are:

- Apple juice: (high in malic acid) or ortho-phosphoric acid, which acts as a solvent in the bile to weaken adhesions between solid globules.

- Epsom salt: (magnesium sulfate), taken by mouth and by enema, which allows magnesium to be absorbed into the bloodstream, relaxing smooth muscles. Large solid particles which otherwise might create spasms are able to pass through a relaxed bile duct.

- Olive oil: unrefined, which stimulates the gall bladder and bile duct to contract powerfully, thus expelling solid particles kept in storage for years.

- Coffee enemas: which consist of a coffee solution retained in the colon. They activate the liver to secrete its waste into the bile, enhancing bile flow and further relaxing the bile duct muscle.

For full instructions on preparing the Liver-Gallbladder Flush, visit http://curezone.com/cleanse/liver/kelley.asp.

### Further Reading and References

- Dr. William D. Kelly's Nutritional-Metabolic Therapy, http://educate-yourself.org/cancer/kellysmetabolictherapy.shtml

- *The Amazing Liver & Gallbladder Flush* by Andreas Moritz (2007)

# Index